OPERATIVE SURGERY

Sir Roy Calne, FRS
Professor of Surgery,
University of Cambridge
Department of Surgery
Addenbrooke's Hospital
Cambridge

Stephen G. Pollard, BSC, FRCS
Clinical Lecturer and Honorary
Senior Registrar in Surgery
University of Cambridge
Department of Surgery
Addenbrooke's Hospital
Cambridge

Gower Medical Publishing
LONDON • NEW YORK

Distributed in the USA and Canada by:
J B Lippincott Company
East Washington Square
Philadelphia
PA 19105
USA

Distributed in the UK and Continental Europe by:
Gower Medical Publishing
Middlesex House
34-42 Cleveland Street
London W1P 5FB
UK

Distributed in Australia and New Zealand by:
Harper and Row (Australia) Pty Ltd
PO Box 226
Artarmon
NSW 2064
AUSTRALIA

Distributed in Southeast Asia, Hong Kong, India and Pakistan by:
Harper and Row (Asia) Pte Ltd
37 Jalan Pemimpin 02-01
Singapore 2057

Distributed in Japan by:
Nankodo Co Ltd
42-6 Hongo 3-chome
Bunkyo-ku
Tokyo 113
JAPAN

A slide atlas of Operative Surgery based on the contents of this book, is available. In the slide atlas format, the material is split into volumes, each of which is presented in a binder together with numbered 35mm slides of each illustration. Each slide atlas volume also contains a list of abbreviated slide captions for easy reference when using the slides. Further information can be obtained from:

Gower Medical Publishing
Middlesex House
34-42 Cleveland Street
London W1P 5FB

Gower Medical Publishing
101 5th Avenue
New York, NY 10003
USA

Project editors:	Samantha J. Robinson
	Alan R. Burgess
Design:	Louise Jayne Bond
	Nancy Elizabeth Chase
Illustration:	Kevin Marks
Paste-up:	Clare Gillmore
	Olgun Horatio Hassan

British Library Cataloguing in Publication Data:
Calne, Roy Yorke *1930*
    Operative surgery.
    1. Medicine. Surgery. Operations. Techniques
    I. Title II. Pollard, Stephen
    617.910028

ISBN 0-397-44628-4

Library of Congress Cataloguing-in-Publication Data:
Operative surgery/[edited by] Sir Roy Y. Calne, Stephen G. Pollard.
    p. cm.
    Includes index.
    ISBN 0-397-44628-4
    1. Surgery, Operative. I. Calne, Roy Yorke. II. Pollard,
Stephen.
    [DNLM: 1. Surgery, Operative. WO 500 0603]
RD32.0585 1991
617.9—dc20

Originated in Hong Kong by Mandarin Offset
Typesetting by M to N Typesetters, London
Text set in Baskerville; captions set in Univers
Produced by Imago, Singapore
Printed in Singapore

Preface

There are many excellent texts on operative surgery each with its own objectives. In this volume we have tried to produce an illustrated account of the common surgical procedures that a surgical resident would be expected to perform on his/her own and, in summary form, an outline of more major procedures in which he/she will probably have to assist.

Most of the operations have been described by our coauthors who are surgical residents at the 'coal face'. Since they are responsible for teaching operative surgery to junior surgical trainees, they ought to know what is required in practice. The diagrams have been faithfully transcribed from operative photographs by Mr Kevin Marks.

The general surgeon's identity is constantly under attack and general surgery with an interest in a speciality or more often a speciality in its own right has become the pattern of surgical development. This is not always to the advantage of patients. A trade union attitude towards certain parts of the body of systems can mean that if a surgeon in that speciality comes across unexpected pathology or anatomical arrangement, he may find it difficult to cope without calling in another sub-specialist who may not be readily available. In most countries it is therefore still regarded as part of the basic training in surgery, that no matter what surgical sub-speciality is the final goal, a general knowledge of anatomy, surgical principles and standard operations is still required.

We have compiled a list of operations performed in a 6-month period in busy teaching hospitals with local district catchment areas in England, the United States and Japan. The types of operation and their frequency of performance are surprisingly similar in these three institutions, both for elective and emergency surgery. The contents of this volume have been selected from this information. From necessity there has been an arbitrary choice to include most general surgical procedures, some urology and trauma, but excluding orthopaedics, plastic surgery, surgery of the newborn and other well-established surgical sub-specialities. We hope that the text will be of use to surgical residents in a practical sense and also in preparation for examinations of surgical Colleges and Boards, and that this book will spare patients from unnecessary disasters. These will be avoided in residents learn and practise good surgical judgment, technique and aftercare. They should operate with confidence within the limits of their expertise, prepared with a sound knowledge of anatomy and never be too proud to seek help before the patient is harmed.

Sir Roy Calne
Stephen G. Pollard

Acknowledgements

We wish to express our thanks to all who have helped produce this long, complicated book, especially the busy surgical residents who have managed to find time to put pen to paper often after nights of emergency operating.

We thank all those in the operating room who at different times have taken photographs on which the drawings have been based and especially thank Sister Wai Kin Celia Chan, Mr Neville Jamieson and Professor Naoshi Kamada for their initial help in arranging the concept of the book.

We are indebted to Kevin Marks for the excellent illustrations, to Louise Bond for her expert design and layout, to Alan Burgess and Samantha Robinson for the long-suffering hours they spent editing and managing the project, and finally to Fiona Foley, UK Managing Director of Gower Medical Publishing, for the unstinting enthusiasm and support she has provided since the inception of *Operative Surgery*.

Finally, we express gratitude to our wives, Patricia Calne and Glenda Pollard, for their patience and understanding over the last three years.

Contents

Contributors

David J. Barron, MB BS
Resident Surgical Officer,
Addenbrooke's Hospital, Cambridge.

Nigel Bleach, FRCS
Senior Registrar in E.N.T.,
Charing Cross Hospital, London.

Terng Fong Chen, FRCS
Research Fellow in Urology, former Rotating Surgical Registrar,
Addenbrooke's Hospital, Cambridge.

C. Richard G. Cohen, BSc, FRCS
Registrar,
Tameside General Hospital, Manchester.

D. St John G. Collier, MS, FRCS, BChD, FDSRCS
Senior Registrar/Clinical Lecturer,
Department of Surgery,
Addenbrooke's Hospital, Cambridge.

Ian Eardley, FRCS
Senior Registrar/Clinical Lecturer,
Department of Urology,
Addenbrooke's Hospital, Cambridge.

Jonathan Forty, MA, FRCS
Research Fellow and former Registrar
in Cardio-thoracic Surgery,
Papworth Hospital, Cambridge.

Robert A. Greatorex, MA, FRCS, BDS
Consultant Surgeon,
Queen Elizabeth Hospital, Kings Lynn, Norfolk,
former Senior Surgical Registrar,
Addenbrooke's Hospital, Cambridge.

Mark Holt, MB, BCh
Resident Surgical Officer,
Addenbrooke's Hospital, Cambridge.

Vivien C. Lees, MA, FRCS
Rotating Surgical Registrar,
Addenbrooke's Hospital, Cambridge.

Harold Lyall, FRCS
Senior House Officer in Plastic Surgery,
Addenbrooke's Hospital, Cambridge.

Robert Macfarlane, MA, FRCS
Senior Registrar in Neurosurgery,
former Rotating Surgical Registrar,
Addenbrooke's Hospital, Cambridge.

Pietro E. Majno, MD, FRCS
Rotating Surgical Registrar,
Addenbrooke's Hospital, Cambridge.

James Pain, MS, FRCS
Senior Registrar,
King's College Hospital, Dulwich, London.

Brian Plaisier, MD
Chief Surgical Resident,
University Hospital, Indianapolis, Indiana USA,
former Visiting Surgical Registrar,
Addenbrooke's Hospital, Cambridge.

Stephen G. Pollard, BSc, FRCS
Senior Registrar/Clinical Lecturer,
Department of Surgery, Addenbrooke's Hospital, Cambridge.

Philip Radford, MA, FRCS
Senior Registrar,
University Hospital, Nottingham,
former Rotating Surgical Registrar,
Addenbrooke's Hospital, Cambridge.

Hugh Thompson, MS, FRCS
Senior Surgical Registrar,
Addenbrooke's Hospital, Cambridge.

Julian Tuson, MA, FRCS
Research Fellow in Surgery, former Rotating Surgical Registrar,
Addenbrooke's Hospital, Cambridge.

Christopher J. Watson, MA, FRCS
Research Fellow in Surgery, former Rotating Surgical Registrar,
Addenbrooke's Hospital, Cambridge.

Introduction

If a surgeon is threatened with an operation on himself, his initial reaction is "lets try conservative treatment and endeavour to avoid surgery". This is because surgeons are acutely aware of the dangers of any operative procedure; even the simplest operation can result in disaster. For example, disconnection of the oxygen supply in a paralysed patient, misplacement or cuff deflation of an endotracheal tube, thiopentone sodium injected into an artery, air entry into the venous system, removal of the wrong limb or organ, or an operation that was not indicated.

If an operation is inevitable, he will be exceedingly careful to select a surgeon who has good judgement and excellent technique. A sympathetic, caring approach will be a bonus, but a gentle, sympathetic, caring surgeon with the most wonderful bedside manner who has poor judgement and operates badly, can be a killer! A surgeon must know his trade which, as with skilled carpentry, follows an apprenticeship that involves working under the supervision of a master. No amount of reading can compensate for observing the master surgeon at work, assisting him and then putting what he has learned into practice.

In the course of training, most residents come in contact with a number of different surgeons and they quickly appreciate that good results can be achieved with a variety of different surgical approaches and techniques. A bad result usually follows a breach of basic rules, lack of knowledge, an attempt to operate too fast for the circumstances, or poor technical ability and judgement. A surgical resident should be a critical observer and learn to avoid the mistakes of the few bad surgeons.

PREOPERATIVE ASSESSMENT

A patient admitted to a surgical ward is almost always anxious and may be frightened or even terrified. For some major procedures it can be comforting for the ward sister to arrange for him to meet a patient who has recovered from a similar operation. For example, a patient fully rehabilitated after an abdominoperineal resection of the rectum, and a visit from a specialist stoma nurse for a patient who is to have a colostomy.

It is important to explain to the patient the exact nature of the operation, what it will involve in terms of the incisions, the pain, and the stay in hospital. If the surgeon is not sure what operation he is going to perform, he should describe the alternatives and ask the patient to delegate the decision to the surgeon at the time of the operation, when it is clear what procedure would be of most benefit to the patient. If it is likely that the patient will be in an intensive care unit (ICU) after operation, it is helpful if an ICU nurse meets the patient and explains the pattern of care in the ICU and the various cannulae likely to be inserted into him. The fullness of the preoperative explanation will depend, to some extent, on the patients own inclinations and intelligence. Some patients like to know everything possible in terms of dangers and pathology, others prefer to be given an outline without going into detail. In all cases, the close relatives should be interviewed and an explanation given to them of the surgeons appraisal of the prognosis and the seriousness of the proposed operation. If a dissection is particularly hazardous, for instance in a parotidectomy, where damage to the facial nerve may result, this must be explained to the patient and the relatives beforehand, although this does not absolve the surgeon from paying due care and attention to avoid this peril.

The anaesthetist's assessment will be extremely important and the surgeon also needs to examine the patient to assess the actual surgical exposure and any technical difficulties. For instance, previous operations or peritonitis may have resulted in adhesions which add to the risks. During special procedures there are important preoperative nursing preparations, for example, bowel wash-outs for large bowel surgery. The outcome following surgery may also be influenced by the physical condition of the patient. Obesity, malnutrition, chronic pulmonary, cardiac, renal or hepatic dysfunction and diabetes are all adverse factors that need to be carefully assessed. In all cases the patient should be as relaxed as possible, clean, with an empty stomach and preferably empty bowels and bladder.

POSITIONING AND CARE OF THE UNCONSCIOUS PATIENT

The anaesthetized patient is vulnerable, being deprived of his protective reflexes. One of the most tragic postoperative complications is a pulmonary embolus, following deep vein thrombosis; therefore great care should be exercised in avoiding undue pressure on the calves and if the patient has a poor peripheral blood supply, pressure points must be specially protected. Perioperative and postoperative subcutaneous heparin is given to patients over 50 years, to women on oral contraceptives, to cases undergoing extensive pelvic dissection and those with a history of previous deep venous thrombosis or pulmonary embolus. In a long operation an unskilled assistant may inadvertently lean on the patient's body and cause damage.

The choice of position and incision will depend on the access required for the procedure in question. Most intra-abdominal procedures are performed with the patient lying supine, at a lateral inclination, or in a head-down or head-up position. A patient will lie on his side for an extraperitoneal approach to the kidney, and a pillow placed under the shoulders to extend the neck facilitates approach to the thyroid.

The anaesthetist must have access to the cannulae that he has inserted, and in major operations he may need to measure urine production during the operation via a catheter draining into a sterile measuring flask at the upper end of the table. It may also be important that the surgeon is able to follow the principal observations of arterial and venous pressure and the electrocardiogram (ECG) on a suitably placed visual monitor.

It is the surgeon's responsibility, in consultation with the anaesthetist, to ensure that the patient is in the most appropriate position for the operation in question. In planning the incision the main consideration is to obtain the best view of the operative field with the minimum trauma to the patient. There is a tendency to try and operate through incisions of inadequate length, which may subject the patient to unnecessary danger and the surgeon to considerable difficulty. It is important to realize that a long incision will heal just as quickly as a short incision and if access through a small incision can only be achieved by excessive traction, this can itself cause damage.

COMMON ABDOMINAL INCISIONS

I will describe the median abdominal, paramedian and subcostal or Kocher's incisions as examples of abdominal incisions (Fig. 1), but in each operation described in the following chapters, special features of incisions with their individual advantages and disadvantages will be considered.

The most effective and one of the cheapest skin disinfectants is tincture of iodine (1% iodine in 70% alcohol). I use this as a routine, substituting Hibitane in spirit for infants and those sensitive to iodine.

THE MEDIAN ABDOMINAL INCISION

Since the linea alba runs from the xiphoid process to the pubic symphysis and is relatively avascular, incisions through it are popular with surgeons because the abdominal cavity can be entered quickly with minimal bleeding, and if the incision requires extension, this can be readily achieved in either direction.

Preparation

Place the patient in a supine position once the skin has been prepared and the operative site draped with towels.

Incision technique

1. Use a knife to make an incision in the skin and superficial fascia; its length depends on the exposure required for the operation in question.

2. Coagulate subcutaneous bleeding points with diathermy forceps and then, keeping strictly to the midline, incise the linea alba.

3. With the exception of patients with portal hypertension and bleeding diatheses, haemorrhage is usually minimal and after cutting the fibrous tissue of the linea alba at one point through its full extent, the parietal peritoneum will be seen as a layer adherent to the linea alba. This is picked up in forceps and incised; opening the peritoneal cavity is followed usually by a slight sucking of air into the abdomen and falling back of adjacent abdominal contents.

4. Using a pair of Mayo scissors, extend the incision in the linea alba through the peritoneum to the full length of the skin incision, taking care to avoid damage to any of the organs (Fig. 2), particularly the bowel which may be adherent to the linea alba as a result of previous surgery or peritonitis.

5. In the upper part of the incision the falciform ligament is attached to the linea alba and it is easy for the surgeon,

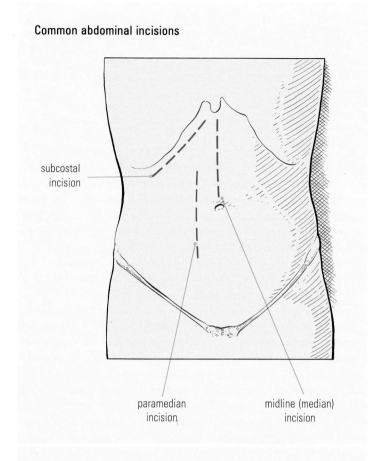

Common abdominal incisions

subcostal incision

paramedian incision

midline (median) incision

Fig. 1

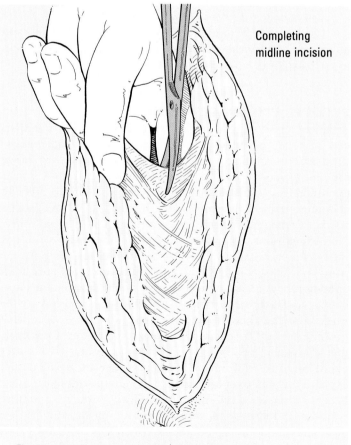

Completing midline incision

Fig. 2

particularly in an obese patient, to start dissecting in a confused way between the layers of the falciform ligament. If the surgeon is aware of the anatomy, he can take avoiding action by cutting the peritoneum just to one side of the falciform ligament, depending on where access is required. It may be necessary to ligate and divide the ligamentum teres and the falciform ligament.

Incision closure

After the operative procedure is completed, closure of the midline incision is usually performed with a non-absorbable monofilamentous synthetic suture such as nylon or a slowly absorbed material like Polydioxamone (PDS). I usually work with a hand-held Moynihan needle swaged to looped nylon (e.g. Ethilon) or PDS, and insert a continuous over-and-over stitch through the edges of cut linea alba starting at each end and tied off in the middle with the cut ends of the suture buried so that they do not stick out through the skin. Skin closure can be performed with either nylon stitches or skin tapes. In obese patients, interrupted absorbable stitches (catgut or Vicryl) are used in the subcutaneous tissue to approximate this layer.

THE PARAMEDIAN INCISION

This has similar exposure characteristics to a median incision, but because the rectus sheath is cut and resutured in front and behind of the rectus muscle, this incision should heal with greater strength and less likelihood of incisional hernia formation than a median incision.

Incision technique

1. Incise the skin and subcutaneous tissues in a vertical direction approximately 4cm from the midline and using diathermy coagulate the bleeding points in the subcutaneous tissue.

2. The anterior rectus sheath, a strong layer of fibrous tissue, then comes into view and is also incised vertically revealing the rectus muscle and its tendonous intersections which are attached to the sheath anteriorly (Fig. 3).

3. Pick up the medial cut edge of the sheath with a series of artery forceps, and use a sharp knife to divide the intersections encountered in the incision so that the rectus muscle is freed from its sheath (Fig. 4).

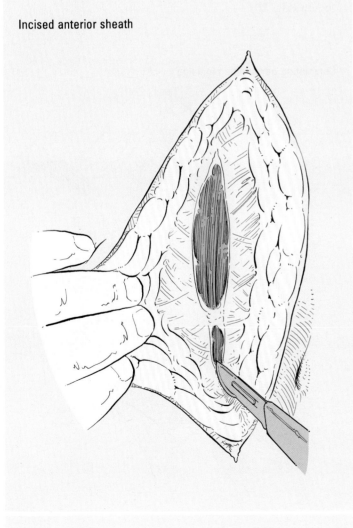

Incised anterior sheath

Fig. 3

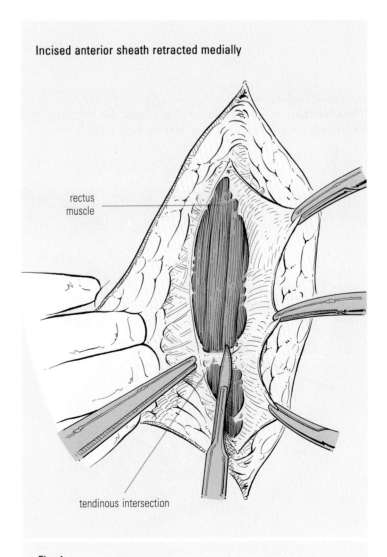

Incised anterior sheath retracted medially

rectus muscle

tendinous intersection

Fig. 4

4. Retract the rectus muscle laterally to reveal the posterior rectus sheath.

5. Pick up the posterior rectus sheath and peritoneum and open them in the same way as in the median incision taking the same precautions (Figs 5 and 6).

Incision closure

Closure of a paramedian incision is performed in two main layers, also with looped nylon or an absorbable material such as PDS. First the edges of the peritoneum and posterior rectus sheath are approximated (Fig. 7). The rectus muscle is then allowed to overlie the suture line and the cut edges of the anterior rectus sheath are sutured together (Fig. 8). The closure of the subcutaneous tissue (Fig. 9) and skin is similar to that described for a median incision.

It can be seen from the illustrations that the rectus muscle overlies and buttresses the two incisions in the rectus sheath. The disadvantage of a paramedian incision is that access to the abdomen on the opposite side to the incision is not quite as easy as with the median incision. Also, making the incision and closing it takes longer.

A median or paramedian incision should be employed if the surgeon performing a laparotomy is not certain of the diagnosis since they can be extended upwards or downwards if necessary.

THE SUBCOSTAL INCISION OF KOCHER

Theodore Kocher, the first surgeon to be awarded the Nobel Prize for Medicine, was Professor of Surgery in Berne and made outstanding contributions in a number of different branches of surgery. He has incisions named after him in the neck for exposure of the thyroid gland, over the hip for operations on the joint, and the right subcostal incision to approach the gall bladder and the right subhepatic fossa of Rutherford–Morison.

Incision technique

1. Make the abdominal incision approximately 4 cm below the costal margin. A common mistake is to cut too close to the costal margin, which can make closure of the incision difficult.

2. Divide the superficial fascia and coagulate the bleeding points. The anterior rectus sheath and the external oblique aponeurosis can now be seen, and at the lateral extremity muscular fibres of the external oblique are observed.

3. Divide this external layer to reveal the internal oblique muscle and the anterior surface of the rectus abdominis muscle. Partially mobilize the rectus with a finger and divide it using cutting diathermy or scissors. A Roberts' forcep deep to the rectus muscle prevents opening into the peritoneum (Fig. 10).

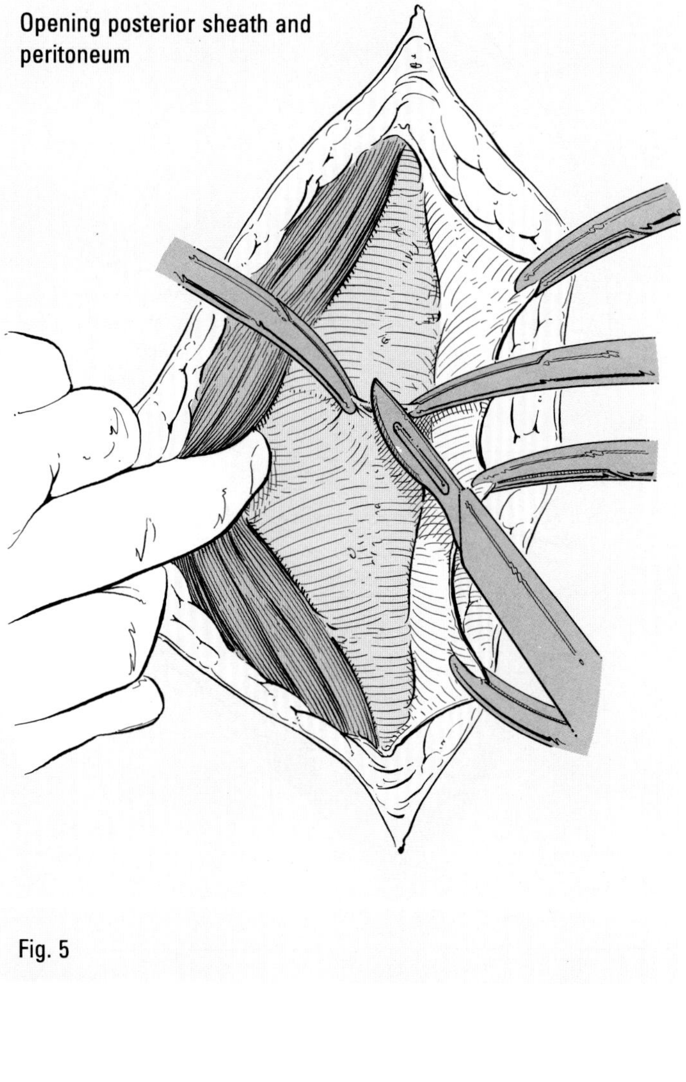

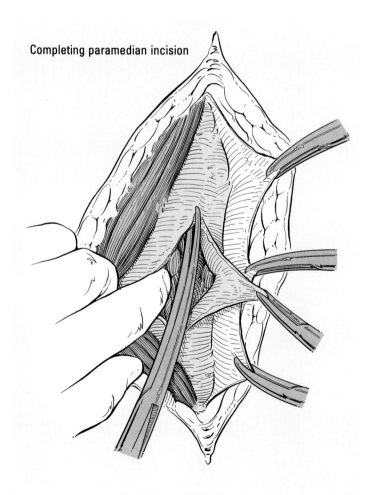

Opening posterior sheath and peritoneum

Completing paramedian incision

Fig. 5

Fig. 6

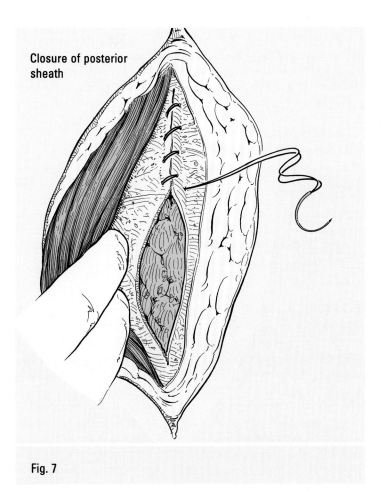

Closure of posterior sheath

Fig. 7

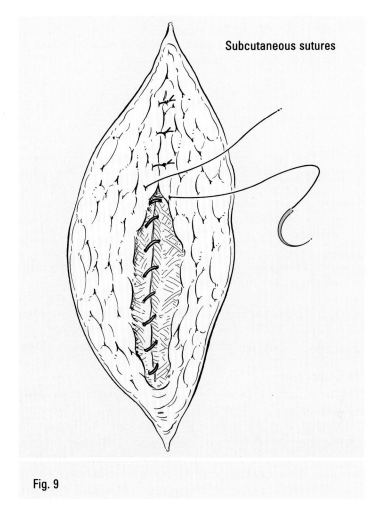

Subcutaneous sutures

Fig. 9

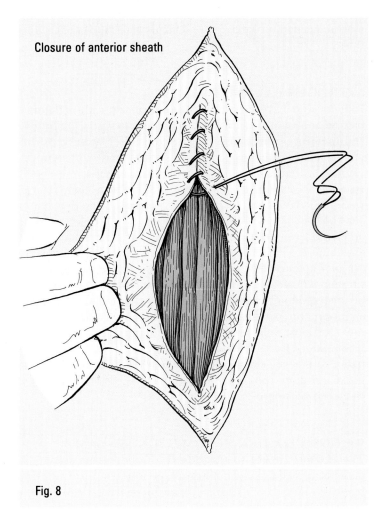

Closure of anterior sheath

Fig. 8

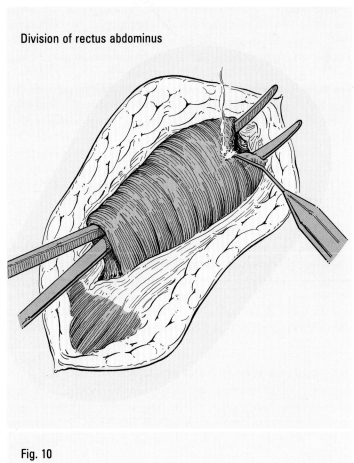

Division of rectus abdominus

Fig. 10

4. Branches of the superior epigastric artery and vein will now be seen. These require either diathermy or suture ligation with absorbable stitches such as Vicryl.

5. When the rectus muscle is fully divided and the posterior rectus sheath is seen, continue the incision through the internal oblique muscle.

6. The eighth and ninth intercostal nerves, with their vessels, passing obliquely between the internal oblique and transversus muscles are revealed. Divide them where they run across the incision; this leads to a partial denervation of the rectus muscle and sensory loss to the skin above the umbilicus.

7. Laterally, separate the fibres to reveal the transversalis fascia and the peritoneum beneath it.

8. Open the peritoneum and extend the incision as for a median or paramedian incision. Again, it is important to avoid a dissection between the layers of the falciform ligament medially.

Incision closure

Closure of a Kocher's incision is similar to closure of a median incision. It requires one layer of looped nylon or absorbable material such as PDS, starting at each end and tied in the middle through all layers of muscle and fascia. The subcutaneous tissue and skin are closed in a similar manner to the other incisions. If the gall bladder or biliary tract are operated on it is customary to drain the peritoneal cavity. For this I use a soft silicone rubber drain, 1cm in diameter, with several side holes cut in it; it drains by a closed system into a sterile bag. The drain is brought out through either a stab incision or via the lateral extremity of a Kocher's incision. In a stab incision the abdominal wall is retracted upwards by means of a pair of Kocher's forceps on the cut edge of the incised abdominal wall musculature and, using a small knife blade, a 1cm incision is made parallel to the intercostal nerves, through the skin and abdominal wall, but not as far as the peritoneum. A pair of Roberts' haemostatic forceps is then passed through the skin incision and pushed through the peritoneum, and used to grasp the obliquely cut end of the drainage tube which is pulled through the abdominal wall under direct vision to avoid catching any other tissues with it. Having positioned the tube so that the holes are all within the peritoneal cavity, it is sutured to the skin with a silk or nylon stitch and left *in situ* until drainage of blood or bile stained haemoserous fluid ceases.

It will be clear from the above description that Kocher's incision requires more dissection and will take longer than either a median or paramedian incision, but it has the advantage of directly overlying the gall bladder and this can facilitate dissection of a diseased gall bladder that might be difficult to see with a median or right paramedian incision.

BACTERIAL WOUND INFECTIONS

With the incisions described above, healing should be by first intention; the skin stitches can be removed between the seventh and tenth day and the patient should be advised not to do any heavy lifting for 3 months, although normal activities such as driving a car or moderate exercise can be permitted after between 2 and 3 weeks. If infection develops in the wound, which is likely if the patient suffered from intra-abdominal sepsis, there will be signs of inflammation with a raised temperature, leucocytosis, redness, swelling of the wound and purulent exudate. The skin sutures surrounding inflamed areas should be removed, the pus cultured and the patient started on broad-spectrum antibiotics, which can be substituted for a specific antibiotic if indicated by the culture.

Perioperative prophylactic antibiotics are used in clean operations involving the vascular system, especially when prosthetic grafts are inserted and in patients where sepsis is suspected or encountered in the course of the operation. The choice of antibiotics will depend on the nature and sensitivities of organisms encountered or suspected of being present. Prophylactic antibiotics should not be given for more than a few days, otherwise resistant bacteria will flourish.

POSTOPERATIVE MANAGEMENT

Postoperatively, it is the responsibility of the anaesthetist to ensure that the patient recovers consciousness and the endotracheal tube remains in place until the patient can breathe and cough spontaneously. If there is danger of vomiting following operations on the abdominal organs it is usually best to leave a nasogastric tube in place until bowel sounds return and flatus is passed *per rectum*. It is most important that the patient is given adequate analgesia and made as comfortable as possible, with attention being paid to his position and pressure points. His mouth should also be kept clean and he must be assisted so he can empty his bladder and bowels when required. Intravenous fluid replacement is continued until the patient can take fluid orally. In seriously ill patients parenteral nutrition may be needed or enteral supplements via a fine-bore feeding tube.

NITROGEN BALANCE

Patients who have been very ill, particularly with abdominal fistulae or prolonged sepsis, will not be able to synthesize protein and therefore cannot heal their wounds after surgery. Such a patient in 'negative nitrogen balance' is a poor risk and definitive surgical procedures should be avoided unless they are absolutely essential, for example draining pus or stopping a haemorrhage. Even if the bowel looks healthy, no attempt should be made at anastomosis unless the patient is in positive nitrogen balance, otherwise even with the most perfect surgical technique the anastomosis will still fall apart. Although the nitrogen balance can be estimated biochemically, an experienced ward sister or surgeon will be able to tell if the patient has achieved this state because suddenly, and it often appears as if it had occurred at an instant, the patient who has previously been sick and wasted starts to look well, feels hungry and can eat. This is often accompanied by a smile when visited rather than a sad countenance. It is at this stage that the patient will probably be able to withstand more complicated operative procedures with a good chance of healing.

WOUND CLOSURE IN COMPLICATED CASES

This section applies to the closure of abdominal wounds in patients with abdominal dehiscence, poor nutrition or suffering from sepsis. In such cases, instead of burying unabsorbable sutures which may cut out through poor quality tissue and provide a nidus for infection, I close the abdomen with one layer of interrupted, deep, approximated nylon sutures with internal tissue loops (Fig. 11). These give a remarkably smooth internal peritoneal suture line that can be felt with a finger prior to closure; the stitches are removed after 6 weeks.

It may be impossible to close grossly infected wounds, especi-ally if there has been tissue loss. The wound then has to be left open with moist antiseptic dressings, for example gauze soaked in half-strength eusol applied two or three times a day, until the patient achieves positive nitrogen balance and can lay down healthy granulation tissue over which skin epithelium can grow. If the defect is large, split-skin grafting may speed the process.

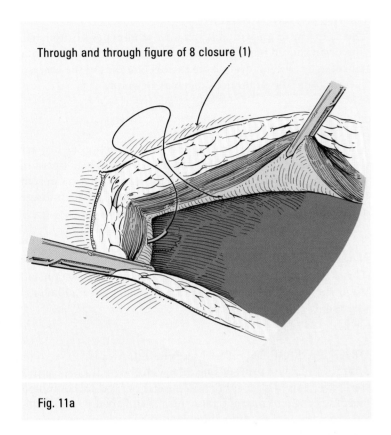

Through and through figure of 8 closure (1)

Fig. 11a

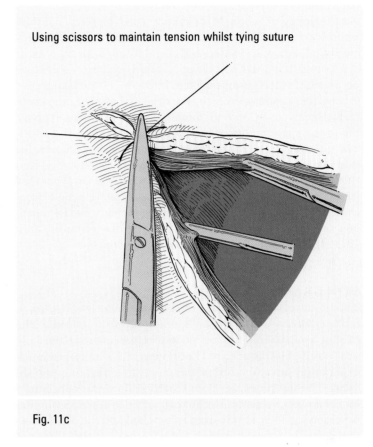

Using scissors to maintain tension whilst tying suture

Fig. 11c

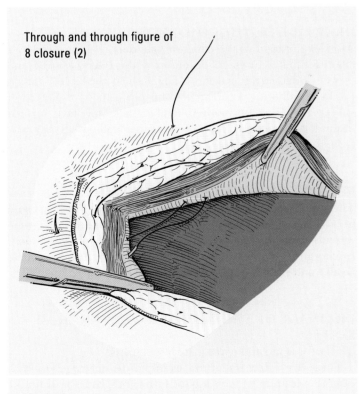

Through and through figure of 8 closure (2)

Fig. 11b

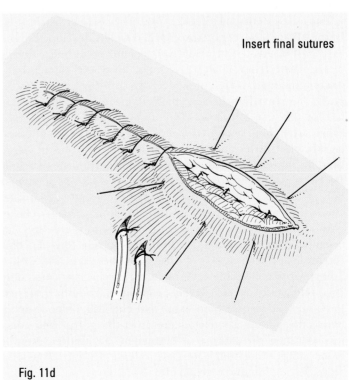

Insert final sutures

Fig. 11d

Healing is usually very slow at first but once started, the process speeds up. The patient may need skilled hospital treatment for weeks or months, before recovering.

MANAGEMENT OF CONTAMINATED WOUNDS

At the end of the 1914–18 war it was agreed by all surgeons who had taken care of casualties that primary closure of a potentially contaminated wound usually resulted in death from overwhelming infection. Many soldiers could be rescued if their wounds were excised until the frank haemorrhage of freshly bleeding tissue was exposed and then left open for 10 days. If the wound was then still clean, delayed primary suture was permissible. Any signs of purulent infection dictated a policy of leaving the wound open with free drainage until healing eventually occurred by second intention with granulation tissue filling the space and later re-epithelialization from the edges. The introduction of antibiotics and new surgical techniques, for example skin grafting, in no way altered the above ground rules developed as a result of the observations of many wounded young men. It is a sad reflection on how little we benefit from experience, that the ground rules had to be relearned by repetition of the same errors in every war that has occurred since 1914–18, including the Falklands engagement.

SKIN GRAFTING

The use of vascularized flaps of skin and underlying tissues to replace defects was practised sporadically from 600 BC. The earliest available description of flap replacement of the nose was recorded by the ancient Hindu surgeons, who gained much experience, since removal of the nose was a common punishment. The technique was popularized in the sixteenth century by the Italian surgeon, Tagliacozzi. After 2–3 weeks the flap developed a blood supply from its new bed and the old connection could be severed, freeing the transposed tissue. Flaps are of great value in covering large defects, especially when bone is exposed.

The use of autologous free skin grafting was described in 1800 by the Milanese surgeon, Baronio, and widely developed in the early half of this century. Survival depends on technical details of the graft removal and placement on a well-vascularized, uncontaminated recipient bed. Both full-thickness (Wolfe) grafts and partial-thickness (Thiersch) grafts have a precarious life for the first 3–4 days before a new blood supply is established, when nourishment depends solely on diffusion of gases, liquids, electrolytes and other vital substances from the tissue fluid on the surface of the graft bed. The advantage of a full-thickness graft is its quality and appearance with its contained normal dermis. However, the defect of the donor site must be closed and may itself need grafting. With a partial-thickness graft sufficient epithelial cells left in the donor site dermis can re-epithelialize the area in 10–15 days (see page 10.7). For this reason split-thickness skin grafts, cut either freehand with a knife or with a mechanical dermatome, are the most commonly used skin grafts. After 3–4 days, capillaries from the graft bed grow into the transplanted tissue and establish a blood supply and connect with vascular elements in the graft, thus safely incorporating the graft as a permanent acquisition. A graft from another individual, unless an identical twin, will be destroyed by an immune reaction after 7–14 days.

DRAINS

The purpose of drainage is to remove potentially dangerous materials from a variety of sites involved directly or indirectly in surgery and to release extravasated blood and body fluids in an abnormal situation or trapped and unable to escape by the normal anatomical route.

DRAINAGE OF AN ABSCESS

This is the most ancient and valuable of all types of drainage. The drain should be large enough to drain thick pus and other debris, and it should drain from the deepest part of the abscess. Suction using the sump principle may be helpful.

URINARY CATHETER

This catheter is used when there is an obstruction of urinary drainage, for operations on the bladder to prevent high pressure developing, and when it is important to measure urinary output (e.g. in a shocked patient). Ureteric and renal pelvis drainage are used for similar reasons in special conditions.

NASOGASTRIC DRAINAGE

This is used in cases of gastric or high intestinal obstruction and when the bowel is paralysed after any major intra-abdominal operation.

DRAINAGE OF THE PERITONEAL CAVITY

A large bore, 1 cm, soft, silicone tube with closed drainage into a sterile bag is used after surgery in cases of peritonitis, continued bleeding or when contamination may be anticipated (e.g. drainage from the region of the duodenal stump, where closure was difficult or unsatisfactory).

DRAINAGE OF THE COMMON BILE DUCT

After exploration of the common bile duct, a drain (usually a latex T-tube) is used to decompress the biliary system and prevent a dangerous leakage of bile. Usually the latex T-tube is removed following a cholangiogram performed 10 days after surgery, when a fibrinous tube-like track will have formed around the emerging limb of the tube, walling off any leak from the peritoneal cavity.

PLEURAL AND PERICARDIAL DRAINS

These are used following operations on the lungs or heart, and in cases of tension pneumothorax and cardiac tamponade when urgent drainage can be life-saving. The end of a pleural drain is submerged underwater in a container beneath the bed to act as a valve and prevent air being sucked into the chest (Fig. 12).

DRAINAGE OF THE CEREBRAL VENTRICULAR SYSTEM

This is for acute and chronic hydrocephalus.

These are a few important examples of drainage. In each case, the drain must have a bore sufficiently large to drain the material in question. The influence of gravity is important, even if there is a marked pressure differential between the space being drained and the outside. Fluid sinks and gas rises (a dictum of Dr Norman Shumway, Surgeon, Stanford, USA), is an essential and continuous thought in the minds of cardiac surgeons at all times, but also important in more mundane drainage procedures. In all cases the possible advantages of gentle suction or sump suction on the drain should be considered and intercostal drains must always be connected to a valve, usually an underwater seal. Siphonage may be utilized but can cause excessive loss if it develops inadvertently, for example, from a long-armed biliary T-tube in the duodenum.

A drain can form a path up which infection can travel, both inside and outside the tube. For this reason care should be taken to clean the skin around the drain and to connect the drain to a bag or bottle as a closed system and to remove the drain as soon as possible. Drains are usually left *in situ* until they stop draining, or the need for which they were originally intended no longer exists (e.g. nasogastric tubes are removed after bowel sounds return and flatus is passed *per rectum*).

Numerous papers appear over the years claiming that drainage is no longer indicated in certain procedures. Although it may be possible to avoid drainage in cases where established teaching would recommend their use, caution should be exercised in abandoning any procedure practised by experienced surgeons where the objective is to increase the safety of the patient. Ask a surgeon having an operation if he would like the usual drainage omitted!

EXPOSURE, ILLUMINATION AND ASSISTANTS

The importance of siting and extent of the surgical incision is central to the safe outcome of an operation. A long incision in the wrong place or too short an incision in the correct site can be disastrous. Most operations are performed near the apex of a cone of exposure, which will be satisfactory only if the view of the operative site is good and appropriate instruments can be manipulated for the job in question. Modern overhead lighting, if properly directed and focused, can reach a small deep target with little disturbance from shadows. However, a point source of light either on the surgeons head or on a malleable, sterlizable, fibre optic stalk will often enhance the view and can be critical when the cone of the operative field is narrow and deep. Experienced, intelligent assistance can be essential to a successful outcome of a difficult operation. A good assistant like a good operating nurse can anticipate the next stage of the operation and facilitate exposure and present layers of tissue at the appropriate time for surgical dissection. Much surgical assistance however involves prolonged and often arduous traction on retractors, requiring no intellectual effort or stimulation. An American anaesthetist, Dr Thompson, having observed this rather unedifying activity of highly selected residents over a 30-year period, designed an adjustable metal frame clamp that can reproduce the retraction efficiently, without wasting the time of a resident and in many cases the surgeon has better access and is not hampered by an assistant standing where he himself may need to be for optimal access. The Thompson retractor (Fig. 13) is an example of many similar mechanical retractors now available. The author has performed an orthotropic liver graft with a Thompson retractor, one surgical assistant and an operating nurse, without any access difficulties; the same number of people as that used for a simple appendicectomy.

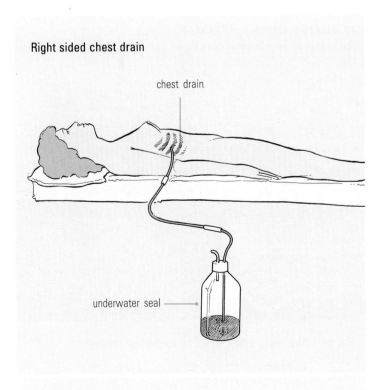

Right sided chest drain

chest drain

underwater seal

Fig. 12

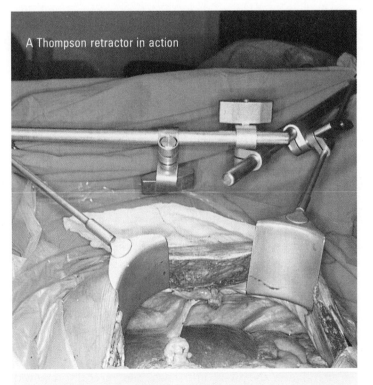

A Thompson retractor in action

Fig. 13

HAEMOSTASIS

With the exception of operating in a bloodless field, for example an exsanguinated limb with a proximal tourniquet, surgical dissection from the skin incision onwards will be accompanied by the division of blood vessels which will shed blood and require the use of swabs, diathermy or packs.

Dabbing the field, not rubbing, will clear the view sufficiently for the bleeding point or vessel to be picked up with fine-toothed dissecting forceps or haemostatic clamps. Diathermy forceps can be used to grasp and coagulate the blood vessels, or they can be applied to the fine-toothed forceps and clamps. With large bleeding points a ligature or, to be more certain, a suture is tied around the vessel secured in forceps or clamps, which are then removed. Blood vessels crossing the operative field may be seen and dealt with before cutting; or a diathermy knife may be used for dissection, but this technique will only coagulate small vessels. An oozing surface or large bleeding vessel may be controlled by temporary packing with pressure applied by hand. After some 10–20 minutes of control, removal of the pack and use of a powerful sucker may permit a sufficiently accurate sighting of the important bleeding point for it to be clamped or sutured. An alternative, happy discovery is that the bleeding point may have sealed itself during the interval. Bleeding from a large vein is particularly worrying, not only is there a danger of exsanguination, but if the pressure within the vein falls too low, air can be sucked into the lumen of the vein causing a fatal embolus by frustrating the function of the chambers of the right side of the heart. If packing does not give control, the vein wall surrounding the hole can often be picked up gently with a Babcock tissue forceps and then a non-absorbable (e.g. Prolene) suture can be inserted around the defect, taking care not to pass the suture through the hollow blades of the forceps, a real hazard!

It may be impossible to control arterial bleeding without proximal control. Obviously it is preferable to obtain control before opening the artery, but unfortunately an arterial wall may be breached before control has been achieved and then management can be difficult. If local pressure on the bleeding point with a dental swab, or any suitable non-traumatic instrument, controls the bleeding temporarily, the surgeon can proceed and dissect carefully above and below so that the artery can be clamped. The main operative incision may need to be enlarged to give safe access. Plunging haemostatic forceps blindly into a pool of blood is likely to lead to disaster, by aggravating the damage. Powerful suction with one or two suckers may be required, whilst rapid blood replacement is taking place. If haemostasis cannot be achieved by the above methods, perhaps in a patient with clotting defects, a contused parenchymatous organ (e.g. the liver), or a large raw dissected surface, careful placement of packs may stop the bleeding. The surgeon should then be delighted and make use of the vital dimension of time, often ignored in surgical practice. The packs should be left undisturbed for approximately 48 hours, whilst the patient treated with broad-spectrum antibiotics, is resuscitated by transfusion and given fresh frozen plasma and platelets until coagulation defects are corrected and the haemodynamic state of the patient restored to as normal a state as possible. Usually a non-shocked patient can then be taken back to the operating theatre and with skilled anaesthesia and experienced surgeons in attendance, the packs are slowly and carefully removed. Irrigation with warm saline may free packs that seem to be stuck by clot to the patient. Often the surgeon is surprised and

gratified to find that no more bleeding occurs, or only a few bleeding vessels are present and these can easily be dealt with. Occasionally a more major procedure is necessary, but the patient has the advantage of a non-shocked state, normal coagulable blood and a rested surgical team.

Bleeding is certainly the chief enemy of the surgeon and dealing with it successfully requires sound judgement, quick and careful action and the exploitation of time for the application of effective haemostatic measures.

CHOICE OF INSTRUMENTS AND SUTURE MATERIALS

The chief surgical instruments are the surgeon's eyes and fingers. Many tissues, organs and pathological lesions can be seen with good exposure, but frequently both the normal anatomy and abnormal changes can only be assessed by careful educated palpation which will provide sufficient information on which to plan the operation (e.g. the degree of mobility of a tumour may determine whether it can be removed). A good surgical technician is usually familiar with a limited repertoire of instruments which are to him like good old friends, efficient and reliable. A surgeon demanding numerous instruments that can only with difficulty be found in a number of catalogues is usually a poor technician. In general the lightest, most atraumatic and smallest instrument and suture that will perform the function required is the best, but to use a fine instrument or suture for thick or hard tissue is a travesty of good surgical technique that will damage the instruments and break the suture. I will give a list of the instruments I use in Figs 14–18, but this is only the opinion of one surgeon.

For ligatures I use an absorbable material such as Vicryl or catgut, or a non-absorbable silk thread. For suturing absorbable catgut, Vicryl or Polydioxamone (PDS), and non-absorbable nylon, Ethibond or Prolene are suitable.

METHODS OF DISSECTION

The purpose of surgical dissection is to reveal sufficient of the

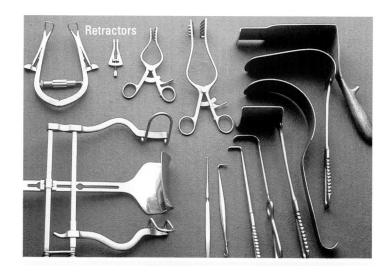

Fig. 14 **Top row:** Jolles, Alms, Weisslander, Travers

Bottom row: Balfour, Gillies skin hooks, Kilner 'cats paw', small and medium Langenbeck, Morris, Deaver, Kelly, St Mark's.

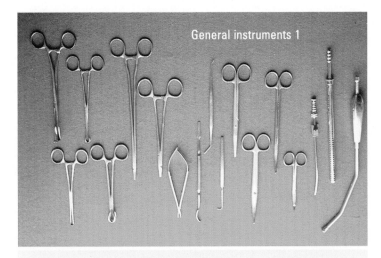

Fig. 15   Tissue holder (Duval, Allis, Babcock, Lane), needle holders (Sarot, Mayo-Hegar, Castroviejo), MacDonald dissector, Watson-Cheyne dissector, Graefe muscle hook, scissors (straight Mayo, curved Mayo, Metzenbaum, Kilner), suckers (American pattern, Pool sump, Yankauer).

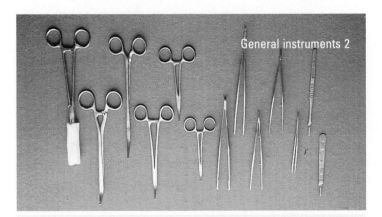

Fig. 16   Rampley sponge holder, artery forceps (Moynihan, Roberts, Birkett, Cryle, Mosquito), dissecting forceps (Lane, DeBakey, MacIndoe, Gillies, Watchmaker's), Bard-Parker scalpel handles.

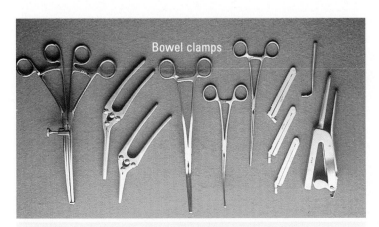

Fig. 17   Lane twin-clamp, large Payr, small Payr, Hayes, curved Doyen, straight Doyen, set of Zachary-Cope clamps.

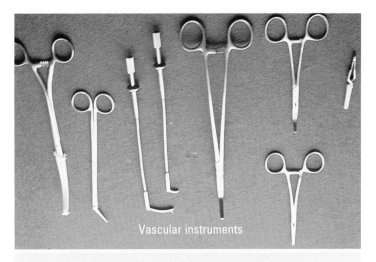

Fig. 18   Crafoord clamp, Potts scissors, large and small Zeppelin clamps, Satinsky clamp, straight and curved Cooley paediatric clamps, Blalock 'bulldog' clamp.

anatomy relevant to the operative procedure; no more and no less. Dissection can be sharp with a knife or scissors, or blunt with a probe, dental swab or the surgeon's finger. Anatomical identification is an essential prerequisite to sharp dissection, and gentle, blunt dissection will help separate tissue planes and define anatomy. A combination of the two techniques is usually necessary to enable completion of the operation.

SURGICAL HAZARDS EXCLUDING HAEMORRHAGE

Most surgical errors occur following damage to important structures (e.g. the common bile duct, the ureter, nerves and blood vessels, which may be cut, bruised or ligated). Failure to define the relevant anatomy due to ignorance, poor exposure or abnormal anatomy, perhaps distorted by pathology, are relevant factors often aggravated by the surgeon trying to operate too fast under the circumstances encountered.

Pus, and infected blood and tissue fluids can be hazardous, not only to the patient but also to the surgical and nursing staff. Bacteria can be identified by culture and antibiotic prophylaxis and treatment is usually effective. Viruses however are more dangerous. All those working in operating theatres should be vaccinated against hepatitis B, but this gives no protection against hepatitis C. The transference of the new hazard HIV during an operation is often said to be unlikely, but the AIDS virus is subject to frequent mutations and since the disease is usually spread by blood innoculation it would be unwise to minimize the potential danger of operating on patients with HIV antigenaemia. Precautions similar to those for hepatitis should always be taken.

ANASTOMOSES

The joining together end-to-end, side-to-side or end-to-side of tubular anatomical structures is called an anastomosis. The success of an anastomosis, whatever the site, depends on an adequate blood supply and a patient in positive nitrogen balance. Interrupted sutures interfere less with the blood supply, but are not quite as sound at sealing together the joined ends as a continuous suture. Non-absorbable sutures give security but if infected can cause prolonged inflammation, and continuous non-absorbable sutures will inhibit growth which may be important when operating on a child. Long lasting, but eventually absorbable modern synthetic sutures (e.g. PDS and Maxon) seem to have the advantages of security and eventual disappearance. Multiple metal staples, which are becoming popular, are dispensed in a disposable cartridge and applied by a mechanical device called a stapling gun. Once the dissection is complete to prepare the ends to be joined, the actual anatomosis is performed instantaneously by squeezing the trigger of the gun.

Endothelial lined blood vessels require careful end-to-end apposition to avoid any tendency to eversion, so that only endothelium is exposed to the lumen. A mattress-everting stitch may help achieve endothelial apposition; any other tissue in contact with blood acts as a nidus for clot formation. There are many methods of anastomosing blood vessels, all derived from the original triangulation technique of Alexis Carrel shown in Fig. 19. I often use one suture starting at the furthermost point and depending on the ease of sighting, either drawing together the walls immediately, or gradually pulling them into approximation if access is difficult. This is sometimes called parachuting because of the multiple, long lengths of suture material like

Triangulation of a tube

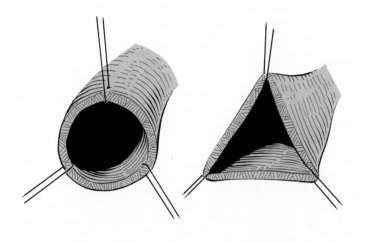

Fig. 19

Anterior layer

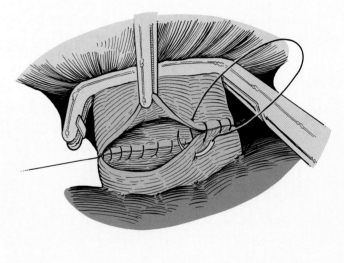

Fig. 20b

Posterior layer of vascular anastomosis (suprahepatic inferior vena cava in a liver transplant)

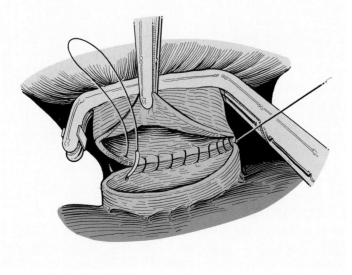

Fig. 20a

Completed anastomosis

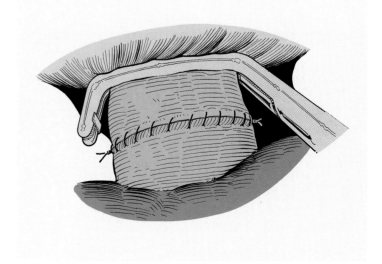

Fig. 20c

parachute strings, but they can easily be fouled with one another to produce an entangled 'cat's cradle'. It is often easy to suture the furthermost wall from within the lumen so that endothelial apposition can be observed with each stitch (Fig. 20). The nearer wall is sutured from outside.

With epithelial lined tubes, for example oesophagus, stomach, small and large bowel, ureter, bile duct, trachea and bronchus, the epithelium should not be permitted to pout externally since this may lead to leakage of luminal contents. The American surgeon, Connell, is said to have learned his stitch from his mother, an accomplished seamstress. It is effective in preventing eversion of the epithelium (Fig. 21). An interrupted equivalent was described by Grey–Turner which can be inserted horizontally or vertically (Fig. 22). The stomach, small bowel

Connell stitch

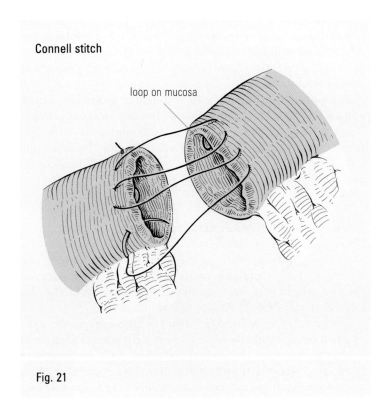

loop on mucosa

Fig. 21

Grey Turner's suture (2)

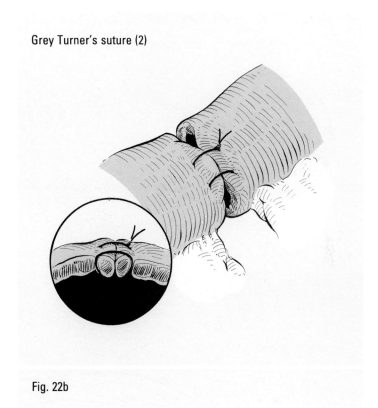

Fig. 22b

Grey Turner's suture (1)

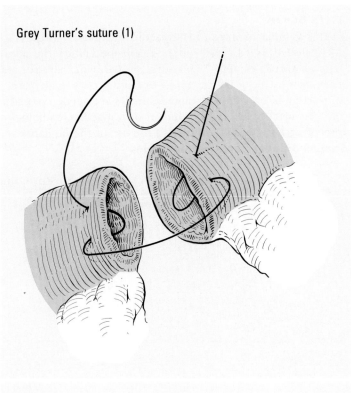

Fig. 22a

Alternative interrupted inverting suture

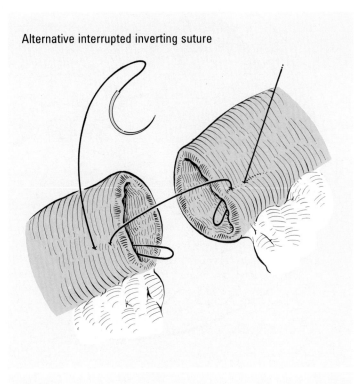

Fig. 22c

Bowel anastomosis in 2 layers

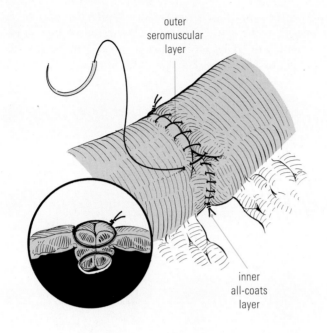

outer
seromuscular
layer

inner
all-coats
layer

Fig. 23

Nephrostomy tube

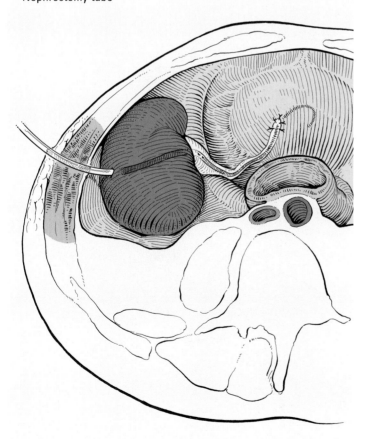

Fig. 24

and proximal large bowel have good blood supplies, so two layers of sutures, an inner all-coats, inverting, continuous layer and a seromuscular Lembert's stitch, continuous or interrupted (Fig. 23), usually give satisfactory results; an absorbable material, such as PDS, is a good suture material for these anastomoses. However, the oesophagus, rectum, trachea, bronchus, common bile duct and ureter all have relatively precarious blood supplies and one layer of sutures with a tendency to inversion can give good results. Fine interrupted absorbable (e.g. PDS) stitches are satisfactory for the biliary and urinary tracts, and may find favour for use in the oesophagus, rectum, trachea and bronchus, where at present non-absorbable sutures are recommended. A few extra interrupted adventitious sutures may take tension off the main anastomotic suture line.

Temporary indwelling soft atraumatic stents are usually employed following anastomosis of the bile duct or ureter, a T-tube for the former (see page 4.12) and a nephrostomy, transvesical tube or double-J ureteric stent for the latter (Fig. 24). The stents are removed when anastomotic healing has been confirmed radiographically.

WOUND DRESSING AND CARE

Before skin closure, application of antibiotic powder to the wound or spraying with an organic iodide compound (e.g. Betadine) may eliminate small numbers of contaminating bacteria which may have reached the wound from the skin edge, atmosphere or the surgical manipulations.

The gaps between the skin stitches or clips are quickly occluded in a clean wound by fibrin. A very light absorbent dressing is usually placed on the wound and fixed there by atraumatic strapping. Modern translucent non-occlusive dressings have the advantage of permitting observation of the wound without disturbing it until the stitches or clips are removed.

THIS BOOK

In this volume neonatal, orthopaedic and plastic surgery are not included, but to each of these sub-specialities, the above general principles apply. Of course, instruments, sutures and delicacy must be scaled down in operating on the neonate, a knowledge of burn injuries and aesthetics are needed in plastic and reconstructive surgery, and in orthopaedics, radiological interpretation, physiotherapy and the use of the implants and fixation techniques are very important.

Professor Sir Roy Calne

1

Head and Neck Surgery

Excision of Sebaceous Cyst

Sebaceous cysts, more properly named pilar or epidermoid cysts, occur on hair-bearing regions of the body, particularly the scalp. Apart from cosmetic considerations they can be inconvenient and may become infected, so surgical removal is generally advisable.

PREOPERATIVE ASSESSMENT
1. Confirm the diagnosis with a careful clinical examination.
2. In infected cases, perform a simple incision and drainage, and attempt to avulse as much of the lining of the cyst as possible with an artery forceps. An elective excision of the cyst can be performed later if it recurs.
3. Is there any history of sensitivity to local anaesthetic agents?

RELEVANT ANATOMY
Pilar or epidermoid cysts arise from the pilosebaceous apparatus following blockage of the mouth of the follicle, which as a result becomes filled with broken down keratin (sebum). Cysts lie within the dermis of the skin, are not tethered deeply, but are attached to the epidermis; this point of attachment is generally marked by a small punctum on the skin surface (Fig. 1.1).

OPERATION
Preparation
The patient is positioned either prone, supine or on their side to expose the area of the cyst, which has been shaved. A water-soluble gel can be used to flatten the hair around the cyst to keep it out of the wound. Do not be tempted to have the patient seated, as they may suffer a vasovagal attack. Cleanse and drape the area and infiltrate around the cyst and along the proposed line of the skin incision with a local anaesthetic agent such as 1% lignocaine.

Incision
Make an elliptical incision over the dome of the cyst, adjusted to allow comfortable approximation of the skin edges when the cyst has been removed (Fig. 1.2).

Operative technique
1. Deepen the incision until the cyst wall is reached; the wall is smooth and shiny and easy to identify. Take care to avoid puncturing the cyst which will make subsequent dissection more difficult.

2. Grasp the skin ellipse with an Allis tissue-holding forceps and use it to apply traction to the cyst.

3. With curved Kilner's scissors, dissect the cyst from the

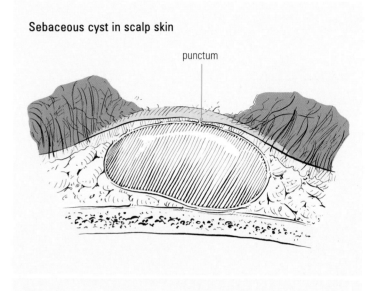

Sebaceous cyst in scalp skin

punctum

Fig. 1.1

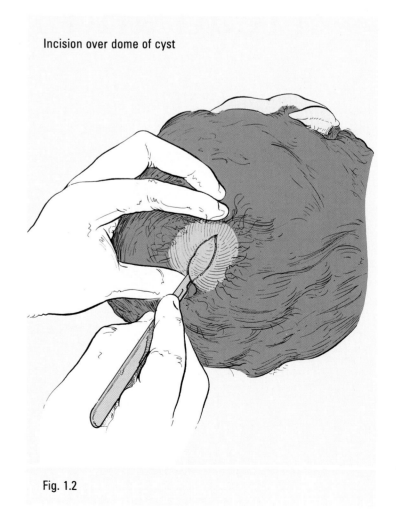

Incision over dome of cyst

Fig. 1.2

1.2

surrounding subcutaneous tissues on one side whilst draw-ing the cyst to the other side (Fig. 1.3). It is essential to keep close to the surface of the cyst at all times. The plane is relatively bloodless. Repeat this, drawing the cyst to the other side until it is completely free. Send the specimen with the attached ellipse of skin for histological analysis.

Dissection kept close to cyst wall

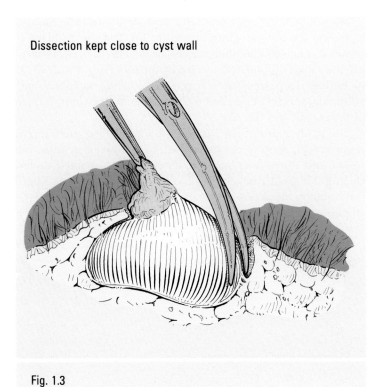

Fig. 1.3

4. Stop bleeding from the scalp edge with diathermy or fine catgut sutures.

Wound closure and dressing
Close the wound with interrupted non-absorbable sutures such as silk. If the operation was on the scalp apply a plastic spray dressing; elsewhere cover it with a waterproof sticking plaster.

POSTOPERATIVE CARE
This procedure is generally performed as a day-case. Advise the patient to keep the area dry until the sutures are removed. If the wound is on the scalp, the hair can be washed in warm water on the day of the operation to remove any blood, but then kept dry for a further week, when the sutures can be removed.

SPECIAL OPERATIVE HAZARDS
Rupture of the cyst; this makes removal more difficult since the cyst collapses and the sebum obscures the operative field.

COMPLICATIONS
1. Recurrence of the cyst, which may occur if the cyst ruptures and part of the wall remains.
2. Wound infection or wound haematoma; these can be reduced by preventing hair from falling into the wound and by ensuring good haemostasis before wound closure.

Lymph Node Biopsy

A lymph node biopsy from the neck should only be performed after careful examination and investigation has failed to elicit an underlying local primary tumour (e.g. in the nasopharynx, tongue or larynx), distant primary tumour (e.g. in the stomach or breast etc.), or source of infection (e.g. a dental abscess, chronic tonsillar infection or pulmonary tuberculosis). HIV infection *per se* is not an indication for lymph node biopsy although a histological diagnosis of tuberculosis or lymphoma may be required in such cases. Lymph node biopsy is a procedure that requires consideration of the anatomy before surgery begins.

PREOPERATIVE ASSESSMENT

1. Confirm the diagnosis; a firm mass in the anterior triangle may be a congenital branchial cyst, while a mass in the cheek may be a lesion in the parotid. An ultrasound scan is indicated if doubt exists.
2. Tumours of the nasopharynx, tongue base and oropharynx, supraglottic larynx and pyriform fossa often present as neck node metastases. Therefore, a full ENT examination (to include dentition, tongue and oral cavity, nasopharynx, and larynx and hypopharynx) is essential. This examination may prove to be inadequate, necessitating full endoscopy of the upper airway, pharynx and oesophagus under general anaesthetic prior to excision biopsy of the node.
3. Thyroid ultrasound and ⁹⁹technetium scanning is indicated if a primary thyroid tumour is suspected.
4. Non-head and neck tumours may metastasize to the neck (e.g. from the oesophagus, stomach, pancreas, breast, bronchus or a distant malignant melanoma). Appropriate investigations should be performed as dictated by presenting symptoms (e.g. fibreoptic bronchoscopy or endoscopy, chest X-ray, mammography etc.).
5. Fine needle aspiration cytology may be diagnostic, but depends on expert interpretation of the sample obtained. However, thyroid carcinoma, squamous or adenocarcinoma, lymphoma and tuberculosis can all be diagnosed in this fashion, which may obviate the need for excision.
6. If tuberculosis is suspected then chest X-ray, sputum bacteriology and Mantoux testing may obviate the need for biopsy.

RELEVANT ANATOMY

The lymphatic drainage of the head and neck is to nodes arranged in superficial and deep groups, the main final pathway being via the deep cervical nodes surrounding the internal jugular vein.

Superficial nodes draining the scalp, face and external ear are arranged in occipital (apex of the posterior triangle), post-auricular, pre-auricular and parotid groups; with the latter lying deep to the parotid fascia on the surface of the gland (Fig. 1.4). The superficial ring is completed by the submandibular and submental nodes, and there are additional superficial nodes along the external jugular vein.

The submental nodes drain the anterior floor of the mouth, including the tongue, gums and lower lip, and the drainage is bilateral. The submandibular nodes lie deep to the fascia covering the salivary gland and receive lymphatics from a wide area, including deep structures (e.g. nasal cavity, maxillary and ethmoidal sinuses), as well as the tongue and oropharynx, floor of the mouth and the face.

The main nodes of the head and neck lie along the internal jugular vein, deep to sternomastoid, in two major groups; the upper and lower deep cervical. There are two named nodes, the jugulodigastric below the posterior belly of digastric where the common facial vein enters the internal jugular vein, and the jugulo-omohyoid above the inferior belly of omohyoid where it crosses the internal jugular vein deep to sternomastoid (Fig. 1.5).

The supraclavicular nodes correspond to the postero-inferior nodes of the deep cervical chain which project into the posterior

Superficial lymph node groups

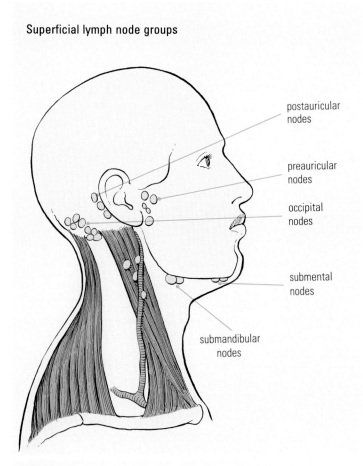

postauricular
nodes

preauricular
nodes

occipital
nodes

submental
nodes

submandibular
nodes

Fig. 1.4

triangle, behind the posterior border of sternomastoid. The lateral nodes of the upper deep cervical group appear in the posterior triangle in close relation to the accessory nerve.

A further group of deep nodes is arranged around the larynx and trachea (pre- and paratracheal nodes) and pharynx (retro-pharyngeal nodes).

OPERATION
Preparation
A preliminary direct laryngoscopy, pharyngoscopy, oesophago-scopy, bronchoscopy and examination under general anaesthetic of the nasopharynx, with biopsies as necessary, are performed with the patient supine and the head extended on a flexed neck. A suitable tooth guard is required to prevent dental injury. If no head and neck primary tumour is found then excision biopsy is performed.

Place the patient supine with the head supported on a ring and a sandbag under the shoulders to extend the neck. The head is turned to the side opposite the lesion and the skin prepared and draped in the usual fashion.

Incision
The site and type of incision depends on the position of the enlarged node. Incisions in, or parallel to, a skin crease are always preferred, except in high masses which should be excised via a formal superficial parotidectomy approach to preserve the facial nerve. Typical incisions are shown in Fig. 1.6. A node in the submandibular regions should be excised via an incision low enough to avoid damage to the marginal mandibular branch of the facial nerve; the approach is similar to that employed for the excision of the submandibular salivary gland.

Operative technique
The techniques used for superficial and for deep nodes (e.g. those that lie along the internal jugular vein deep to sterno-mastoid differs only in the methods of providing adequate exposure. Excision is similar for both. The nodes in the anterior triangle are approached in a similar fashion to the excision of a branchial cyst (see page 1.7).

Superficial nodes
1. Deepen the incision to include platysma in the skin flaps. If the node is superficial then it will become immediately apparent. Close dissection with McIndoe scissors, opening the curved blades parallel to the surface of the node, will define a plane. The node should be handled gently with non-toothed dissecting forceps or Babcock tissue forceps to prevent rupture.

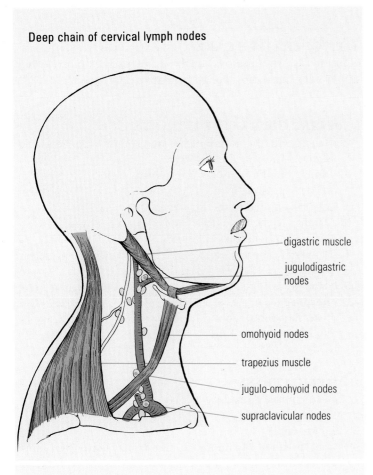

Deep chain of cervical lymph nodes

digastric muscle

jugulodigastric nodes

omohyoid nodes

trapezius muscle

jugulo-omohyoid nodes

supraclavicular nodes

Fig. 1.5

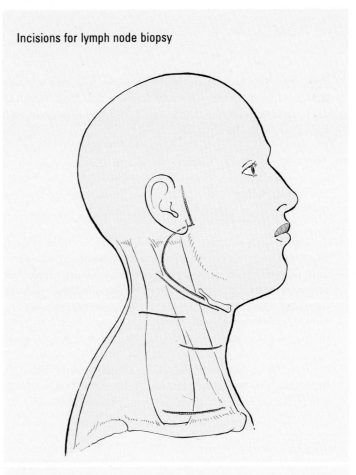

Incisions for lymph node biopsy

Fig. 1.6

Excision of lymph node

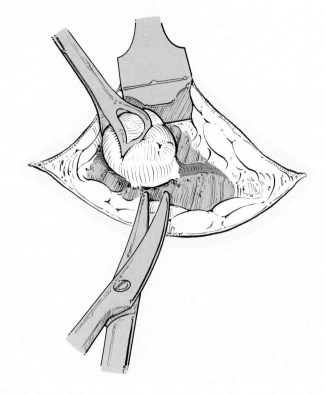

Fig. 1.7

nodes around the internal jugular vein. Identify and preserve the accessory nerve and, in higher nodes, the hypoglossal nerve.

2. Submandibular nodes. These nodes are deep to the fascia of the submandibular salivary gland. Incise this fascia at the level of the hyoid bone and reflect it upwards in the superior flap to avoid damage to the mandibular nerve (see page 1.28). Often, however, submandibular nodes are enlarged upper deep cervical nodes or jugulodigastric nodes which lie more superficially, close to the common facial vein (which may require ligation) and overlie the hypoglossal nerve and external carotid artery.

3. Supraclavicular nodes. These are part of the inferior deep cervical group which project into the posterior triangle, and are related to the internal jugular vein close to its junction with the subclavian vein. They lie in fatty tissue superficial to the trunks of the brachial plexus and phrenic nerve. Deep dissection and excessive traction through a small incision in the supraclavicular region is therefore to be avoided.

Wound closure and dressing
1. If a large node mass has been excised then occasionally a small suction drain may be required for 24 hours.
2. Close the wound using absorbable braided sutures (e.g. Vicryl) for the subcutaneous layers, with a subcuticular or an interrupted monofilament suture for the skin.
3. Send the nodes for histological examination. They are usually sent fresh rather than in a fixative.

POSTOPERATIVE CARE
Routine care with removal of the drain after 24 hours (where applicable) and removal of sutures after 5 to 7 days.

SPECIAL OPERATIVE HAZARDS
1. Damage to the facial nerve may occur when excising nodes in the parotid region.
2. Damage to the marginal mandibular branch of the facial nerve is possible if the incision is misplaced or excessive traction applied to the upper flap.
3. Damage to the hypoglossal nerve may result when dissecting upper deep cervical nodes.
4. Damage to the accessory nerve can occur in the posterior triangle.
5. Damage to the subclavian vein or internal jugular vein, the phrenic nerve or brachial plexus may occur when dissecting too deeply during excision of supraclavicular nodes.

2. Progressive dissection around the node will free it from surrounding structures. Gentle traction will then allow the deep surface to be mobilized (Fig. 1.7); blunt dissection with Lahey swabs is often useful.

3. There is invariably a feeding vessel and draining vein forming a vascular pedicle which may tether the node. Ideally this should be defined, diathermized and divided to free the node.

4. Enlarged nodes in the posterior triangle are often closely related to the accessory nerve which must be clearly identified and preserved. It passes obliquely downwards from the posterior border of sternomastoid (which should be defined by sharp dissection) to the anterior border of trapezius. The nerve is correspondingly smaller in children and is easily damaged, especially if stretched over a large mass of nodes.

5. If care is taken then the node will be delivered intact, although malignant nodes may be very friable and/or extremely large in which case only partial excision may be possible.

Deep nodes
1. Deep cervical nodes. Define the anterior border of sternomastoid by incising the deep cervical fascia; the dissection then proceeds medial to the muscle, exposing the enlarged

COMPLICATIONS
1. Specific nerve damage as above.
2. Wound infection.
3. Haematoma.
4. Local spread of squamous carcinoma may occur after biopsy of a cervical node in a case with an unsuspected head and neck primary tumour, compromising further surgery (such as block dissection) and adversely affecting prognosis.

Excision of Branchial Cyst

Branchial cysts are congenital lesions which present as an intermittent or continuous swelling in the neck that may become infected. The contents are usually fluid but can be solid.

PREOPERATIVE ASSESSMENT

1. Differentiate a branchial cyst from a malignant cervical node and a pharyngeal pouch. CT scanning may clarify the diagnosis, and a full ENT examination must be performed if doubt exists.
2. Ensure that the lump is not within the lower pole of the parotid gland. Rarely, branchial remnants occur here and require parotidectomy for their removal.
3. Treat an acutely inflamed or infected lesion with intravenous antibiotics and electively excise it after 4–6 weeks. Gross suppuration requires incision and drainage but this makes subsequent definitive surgery more difficult.
4. Examine carefully for evidence of an external communication which appears as a dimple along the anterior border of sternomastoid low down in the neck.

RELEVANT ANATOMY

There are several popular theories regarding the origin of branchial cysts (Fig. 1.8), these include that it is (i) a remnant of the second pharyngeal pouch (explaining the internal connection with the tonsillar fossa which is sometimes seen); (ii) a persistent cervical sinus of His, a cystic space over the second, third and fourth branchial clefts following the downgrowth of the second arch mesoderm which fuses with the fifth arch; and (iii) an epithelial inclusion in a cervical lymph node.

Anatomically, a typical cyst appears from behind the anterior border of the upper third of sternomastoid. An external opening, when present, is visible low in the neck, often at the sternal notch, anterior to sternomastoid. The deeper part of the cyst lies under sternomastoid and overlies the carotid sheath which contains the carotid artery, internal jugular vein and vagus nerve. Closely related to the cyst is the accessory nerve entering the deep surface of sternomastoid. Superiorly, the hypoglossal nerve loops down on the surface of the internal and external carotid arteries deep to the common facial vein. A proximal extension or internal connection when present passes between the internal and external carotid arteries over the hypoglossal and glossopharyngeal nerves deep to the posterior belly of digastric to open into the tonsillar fossa.

OPERATION

Preparation

The operation is performed under a general anaesthetic. The patient is placed supine with a sandbag under the shoulders and the neck extended with the occiput supported on a head ring. Venous engorgement is reduced by applying head-up tilt and the head is rotated away from the side of the lesion. The skin of the neck is cleansed and draped so as to cover the anaesthetic tubing.

Incision

Make a transverse skin crease incision over the cyst, long enough to raise adequate skin flaps to expose the cyst, and low enough to avoid damage to the mandibular branch of the facial nerve (Fig. 1.9). The incision is deepened through platysma.

Operative technique

1. Grasp the subcutaneous tissue of the upper and lower flaps with Allis tissue forceps and elevate the tissue to expose the deep cervical fascia which is opened with scissors along the anterior border of sternomastoid (Fig. 1.10). Avoid damage to the external jugular vein and the great auricular nerve.

2. Expose the shiny wall of the cyst by dissecting it free from sternomastoid which is retracted laterally with a Langenbeck retractor, and grasp the cyst with a Babcock's forceps. Avoid

Embryological anatomy

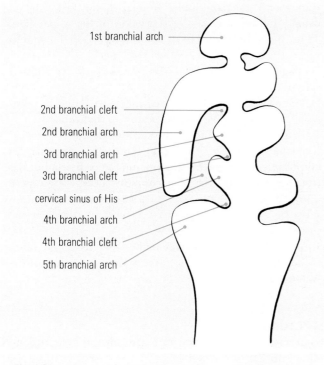

1st branchial arch

2nd branchial cleft
2nd branchial arch
3rd branchial arch
3rd branchial cleft
cervical sinus of His
4th branchial arch
4th branchial cleft
5th branchial arch

Fig. 1.8

1.7

Incision to remove branchial cyst

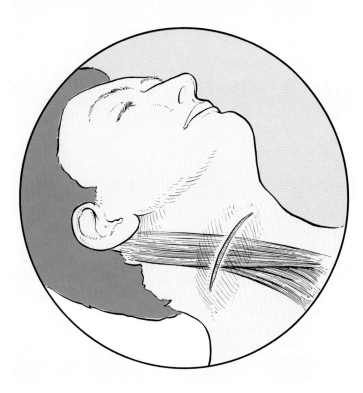

Fig. 1.9

Exposure of cyst

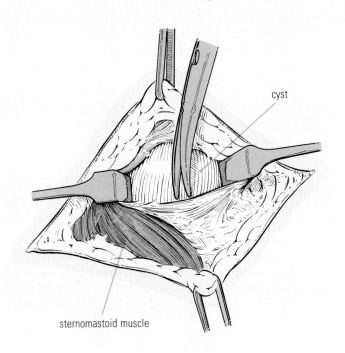

cyst

sternomastoid muscle

Fig. 1.10

damage to the accessory nerve which enters the deep surface of the upper part of sternomastoid.

3. With traction on the cyst free it from the underlying carotid sheath by careful sharp dissection, and then continue the dissection cranially until the upper limit, which is variable, is reached. Deep to the cyst identify the hypoglossal nerve looping below the posterior belly of digastric over the internal and external carotid arteries (Fig. 1.11); further cranially the cyst extends between the internal and external carotid arteries to overlie the glossopharyngeal nerve on the surface of the middle constrictor of the pharynx (Fig. 1.12). Access can be improved by ligation and division of the common facial vein and excision of a portion of the posterior belly of digastric, if the cyst extends this far up.

4. At its upper limit there may be a communication with the tonsillar fossa of the oropharynx (Fig. 1.12). Excise the track and close any resulting hole in the oropharynx with interrupted catgut sutures or a purse string.

Wound closure and dressing

Carefully ensure complete haemostasis, avoiding the use of diathermy close to important nerves. Insert a fine suction drain and repair the deep fascia and platysma with interrupted catgut sutures, and close the skin with interrupted 3/0 nylon sutures or Michelle clips. Cover the wound with a light dressing.

POSTOPERATIVE CARE

Nurse the patient in the semi-sitting position for the first 24 hours to reduce any venous ooze. The drain can be removed after 24–48 hours and the sutures or clips after 3–4 days.

SPECIAL OPERATIVE HAZARDS

1. Damage to the mandibular branch of the facial nerve, usually following excessive retraction of the upper flap. This causes the corner of the mouth to droop but should recover if the nerve has not been divided.
2. Damage to the hypoglossal nerve causing paralysis of that side of the tongue.
3. Damage to the accessory nerve causing weakness or paralysis of sternomastoid and trapezius on that side.
4. Damage to the contents of the carotid sheath.
5. External opening in the neck; in which case make an elliptical incision around the opening and dissect out the track which follows the same course as a cyst. Often these openings are low in the neck and a second, parallel incision must be made higher up in the neck to complete the dissection.
6. Rupture of the cyst, which makes the dissection more difficult. It is important not to leave any fragments of the wall behind.

COMPLICATIONS

1. Recurrence due to failure to excise all the cyst; this may follow rupture of the cyst.
2. Wound haematoma and infection.
3. Specific nerve palsies (see above).

Dissection proceeding cranially

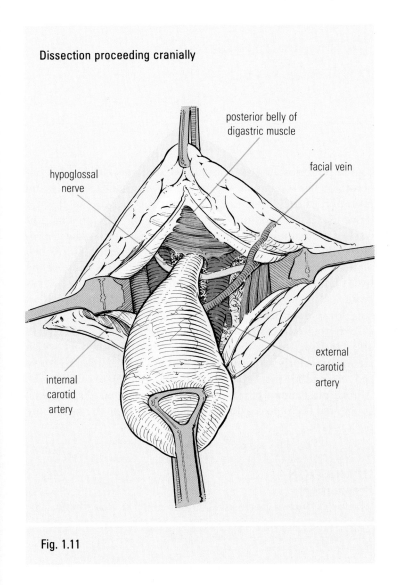

Fig. 1.11

Labels: posterior belly of digastric muscle; facial vein; hypoglossal nerve; external carotid artery; internal carotid artery

Division of digastric to expose apex of extensive cyst

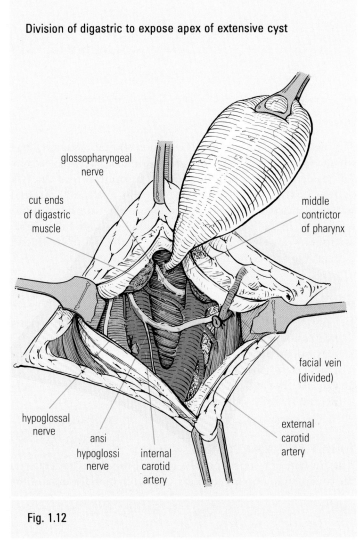

Fig. 1.12

Labels: glossopharyngeal nerve; cut ends of digastric muscle; middle contrictor of pharynx; facial vein (divided); hypoglossal nerve; ansi hypoglossi nerve; internal carotid artery; external carotid artery

1.9

Excision of Thyroglossal Cyst

Thyroglossal cysts are relatively common midline cystic swellings which are diagnosed clinically. They should be excised electively for cosmetic reasons, and because of discomfort and the risk of infection. A small percentage present as acutely infected swellings which should be treated vigorously with intravenous antibiotics; incision and drainage should be avoided if possible as this may cause fibrosis and tethering of the cyst or produce a discharging fistula, both of which complicate excision.

PREOPERATIVE ASSESSMENT
1. Confirm that the lesion is cystic and moves up on tongue protrusion and swallowing.
2. Ultrasound may confirm the diagnosis and also define a patent thyroglossal duct passing superiorly.
3. Confirm normal thyroid function preoperatively. A [99]technetium thyroid scan may also be of benefit.

RELEVANT ANATOMY
The thyroid develops from the floor of the pharynx, between the tuberculum impar anteriorly (first arch mesoderm) and the copula posteriorly (second and third arch mesoderm); this site of origin later becomes the midline foramen caecum in the posterior third of the tongue. From this origin the thyroid descends in the midline, superficial to the oesophagus and trachea, remaining connected to the pharynx by the thyroglossal duct, which later solidifies and then regresses. The course of thyroid descent lies in close proximity to the body of the hyoid bone, passing initially anteriorly, then looping upwards posterior to the body, before descending to its final position anterior to the trachea in the neck (Fig. 1.13).

A thyroglossal cyst may appear anywhere along this course and be associated with a persistent thyroglossal duct which passes superiorly from it to the tongue base. Ninety-five percent are midline cysts, the remainder presenting to the left side. All are intermittently related to the hyoid bone. An external congenital thyroglossal duct fistula opening onto the skin of the neck is rare.

OPERATION
Preparation
The procedure is performed under general anaesthetic. The

Course of descent of thyroid gland showing commoner sites of thyroglossal cyst

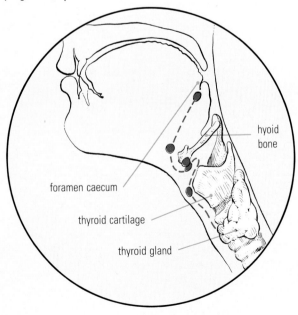

foramen caecum

thyroid cartilage

thyroid gland

hyoid bone

Fig. 1.13

Site of incision

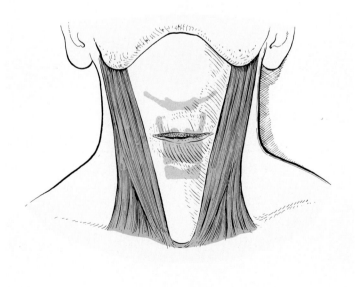

Fig. 1.14

patient is positioned as for a thyroidectomy, supine on the operating table with a sandbag beneath the shoulders to extend the neck and the occiput supported on a head ring. Standard skin preparation is performed and the patient is draped with a head towel to exclude the mouth from the operating field. The endotracheal tube and anaesthetic connections should pass superiorly over the head of the table. The table should be tilted head-up (reverse Trendelenberg) to reduce venous congestion.

Incision

Make a horizontal skin crease incision directly over the cyst which should be long enough to allow elevation of an adequate superior flap for subsequent dissection (Fig. 1.14). Excision following infection, or in the presence of a fistula should include an ellipse of skin around the opening or any tethered area.

Operative technique

1. Deepen the incision through platysma, and elevate the upper and lower flaps for adequate access. Divide the anterior jugular veins between clamps and ligate them.

2. Locate the cyst, which should appear directly, and gently dissect it free from the surrounding tissues and underlying strap muscle using McIndoe scissors and non-toothed forceps.

3. Once mobilized gently retract the cyst with a Babcock tissue forceps. Use bipolar diathermy to keep the operative field dry and small Langenbeck or self-retaining retractors to maintain exposure (Fig. 1.15). Rarely, there will be an extension of the track downwards to the thyroid isthmus which, if present, must be excised.

4. Careful retraction and dissection will define the thyroglossal duct passing upwards to the hyoid bone. A high cyst will overlie the hyoid and be firmly adherent to it making separation impossible. The hyoid bone is very mobile and is palpated and then held firmly with an Allis forceps to allow sharp dissection onto the body of the bone to free the muscle attachments and thyrohyoid membrane. Further dissection with Lahey swabs isolates the central portion of the hyoid which is removed in continuity with the cyst and duct (Sistrunk's procedure) using fine bone-cutting forceps or heavy Mayo scissors. Care must be taken to avoid penetrating the mucosa deep to the hyoid (Fig. 1.16).

5. Downward retraction using an Allis forceps on the 2-cm segment of hyoid bone will define a conical core of muscle,

Mobilization of cyst

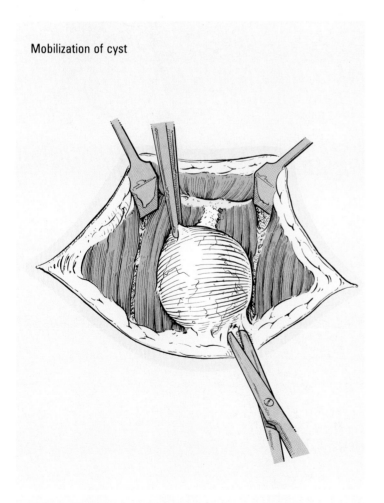

Fig. 1.15

Excision of the middle third of the hyoid bone

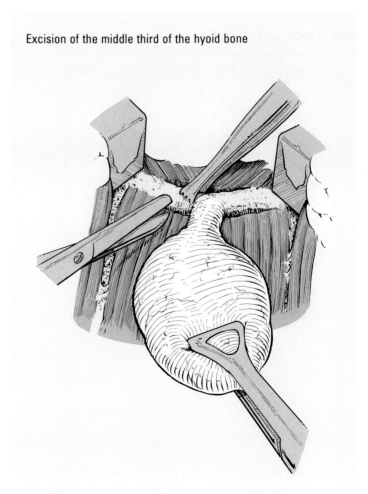

Fig. 1.16

or obvious duct, passing superiorly into the tongue base. Dissect the duct to its apex and excise it in continuity to avoid recurrence (Fig. 1.17), taking care to avoid opening the mucosa of the mouth. The specimen comprises the excised cyst, the duct and the central portion of the hyoid bone. Some surgeons recommend digital pressure onto the tongue base from within the mouth to aid the final dissection, but this increases the risk of postoperative infection by introducing intra-oral flora into the operating field. It is not therefore recommended and if performed it is best done by the anaesthetist or adequate antibiotic cover should be employed.

6. If a defect in the tongue base communicating with the oropharynx occurs in the course of excising the duct superiorly, close it with an absorbable (e.g. catgut) suture.

Wound closure and dressing

1. Perform careful haemostasis using bipolar diathermy, and insert absorbable sutures to approximate the muscles of the tongue base in order to prevent haematoma.
2. Place a fine suction drain via a separate stab incision and commence suction prior to wound closure to prevent blockage of the drain with blood clot.
3. Close the wound in two layers using a fine absorbable suture for the subcutaneous tissues (including the platysma), then subcuticular monofilament suture and adhesive strips for the skin.

POSTOPERATIVE CARE

The patient can eat and drink the next day. The suction drain remains for 24–48 hours and the sutures are removed after 7 days.

SPECIAL OPERATIVE HAZARDS

1. Drainage to the thyrohyoid membrane when dividing the hyoid bone.
2. Opening the mucosa and entering the mouth.

COMPLICATIONS

1. Haematoma in the neck due to excessive dissection and inadequate haemostasis in the tongue base and/or failure of the suction drain.
2. Recurrence due to failure to excise the body of the hyoid bone or to dissect the duct superiorly in the tongue base.

Excision of the proximal duct

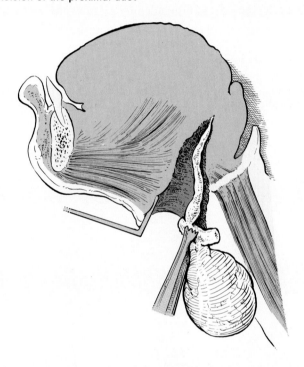

Fig. 1.17

Thyroidectomy

A thyroidectomy may be performed for medically uncontrollable thyrotoxicosis, for suspected thyroid malignancy or for the pressure symptoms or cosmetic appearance of a large multinodular goitre. For thyrotoxicosis or a multinodular goitre a subtotal thyroidectomy is performed. The management of a solitary thyroid nodule is controversial, but in general is treated by a total lobectomy, although some would advocate a total thyroidectomy for follicular carcinoma.

PREOPERATIVE ASSESSMENT
1. Check thyroid function tests (T3, T4 and TSH) and thyroid auto-antibodies.
2. Ensure that an ENT surgeon has examined the vocal cords.
3. Use X-rays of the chest and thoracic inlet to look for tracheal deviation or stenosis. Also X-ray the neck in patients with rheumatoid arthritis or cervical spondylosis.
4. Perform an ECG in patients who are or have been thyrotoxic.
5. Ensure than when operating for thyrotoxicosis, the patient has been rendered euthyroid medically. Vascularity of the thyroid gland in thyrotoxic patients can be reduced by pretreatment with either Lugol's iodine (a mixture of 5% iodine and 10% potassium iodide in water) at a dose of 0.5 ml t.d.s. or potassium iodide 15 mg t.d.s. for 10 days. Propranolol can be given to reduce the cardiotoxic complications of severe thyrotoxicosis.
6. Forewarn the patient of the risk and implications of recurrent laryngeal nerve palsy and hypothyroidism.
7. If the nature of a thyroid swelling is in doubt consider arranging for frozen section facilities to be available for use peroperatively.

RELEVANT ANATOMY
The thyroid gland lies in the neck enclosed within the pretracheal fascia. It has two pear-shaped lateral lobes joined anteriorly by an isthmus which overlies the second, third and fourth tracheal rings (Fig. 1.18). The lateral lobes lie on either

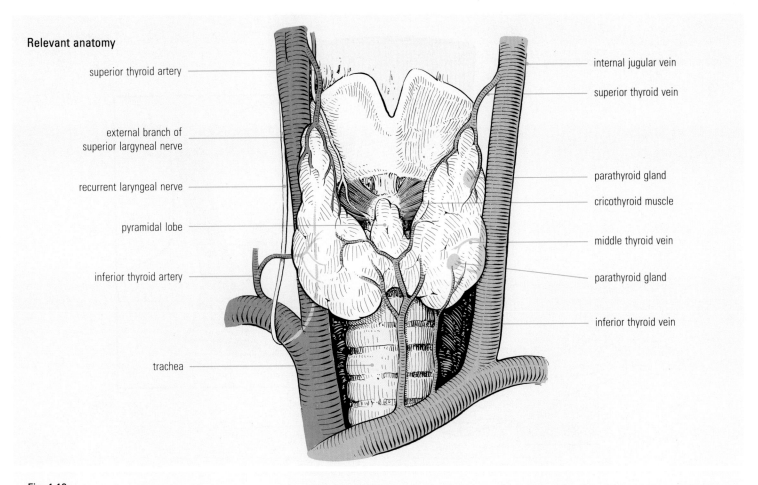

Relevant anatomy

superior thyroid artery

external branch of superior largyneal nerve

recurrent laryngeal nerve

pyramidal lobe

inferior thyroid artery

trachea

internal jugular vein

superior thyroid vein

parathyroid gland

cricothyroid muscle

middle thyroid vein

parathyroid gland

inferior thyroid vein

Fig. 1.18

of the larynx and upper trachea, the upper poles lying immediately lateral to the cricothyroid muscles. Posterior to the lateral lobes lies the carotid sheath with its contained common carotid artery, internal jugular vein and vagus nerve. There is frequently a small projection from the gland extending upward from the midpart of the isthmus. This represents the caudal end of the thyroglossal duct and is known as the pyramidal lobe. Anteriorly the gland is covered by the paired strap muscles; the sternothyroid muscles are in contact with the gland and are covered by the sternohyoid muscles. The strap muscles are supplied by nerves from the ansa hypoglossi. Laterally lie the sternomastoid muscles and superficially are the subcutaneous tissues containing the paired anterior jugular veins, platysma, and the skin.

The arterial supply of the thyroid is from the superior and inferior thyroid arteries. The superior arteries descend from their origin on the external carotid artery and pierce the pretracheal fascia to enter the apex of the upper pole of each lateral lobe. They are closely related to the external branch of the superior laryngeal nerve which supplies the cricothyroid muscle. The inferior thyroid arteries arise from the thyrocervical trunk (a branch of the subclavian artery), pass behind the carotid artery, pierce the pretracheal fascia, and then divide into several branches before entering the posterior border of the middle or lower part of each lobe. Having ascended in the tracheo-oesophageal groove the recurrent laryngeal nerve lies close to the inferior thyroid artery, and although the nerve generally lies behind the artery, it can lie in front of or even pass between its branches before entering the cricopharyngeus muscle. The recurrent laryngeal nerve is sensory to the larynx and supplies all the intrinsic muscles of the larynx except for cricothyroid. A small artery, the thyroidea ima, occasionally ascends from the aortic arch or brachiocephalic trunk to enter the isthmus.

The venous drainage from each lobe is via the superior, middle and inferior thyroid veins. The superior thyroid vein drains the upper part of the lobe, lies alongside the superior thyroid artery and drains into the internal jugular or common facial vein. The middle thyroid vein, which may be multiple, runs laterally from each lobe to join the internal jugular vein. The inferior thyroid veins drain the isthmus and lower poles of each lobe and form a plexus in the pretracheal fascia which drains into the brachiocephalic vein.

The four parathyroid glands are intimately related to the thyroid gland. Each is 2–3 mm in diameter, brownish in colour and usually sited behind the upper and lower poles of each lobe within the pretracheal fascia. Ectopic parathyroid tissue is not uncommon and may be located outside the pretracheal fascia

Position of patient and site of incision

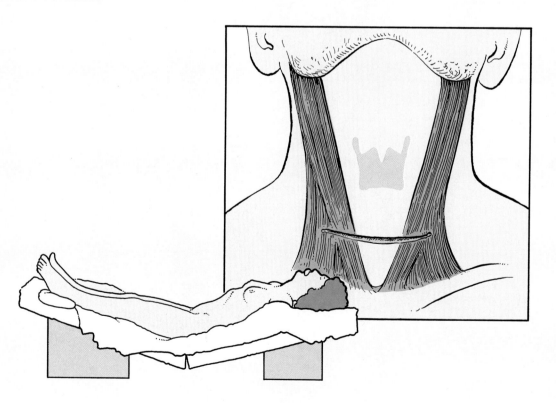

Fig. 1.19

1.14

around the thyroid gland or in the superior mediastinum. When performing a total thyroidectomy it is important to identify and preserve some parathyroid tissue or hypocalcaemia will ensue.

OPERATION
Preparation
The patient's hair is covered with a theatre cap or polythene bag which is taped to the skin along the hairline. A general anaesthetic is given and the patient placed supine with head-up tilt of about 20°; break the table in the middle so that the patient is in a semi-sitting position and will not slide down the table. Place a sandbag or inflatable cushion under the shoulders and extend the neck, supporting the occiput on a head ring (Fig. 1.19). Avoid overextending the neck if there is cervical spine disease. Cleanse the skin from the lower lip to the nipples, position a double head-towel beneath the head and neck, and use the upper towel to enclose the head, face and anaesthetic tubing. Place further drapes over the upper chest and along each side leaving the neck displayed from the chin to the sternal notch.

Incision
Irrespective of what operation is planned, the same incision is employed. Using a piece of 00 linen thread held taut, mark the site of the skin incision by cheese-wiring it into the skin approximately 2 cm above the sternal notch. If possible site it in an existing skin crease. To aid accurate skin closure at the end of the operation draw three vertical lines across the indentation mark with ink. Make a symmetrical skin incision along the indentation to beyond the medial border of sternomastoid and deepen it through platysma.

Operative technique
1. Using three Allis forceps applied to the subcutaneous tissue (but not the skin) of the upper flap, an assistant lifts the upper flap vertically. Then, by a mixture of sharp dissection with a knife or scissors and blunt dissection with a gauze swab, dissect the flap of skin with platysma from the underlying strap muscles and sternomastoid (Fig. 1.20) as far as the upper border of the thyroid cartilage; this is recognized by the easily palpable notch. If the anterior jugular veins are damaged, ligate with 3/0 catgut and divide them completely. Mobilize the upper flap along its entire width.

2. Leaving the central Allis forceps on the upper flap to maintain its upward retraction, resite the other two on the subcutaneous tissue of the lower flap which is then mobilized as far as the sternal notch. It is unnecessary to dissect the lower flap too far laterally.

3. Apply four small wound towels, from the end of the incision to the centre of one of the flaps, and insert a Joll's thyroid retractor, with its clips in the midpoint of each flap so as to secure the wound towels, and wind it open. Use a further two towel clips to secure the wound towels to the ends of the incision to create a diamond-shaped operative field (Fig. 1.21).

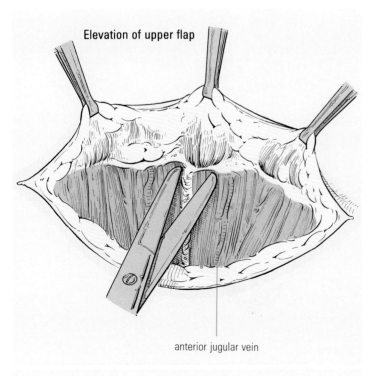

Elevation of upper flap

anterior jugular vein

Fig. 1.20

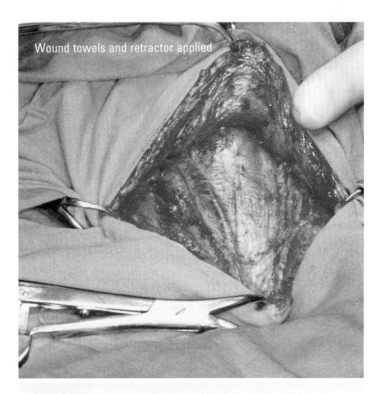

Wound towels and retractor applied

Fig. 1.21

4. Mobilize the medial borders of sternomastoid from the underlying strap mucles. Using a mosquito forceps, pick up the pretracheal fascia in the midline and incise it with diathermy and then scissors (Fig. 1.22).

5. Decide which lobe to approach first if both are to be operated on and stand on the opposite side of the patient. Grasp the strap muscles with Babcock's forceps which an assistant lifts to display the plane on the deep surface of the muscles (Fig. 1.23). It is very important to enter the plane between the strap muscles and the thyroid gland; further dissection in the wrong plane will be very bloody and make the operation impossible until the correct plane is established. When the correct plane is entered the veins of the thyroid fill and bulge visibly. The muscle may be very adherent to the gland. A large goitre may have displaced the medial border of the strap muscles from the midline and the muscles may become paper thin from stretching. The entire length of the sternothyroid should be gently separated from the underlying gland. If the goitre is very large and access difficult, divide the strap muscles high up (to retain the innervation) between Kocher's forceps after mobilizing the gland as fully as possible. Transfix the strap muscles with 00 catgut (Fig. 1.24).

Enter plane between thyroid gland and strap muscles

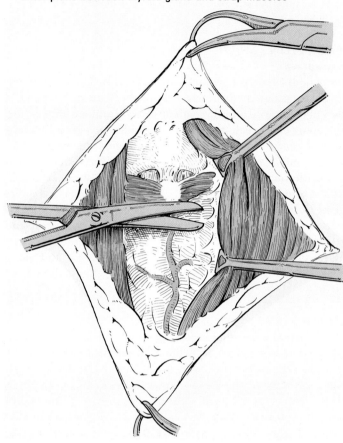

Fig. 1.23

Division of pretracheal fascia

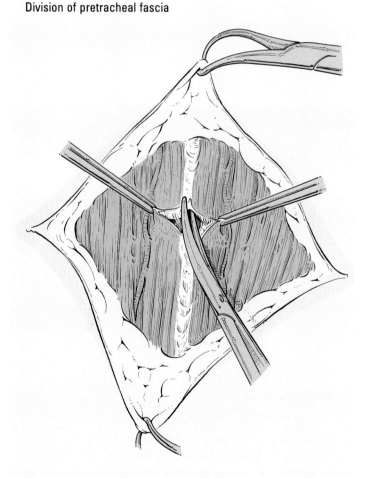

Fig. 1.22

Division and transfixion of strap muscles

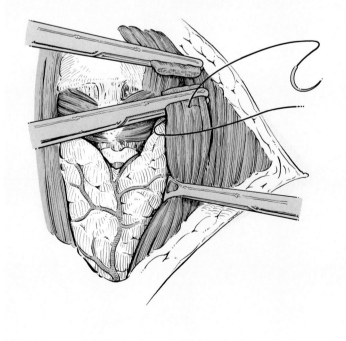

Fig. 1.24

Ligation of middle thyroid vein

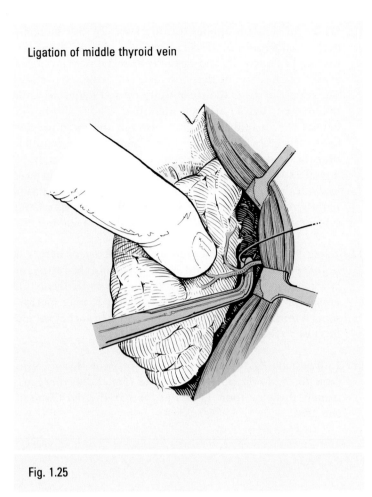

Fig. 1.25

6. With the strap muscles and sternomastoid drawn laterally by an assistant, and using two small Langenbeck's retractors, identify, ligate and divide the middle thyroid vein entering the internal jugular vein (Fig. 1.25). There may be more than one. Continue to mobilize cranially, freeing the lateral side of the upper pole.

7. Define the plane between the medial border of the upper pole of the thyroid and cricothyroid muscle and free the posterior aspect of the gland at this point. Insert a Kocher's grooved director into this plane under the upper pole and slide an aneurysm needle loaded with a 00 linen tie along the groove in the instrument and tie it around the glandular tissue of the upper pole.

8. Whilst the assistant draws the upper pole down by traction on this ligature, pass two further ligatures around the upper pole pedicle and tie them or transfix the pedicle. Avoid tying the pedicle too high, endangering the external laryngeal nerve which lies on the surface of the middle constrictor, deep to the vessels, entering the cricothyroid muscle.

9. Divide the pedicle with a knife, cutting down into the groove of the grooved director, leaving the lowest ligature on the gland (Fig. 1.26); the doubly tied upper pole vessels will retract out of site into the neck.

Division of upper pole pedicle

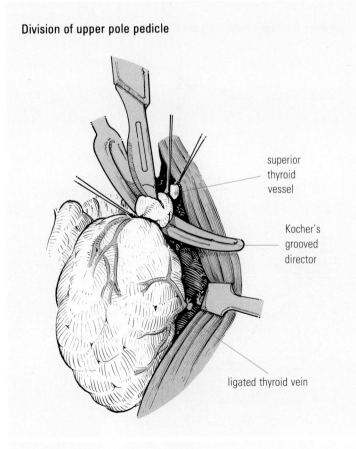

superior thyroid vessel

Kocher's grooved director

ligated thyroid vein

Fig. 1.26

Ligation of inferior thyroid artery

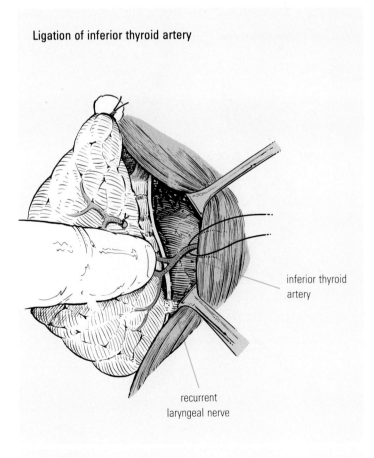

inferior thyroid artery

recurrent laryngeal nerve

Fig. 1.27

1.17

Ligation of inferior thyroid vein

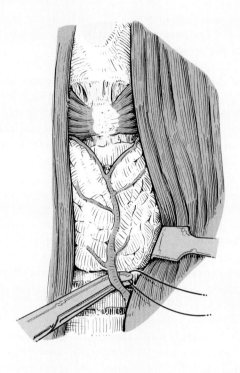

Fig. 1.28

10. Whilst an assistant applies traction laterally with Langenbeck's retractors on the strap muscles, firmly draw the thyroid lobe medially and carefully dissect down the lateral aspect of the lobe in the loose areolar tissue. Reposition the retractors over the carotid artery and continue until the inferior thyroid artery is identified. The artery passes behind the carotid artery and through the loose areolar tissue which lies lateral to the lobe. Follow the artery until it branches and identify the recurrent laryngeal nerve; this is a white structure with a fine vessel visible on its surface, and it feels firm when rolled under the finger. The inferior parathyroid gland is closely related to the point where the inferior thyroid artery and recurrent laryngeal nerve cross.

11. Using 00 linen ligate the inferior thyroid artery before it branches lateral to the gland and thus clear of the recurrent laryngeal nerve (Fig. 1.27). It is not necessary to divide this vessel for a subtotal thyroidectomy but it is when performing a total lobectomy; the division of the branches should be close to the gland and clear of the nerve.

12. Individually ligate and divide each inferior thyroid vein close to the lower pole of the gland (Fig. 1.28); there are usually three or four. Look out for parathyroid tissue in this area.

Division of thyroid isthmus

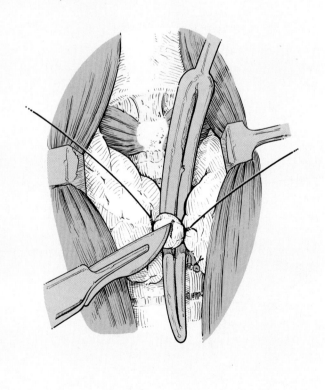

Fig. 1.29

Division of thyroid lobe for a subtotal lobectomy

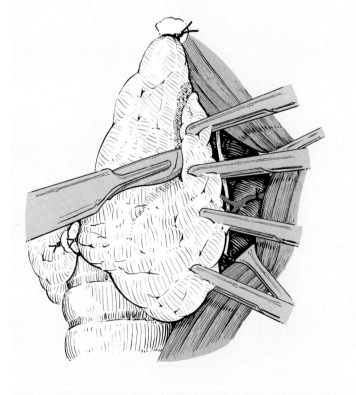

Fig. 1.30

For a subtotal thyroidectomy

13. Complete the mobilization of the other lobe of the gland.

14. Mobilize the isthmus from the trachea by blunt dissection, freeing a pyramidal lobe if present. Pass a grooved dissector behind the isthmus, pass two ligatures around it, and having tied them, divide the isthmus between them with a knife by cutting down onto the grooved director so as to protect the trachea (Fig. 1.29).

15. Draw the divided isthmus to the sides by gentle traction on the ligatures and free the medial attachments of each lobe to the trachea.

16. Apply a series of artery forceps to the lateral side of the gland so as to leave about 5 cm³ of gland, the parathyroid glands and the recurrent laryngeal nerve when everything in front of the clips is removed. Cut cleanly with a scalpel obliquely down to the trachea through the gland (Fig. 1.30) leaving the clips attached to the remnant.

17. The cut surface of the remnant may bleed considerably. Draw the clips medially and suture the cut edge of the remnant to the trachea with a continuous 00 catgut stitch (Fig. 1.31).

For a total lobectomy

13. Having carefully identified and preserved the recurrent laryngeal nerve and if possible the parathyroid glands, dissect the lobe completely free from these structures and from the surface of the trachea, working from lateral to medial (Fig. 1.32). Pick up bleeding points with fine haemostats and ligate with 3/0 catgut. Do not use diathermy in the vicinity of the nerve. If bleeding makes identification of the recurrent laryngeal nerve difficult pack the area with a dry swab for 5 minutes, then apply a saline-soaked swab. This will make the nerve appear whiter than the surrounding tissue. Divide the branches of the inferior artery close to the gland.

14. Dissect the isthmus from the trachea and place a Spencer-Wells or Kocher's clamp across it. Divide the isthmus to free the affected lobe and suture the cut end of the remaining isthmus to the trachea with 00 catgut to prevent bleeding.

Wound closure and dressing

Check all bleeding has stopped. Insert a corrugated or fine suction drain into the space previously occupied by each removed lobe. Bring the drain out between the strap muscles in

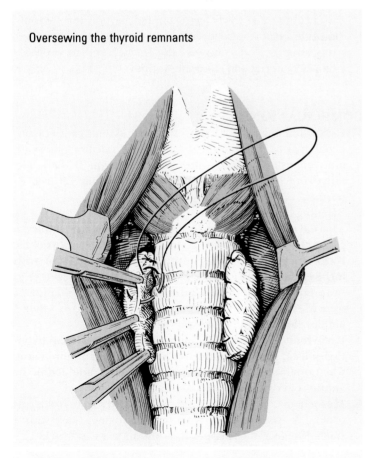

Oversewing the thyroid remnants

Fig. 1.31

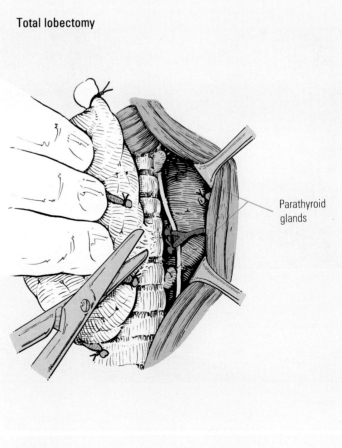

Total lobectomy

Parathyroid glands

Fig. 1.32

1.19

the midline of the neck and out through the opposite end of the wound. Repair the strap muscles if they had been divided with catgut and loosely approximate the strap muscles in the midline with 3/0 catgut. Close the skin with Michelle clips, or subcuticular monofilament polypropylene, realigning the ink marks made at the beginning (Fig. 1.33). Apply a gauze dressing held in place with straps of adhesive plasters.

POSTOPERATIVE CARE

Nurse the patient in the semi-sitting position for the first 24 hours to keep venous pressure in the neck low and thus reduce the risk of venous oozing. In the event of a reactionary haemorrhage urgent action must be taken since an expanding haematoma confined behind the strap muscles can buckle the trachea and threaten the airway by pressure and laryngeal oedema, particularly if it has been softened by the pressure of a large goitre. If the situation is not critical return the patient to the operating theatre and formally re-explore the neck, evacuating haematoma and securing haemostasis. If the patient is becoming asphyxiated, reopen the incision on the ward to allow immediate decompression of the trachea. In such cases there may be considerable oedema of the larynx necessitating a tracheostomy as a life-saving manoeuvre.

Check the serum calcium level daily for the first 2 days and thereafter if it is subnormal or falling since removal or bruising

of the parathyroids can cause hypocalcaemia from reduced levels of parathormone. Remove the drains after 24 hours and alternate clips on days 3 and 4 or a subcuticular suture on day 4.

SPECIAL OPERATIVE HAZARDS

1. Bleeding, particularly from a torn middle thyroid vein following clumsy dissection. If the bleeding point cannot be seen and picked up with a haemostat and ligated, first insert a gauze swab for a few minutes and await control of the bleeding. Divide the strap muscles to improve access if need be. Bleeding also occurs when the dissection is in the wrong plane, between the sternothyroid and sternohyoid muscles. In addition a slipped tie on the superior pedicle can cause severe bleeding which is usually out of sight, so always doubly ligate this pedicle.

2. Damage to the recurrent laryngeal nerve; this causes hoarseness of the voice which will recover if due to a neuropraxia, but not if the nerve has been divided, in which case laryngoscopic Teflon (PTFE) injections may be required to stiffen the paralysed vocal cord and allow apposition of the cord on the opposite side. Very occasionally the nerve is not recurrent and does not lie in the tracheo-oesophageal groove.

3. Damage to the external laryngeal nerve; this results in little disability except in opera singers who may be unable to reach very high notes.

4. Retrosternal goitre; most can be removed through the standard incision, delivering the lower part of the goitre into the neck by traction from above. Only very rarely is it necessary to divide the sternum.

5. Anaplastic tumours; if an aggressive invasive tumour is encountered which has extended beyond the thyroid capsule, do not proceed with thyroidectomy. Merely excise the isthmus to decompress the trachea and to provide biopsy material and close the wound.

COMPLICATIONS

1. Hypocalcaemia may be manifest acutely as tetany with carpopedal spasm. Treat with 20 ml of 10% calcium gluconate intravenously followed with 5 mg of vitamin D daily and dihydrotachysterol until the plasma calcium returns to normal.

2. Bleeding (see Postoperative Care).

3. Thyroid crisis, a rare complication, is seen in patients undergoing thyroidectomy for poorly controlled thyrotoxicosis. Block further thyroxine output from the remnant with intravenous potassium iodide and give a ß-blocker (e.g. propranolol) to block the cardiotoxic effects. If the temperature rises relentlessly administer sedation and cortisol and employ fanning and tepid sponging.

4. Recurrent thyrotoxicosis is more difficult to treat than hypothyroidism, so in general leave less rather than more tissue when operating for thyrotoxicosis. Ablative radio-iodine or antithyroid drugs are used to treat it.

5. Myxoedema, a common end-point of many thyroid disorders, is easily treated with oral thyroxine. Start with a small dose (e.g. 0.05 mg per day) and increase gradually.

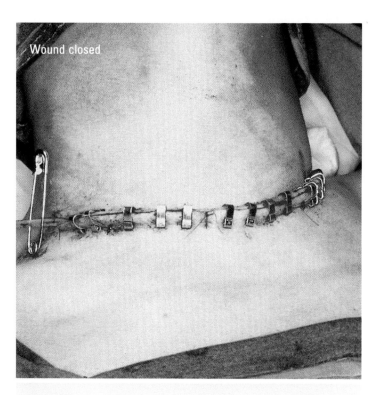

Fig. 1.33

Parathyroidectomy

Surgical exploration of the parathyroid glands may be indicated for cases of hypercalcaemia due to primary, secondary, or tertiary hyperparathyroidism. Primary hyperparathyroidism is due to either a secreting parathyroid tumour (80%) or glandular hyperplasia (20%). Tertiary hyperparathyroidism occurs when chronic glandular stimulation (secondary hyperparathyroidism) such as occurs in chronic renal failure leads to autonomous hypersecretion.

PREOPERATIVE ASSESSMENT
1. Confirm the diagnosis of hyperparathyroidism; serum and urinary calcium are elevated, serum phosphate lowered and serum parathyroid hormone levels elevated, or inappropriately normal.
2. Assess renal function. Hyperparathyroidism occurs in chronic renal failure and hypercalcaemia can cause polyuria, nephrocalcinosis and renal calculi.

Common position of parathyroid glands (viewed from behind)

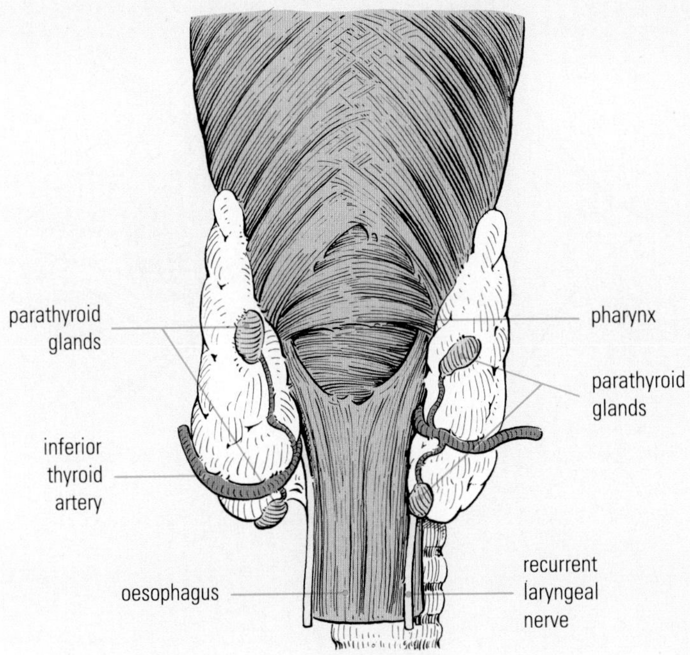

parathyroid glands

inferior thyroid artery

oesophagus

pharynx

parathyroid glands

recurrent laryngeal nerve

Fig. 1.34

3. Familial screening may be appropriate since hyperparathyroidism is a feature of multiple endocrine neoplasia (MEN) syndromes.
4. Ensure than an ENT surgeon has screened the vocal cords and forewarn the patient of the small risk and the implications of recurrent laryngeal nerve palsy.
5. Arrange with the histology department for frozen section facilities to be available for use peroperatively.
6. Some surgeons inject methylene blue intravenously prior to the operation. The parathyroids preferentially take up the dye and this manoeuvre may assist in their identification during the operation.
7. Draw a large outline of the thyroid gland on a board or a piece of paper to mark the relative positions of excised specimens.

RELEVANT ANATOMY
There are two pairs of parathyroid glands which are generally related to the posterior surface of the upper and lower poles of the lateral lobes of the thyroid gland, the latter being closely related to the recurrent laryngeal nerve (Fig. 1.34) (see page 1.13 on thyroidectomy for a full description of the relevant anatomy of the thyroid). It is not uncommon for parathyroid tissue to be ectopic and this need not be the same on both sides. The superior gland may lie deep to the thyroid, related to the pharynx or oesophagus. The inferior gland may lie more lateral, as far as the carotid sheath or more caudal, related to the inferior thyroid veins, either low in the neck or in the superior mediastinum, close to or even within the superior horns of the thymus gland. A normal parathyroid gland is brownish yellow in colour and softer than thyroid tissue due to its greater vascularity. They are on average about 0.5 cm across and are enclosed within a thin envelope. Parathyroid tumours are also yellowish brown, but larger and usually darker than the normal glands. Even when in an ectopic position the parathyroid glands generally retain their blood supply from the inferior thyroid arteries.

OPERATION
Preparation
The patient is positioned as for thyroidectomy (see page 1.15).

Incision
A collar incision is made as for thyroidectomy (see page 1.15).

Operative technique
1. Select which side of the thyroid to explore first and expose that lateral lobe by dissection from the overlying strap muscle; divide the middle thyroid vein. This is fully described in steps 1 to 6 of thyroidectomy.

Placing a ligature around the
inferior thyroid artery

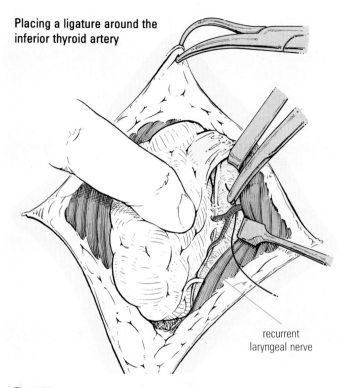

recurrent
laryngeal nerve

Fig. 1.35

2. Draw the thyroid lobe medially and free it from the loose
areolar tissue on its lateral side. Identify the inferior thyroid
artery lateral to the gland, and place a strong ligature around
it which is left untied (Fig. 1.35). Find the recurrent laryngeal
nerve as it ascends in the tracheo-oesophageal groove; it will
be closely related to the inferior thyroid artery.

3. Carefully examine the posterior surface of the thyroid for
the superior parathyroid gland. This is usually applied to
the posterior surface of the lower part of the upper pole of
the lateral lobe (Fig. 1.36). If it is not visible search further
cranially and posteriorly, on the side wall of the larynx,
pharynx and cervical oesophagus (Fig. 1.37). In order to
clearly see this area it is sometimes necessary to divide the
superior thyroid artery and vein so as to mobilize the upper
pole as described in steps 7, 8 and 9 of thyroidectomy (Fig.
1.19, on page 1.14).

4. Search for the inferior parathyroid gland which commonly
lies on the posterior aspect of the lower pole of the thyroid
close to the junction of the inferior thyroid artery and recurrent laryngeal nerve (Fig. 1.38). If it is not visible here

Common site for superior gland

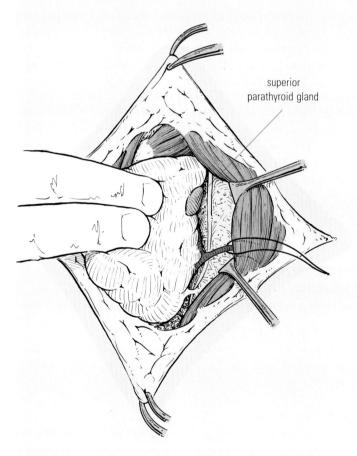

superior
parathyroid gland

Fig. 1.36

Superior gland on side of pharynx

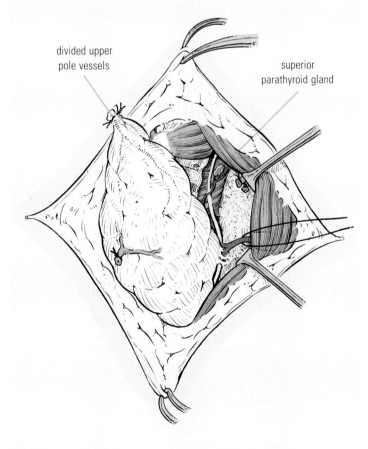

divided upper
pole vessels

superior
parathyroid gland

Fig. 1.37

dissect the tissues around the inferior thyroid veins, which are divided to improve access, and continue down into the superior mediastinum, identifying the paler thymus gland (Fig. 1.39). The inferior parathyroid gland may be related to the inferior thyroid veins or adjacent to or even within the thymus. Explore in the loose areolar tissue as far laterally as the carotid sheath.

5. Repeat the entire procedure on the other side.

6. Having located the parathyroid glands, the exact procedure depends upon the findings. Completely remove an obvious adenoma, leaving the three remaining glands if normal; take a biopsy from one. With hyperplasia affecting all four glands either remove three glands completely and bisect the fourth (which should be the most normal of the four), excising the half furthest from the vascular pedicle and mark it with a metal clip. Alternatively remove all four, keeping half of one gland wrapped in a saline-soaked swab. At the end of the operation an incision is made in the forearm and deepened into the brachioradialis muscle, and this half of a gland is sliced up and placed within the muscle

belly where it will hopefully function as an autograft. Each piece of tissue which is removed is carefully labelled and numbered, and the position it was removed from is marked on the diagram. Each specimen is sent for frozen section examination.

Wound closure and dressing

The wound is drained, closed and dressed as for a thyroidectomy (see page 1.19).

POSTOPERATIVE CARE

Make meticulous notes of the operation and sites of excised and remaining parathyroid tissue. The patient is nursed in the semi-sitting position to reduce venous pressure and carefully observed for evidence of bleeding into the neck. The serum calcium level will normally fall to within normal limits within 1–2 days, and may become subnormal, requiring calcium and vitamin D supplements and liaison with the referring endocrinologist is recommended. Drains are removed after 24 hours and the clips are removed after 3 or 4 days. The patient is

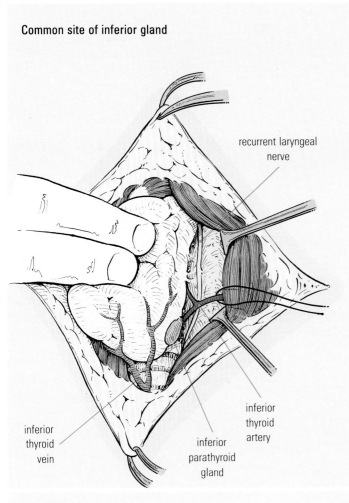

Common site of inferior gland

recurrent laryngeal nerve

inferior thyroid vein

inferior parathyroid gland

inferior thyroid artery

Fig. 1.38

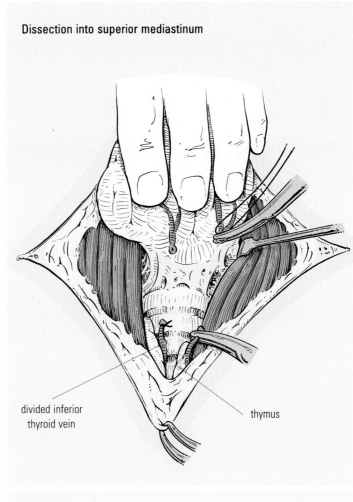

Dissection into superior mediastinum

divided inferior thyroid vein

thymus

Fig. 1.39

allowed home when their serum calcium can be managed on an outpatient basis.

SPECIAL OPERATIVE HAZARDS

1. Inability to find all four parathyroids despite extensive searching. If an obvious adenoma and at least one normal gland have been found, carefully excise the adenoma completely and close the wound. If no abnormal tissue has been found, or all glands so far found are hyperplastic, mobilize the upper horns of the thymus gland from the superior mediastinum and excise them. Excise all the loose areolar tissue from behind the lateral lobes, as far laterally as the carotid sheath. Remember that there may be three glands on one side and one on the other. It is not policy in our unit to perform either a sternotomy or a 'blind' total thyroid lobectomy.
2. Damage to the recurrent laryngeal nerve (see page 1.20).
3. Bleeding (see page 1.20).

COMPLICATIONS

1. Hypocalcaemia. This may be due to suppression of remaining parathyroid tissue by an adenoma, increased uptake by rarefied bone or parathyroid gland damage at the time of surgery (temporary or permanent). It may be manifest as pretetanic symptoms, overt tetany or be noted biochemically. Treat initially with oral calcium supplements. If this is insufficient add oral vitamin D. The serum calcium must be carefully monitored and these measures withdrawn if and when they become unnecessary.
2. Hypercalcaemia. If noticed early in the postoperative period this infers a failure to remove hypersecreting parathyroid tissue (or failure to establish the correct diagnosis preoperatively). Late recurrence may be due to regrowth of an incompletely excised adenoma or hyperplastic gland, or rarely the development of neoplasia in a previously normal gland. The autograft placed in the forearm can become overactive but is easily accessible for excision.

The management of hyperparathyroidism following parathyroidectomy must be referred to a specialist unit with facilities for localization of remaining parathyroid tissue (e.g. ultrasound and angiography of the neck, CT of the mediastinum and selective venous sampling from the neck veins for parathyroid hormone) and the surgical expertise to perform what can be extremely demanding surgery.

Parotidectomy

Superficial parotidectomy is generally undertaken for either parotid tumours which are confined to the superficial lobe, or calculous disease where the stone is not accessible through the mouth. Total parotidectomy is indicated for those tumours which involve the deep lobe and may be performed with either conservation or sacrifice of the facial nerve, depending on the relationship between the nerve and the tumour. It is important to excise all parotid tumours with a margin of normal tissue because of their strong tendency for local recurrence.

PREOPERATIVE ASSESSMENT
1. Establish if there is any facial nerve palsy. Warn the patient of the risk of palsy after the operation.
2. Palpate the deep lobe intra-orally.
3. The duct system can be visualized with a sialogram.

RELEVANT ANATOMY
The facial nerve (Fig. 1.40) divides the parotid gland into a superficial and a deep lobe. The main trunk of the facial nerve lies close to the posterior limit of the gland, between the posterior belly of digastric and the mastoid process in close proximity to the stylomastoid artery. Having entered the gland it divides into upper and lower trunks, which then divide into the temporal, zygomatic, buccal, mental and cervical branches. Their fine branches spread out in a fan-like manner, from posterior to anterior, and as they spread out they become more superficial. Their pattern has been likened to a goose's foot (*pes anserinus*).

OPERATION
Preparation
Shave 5 cm around the ear in all directions and place the patient in a head-up tilt, with the neck extended and rotated away from the side to be operated. The skin is cleansed, and drapes applied to expose the cheek, ear and side of the neck.

Incision
The parotid is approached through an S-shaped incision which starts in front of the tragus, and then curves under the pinna to the mastoid process before continuing forward in the upper skin crease of the neck (Fig. 1.41). Place stay sutures in the skin edges for retraction.

Relevant anatomy

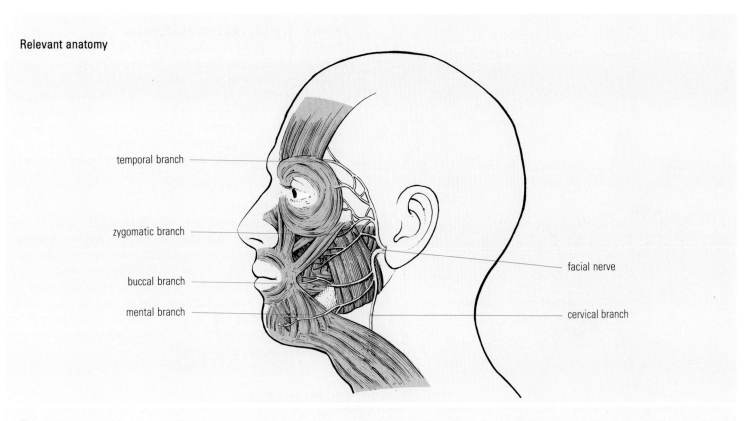

temporal branch

zygomatic branch

buccal branch

mental branch

facial nerve

cervical branch

Fig. 1.40

The greater auricular nerve may be removed and kept in a saline-soaked swab for use as a cable graft if the facial nerve has to be removed. Deepen the incision along the anterior border of sternomastoid to expose the posterior belly of the digastric and stylohyoid muscles, working up towards the mastoid process. Deepen the incision in front of the ear by blunt dissection

until the bony external auditory meatus is reached. Carefully divide the tissues between these two incisions in front of the mastoid process, where the facial nerve will be encountered, lying below and in front of the auditory meatus, just deep to the stylomastoid artery.

Operative technique
1. To perform a superficial parotidectomy follow the facial nerve forwards in the gland substance and develop the plane between the superficial and deep lobes by passing a blunt dissector or haemostat along each branch of the nerve in turn, and divide the intervening tough parotid tissue. Each time a bifurcation is encountered follow the superior branch.

2. When the anterior border of the gland is reached the superficial lobe can be reflected forward off the facial nerve (Fig. 1.42).

3. Now dissect the superficial surface of the gland from the overlying skin flap. Divide the parotid duct as far forward as possible and ligate it with catgut.

Wound closure
It is only necessary to close the skin, usually over a fine suction drain, with fine interrupted nylon sutures. Apply a gauze dressing.

POSTOPERATIVE CARE
Remove the drain after 24–48 hours, and the sutures after 5 days.

Position of patient's head and incision

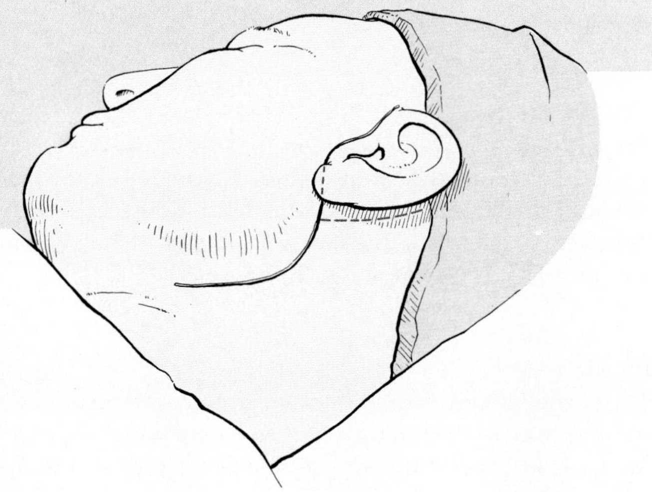

Fig. 1.41

Superficial lobe of parotid reflected forward off the facial nerve

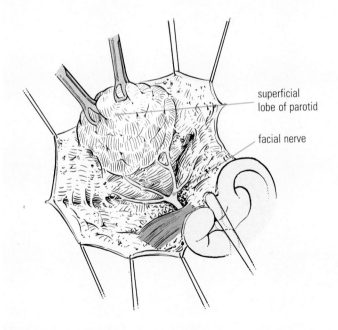

superficial lobe of parotid

facial nerve

SPECIAL OPERATIVE HAZARDS
1. The facial nerve is particularly at risk of being damaged as its filamentous branches can be difficult to see, and their position may have become distorted by the tumour. A low voltage nerve stimulator can be used to locate the branches of the nerve, and Faradic stimulation adjacent to the nerve will elicit a contraction in the corresponding muscles of facial expression. If a branch of the nerve is divided, perform a primary repair, or interpose a segment of the auricular nerve as a cable graft using microsurgical techniques.
2. Damage to the jugular vein.
3. Tumour in the deep lobe, in which case this lobe can be removed between the branches of the facial nerve following mobilization. This requires the external carotid artery to be ligated and divided. With a tumour involving the nerve itself then some or all of its branches must be sacrificed to allow adequate clearance of the tumour. If this is necessary the divided nerve can be repaired by end-to-end apposition or by an interposition graft using a segment of the auricular nerve.

COMPLICATIONS
1. Salivary fistula.
2. Local recurrence of pleomorphic adenoma.
3. Frey's syndrome.

Fig. 1.42

Submandibular Duct and Gland Surgery

Stones that are palpable in the anterior part of the submandibular duct can be removed intra-orally, while those in the posterior part of the duct adjacent to the gland require the removal of the gland, as do calculi within the gland. Both intra-oral stone removal and excision of the gland are described in this chapter.

PREOPERATIVE ASSESSMENT

1. Prior to surgery, use intra-oral radiography of the floor of the mouth to show any radio-opaque calculi and sialography to reveal obstructions of the duct and disease within the gland.
2. Whilst most tumours are pleomorphic adenomas and are treated by wide excision of the gland, a small percentage are carcinomas which require a wider excision with, in some instances, resection of part of the mandible and block dissection of the neck.
3. Sialectasia, with irregular beaded dilatation of the salivary gland ducts, can be seen on a sialogram and the patient presents with recurrent pain and infection. Excision of the gland will be necessary.

RELEVANT ANATOMY

The floor of the mouth is formed from the right and left mylohyoid muscles which arise from the inner aspect of the mandible and extend inferiorly to the hyoid; the muscles meet as a midline raphé.

The submandibular gland consists of a superficial part which lies between the mandible and the mylohyoid and wraps around the posterior border of the muscle to form a deep part in the floor or the mouth, from which the submandibular duct arises. This duct passes forward in the floor of the mouth and opens into the oral cavity at a papilla adjacent to the frenulum of the tongue.

The gland is indented posteriorly by the common facial vein and superiorly by the facial artery which lies between it and the mandible. Inferiorly the gland protrudes below the mandible and at this point it is crossed by the mandibular branch of the facial nerve (Fig. 1.43). Medially the gland is related to the hyoglossus and hypoglossal nerve. Running on the inner surface of the mylohyoid muscle is the lingual nerve which passes under the submandibular duct from lateral to medial and contains the sensory apparatus of the anterior two-thirds of the tongue (Fig. 1.44).

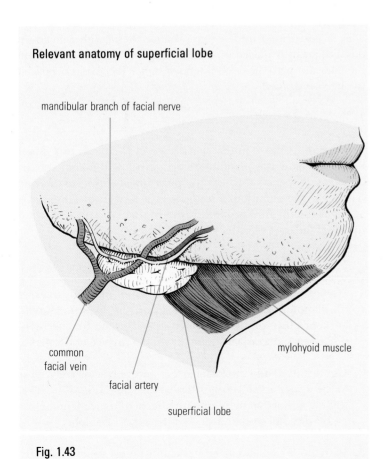

Relevant anatomy of superficial lobe

mandibular branch of facial nerve

common facial vein

facial artery

superficial lobe

mylohyoid muscle

Fig. 1.43

Relevant anatomy of deep lobe and duct

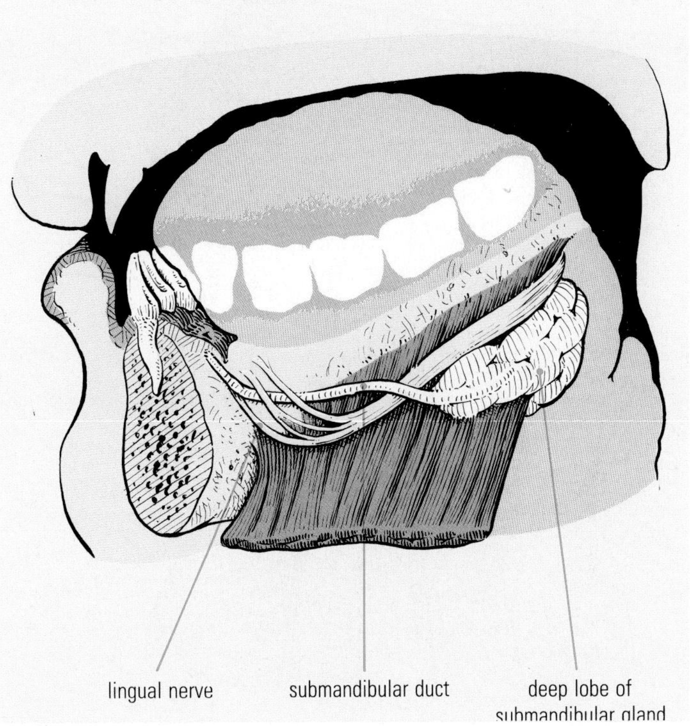

lingual nerve   submandibular duct   deep lobe of submandibular gland

Fig. 1.44

Submandibular duct controlled with stay suture

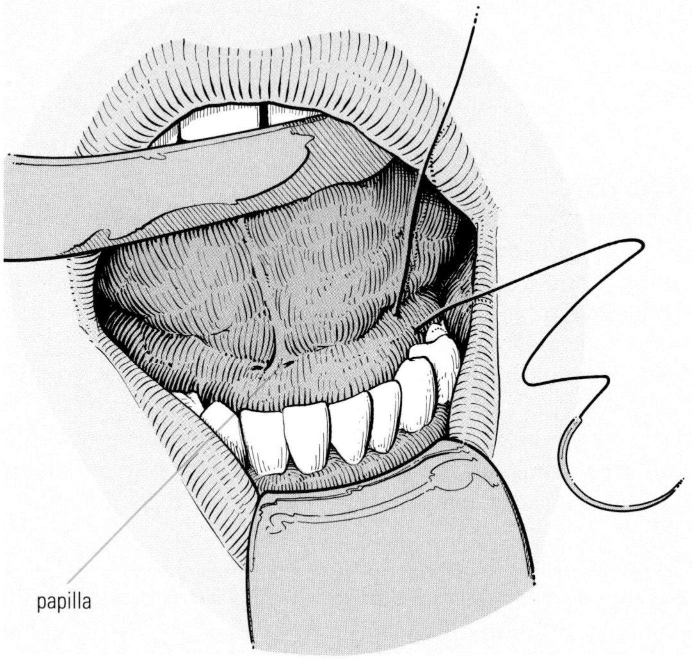

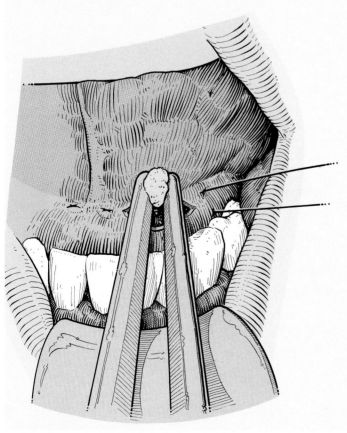

papilla

Fig. 1.45

Removal of stone from duct

Fig. 1.46

OPERATION
REMOVAL OF A STONE FROM THE SUBMANDIBULAR DUCT
Preparation

During this operation, which can be performed under general or local anaesthesia, the mouth is held open with a gag. Prior to the incision the stone is palpated within the duct to reveal its position. The tongue is then retracted and a suture is placed around the duct between the stone and the gland. Gentle traction is exerted on this suture in order to prevent the stone slipping back up the duct (Fig. 1.45).

Incision

Using a scalpel incise the duct over the stone.

Operative technique

1. Lift the stone out of the mouth with forceps (Fig. 1.46). No sutures are required.

2. If the stone is impacted at the papilla, it should be milked back so that the incision into the duct does not encroach onto the papilla.

3. If it is impossible to milk the stone back and the incision involves the papilla, a stomatoplasty is necessary to prevent stenosis. This entails suturing the cut edges of the papillary end of the duct to the floor of the mouth with interrupted 4/0 catgut.

EXCISION OF THE GLAND
Preparation

This is performed under general anaesthesia with a head-up tilt. The head is placed on a head ring and turned away from the operator with the neck extended. Once the skin is prepared the head is draped.

Incision

An incision is made in the skin crease of the neck, two finger breadths below the mandible, starting below the angle of the jaw. It is deepened through the platysma at this level to avoid damage to the mandibular branch of the facial nerve (Fig. 1.47) and an assistant applies gentle, upward traction with a retractor to reveal the lower border of the gland.

Operative technique

1. Mobilize the superficial lobe of the gland upwards towards the mandible. For tumours of the gland, the dissection should be kept clear of the glandular tissue itself; for calculous disease or sialectasia it should be on the surface of the gland.

2. Ligate and divide the facial artery and vein separately, close to the upper and lower borders of the gland (Fig. 1.48), thus leaving a short segment of each attached to the gland before mobilizing the deeper aspect of the superficial lobe.

3. With posterior and lateral traction on its superficial part, separate the deeper aspect of the gland from the posterior

Line of incision for excision of gland

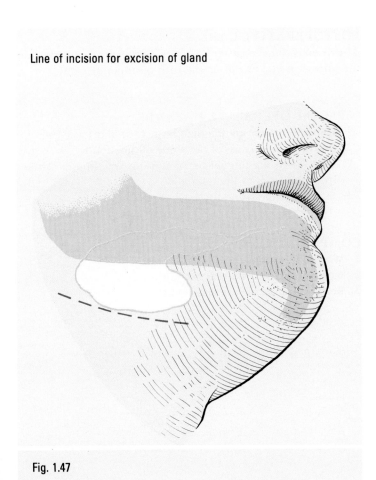

Fig. 1.47

border and deep (lingual) surface of the mylohyoid muscle (Fig. 1.49). The deep lobe is then dissected free from the underlying hyoglossus muscle with blunt dissection; care must be taken as it is closely related to the ribbon-like lingual nerve. The dissection continues until the gland is only attached by its duct (Fig. 1.50).

4. Mobilize the duct forward along the floor of the mouth before ligating it with catgut and dividing it as far anteriorly as possible. Care must be taken to avoid damage to the lingual nerve, which crosses the duct at this level.

5. In cases of malignant disease, extend the margins of resection to allow complete excision of the tumour. This commonly requires *en bloc* resection of part of the mylohyoid and other adjoining structures, such as the digastric and hyoglossus muscles, and the mandible. It is occasionally necessary to sacrifice the lingual nerve.

Wound closure and dressing
1. Close platysma with catgut after the insertion of a fine-bore suction drain.
2. The skin is closed with interrupted nylon sutures or clips and a light non-occlusive dressing is applied.

Ligation and division of facial artery above submandibular gland

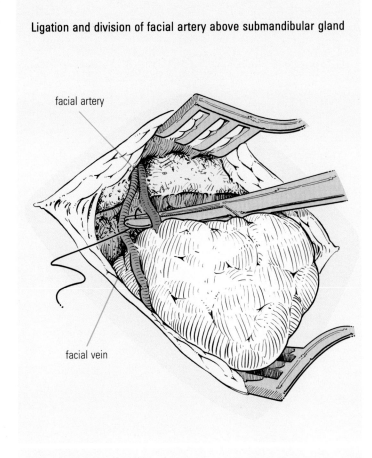

facial artery

facial vein

Fig. 1.48

Freeing the deep lobe from the inner surface of the mylohyoid muscle

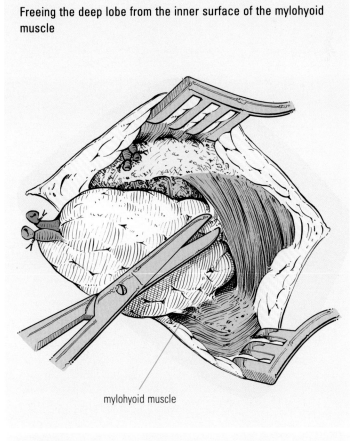

mylohyoid muscle

Fig. 1.49

1.29

Display lingual nerve and its close relation to the duct

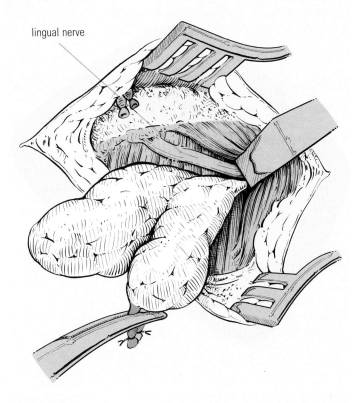

lingual nerve

Fig. 1.50

POSTOPERATIVE CARE

The drain is removed after 24 hours if drainage is minimal and the sutures are taken out on the fifth postoperative day.

SPECIAL OPERATIVE HAZARDS

1. Damage to the mandibular branch of the facial nerve, producing weakness of the angle of the mouth.
2. Damage to the lingual nerve causing anaesthesia of the ipselateral half of the tongue.
3. Haemorrhage from the facial artery.

COMPLICATIONS

1. Wound infection.
2. Dry mouth after bilateral excision.
3. Recurrence in cases of malignancy.

Elective Tracheostomy

Elective tracheostomy implies the intubation of the trachea in a patient who is already ventilated in the controlled environment of the operating room under general anaesthesia.

The indications for tracheostomy include access to an otherwise obstructed airway, reduction of the dead space to facilitate weaning from a ventilator, and for long-term elective ventilation. Sometimes tracheostomy is undertaken for tracheal toilet but often this function can be performed satisfactorily via the much less invasive minitracheotomy (see page 1.34).

A typical tracheostomy tube is the Portex device shown in Fig. 1.51. This is a curved plastic tube with a short intratracheal length to allow the tip to lie above the carina. It has a relatively large low pressure balloon cuff which is inflated to form a seal within the trachea. The pilot tube has a second balloon in series with the main one so that inflation pressure can be palpated. (It is, however, better practice to formally measure this pressure in patients who are intubated for any length of time.)

PREOPERATIVE ASSESSMENT
1. Identify the indications, such as access, long-term ventilation or reduction of dead space.
2. Ascertain whether there are coagulation defects.
3. Check ventilation in conjunction with the anaesthetist.

RELEVANT ANATOMY
The trachea is easily exposed just above the sternal notch. Beneath skin and platysma the trachea is overlain by the strap muscles and in part by the thyroid isthmus. The strap muscles are arranged here in two layers; the more superficial are the sternohyoid muscles running from the hyoid bone to the back of the sternum and clavicles. In their lower part, where they overlie the trachea, they diverge a little from the midline. Deep to these are the broader sternothyroid muscles running, as their name suggests, from the thyroid cartilage to a more caudal insertion on the sternum. When the strap muscles are separated in the midline the trachea is exposed as it enters the chest. The second, third and fourth tracheal rings are also covered by the thyroid isthmus which, with the intervening pretracheal fascia, is adherent to them. In a small number of individuals a thyroidea ima artery which arises from the aortic arch runs up to the isthmus; this anatomy is shown in Fig. 1.52.

OPERATION
Preparation
Move the patient to the operating room where all the facilities are available. Ensure that a selection of tubes are present and that a syringe to inflate the balloon and a catheter mount are available.

With the help of the anaesthetist place the ventilated patient in the thyroid position, then prepare the skin and drape as you

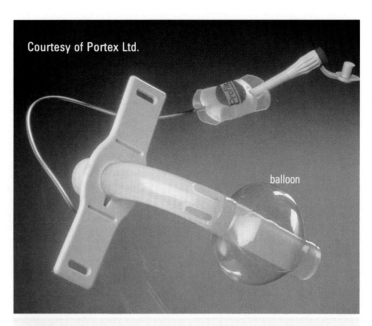

Courtesy of Portex Ltd.

balloon

Fig. 1.51

Relevant anatomy

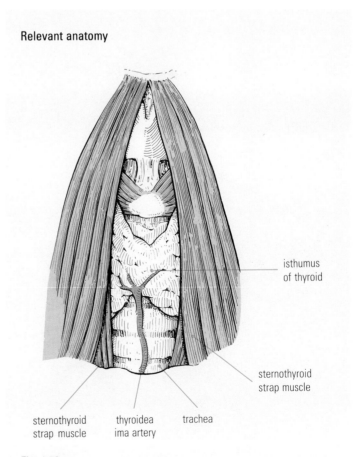

isthumus of thyroid

sternothyroid strap muscle

sternothyroid strap muscle

thyroidea ima artery

trachea

Fig. 1.52

would for a thyroidectomy (see page 1.15).

Select a suitably sized tracheostomy tube; the size of endotracheal tube already in place will help with this. Check that the obturator can be withdrawn from the tube, that the balloon inflates, does not leak, and deflates, and that the catheter mount fits both the tracheostomy tube and the anaesthetic tubing from the ventilator. Lubricate the tube with a water-soluble jelly such as K-Y before proceeding.

Incision
Make a transverse skin incision 2cm above the sternal notch and deepen this through platysma to expose the strap muscles.

Operative technique
1. Open the connective tissue in the midline using sharp and blunt dissection with scissors (Fig. 1.53) and hold the muscles apart with a small retractor.

2. Open the exposed pretracheal fascia with a knife or scissors, and get the assistant to retract the thyroid isthmus in a cephalic direction (Fig. 1.54). Sometimes this needs to be divided for adequate access to the trachea.

3. At this stage pay meticulous attention to haemostasis so as to avoid aspiration of blood.

4. After warning the anaesthetist, create a tracheostomy by cutting a circular window through the second and third tracheal rings (Fig. 1.55); avoid the first as damage to this

Incision of pretracheal fascia

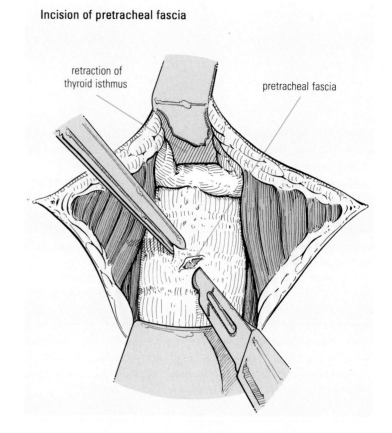

retraction of thyroid isthmus

pretracheal fascia

Fig. 1.54

Separation of strap muscles in the midline

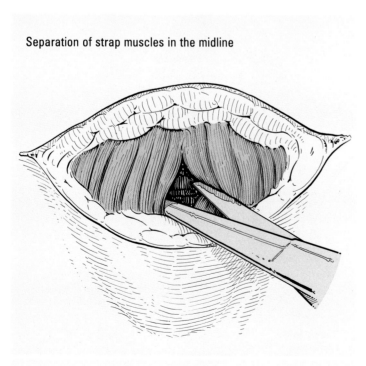

Fig. 1.53

Excision of a disc of trachea

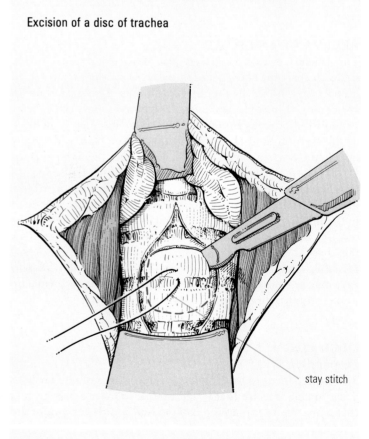

stay stitch

Fig. 1.55

can later lead to tracheal stenosis. Using an inverted U-flap with the apex sutured to the lower skin edge has the advantage of easing resiting of a displaced tube but is associated with delayed healing when the tube is no longer needed. In an infant make a vertical incision only.

5. Pass a non-absorbable suture through a ring as this will help with the removal of the window.

6. Ask the anaesthetist to withdraw the endotracheal tube only so far as to allow the surgeon to insert the tracheostomy tube with its cuff deflated. When this is in place the endotracheal tube is completely withdrawn, the catheter mount is attached to the tracheostomy tube and passed to the anaesthetist who now reconnects the ventilator.

7. With a one-way valve in place on the end of the pilot tube inflate the cuff just enough to prevent an air leak (Fig. 1.56). Use suction to clear the airway of secretions and blood.

Wound dressing
Place a dry dressing around the wound and tie the tube firmly in place with tapes (Fig. 1.57). The skin wound is left open to prevent surgical emphysema in the event of an air leak.

POSTOPERATIVE CARE
Once back on the ward the oxygen supplied to the tracheostomy must be humidified, and the tube should be sucked out regularly and changed when secretions begin to form a crust on it. The Portex tube may be changed for a valved silver speaking tube as part of a weaning process once the patient is able to breath air spontaneously. Later this tube will be removed and a dry dressing applied while the tracheostomy closes spontaneously.

SPECIAL OPERATIVE HAZARDS
1. Haemorrhage from small or large vessels (especially veins).
2. Failure to intubate the trachea.
3. Preoperative airway obstruction by secretions or blood.

COMPLICATIONS
1. Delayed haemorrhage (classically from the innominate artery).
2. Blocked or displaced tube.
3. Tracheo-oesophageal fistula if the cuff is over-inflated for long periods of time.
4. Tracheal stenosis after the tube has been removed.

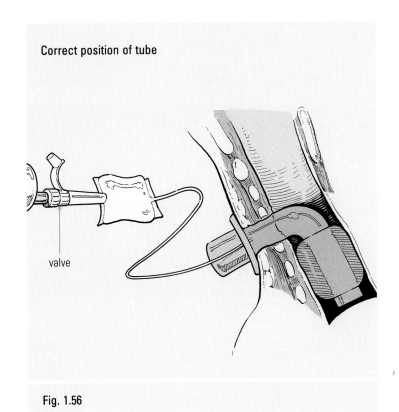

Correct position of tube

valve

Fig. 1.56

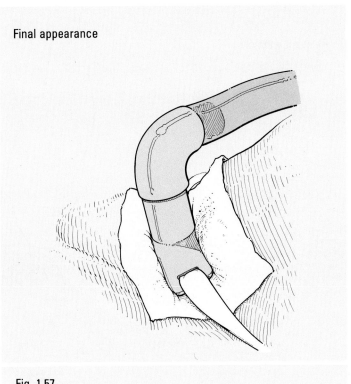

Final appearance

Fig. 1.57

Insertion of Minitracheotomy Tube

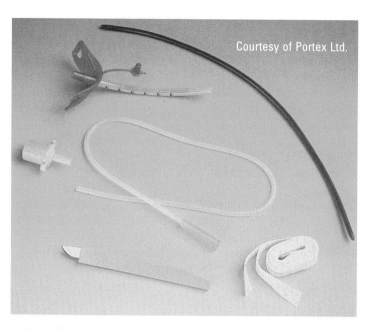

Courtesy of Portex Ltd.

Fig. 1.58

The Portex minitracheotomy tube is a plastic, 4-mm diameter tube which can be inserted into the airway via the cricothyroid membrane under local anaesthestic to provide access for airway suction or even, under exceptional circumstances, to provide an emergency airway.

The device is conveniently packaged with a guarded blade, an obturator, a suction catheter, tapes to fasten the tube and a catheter mount. The external end can be spigotted so that when not in use the airway remains uncompromised (Fig. 1.58).

It is of enormous value in aiding patients clear secretions in the postoperative period when a painful incision may prevent expectoration, even with the help of good physiotherapy. It is especially useful after lateral thoractomy, which is a relatively painful approach to the chest.

PREOPERATIVE ASSESSMENT
1. Ensure that suction apparatus is available.

Relevant anatomy

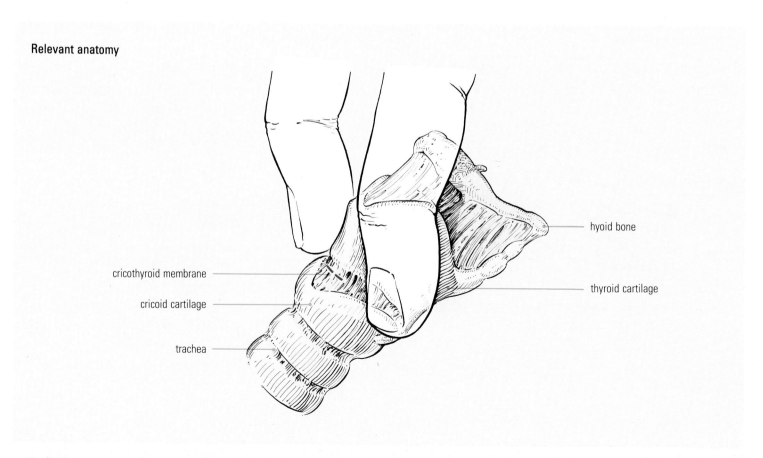

hyoid bone

cricothyroid membrane

cricoid cartilage

thyroid cartilage

trachea

Fig. 1.59

2. Has previous surgery been performed in the neck?

3. Check the coagulation status.

RELEVANT ANATOMY

The cricothyroid membrane is an oval sheet of fibrous tissue connecting the anterior surfaces of thyroid and cricoid cartilages, with its long axis lying horizontally. It is partially overlain by the sternohyoid muscles and, deeper, the sternothyroid muscles. However, these diverge in this region and this feature, and the more caudal position of the thyroid isthmus, means that the membrane can usually be easily palpated as a depression between the thyroid and cricoid cartilages (Fig. 1.59).

Although a vein may occasionally overlie the membrane, it is usually possible to pass a blade and then the tube into the airway through the membrane without damage to other neck structures.

Since the membrane lies below the vocal cords these are not injured by the procedure and can still approximate to allow the patient to speak or cough for himself between suctioning.

OPERATION
Preparation

This procedure can often be performed with local anaesthetic in the ward but if the surgeon is inexperienced, the patient is unco-operative or some other complicating factor is present (e.g. a 'thick' neck, previous neck surgery, or the patient has been anticoagulated) do not hesitate to summon the help of an anaesthetist and take the patient to the operating theatre.

Place the patient in the 'thyroid' position with the neck extended, and clean and drape a generous area of skin. Standing on the right of the patient, fix the larynx with your left hand having first identified with certainty the cricothyroid membrane, and then raise a bleb in the skin overlying the membrane and carefully infiltrate the deeper tissues with 1% plain lignocaine until the membrane itself is reached. As you penetrate this the patient will cough. Wait for the anaesthetic to take effect and then confirm your impression of the anatomy. Lubricate the obturator so that the tube can easily slide over it into the trachea.

Incision

Take the guarded blade and insert this to the hilt transversely into the membrane. Keep the larynx and overlying skin firmly fixed with the left hand (Fig. 1.60).

Operative technique

1. Withdraw the blade and in a single movement insert the obturator and tube into the airway, keeping the incisions in the skin and the membrane in line (Fig. 1.61).

2. Pass the tube fully into the trachea, withdraw the obturator and immediately suck out the airway as its patency may be significantly compromised.

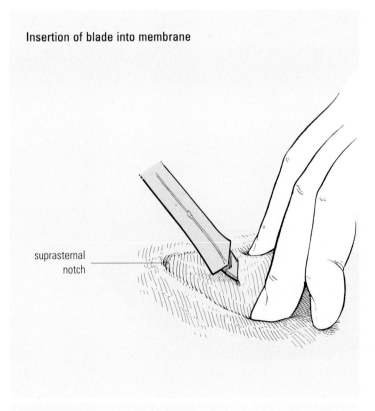

Insertion of blade into membrane

suprasternal notch

Fig. 1.60

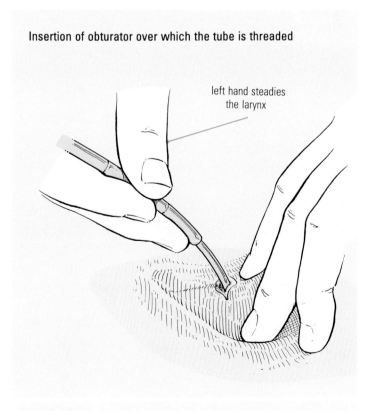

Insertion of obturator over which the tube is threaded

left hand steadies the larynx

Fig. 1.61

Minitracheotomy tube secured in position

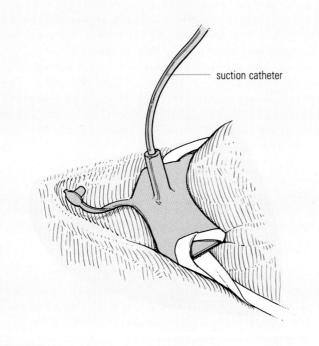

suction catheter

Fig. 1.62

3. Spigot the tube and fasten it in place with linen tapes as for a tracheostomy tube (Fig. 1.62).

POSTOPERATIVE CARE

Arrange intensive physiotherapy and for the dressing to be changed daily. When the tube is no longer needed it is simply withdrawn and a dry dressing is applied.

SPECIAL OPERATIVE HAZARDS

1. Haemorrhage from an overlying vein.
2. Failure to enter the airway.
3. Bleeding into the airway during insertion leading to airway obstruction, or a haemotoma in the soft tissues of the neck.

COMPLICATIONS

1. Blockage of tube with secretions.
2. An air leak when the minitracheotmy tube is removed will close spontaneously.

2

Cardiothoracic Surgery

Resuscitation of the Shocked Patient

Shock can be defined as a condition of tissue underperfusion by blood and follows cardiac insufficiency (e.g. following myocardial infarction), loss of circulating volume (e.g. haemorrhage), or redistribution and lowered resistance to regional blood flow (septicaemic shock in overwhelming infection). This leads to secondary effects as metabolic substrates are exhausted, toxins accumulate and the hypoxic tissues fail.

The response of tissues to underperfusion leads to the clinical manifestations and consequences of shock. Peripheral vasoconstriction causes a pallid appearance and all tissues begin to undergo anaerobic glycolysis with the production of significant amounts of lactate which compounds the problem with its direct myocardial depressant action. Spasm of precapillary sphincters and venules especially in the splanchnic circulation leads to hypoxic damage and later to stasis of the blood. The damaged bowel may become necrotic or at least cease to prevent bacterial entry from the gastrointestinal tract with consequent bacteraemia and endotoxaemia. Renal plasma flow and glomerular filtration rates are depressed with consequent oliguria; if underperfusion is prolonged acute tubular necrosis may follow with subsequent renal failure. Coronary circulation and myocardial oxygenation is inadequate and there is additional direct depression of cardiac action by metabolites and toxins. However, perfusion of the brain and heart is maintained at the expense of other tissues but if shock is untreated or becomes irreversible even these are compromised. When cerebral circulation fails the brain's extreme sensitivity to hypoxia leads to rapid loss of consciousness and death supervenes.

THE MANAGEMENT OF SHOCK

Priority is given to monitoring and the restoration of an adequate supply of oxygenated blood to the tissues. The underlying aetiology is then treated.

Monitoring

The importance of appropriate monitoring of the acutely ill patient cannot be overemphasized and if surgery is not an immediate necessity the intensive care unit is the best place to resuscitate the patient. If surgery is required it is safest to undertake this on a patient who is in as stable a condition as possible. The following variables should be monitored: pulse rate, blood pressure and respiratory rate; peripheral (big toe) and core (rectal) temperatures; urine output (urethral catheter); conscious level; blood gases; electrocardiogram (rhythm and electrolyte changes); central venous pressure (neck line); cardiac output and derived systemic and pulmonary resistances (Swan-Ganz catheter); and routine radiology and laboratory measurements.

Treating the effects of shock

Hypovolaemia is treated with volume replacement. The choice of fluid should be made with care; in general large volumes of crystalloid are hazardous and may result in pulmonary oedema (a contributing factor to shock lung). Unless specific electrolyte disturbances require treatment the volume is best replaced with blood or a colloid substitute (e.g. gelatin polypeptides). The amount of fluid given should be controlled according to accurate monitoring of cardiac filling pressures; the central venous or right atrial pressure via a neck line, and the left atrial pressure via a Swan-Ganz catheter. It is advisable to warm large volumes given rapidly, filter blood, and consider possible complications of supporting a circulation with transfused blood (e.g. hypocalcaemia).

Vasoconstrictors such as metaraminol (e.g. Aramine) or adrenaline may be used in the treatment of vasodilatation contributing to central underperfusion, but in general it should be possible to manage this problem with volume replacement. In addition, such agents may lead to vasconstriction of central vessels such as renal arteries compounding the patient's condition.

Inotropic support of the heart should always be instituted when it fails to support an adequately filled circulation; dopamine and dobutamine are useful agents but they may cause a

Compression of sternum

Fig. 2.1

tachycardia (dopamine especially) which if marked may, paradoxically, reduce cardiac output. Dopamine may also be used in low dose ($2-5\,\mu g\,kg^{-1}\,min^{-1}$) to stimulate renal blood flow and promote urine production. The pharmacological armoury for managing the acutely ill as well as the shocked patient should also include agents such as isoprenaline (a positive chronotrope and pulmonary vasodilator) and nitroprusside (a vasodilator and cardiac afterload reducer).

Ventilation of the severely shocked patient should be considered as this will optimize oxygenation, control acidosis and reduce the energy requirement and metabolic load placed on the injured body by the effort of breathing.

Treating the cause of shock

Haemorrhage is controlled, infection is treated with the appropriate antibiotics, sepsis is drained, dead tissue is debrided, and the extent and severity of cardiac infarction or decompensation is minimized with drugs or surgical correction.

CARDIAC ARREST

It is important firstly to establish the diagnosis (the patient is unconscious, not breathing and has no cardiac output) and then to decide whether resuscitation is warranted (from the duration of arrest, the age and general condition of patient and the probable cause). Once the decision to resuscitate has been taken, the principles are to establish an airway, to support ventilation, to provide cardiac output and to support the body pharmacologically, in that order.

Principles of treatment

1. Establish an airway with the patient supine and the neck extended. Support the lower jaw with one hand to keep the tongue out of the airway. Clear debris and mucous from the pharynx. If the airway cannot be cleared perform a cricothyroid stab or a tracheostomy. Once established the airway can be held open with a Brook oropharyngeal tube, if available, or with a cuffed endotracheal tube if the surgeon is competent at intubation or an anaesthetist is present.

2. Commence artificial ventilation; expired air mouth-to-mouth breathing is simple and effective. Alternatively, use an Ambu bag and a face mask over an oropharyngeal airway or formal ventilation via an endotracheal tube.

3. Provide cardiac output by external cardiac massage. Intermittently compress the heart between sternum and vertebrae (Figs 2.1 and 2.2) by depressing the sternum vigorously with both hands approximately 60 times a minute. Pause after every fifth compression to allow ventilation of the lungs. Placing the patient on a hard surface rather than a soft mattress will make massage more efficient.

4. Administer sodium bicarbonate (100 ml of an 8.4% solution) to counter the inevitable acidosis which will be present. Peripheral lines are difficult to place in the absence of a circulation and drugs administered through them will take a long time to reach the heart; a central line is more useful. A technique for central line placement is described later in this chapter.

5. Connect an ECG monitor and treat the underlying cardiac rhythm. Pharmacological management of cardiac dysrhythmias is not within the scope of this chapter but asystole can be treated with adrenaline and calcium gluconate, and ventricular fibrillation by DC cardioversion assisted if necessary by boluses of lignocaine. Heart block is overcome by ventricular pacing (via a wire introduced into the right ventricle through a central line or by a transoesophageal impulse).

Whilst priority is given to these supportive measures the cause of the arrest must be ascertained and treated to allow successful resuscitation. Cardiac tamponade or tension pneumothorax is drained and relieved, a pulmonary embolus is thrombolysed or removed and metabolic abnormalities are corrected.

PLACEMENT OF A CENTRAL VENOUS LINE
Relevant Anatomy

Cannulation of the right internal jugular is preferred to the left since this provides a more direct route for the cannula to pass into the right atrium. The internal jugular vein emerges from the posterior part of the jugular foramen and runs inferiorly through the neck, at first behind the internal carotid artery then lateral and anterior to this and the common carotid artery. The artery, vein and vagus nerve are enclosed within the carotid sheath which is very thin over the vein to allow it to expand. In its lower part the vein is overlain by the sternomastoid muscle. On the left side the jugular vein joins the subclavian vein to form the innominate vein which passes transversely in front of the aortic arch and great vessels to join the superior vena cava on the right. The right internal jugular vein thus has a more direct path into the superior vena cava.

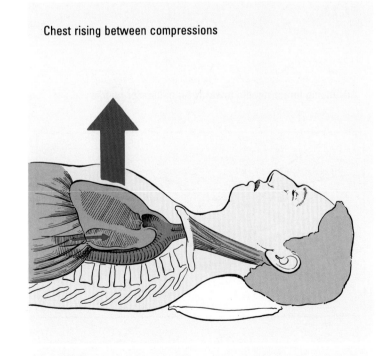

Chest rising between compressions

Fig. 2.2

Preparation

The patient is placed supine with slight head-down tilt to fill the internal jugular vein, and the head is turned to the left (Fig. 2.3). The skin of the right side of the neck is prepared and towels are placed around the sterile field.

Technique

1. Insert an 18G needle between the sternal and clavicular heads of the sternomastoid muscle 2 cm above the clavicle in

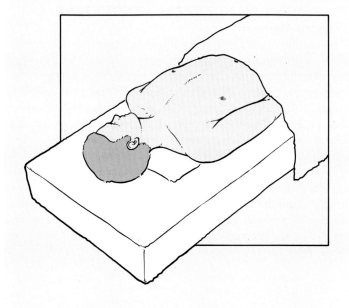

Position of the patient

Fig. 2.3

a posterior direction until blood is seen to well from its hub; flow and colour will distinguish between a needle in the internal jugular vein and the carotid artery.

2. Now insert a larger needle from a more cephalad position aiming for the tip of the first needle which is known to lie in the jugular vein (Fig. 2.4). Aspirate using the attached syringe as the needle is advanced, until it enters the vein.

3. Introduce a guide wire into the vein through the lumen of the large-bore needle and withdraw both needles leaving the wire *in situ*. Pass a dilator over the guide wire (Fig. 2.5).

4. Remove the dilator, again leaving the wire in place, and pass a single or double-lumen catheter over the guide wire into the vein. Remove the guide wire, pass the catheter into the right atrium and check that it remains within the venous system by aspirating from it with an attached syringe. Suture the catheter in place, flush with heparinized saline and attach it to a controlled infusion or monitoring apparatus as desired.

5. Use a chest X-ray to confirm the position of the radio-opaque marker of the catheter within the right atrium.

SPECIAL OPERATIVE HAZARDS OF CENTRAL VENOUS CANNULATION
1. Haemorrhage.
2. Pneumothorax.
3. Air embolus.

COMPLICATIONS OF CENTRAL VENOUS CANNULATION
1. Line sepsis.
2. Line fracture with embolization.
3. Thrombosis.

Advancing larger needle towards tip of smaller needle

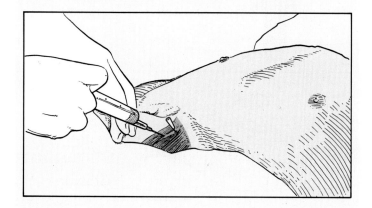

Fig. 2.4

Introducing dilator over guide wire

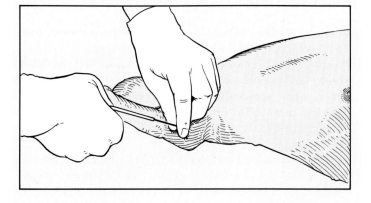

Fig. 2.5

Rigid Oesophagoscopy

Rigid oesophagoscopy should be seen as an adjunct to the use of the flexible instrument. Its advantage lies in the ease with which procedures such as removal of impacted foreign bodies, dilatations and biopsies can be performed with it and the feel that is obtained when assessing tumours. Its limitations include the need for general anaesthesia and the inability to pass the scope any distance beyond the gastro-oesophageal junction. A rigid oesophagoscope and bougies are shown in Fig. 2.6.

PREOPERATIVE ASSESSMENT
1. Perform barium swallow, oesophageal manometry and pH studies.
2. Check for loose teeth or crowns.
3. X-ray the neck if disease of the cervical spine is suspected (e.g. rheumatoid arthritis).

RELEVANT ANATOMY
The oesophagus is about 25cm long and its entire length is easily within the reach of the rigid scope. It is normally indented by structures from without and these should not be mistaken for pathological findings. They include vertebral bodies, especially if osteophytes are present, the arch of the aorta, and the left main bronchus.

PROCEDURE
RIGID OESOPHAGOSCOPY
Preparation
Display a recent barium swallow. The anaesthetist induces general anaesthesia, and passes a cuffed single lumen tube for ventilation and to protect the airway; this is not tied in place so it can be manoeuvred out of the way. After arranging the patient on the table so that the neck is flexed but can easily be extended on the head support, wrap a towel around the head to protect the face and eyes leaving the mouth exposed. Lubricate the oesophagoscope with a lubricating jelly (e.g. K-Y).

Operative technique
1. Holding a swab in your left hand to protect the upper gum or teeth, insert the scope with your right hand, looking down the instrument as it is advanced (Fig. 2.7). Rest the oesophagoscope on the thumb of your left hand to protect the patient.

2. Ensure the lip of the instrument is at the front and the bevel faces backwards.

3. Advance in the midline but do not force the instrument; the pharynx and oesophagus are very fragile. Deflate the oeso-

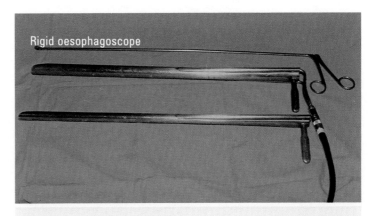

Rigid oesophagoscope

Fig. 2.6

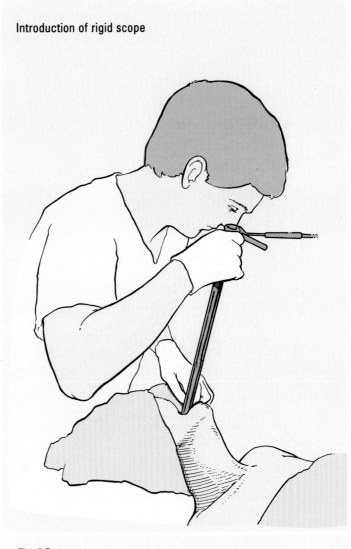

Introduction of rigid scope

Fig. 2.7

Tube advanced

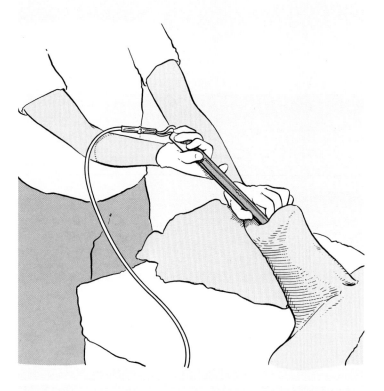

Fig. 2.8

Visualization of the oesophagus

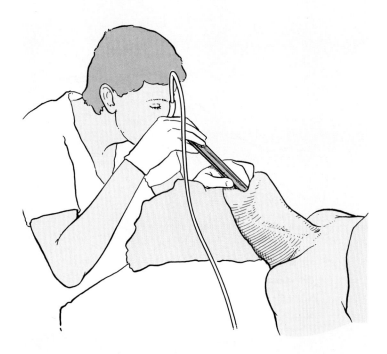

phagus, extending the patient's neck as this is done (Fig. 2.8). As you progress you will complete this extension so that the oesophagus, pharynx and mouth lie in a straight line. A rolled-up pillow behind the patient's shoulders can help.

4. Advance, but as with any endoscopic procedure, do so only when the lumen ahead can be seen (Fig. 2.9). The pulsation in the aorta can be felt as the oesophagoscope passes it, and at the gastro-oesophageal junction the surgeon will notice the relatively featureless lining of the oesophagus give way to the gastric mucosa. Beyond this point the oesophagus has to be regularly sucked clear of secretions and debris.

5. During the procedure note the appearance of the mucosa and the level (measured from the incisors) of any changes (inflammation, bleeding, ulceration or neoplasia). Dilate strictures if appropriate (see later in this chapter) and biopsy lesions or areas of interest with long handled forceps.

6. When the procedure has been completed withdraw the scope and allow the patient to recover.

OESOPHAGEAL DILATATION
Perform this before any biopsies are taken to minimize the risk of perforating the oesophagus.

Ensure that the narrowed lumen of the oesophagus seen through the oesophagoscope is directly ahead. Sequential dilatation involves advancing, consecutively, 10 Fr through to 24 Fr gum elastic bougies which have been softened in warm water and lubricated; other types of dilator are available but are in general less safe. Never force a dilator and if it cannot be passed summon help as a ruptured oesophagus can be a fatal complication.

After the oesophagoscope has been withdrawn flex the neck again and insert a 50 or 60 Fr Hurst–Maloney bougie and allow it to cross the stricture under its own weight (these are soft, tapered and mercury filled and are shown alongside the oesophagoscope in Fig. 2.6).

POSTOPERATIVE CARE
A chest X-ray is taken before the patient drinks and if there is any doubt as to the integrity of the oesophagus arrange a barium swallow to exclude a leak.

SPECIAL OPERATIVE HAZARDS
1. Oesophageal perforation.
2. Damage to incisors and crowns.

COMPLICATIONS
1. Oesophageal pain.
2. Recurrence of stricture.

Fig. 2.9

Rigid bronchoscopy gives good access to the proximal airways for removal of foreign bodies, clearance of sputum plugs, tumour assessment and biopsy, and endobronchial cautery but a general anaesthetic is required. Flexible instruments can be used with local anaesthetic, can visualize more distal bronchial divisions and permit transbronchial biopsy (e.g. of a tumour, or the lung following transplantation). In the assessment of tumour operability endoscopic viewing and biopsy of a bronchial tumour can be supplemented by superior mediastinoscopy in cases where CT scanning has demonstrated the presence of enlarged lymph nodes.

PREOPERATIVE ASSESSMENT
1. Investigate tumours using radiological techniques including chest X-ray, tomography and CT scanning.
2. Perform anaesthetic assessment including a check for loose teeth and crowns.
3. Exclude cervical spine disease with an X-ray of neck if indicated (e.g. history of rheumatoid arthritis).

RELEVANT ANATOMY
The trachea and major bronchi of the branching airway through which the bronchoscope is advanced are held open by cartilaginous rings which are incomplete posteriorly where the tubes are membranous and muscular. The airway is lined with a respiratory mucous membrane surfaced with a ciliated columnar epithelium.

The airway is guarded by the epiglottis which overlies the opening to the larynx. The vocal cords lie in an anteroposterior plane in the larynx, and after passing these the bronchoscope enters the trachea (at the level of C6). The trachea bifurcates about 5 cm below the level of the manubriosternal junction, the carina forming a sharp ridge at this point (Fig. 2.10a). The left and right main bronchi now pass off into their respective hila, the left making a more acute angle to the trachea than the right.

The basic arrangement is for the bronchi to supply two pulmonary lobes on the left and three on the right. As the bronchoscope is passed into the left side a secondary carina is encountered where the main bronchus gives rise to the left upper lobe bronchus (itself dividing into upper and lingular divisions). The left main bronchus continues as the lower lobe bronchus which gives off the apical lower lobe branch and then divides into three basal branches. The right main bronchus descends at a steeper angle and gives rise to the upper lobe bronchus laterally and then continues as the intermediate bronchus until it gives off the middle lobe bronchus anteriorly. It terminates in the lower lobe divisions (Fig. 2.10b). Differences in this pattern can be caused by distortion resulting from extrinsic disease or congenital variation.

The mediastinoscope is used to examine the contents of the anterior part of the superior mediastinum. This is bounded

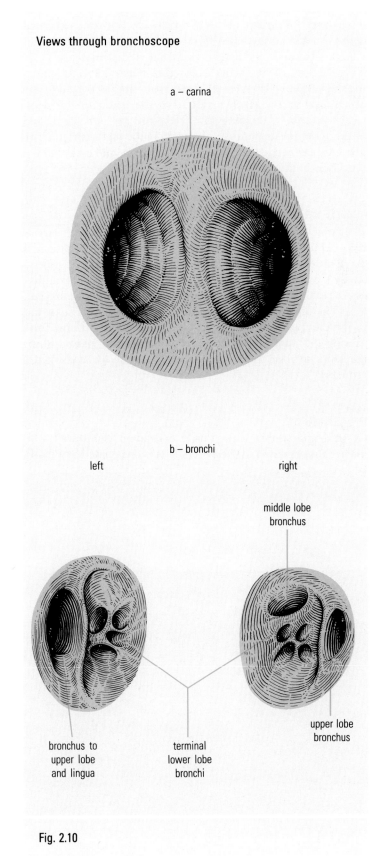

Views through bronchoscope

a – carina

b – bronchi

left   right

middle lobe bronchus

bronchus to upper lobe and lingua

terminal lower lobe bronchi

upper lobe bronchus

Fig. 2.10

superiorly by the thoracic inlet and inferiorly by the tracheo-bronchial angles. Anteriorly lies the sternum, and lateral to the trachea are the great vessels of the neck. The brachiocephalic vein crosses in front of the trachea and further inferiorly the aorta gives rise to the innominate artery as it crosses anterior to the carina. Thus both innominate vessels overlie the airway. The recurrent laryngeal nerves are adjacent to the proximal trachea. Nodes in pre- and paratracheal positions and those at the tracheobronchial angles may be biopsied with the media-stinoscope. Precarinal nodes are in reach but the subcarinal nodes can be biopsied only if they are exceptionally large.

Access to this compartment with the mediastinoscope is via the neck, the trachea being exposed in much the same way as for tracheostomy. Passage into the mediastinum is behind the pretracheal fascia which arises from the hyoid in the neck, passes inferiorly, dividing to enclose the thyroid gland, and blends with the adventitia of the aorta in the mediastinum. The procedure of mediastinoscopy requires deliberate entry behind this fascia in the neck.

RIGID BRONCHOSCOPY

The apparatus (Fig. 2.11) consists of a rigid tube which carries a fibreoptic light within its lumen and to which can be attached the Sanders venturi ventilation system. This system injects oxygen axially down the bronchoscope, its gas-entraining effect resulting in the lungs being inflated with an air–oxygen mix. The anaesthetist uses this device intermittently so as not to inhibit the bronchoscopist. Fibreoptic end- (0°) and side-viewing (90°) and illuminating telescopes can be passed down the bronchoscope to give good views into the divisions of the bronchi.

Preparation

General anaesthesia with muscle relaxation is induced with intravenous agents and the patient is pre-oxygenated by a mask.

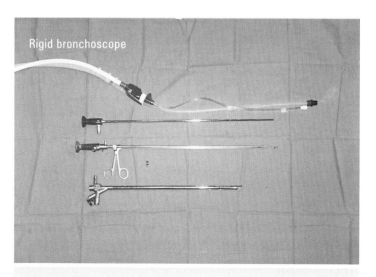

Rigid bronchoscope

Fig. 2.11

Introduction of bronchoscope

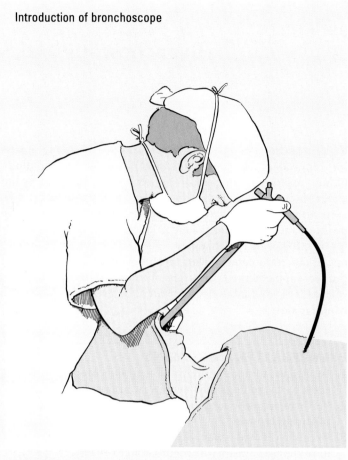

Fig. 2.12

The use of a digital pulse oximeter to monitor oxygen saturation is recommended.

The patient has a green towel wrapped around the upper part of the head to protect the eyes and is positioned supine with the head supported on a pillow and the chin pointing directly upwards. Guard the upper teeth with a folded and lubricated swab held in the left hand and insert the broncho-scope into the mouth using the right hand with the bevel facing backwards (Fig. 2.12).

Procedure

1. Look down the bronchoscope. Manoeuvre it over the back of the tongue and angle it forwards. See the epiglottis and lever this upwards with the tip of the instrument to visualize the vocal cords. Turn the bronchoscope through 90° so that it will pass easily between them, and then return it to its original orientation.

2. At all times rest the instrument on the thumb of your left hand to protect the upper teeth.

3. Extend the neck so that the bronchoscope points directly down the trachea (Fig. 2.13). The anaesthetist will now attach

the Sanders injector and start intermittent ventilation. The trachea is distinguished by its cartilaginous rings and should not be confused with the oesophagus.

4. Examine the bronchial tree; an impression of what is normal will develop with practice. Note the colour and texture of the mucosa, and the position of tumours with a view to assessing what resection is needed for their removal (is a pneumonectomy required or can a lobectomy be performed?). Fibreoptic telescopes give a better the view of the more terminal divisions.

5. Develop a routine to examine the airway. Look at the trachea and carina and then turn the patient's head to the right and pass the bronchoscope into the left main bronchus or to the left to enter the right main bronchus. Assess the normal side first. Use the 90° telescope to see into the bronchial division to the right and left upper lobes, the middle lobe on the right and other angled bronchi. Gentle inflation by the anaesthetist will open the airway and help clear condensation from the telescopes.

6. Take biopsies either with biopsy forceps alone for larger lesions or with the telescopes for less accessible ones. Biopsy sites usually stop bleeding very quickly but haemostasis can be helped by dipping a cotton bud in 1:1,000 adrenaline and applying it to the biopsy site for a few minutes using biopsy forceps.

7. Removing foreign bodies is not easy. Intense swelling of the mucosa can hide the object and biological material (peanuts are the worst offenders), excite a strong inflammatory response and often crumble when grasped. Be prepared to perform a thoracotomy and bronchotomy to retrieve the object if endoscopy fails.

POSTOPERATIVE CARE
A postoperative chest X-ray is taken and examined.

SPECIAL OPERATIVE HAZARDS
1. Damage to teeth or crowns.
2. Failure to intubate the trachea, in which case withdraw the bronchoscope, allow the anaesthetist to reoxygenate the patient and try again.
3. Haemorrhage from biopsy sites.
4. Damage to a bronchus.
5. Dislodging a foreign body or friable tumour into the more distal airways.

SUPERIOR MEDIASTINOSCOPY
The mediastinoscope is a short device which has a light source attached and a handle to facilitate manipulation. It has a split along its length to allow easier passage of instruments, swabs and a combined diathermy device and sucker.

Preparation
Display the CT scan and make sure you can identify the nodes to be biopsied. Rigid bronchoscopy is performed as described above. The intubated patient is then transferred to the operating theatre, positioned supine and draped with towels as for a thyroidectomy (see page 1.12). Position the whole table slightly head-up to reduce venous engorgement; this will make it easier to look down the mediastinoscope later.

Incision
Stand on the patient's left and make a short transverse skin crease incision about 2 cm above the sternal notch and deepen this through platysma to the strap muscles.

Procedure
1. Separate the strap muscles in the midline and expose the trachea which is covered with pretracheal fascia and partly overlain by the thyroid isthmus.

2. Retract the thyroid in a cephalad direction and open the fascia, ensuring careful haemostasis.

3. Insert your right index finger into the mediastinum behind the fascia and identify the structures that you feel (e.g. the sternum, aorta, innominate artery and each bronchus). The nodes being sought may also be felt but palpation will not identify the soft great veins or the roof of the left atrium, all of which are within reach.

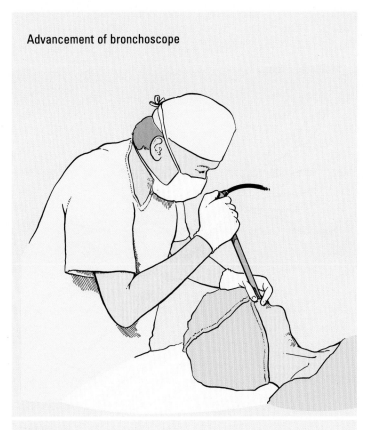

Advancement of bronchoscope

Fig. 2.13

Insertion of mediastinoscope

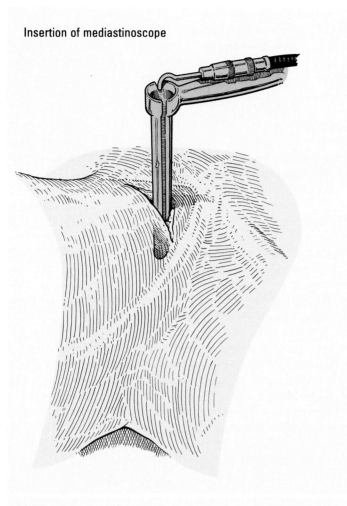

Fig. 2.14

Mediastinoscopy

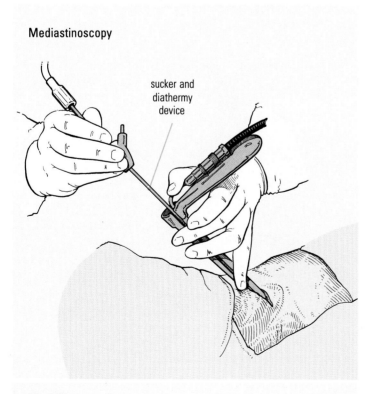

sucker and diathermy device

Fig. 2.15

4. Insert the mediastinoscope with the bevel facing down and ease it into the chest (Fig. 2.14). Further extension of the patient's head may help. Use the sucker and diathermy device as a probe to dissect out the nodes required (Fig. 2.15). Before taking a biopsy attempt to aspirate the target with a syringe and long spinal needle. Beware of the great veins stretched ribbon-thin over the nodes.

5. Take your biopsies and achieve haemostasis with the diathermy device. On rare occasions haemorrhage may precipitate thoracotomy.

Wound closure and dressing
Close the wound in layers with absorbable sutures (e.g. Vicryl) and the skin with a subcuticular stitch. Apply a dry dressing.

POSTOPERATIVE CARE
Arrange a postoperative chest X-ray.

SPECIAL OPERATIVE HAZARDS
1. Damage to major blood vessels.
2. Biopsy of the roof of the left atrium.
3. Damage to recurrent laryngeal nerves.
4. Pneumothorax.
5. Haemorrhage following biopsy, which can on rare occasions require thoracotomy.

Ivor Lewis Oesophagectomy

Treatment of carcinoma of the oesophagus is difficult. The tumour has often spread extensively into adjacent structures or regional lymph nodes, or even metastasized at the time of diagnosis, and often no more than palliative oesophageal intubation is warranted (see page 2.16). However, it should be remembered that the quality of swallowing with an oesophageal tube in place is poor so it is not unreasonable to resect a tumour even when a cure is improbable; many patients survive for a significant time able to eat a normal solid diet after oesophagectomy.

Oesophageal tumours, like gastric ones, tend to spread through the submucosal layers leaving the lumenal surface intact. A thoraco-abdominal approach is indicated for a tumour of the lower oesophagus or at the gastro-oesophageal junction (see page 5.10). A middle third tumour will necessitate a two-stage (Ivor Lewis) oesophagectomy with gastric replacement of the oesophagus; this is the subject of this chapter. For more proximal tumours a three-stage procedure with a cervical anastomosis will be needed. Blind oesophagectomy with abdominal gastric mobilization, blunt thoracic dissection without thoracotomy and cervical anastomosis may gain popularity in the future.

PREOPERATIVE ASSESSMENT
1. Confirm the diagnosis and the extent of disease using a barium swallow, oesophagoscopy and biopsy (see page 2.5), chest X-ray and CT scanning of chest and abdomen.
2. Correct dehydration and electrolyte abnormalities which result from the patient's dysphagia.
3. Explain to the patient that palliative intubation may be found to be more appropriate during the operation.
4. Arrange a visit to the intensive care unit.

RELEVANT ANATOMY
The oesophagus is 25–26cm long and extends from the cricopharyngeus muscle in the neck to the stomach just below the diaphragm. It has a muscular wall arranged in inner circular and outer longitudinal layers which are striated in the upper third and progressively become smooth muscle in the lower part. There is no serosa except around the short intra-abdominal segment.

As the oesophagus passes through the superior mediastinum it lies behind the left main bronchus and then in front of the aorta. It continues down through the posterior mediastinum on the vertebral bodies just to the left of the midline to pierce the diaphragm surrounded by sweeping fibres of the diaphragmatic crura. A short intra-abdominal segment leads to the stomach at the angle of His. Important relationships are to the thoracic duct and aorta on the left. On the right it is crossed by the azygos vein as it drains into the superior vena cava. On both sides the oesophagus is covered with parietal pleura in the thorax, and in the abdomen it is covered with peritoneum.

The vagus nerves reform from the oesophageal plexuses to accompany the oesophagus as it enters the abdomen.

The cervical oesophagus is supplied by the inferior thyroid arteries, the thoracic part by segmental branches from the aorta and the lower third and abdominal part from branches of the left gastric artery. Accompanying venous drainage permits a portal-systemic venous connection. Lymphatic drainage in the thorax is to the pre-aortic nodes and from the lower third it is to the coeliac nodes around the left gastric artery.

The gastric anatomy is covered on page 5.22.

OPERATION
This is a two-stage operation; an abdominal procedure followed by a thoracic procedure.

ABDOMINAL PROCEDURE
Preparation
The anaesthetized patient is placed supine and intubated and ventilated with a double-lumen endotracheal tube to allow selective deflation of the right lung later in the operation. A nasogastric tube is sited with its tip in the upper oesophagus. The skin of the abdomen is prepared and draped.

Incision
Make a short left subcostal incision (see the Introduction).

Operative technique
1. Perform a laparotomy through the incision. If extensive lymphatic (lesser curve and coeliac), local or metastatic (hepatic) spread precludes resection consider palliative intubation (see page 2.16). Otherwise extend the incision bilaterally and proceed to mobilize the stomach.

2. Divide the gastrocolic omentum taking care to preserve the gastro-epiploic arcade with the greater curve. Preserve the right gastro-epiploic artery, but divide the left gastro-epiploic artery. Separate the stomach from the spleen, dividing the short gastric vessels.

3. Divide the left triangular ligament of the liver and retract the left lobe of the liver to expose the lesser omentum and the hiatus (see page 5.4 in Nissen Fundoplication).

4. Divide the lesser omentum and free the gastro-oesophageal junction completely at the hiatus (see page 5.29 in Total Gastrectomy).

5. Retract the stomach in a cephalad direction, divide any adhesions within the lesser sac between the stomach and the

pancreas, and identify and divide the left gastric artery. This vessel should be oversewn with a non-absorbable suture (e.g. 4/0 Prolene) for security. Aberrant hepatic branches from the left gastric artery should be identified and preserved.

6. Free the stomach completely and ensure that the pylorus can be brought up to the hiatus without tension. Examine the stomach and ensure that its blood supply is adequate.

7. Perform a longitudinal pyloromyotomy (see page 5.10) to facilitate gastric emptying since the vagi have been divided.

Wound closure and dressing
Close the abdomen with monofilament nylon and interrupted skin sutures. Apply a dry dressing.

THORACIC PROCEDURE
Preparation
The patient is turned to the full lateral position with the right side uppermost and the skin prepared and draped as for a thoracotomy (see page 2.19).

Incision
Perform a right posterolateral thoracotomy above the sixth rib. The anaesthetist deflates the right lung.

Operative technique
1. Divide the pulmonary ligament and retract the lung anteriorly. Divide the azygos vein between ties (Fig. 2.16).

2. Open the pleura over the oesophagus and mobilize it with diathermy, ligating the larger segmental vessels to it from the aorta. Continue the mobilization to about 5 cm above the tumour. The blood supply is tenuous so do not over mobilize; resection occurs at the limit of your dissection. Now free the oesophagus down to the hiatus.

3. Draw the mobilized stomach into the chest through the hiatus and check that it is still well vascularized. Place a linear stapler across the upper stomach from the angle of His to a point on the lesser curvature that will give maximal clearance of the tumour and divide the stomach between the staples. Oversew the staple line (Fig. 2.17) taking care not to twist the stomach tube that has been created.

4. Draw the oesophageal segment to be resected out of the chest so as to expose the posterior wall of the disease-free oesophagus at the upper limit of the mobilization. Draw the stomach up to this point and place three interrupted non-absorbable sutures (e.g. 3/0 Prolene) between the oesophagus (muscular suture) and a point on the stomach about 2 cm from the apex of the gastric tube (seromuscular suture). These are left long and untied (Fig. 2.18).

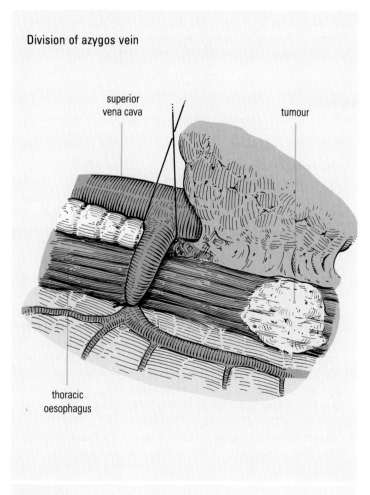

Division of azygos vein

superior vena cava

tumour

thoracic oesophagus

Fig. 2.16

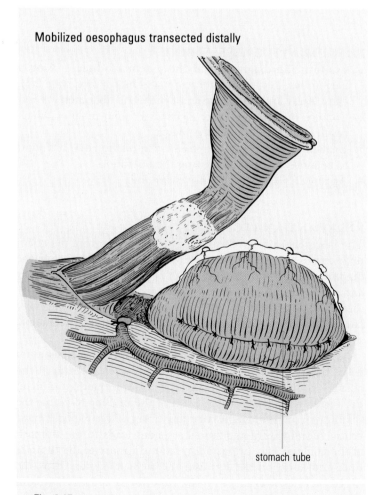

Mobilized oesophagus transected distally

stomach tube

Fig. 2.17

5. Incise the stomach (a 2.5 cm gastrotomy) just distal to these sutures and hemisect the oesophagus just above them; avoid soiling the thoracic cavity with gastric contents. Tie the sutures leaving the outer two as stays on the anastomosis.

6. Perform an all-layer anastomosis between the two segments of bowel with a continuous non-absorbable suture (e.g. 3/0

Prolene). Interrupting this at two or three points around the anastomosis will prevent narrowing as the suture is pulled up. It is important to get a good bite of the submucosa with each pass of the suture as this is the layer which gives the anastomosis strength. Complete the anterior layer of the anastomosis after fully transecting the oesophagus and removing the specimen. As the anastomosis is closed ask the anaesthetist to advance the nasogastric tube so it can be placed well down into the gastric remnant. Oversew the anastomosis with a series of interrupted non-absorbable (e.g. Prolene) musculo-seromuscular stitches to compliment the three placed earlier in the posterior layer (Fig. 2.19).

Wound closure and dressing

Place two chest drains, one basal and one apical, and close and dress the wound in the usual way after the anaesthetist has reinflated the lung (see page 2.21).

POSTOPERATIVE CARE

The patient, who is transferred to the intensive care unit and ventilated overnight, should be nursed at a 45° angle and the nasogastric tube aspirated hourly to reduce the likelihood of reflux. The intercostal drains are not placed on suction unless a persistent air space is detected on X-ray. The following day the patient is extubated and transferred to the ward if well. Allow drinking after 3 days and, if bowel sounds have returned, eating after a week provided there is no evidence of an anastomotic leak. The nasogastric tube is removed once free fluids are tolerated.

If an effusion is seen on the daily chest X-ray or if there is persistent fever with a significant leukocytosis suspect a leak and perform a meglumine diatrizoate (e.g. Gastrografin) swallow. Some leaks may be managed semi-conservatively with parenteral antibiotics and nutrition, drainage and keeping the patient nil-by-mouth. Others may require operative decortication of a thoracic empyema and repair.

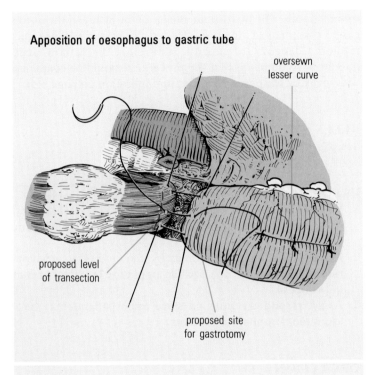

Apposition of oesophagus to gastric tube

overseen lesser curve

proposed level of transection

proposed site for gastrotomy

Fig. 2.18

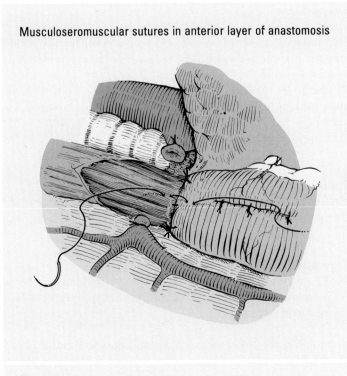

Musculoseromuscular sutures in anterior layer of anastomosis

Fig. 2.19

SPECIAL OPERATIVE HAZARDS

1. Inoperable tumour.
2. Damage to the spleen which may be treated with local repair, but splenectomy is usually safest.
3. Thoracic soiling with gastric contents.
4. Damage to the thoracic duct resulting in chylothorax.

COMPLICATIONS

1. Aspiration and pneumonitis can be reduced by ensuring the patient sleeps and is nursed at all times at 45°.
2. Anastomotic leakage, mediastinitis and empyema.
3. Anastomotic stricture. Early dysphagia is due to oedema or too small an anastomosis. Later symptoms can be due to an inflammatory stricture resulting from the reflux of bilious gastric contents into the oesophageal remnant or malignant recurrence. These are managed by endoscopic dilatation or palliative oesophageal intubation.
4. Delayed gastric emptying due to inadequate pyloromyotomy; formal pyloroplasty may be needed.
5. Chest infection which can be avoided with aggressive physiotherapy.
6. Post-thoracotomy pain.

Heller's Operation for Achalasia of the Oesophagus

Achalasia is characterized by progressive dilatation of the oesophagus above the lower segment which fails to relax. The physiological features are spasticity of the lower oesophageal sphincter, both at rest and during swallowing, and failure of the oesophageal contractions to be propulsive. As the oesophagus fills, food passes into the stomach either due to the effect of gravity or as the pressure of the unco-ordinated oesophageal contractions overcomes the spasm in the distal oesophagus. Reflux and overflow with bronchial aspiration can lead to pulmonary infection.

The smoothly tapered appearance of the oesophagus on barium swallow is distinctive but preoperative diagnostic studies are directed to excluding a physical obstruction. Oesophago-scopy is useful and it should be noted that a large bougie will pass with ease through the lower oesophagus. In addition, oesophageal manometry will demonstrate contractions within the oesophagus, but although they are of sizeable amplitude they do not result in peristalsis.

Treatment is aimed at disrupting the lower oesophageal sphincter either by hydrostatic dilatation or by myotomy of the gastro-oesophageal junction (Heller's operation). Since this myotomy destroys the intrinsic anti-reflux mechanism some operators recommend that the procedure should be combined with a gastric wrap (see Nissen's fundoplication on page 5.5).

RELEVANT ANATOMY
See page 2.11.

PREOPERATIVE ASSESSMENT
1. Exclude mechanical obstruction using barium swallow and endoscopy. A smoothly tapered oesophagus is characteristic on a barium swallow.
2. Demonstrate abnormal motility by manometry; in achalasia the contractions are of a sizeable amplitude but do not result in peristalsis.
3. Assess respiratory function since these patients may have aspirated oesophageal contents.

OPERATION
Thoracic or abdominal approaches are possible but surgery through the chest is described here.

Preparation
As with any oesophageal procedure assessment must be complete and a recent barium swallow should accompany the patient into the operating theatre. The surgeon performs preoperative oesophagoscopy.

The anaesthetist then inserts a double-lumen endobronchial tube so that the left lung may be deflated during surgery. The patient is firmly fixed in the full lateral position with the left side uppermost.

Incision
Perform a left posterolateral thoracotomy above the seventh rib (see page 2.19).

Operative technique
1. The anaesthetist deflates the left lung. Divide the inferior pulmonary ligament and ask the assistant to retract the lung upwards.

2. Mobilize the lower oesophagus and gastric fundus as described for a transthoracic Nissen's fundoplication, taking care to minimize disruption of the hiatus and the vagus nerves which should be preserved (see page 5.4).

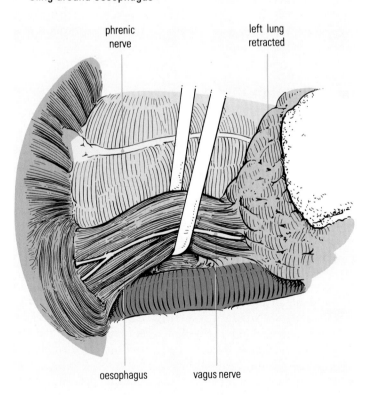

Sling around oesophagus

phrenic nerve

left lung retracted

oesophagus   vagus nerve

Fig. 2.20

3. With a sling around the oesophagus (Fig. 2.20), support the lower segment of the oesophagus and the proximal stomach over the fingers of the left hand. Divide the muscle of the lower 5 cm of the oesophagus longitudinally with careful strokes of a scalpel, gradually deepening the incision through the muscle until the mucosa pouts through (as in a Ramstedt's operation) (Fig. 2.21). Extend the myotomy down onto the stomach. Care must be taken to divide all strands of muscle over the mucosa and this clearance is completed by sweeping the muscle coat laterally on either side.

4. Carefully examine the mucosa for holes and repair any that are seen with a fine suture.

5. Perform a Nissen-style gastric fundoplication if it is believed that interference with the hiatus will result in gastro-oesophageal reflux (see page 5.4).

Wound closure and dressing
Insert a single chest drain, reinflate the lung and close the chest (see page 2.21). Apply a dry dressing to the wound.

POSTOPERATIVE CARE
A nasogastric tube is not used and the patient is allowed to drink and then eat as soon as bowel sounds are heard. The drain is removed on the first postoperative day provided that there is no air leak.

Performing cardiomyotomy

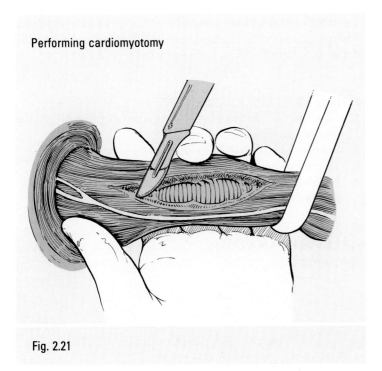

Fig. 2.21

SPECIAL OPERATIVE HAZARDS
1. Perforation of the mucosa, which leads to mediastinitis if it is not recognized and repaired.
2. Incomplete myotomy.
3. Air leak as a result of damage to the left lung.
4. Damage to the vagus nerves leading to failure of gastric emptying.

COMPLICATIONS
1. Oesophageal reflux sometimes results.
2. Late development of malignancy.

Although intra-oesophageal tubes can be used for brief periods to stent benign strictures their main use is for palliation of oesophageal cancer and it is in this context that they will be discussed here.

Oesophageal tumours are generally aggressive and at the time of diagnosis have usually spread not only through the oesophageal wall but also into regional lymphatics. This does not preclude resection of the tumour but does mean that cure in these cases is a rare result and oesophagectomy might be viewed as a palliative procedure in itself.

If the tumour cannot be resected and symptoms of dysphagia are severe then palliation may be achieved by oesophageal intubation. However, this alternative to oesophagectomy should not be undertaken lightly since although intubation is easy and relatively safe and resection is unlikely to improve life expectancy there is no doubt that quality of life after oesophagectomy is superior to that with an oesophageal tube, the acceptability of oesophageal intubation being limited by the need to eat near liquid food and frequent obstructions within the tube.

Various types of tube exist but they can be divided into two categories; those which are pushed into place endoscopically, such as the Atkinson tube, and those which are pulled into place operatively such as the Mousseau–Barbin or some types of Celestin tube. Operatively placed tubes are probably easier to seat satisfactorily within a tumour but do require an anaesthetic. The placement of a Celestin tube is described here and this device is pictured with its introducer in Fig. 2.22.

PREOPERATIVE ASSESSMENT
1. Confirm the presence of the tumour using radiography, oesophagoscopy and biopsy.
2. Confirm unresectability on scans or at laparotomy.
3. Ascertain whether the symptoms warrant palliation.
4. Ascertain during oesophagoscopy that the tumour is physically able to accept and retain a tube.

RELEVANT ANATOMY
See page 2.11.

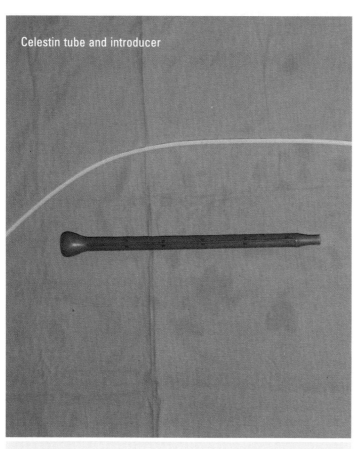

Celestin tube and introducer

Fig. 2.22

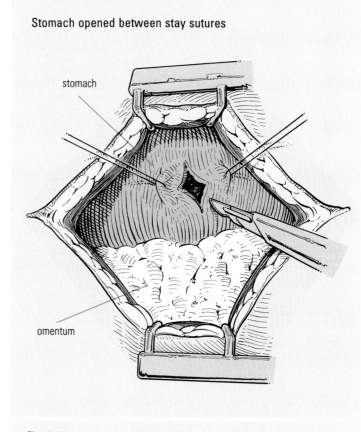

Stomach opened between stay sutures

stomach

omentum

Fig. 2.23

OPERATION
Preparation
Display the barium swallow, perform a rigid oesophagoscopy on the anaesthetized patient to assess how easy it will be to pass a tube across and seat it on the tumour, and select the size of tube that will be used. Then place the patient supine on the operating table and prepare and drape the abdomen.

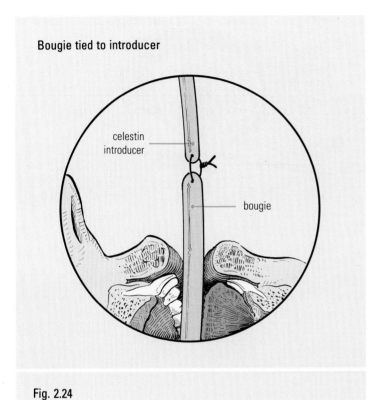

Bougie tied to introducer

celestin introducer

bougie

Fig. 2.24

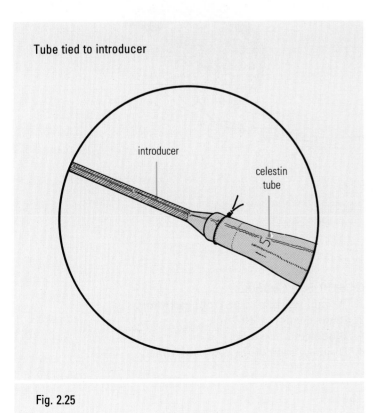

Tube tied to introducer

introducer

celestin tube

Fig. 2.25

Incision
Open the abdomen through a left subcostal incision unless the costal angle is small in which case a left paramedian incision is used.

Operative technique
1. Examine the abdominal contents paying particular attention to the direct invasion of the tumour into adjacent structures, lymphatic spread especially to coeliac nodes, and liver metastases. If the tumour is resectable, extend the incision and proceed to mobilize the stomach as described elsewhere (on page 5.11).

2. If it is decided that palliative intubation is appropriate make a small gastrotomy between two stay sutures and stop any bleeding (Fig. 2.23).

3. Feel inside the stomach with a finger and identify the lumen of the gastro-oesophageal junction. Pass a lubricated gum elastic bougie up through the stricture, ensuring that the tumour is not perforated. The anaesthetist grasps the end of the bougie in the pharynx with a pair of Magill forceps.

4. The anaesthetist ties the end of the Celestin introducer to his end of the bougie (Fig. 2.24). Meanwhile the surgeon inserts the other end of the introducer into a Celestin tube and places a strong tie around it (Fig. 2.25).

5. Now simply draw first the bougie, then the introducer, and finally the Celestin tube into the mouth, pharynx and oeso-phagus (Fig. 2.26). Firm resistance is felt as the funnelled end of the tube passes through the cricopharyngeus muscle; do not be deceived into thinking this is the tumour.

6. Seat the tube well down onto the tumour and confirm that you cannot pull it through.

7. Cut the tube off so that its distal end can return into the stomach (Fig. 2.27), and fix the tube in place within the stomach with a suture.

8. Close the gastrotomy in two layers with a non-absorbable suture (e.g. 3/0 Prolene).

9. If a lumen cannot be found through the tumour it may be appropriate to create a feeding jejunostomy.

Wound closure and dressing
Close the abdominal incision in layers and apply a dry dressing.

POSTOPERATIVE CARE
The patient is started on fluids when bowel sounds are heard and this progresses to a semi-liquid diet over the next few days. Fizzy drinks such as soda water are used to clear the tube of any food blockages. Should such a blockage persist the tube may be cleared with slow sips of dilute hydrogen peroxide.

The patient and his family should be advised and instructed in food preparation by a dietician and on the inoperable nature of the tumour by the surgeon, as he feels appropriate.

Introduction of tube

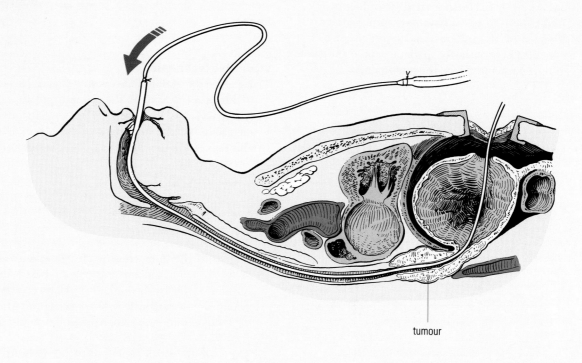

tumour

Fig. 2.26

Tube in place

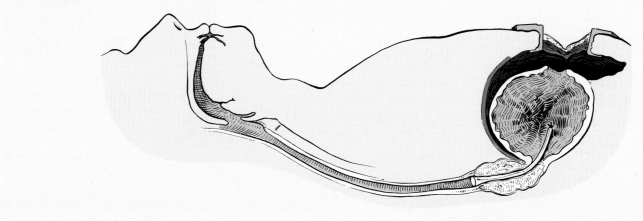

Fig. 2.27

SPECIAL OPERATIVE HAZARDS
1. Perforation of the tumour with resultant mediastinitis.
2. Failure to find a lumen.

COMPLICATIONS
1. Wound sepsis/leakage from gastrotomy.
2. Regurgitation of the tube.
3. Blockage of the tube.
4. Disintegration of the tube with time.

Posterolateral Thoracotomy

Whilst there are many approaches to the thoracic structures, the two most useful incisions are the posterolateral thoracotomy, which exposes the lungs, oesophagus and the thoracic aorta on the left, and the midline sternotomy giving access to the anterior mediastinum and the pericardium (see page 2.28). An anterior thoracotomy is valuable for limited intrathoracic procedures, for example lung biopsy or pericardial fenestration, and an anterior mediastinotomy in conjunction with mediastinoscopy can yield valuable information in the diagnosis of mediastinal tumours and the staging of thoracic disease.

RELEVANT ANATOMY

To perform a posterolateral thoracotomy, muscles must be divided and this makes the incision a relatively painful one. The morphological outer layer of the body musculature is adapted around the chest to form those muscles which attach the upper limb girdle to the thorax. The middle layer forms the intercostal muscles and the inner one makes up an incomplete lining to the thoracic cavity.

When performing a posterolateral thoracotomy, the latissimus dorsi muscle and a small part of the trapezius muscle posteriorly are encountered and have to be divided. Deep to these is the serratus anterior muscle at the front end of the incision. This muscle is continued posteriorly as the thoracolumbar fascia which when opened reveals the ribs beneath. Sometimes it is necessary to divide part of the serratus anterior muscle to improve access in the chest. This should be done as far inferiorly as possible to avoid damage to the muscle's nerve supply, the long thoracic nerve, and producing a 'wing scapula'.

The intercostal muscles are easily stripped from the adjacent rib; separating them from the upper surface of a rib protects the neurovascular intercostal bundle. It is not necessary to resect ribs but access is greatly improved if the posterior segment of the rib below the chosen space is excised. The part beneath the erector spinae muscle, which runs longitudinally over the posterior aspect of the ribs, is selected. It is important not to divide this muscle as this may lead to the later development of a scoliosis.

Figure 2.28 shows the anatomy seen during posterolateral

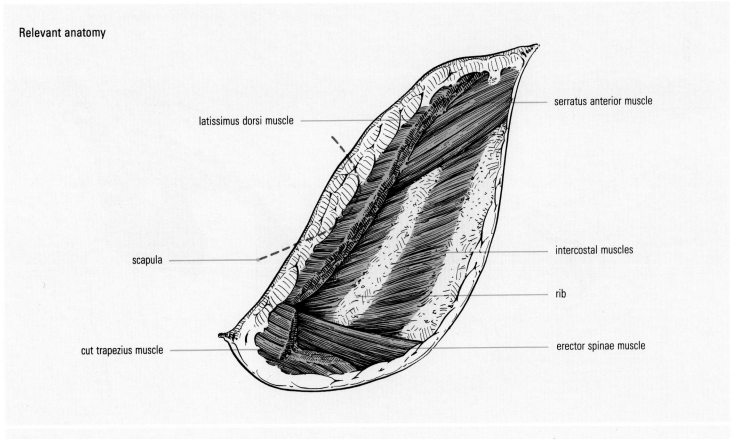

Relevant anatomy

latissimus dorsi muscle

serratus anterior muscle

scapula

intercostal muscles

rib

cut trapezius muscle

erector spinae muscle

Fig. 2.28

thoracotomy. The pleura lies immediately beneath the intercostal muscles and is usually thin enough to be opened with a finger, but if not, it is opened by a small cut with a scalpel. This allows the compliant lung to fall away from the chest wall.

The intercostal space that is opened is chosen according to the procedure to be carried out: the fifth rib approximately overlies the oblique fissure on each side and therefore a thoracotomy is performed above the fifth rib for an upper lobectomy, and above the sixth rib for either a lower lobectomy, a pneumonectomy or a middle lobectomy on the right; access to the lower oesophagus is above the seventh rib on the left and the anastomosis in an Ivor Lewis oesophagectomy at the level of the azygos vein is performed from above the sixth rib on the right; aortic arch surgery can be attempted from above the fourth rib on the left; and a thoracic incision can be extended across the cartilage of the costal margin and down into the diaphragm as a thoraco-abdominal incision to give access to the abdomen.

OPERATION
Preparation
To ensure that the operation is performed on the correct side, display a chest radiograph. The patient is anaesthetized and an appropriate double-lumen endobronchial tube is inserted to allow deflation of the lung on the side to be operated upon.

Place the patient in a full lateral position and fix him firmly there with the arm supported as shown in Fig. 2.29. Prepare the skin and drape the patient so that the landmarks shown in Fig. 2.28 are easily palpable. Stand at the patient's back.

Procedure
1. Commence the incision posteriorly, midway between the spinous processes of the vertebrae and the medial border of the scapula, and extend it forwards in the line of the ribs two to three finger breadths below the tip of the scapula. Carry this line anteriorly with a slight inferior curve as far as needed to give adequate exposure (Fig. 2.29).

2. With a blend of cutting and coagulation diathermy, deepen the incision through fat and fascia until the latissimus dorsi muscle is reached.

3. Cut through the muscle posteriorly, insert the index finger of your left hand beneath it and progress anteriorly with cutting diathermy, taking care not to damage the serratus anterior muscle which lies immediately deep to latissimus dorsi (Fig. 2.30). At the posterior end of the incision it may be necessary to incise a few centimetres of the trapezius muscle.

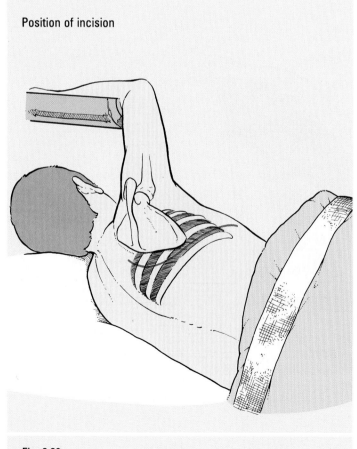

Position of incision

Fig. 2.29

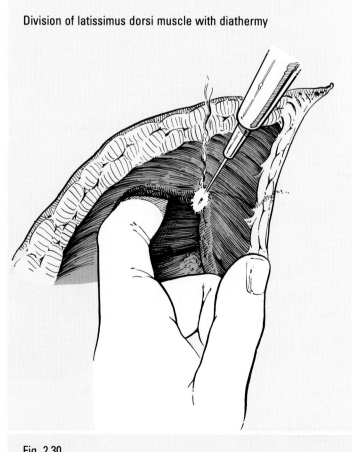

Division of latissimus dorsi muscle with diathermy

Fig. 2.30

4. Cut through the fascia thus exposed posteriorly and extend this cut along the inferior border of the serratus anterior muscle. If it is necessary to divide any of this muscle anteriorly, do so as low as possible.

5. Sweep a hand under the scapula and insert a scapula retractor here to lift the bone away from the chest wall.

6. Identify the chosen rib by counting down from the top; the highest rib which can be felt is the second rib (the first rib can be palpated only with great difficulty and is a flat structure lying within the concavity of the second rib).

7. Using diathermy, cut the periosteum along the superior margin of the selected rib and clear the erector spinae muscle from its posterior end, but do not divide it. Use a rugine to strip the periosteum from the upper border of the rib as far forward as possible beneath the incision (Fig. 2.31). Clear the complete circumference of the rib at its posterior end.

8. Use rib shears (costatome) to excise a segment of rib at the point cleared (Fig. 2.32). The intercostal bundle should be unharmed.

9. Complete the division of the intercostal muscles, which was commenced with the rugine where the periosteum was stripped, using diathermy, and open the pleura with the finger and scalpel, allowing the lung to fall away. The anaesthetist can now deflate the lung.

10. Place towels over the edges of the wound, insert a retractor and then proceed with the operation.

Wound closure and dressing

1. The principles of thoracic drains are discussed on page 8.7 in chest drainage and management of chest trauma. Drains are usually brought out of the chest in the midaxillary line through the lowermost available intercostal space and connected to an underwater seal bottle. They should be sited so that the patient will not kink them when lying in bed. Tie the drains in place and leave an untied mattress suture to close the incision when the drains are removed.

2. Following the intrathoracic surgery, the anaesthetist should reinflate the lung.

3. A simple and effective way to reapproximate the ribs is to place interrupted, heavy-braided nylon sutures (size 5) around the rib above and the rib below (pericostal), and tie

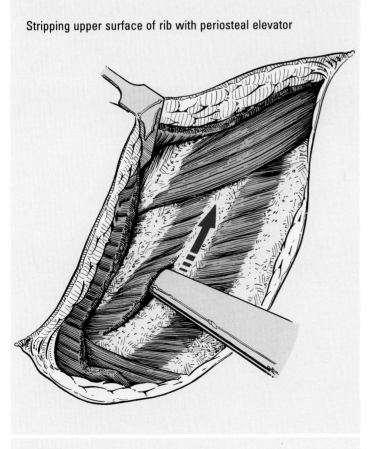

Stripping upper surface of rib with periosteal elevator

Fig. 2.31

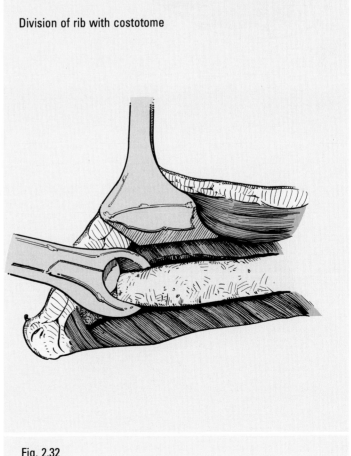

Division of rib with costotome

Fig. 2.32

them in turn to draw the ribs to their normal anatomical position (Fig. 2.33); do not overtighten these sutures. Draw the intercostal bundle out from between the ribs.

Closure with pericostal sutures

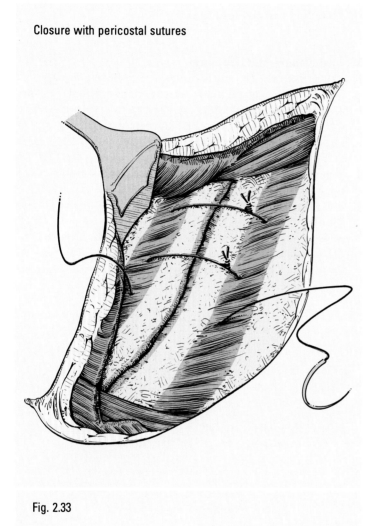

Fig. 2.33

4. Now close the muscles in two layers, fascia and serratus followed by latissimus dorsi and trapezius, with a non-absorbable material. Take care to line the muscles up accurately at this stage and do not bunch the latissimus dorsi muscle as this will lead to an unsightly result.
5. Use an absorbable suture, such as Vicryl, to close first the fascia and then the skin with a subcuticular stitch.
6. Apply a dry gauze dressing to the wound.

POSTOPERATIVE CARE
On return of the patient to the ward, arrange for a chest radiograph to be taken to check that the lung has expanded fully. The timing of drain removal is discussed on page 8.8 in chest drainage and management of chest trauma. Mobilization is limited by the need for suction.

Analgesia is important to allow satisfactory chest physiotherapy and intravenous papaveretum (Omnopon) infusion, intercostal nerve blocks and transcutaneous nerve stimulation may be used. Insertion of a minitracheotomy tube may be of help in patients who are unable to clear their secretions effectively.

Prophylaxis against deep venous thrombosis is routine; subcutaneous heparin is started on admission to hospital and pneumatic calf stimulators peroperatively may be used.

SPECIAL OPERATIVE HAZARDS
1. Damage to the underlying lung. This is particularly a hazard in the presence of pleural adhesions.
2. Damage to the intercostal neurovascular bundle.
3. Incorrect placement of drains which can lead to incomplete expansion of the lung and surgical emphysema.

COMPLICATIONS
1. Wound infection.
2. Haematoma or empyema formation.
3. Postoperative pneumonia.
4. Long-term post-thoracotomy pain.

Principles of Lung Resection

Lung resection is indicated for tumours, some cases of chronic sepsis, and expanding destructive lesions such as bullous disease too extensive to be treated by bullectomy. The extent of resection extends from segmentectomy through lobectomy to pneumonectomy. Open lung biopsy is also possible, as are the endobronchial removal of tumour confined to the mucosa of a larger airway and the 'shelling out' of benign tumours. This chapter will confine itself to the principles of lobectomy and pneumonectomy.

PREOPERATIVE ASSESSMENT

1. Identify the cell type by open or endoscopic biopsy, endoscopic brushing or sputum cytology. Patients with small cell tumours do not benefit from resection.
2. Determine the extent of disease and operability using a chest X-ray, thoracic CT and a liver scan or CT. It should be borne in mind that lymphatic involvement does not always preclude resection (nodes can be cleared along with the resected lung), a proximal tumour at the hilum may be resectable by an intrapericardial pneumonectomy, and chest wall invasion may be resected along with lung tissue.
3. Complete the staging of the tumour where it is required by mediastinoscopy (see page 2.9) and anterior mediastinotomy.
4. Assess lung function formally to determine fitness for a pneumonectomy. The decision whether to perform a lobectomy or pneumonectomy is often taken during the operation.
5. Consider preoperative physiotherapy, antibiotics, bronchodilators and postural drainage in selected patients with chronic lung disease.

RELEVANT ANATOMY

A complete knowledge of the lobar and segmental anatomy of the lung is vital if resections are to be performed safely; the vascular anatomy can be very variable. Each lung is divided into lobes; the upper and lower on the left and the upper, lower and middle on the right. Each lobe and the segments into which it is divided and serviced by a vein (oxygenated blood), an artery (deoxygenated blood) and a bronchus (airway).

Whilst a knowledge of the surface anatomy of the lobes is useful when examining a patient, it should be realized that it is the position of the hilar structures of each lobe that determines the incisions used for lung resections. Each lung is invested in visceral pleura which exists as a loose sleeve inferiorly around the hilum (the pulmonary ligament). Division of this in any resection is a great help as it improves the mobility of the lung (access is always limited through a thoracotomy).

On each side the bronchus lies posteriorly in the upper part of the hilum. The pulmonary artery, a thin-walled and fragile structure, is anterior to the bronchus and the superior and inferior pulmonary veins are more caudally situated. As the bronchus passes into the lung it divides into lobar branches and these in turn produce segmental branches (see page 2.7). The pulmonary arteries give rise to branches which carry blood to the alveoli and correspond to the bronchial divisions (the bronchi themselves have a systemic supply from the aorta). The pulmonary veins carrying oxygenated blood back to the heart travel separately and tend to run between the segments. They terminate as two large pulmonary veins at each hilum; the superior from the upper lobe on the left and upper and middle lobes on the right, and the inferior from the lower lobes on each side.

The phrenic nerves are clearly seen on each side on the mediastinal pleura running to the diaphragm anterior to each hilum. On the right side the azygos vein arches over the hilum into the superior vena cava; it may be divided to improve access in a right pneumonectomy.

OPERATION

Preparation

Perform preoperative bronchoscopy. The anaesthetized patient is then placed in the lateral position and intubated with a double-lumen endotracheal tube in such a way that the side to be operated can be selectively isolated and deflated. If a pneumonectomy is to be performed it is important to use a tube which does not enter or hook onto the bronchus on the operative side.

Incision

Access is via a posterolateral thoracotomy (see page 2.19). The upper lobe is best approached from above the fifth rib; other lobectomies and pneumonectomies are performed through a thoracotomy above the sixth rib.

Operative technique

1. Upon opening the chest, complete the assessment of the extent of the tumour and its operability; do not commit yourself to resection by dividing a vital structure until you are sure the operation is feasible. Check for nodal involvement and, with proximal tumours, feel for invasion of the malignancy along the pulmonary vessels into the heart. Feel the lung tissue for other tumours.

2. Divide the pulmonary ligament and any adhesions between parietal and visceral pleura with diathermy.

3. Open the pleura at the hilum, mobilize the vessels and bronchus to the whole lung and display the structures which will require division during the proposed resection. Use a mixture of sharp and blunt dissection; small vascular branches should be ligated. Ensure that the proposed resection will not compromise the structures to the lobes that will be

left (there may be anomalous vessels). Normally when performing a pneumonectomy the lobar structures are divided outside the pericardium, although tumour clearance can be improved by dividing the vessels within the pericardium (Fig. 2.34).

4. If a lobectomy is to be performed the lobe is separated by sharp dissection along the fissure. Work towards the hilum and coagulate interlobar vessels with diathermy, taking care not to damage the major vessels as you complete this dissection.

5. Divide the vessels and then the bronchus and remove the resected specimen.

6. Either divide the pulmonary veins and arteries between ligatures and then oversew their stumps with a non-absorbable suture (e.g. 4/0 Prolene), or clamp the vessels and close them with an anchored non-absorbable suture (e.g. 4/0 Prolene) (Fig. 2.35).

7. Perform the bronchial resection flush with its carina so as not to leave a sump in which infected sputum may rest as this may later precipitate a bronchopleural fistula. Clamp the bronchus flush and divide it along the clamp with a knife.

Anchored tie

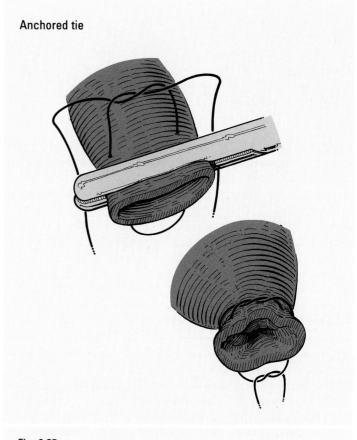

Fig. 2.35

Left intrapericardial pneumonectomy

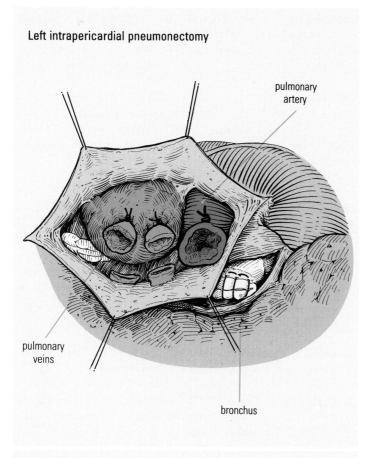

pulmonary artery

pulmonary veins

bronchus

Fig. 2.34

Closure of bronchus

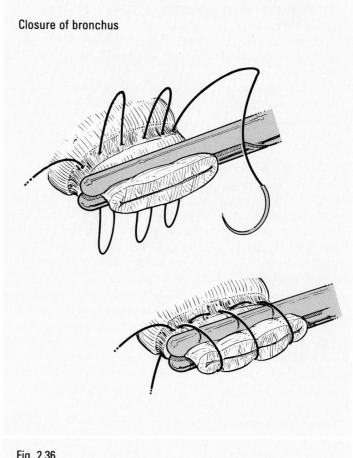

Fig. 2.36

The bronchial closure must be airtight, so a non-absorbable suture (e.g. 3/0 Prolene) is run under the clamp as a machine stitch and then back over-and-over the clamp so that both tails emerge from the same end of the closure (Fig. 2.36). The clamp is now drawn out from the other end as the suture is drawn tight. An alternative is to use a linear stapling device to close the bronchus. Place enough warm water in the chest to cover the stump and ask the anaesthetist to inflate to a pressure of at least 40cm of water. Look for escaping air. Any leak must be repaired.

8. Use the same technique to detect any major air leaks from a remaining lobe; a carefully placed suture with a non-absorbable material (e.g. 4/0 Prolene) will stop most of these.

9. Resect or sample mediastinal lymph nodes. Check haemostasis is complete.

Wound closure and dressing
Insert two intercostal drains after a lobectomy and a single drain after a pneumonectomy and close the chest (see page 2.21). All drains are connected to an underwater seal bottle. Drains are placed on suction following a lobectomy, but are clamped and intermittently released after a pneumonectomy. Apply a dry dressing.

POSTOPERATIVE CARE
Lobectomy drains are placed on 13kPa wall suction. This maintains the lobes in an inflated state and indeed after a day or two the lobectomy space will have disappeared. Drains are not removed until any air leak has ceased and the lung remains inflated. It is important to X-ray the chest regularly including immediately after surgery.

The drain placed in a pneumonectomy space is kept clamped to decrease mediastinal shift as the remaining lung moves the mediastinum across with ventilation. It is unclamped briefly every hour to allow blood to drain; there should of course be no air leak after this operation. This drain is removed when blood loss has stopped, usually on the first postoperative day.

Following a pneumonectomy patients are nursed and instructed to sleep on the side that was operated on so that in the event of a bronchopleural fistula forming they will be less likely to aspirate their space fluid through the bronchial stump into the remaining lung.

Analgesia (a continuous narcotic infusion and indomethacin suppositories) and aggressive physiotherapy with postural drainage are important in preventing chest infection. If the patient has inadequate clearance of sputum place a minitracheotomy tube (see page 1.31).

SPECIAL OPERATIVE HAZARDS
1. Haemorrhage from large pulmonary vessels especially the fragile pulmonary artery.
2. Failure to recognize the anatomy which may result in devascularization of a remaining lobe.
3. Pulmonary vessel slipping out of clamp and retracting inside the pericardium, in which case open the pericardium and control haemorrhage by placing fingers around the hilum within the pericardium.
4. Inoperability due to proximal involvement of the heart.
5. Inadequate closure of the bronchus resulting in immediate bronchopleural fistula and pleural soiling with bronchial contents.

COMPLICATIONS
1. Secondary haemorrhage at about 7 days after surgery.
2. Wound infection. Space infection will result in empyema requiring drainage and decortication.
3. Chest infection, in which case bronchoscopy can be employed to remove plugs of sputum.
4. Bronchopleural fistula after pneumonectomy. If it occurs soon after the operation it is probably due to poor technique, but later it may result from stump infection or malignant recurrence. The emergency treatment of this condition is to lie the patient on the operated side and institute intercostal drainage to prevent aspiration of space fluid through the fistula and soiling of the remaining lung with resultant pneumonitis. The relative merits of repair or chronic drainage may then be considered.
5. Persistent air leak after lobectomy. If the lung is kept inflated it will eventually adhere to the chest wall at which time suction may be stopped thus reducing the leak. Most leaks stop eventually; very few require re-exploration.
6. Persistent post-thoracotomy pain.
7. Herniation of the heart following intrapericardial pneumonectomy is prevented by repairing the pericardial sac with pleura or a patch of synthetic material.
8. Excessive mediastinal shift after pneumonectomy may necessitate instillation of air into the pneumonectomy space to correct the shift.

Management of Pneumothorax

Spontaneous pneumothorax usually results from the rupture of a bullus on the surface of the lung. Often these bullae are small and solitary, and are usually of no significance in relatively young patients. Sometimes, however, especially in the elderly, there is diffuse disease of the lungs.

Many pneumothoraces can be successfully managed with tube drainage, the lung being held expanded against the chest wall until it sticks there and the air leak stops. The insertion and management of intercostal drains is described on page 8.8. However, if there is diffuse lung disease or a large air leak, the pneumothorax may become persistent and occasionally infection may supervene to create an empyema. In these cases, and where there are recurrent or have been bilateral pneumothoraces, surgery is indicated.

The aims of surgery are: to identify the source of the air leak and close it; to allow the lung to fully expand to fill the thoracic cavity; to keep the lung expanded with well-placed drains on suction; to encourage the lung to stick to the chest wall either by irritating the parietal pleura with vigorous swab abrasion (a pleuradesis) or by removing the parietal pleura to strip the wall (a pleurectomy). Pleurectomy is the procedure of choice. The introduction of talc or tetracycline into chest drains to create physical or chemical pleuradesis is unreliable.

If the pneumothorax space becomes infected, an empyema will form and in such circumstances a thick rind will compress the lung beneath. This must be stripped away painstakingly (a decortication) with a combination of sharp and blunt dissection to allow the lung to expand. This is a time-consuming procedure which may involve considerable blood loss.

PREOPERATIVE ASSESSMENT
1. Through the history, examination, and investigation (i.e. X-ray), assess for persistent pneumothorax despite tube drainage, recurrent pneumothorax or metachronous bilateral pneumothoraces.
2. Check for early empyema.
3. Consider the possibility of diffuse lung disease, which would make surgery very difficult.

RELEVANT ANATOMY
The inner surface of the chest wall is lined with a thin sheet of pleura (parietal pleura). The lung is invaginated in this tissue so that the pleura also covers its surface (visceral pleura); the two pleura are continuous at the hilum of the lung. The lung and chest wall are therefore separated by two serous surfaces lubricated by a small amount of pleural fluid and the lung can thus move freely over the inner surface of the chest wall. Movement is also facilitated by a loose sleeve of pleura below the hilum of the lung (the pulmonary ligament) which also permits expansion of the pulmonary vessels.

If air enters the pleural space from outside the chest wall or from within the lung from a ruptured bullus (the result of

dilatation of the alveoli ducts and spaces) the lung is free to drop away from the chest wall since no adhesion is present between the two layers of the pleura. The resulting air space is a pneumothorax. If air continues to enter this space and cannot escape (e.g. if a ruptured bullus acts as a valve allowing air to escape from the lung during inspiration and closing during expiration) the pressure in the space will increase and eventually lead to a shift of the mediastinum (a tension pneumothorax). This is a potentially fatal complication of pneumothorax requiring immediate intercostal drainage.

OPERATION
Preparation
Cross-match two units of blood, or six units if decortication of an empyema is anticipated. The patient is then anaesthetized and a double-lumen endobronchial tube inserted so that the lung on the side to be operated can be deflated. Prophylactic antibiotics are given (e.g. benzyl penicillin and flucloxacillin) and a chest radiograph is displayed.

The patient is positioned and the skin prepared and draped for a posterolateral thoracotomy as described on page 2.20. If there is a chest drain *in situ*, do not remove it as this may lead to a tension pneumothorax. However the drain's tie is divided so that it can later be withdrawn from beneath the drapes once the chest has been opened.

Incision
Perform a posterolateral thoracotomy (see page 2.20) above the fifth or sixth rib but do not open the pleura.

Operative technique
1. Begin by stripping the pleura from the chest wall, working away from the incision in all directions; use fingers or a 'swab on a stick' in a rolling fashion to do this (see Fig. 2.37). Care should be taken at the apex where the subclavian vessels are at risk and inferiorly where the pleura passes over the diaphragm. Ensure that the mediastinum is left undisturbed. It should be noted that the pleura will be adherent where chest drains have been placed.

2. When as much of the pleura as possible has been stripped away from the chest wall it should be opened. The anaesthetist should deflate the lung and any adhesions in the pleural space can then be divided with scissors. Excise the pleural sheets as completely as possible and send them for histological examination.

3. Abrade any remaining parietal pleura with a swab.

4. Examine the lung to find the source of the air leak; bullae

are usually found either at the apex of the lung or along the margins of the interlobar fissures. It is usually adequate to ligate them with strong non-absorbable ties at their base (Fig. 2.38), but some may need to be stapled using 3.5mm staples (see inset to Fig. 2.38).

5. To ensure that the lung is airtight pour warm water into the chest and ask the anaesthetist to hand inflate the lung to a pressure of 40mmHg or more; any leak is revealed by gas bubbles escaping from the lung.

6. Check the chest wall to make sure there is no bleeding. A dental mirror and ball diathermy are helpful for this.

7. Insert an apical and possibly a basal drain if excessive bleeding or an air leak with a basal source is present. The anaesthetist is asked to reinflate the lung.

Wound closure and dressing
The wound is closed as described on page 2.21 and a gauze dressing is applied for the first 24 hours.

POSTOPERATIVE CARE
Chest drains are connected to an underwater seal (see page 8.7) and are placed on 13kPa of suction from a wall unit to maintain expansion of the lung against the chest wall. Drains are left in place until blood loss (if any) has stopped and the cessation of an air leak; typically, they are removed after 2–3 days. Maintained lung expansion is monitored with daily chest X-rays.

Prophylactic antibiotics continue for 48 hours and postoperative chest infection is prevented with regular physiotherapy and analgesia (the wound is a painful one so a continuous Omnopon infusion is appropriate for the first 48 hours). A postoperative hospital stay of 5 days is typical in uncomplicated young patients, though elderly patients with diffuse bullous disease may be in hospital for many weeks with protracted air leaks and other complications.

SPECIAL OPERATIVE HAZARDS
1. Damage to intrathoracic vessels and nerves.
2. Damage to diffusely diseased lung.
3. Bleeding from chest wall.

COMPLICATIONS
1. Infection and empyema requires treatment with prophylactic antibiotics and drainage/decortication.
2. Persistent air leak.

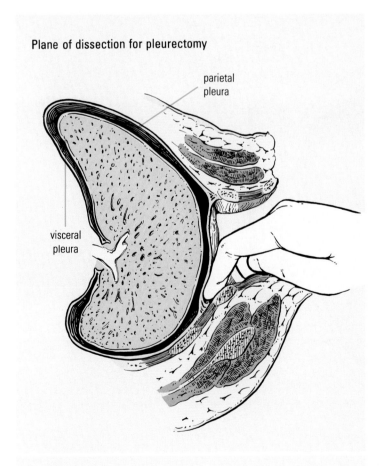

Plane of dissection for pleurectomy

parietal pleura

visceral pleura

Fig. 2.37

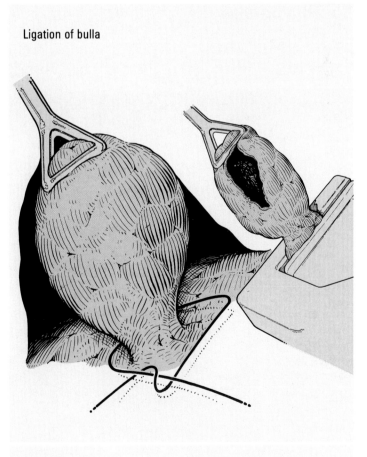

Ligation of bulla

Fig. 2.38

Median Sternotomy

Median sternotomy provides access to all the structures within the anterior mediastinum and those which can extend there from the neck, such as a retrosternal goitre. It is also used as a standard exposure of the pericardium for cardiac surgery.

RELEVANT ANATOMY

Division of the sternum in the midline is a simple procedure with minimal disruption of soft tissues, thus making it relatively free from pain. The bone is covered only by fat and a few pectoral fibres. Cranially, the suprasternal ligament passes from one sternoclavicular joint to the other, and caudally the rectus abdominis muscles, separated in the midline by the linea alba, insert into the thoracic cage. A median sternotomy is facilitated by separation of these muscles for a few centimetres below the xiphisternum.

Immediately deep to the sternum lies a condensation of fascia and fat, and behind this lies the thymus superiorly and the pericardium inferiorly (Fig. 2.39). The latter passes up behind the thymus superiorly. In adults, the thymus is usually atrophic but it still remains relatively vascular with many veins draining into the innominate vein which it surrounds.

The pleurae overlap the pericardium anteriorly and often meet in the midline where they can be easily damaged during splitting of the sternum. If the pericardium is opened, all parts of the heart can be reached and dissection may be carried along the aorta to the great vessels as they leave the chest.

OPERATION
Preparation

The operation is performed with the patient in a supine position, under a general anaesthesia, and with all the appropriate monitoring lines in position; these may include the right atrial

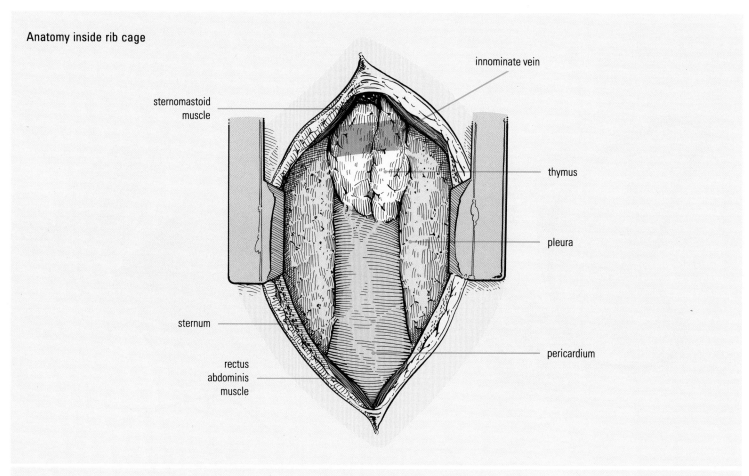

Anatomy inside rib cage

sternomastoid muscle

innominate vein

thymus

pleura

sternum

pericardium

rectus abdominis muscle

Fig. 2.39

and systemic arterial lines, the transfusion lines and a urinary catheter. For cardiac procedures an area of skin from chin to midthigh is prepared and draped. This allows good access to the chest and also permits femoral cannulation if needed. The legs may also be prepared for long saphenous vein harvesting if coronary artery bypass surgery is to be undertaken.

Procedure

1. Stand on the right of the patient and make a midline incision from 1 cm below the suprasternal notch to approximately 6 cm below the xiphisternum (Fig. 2.40). The incision is longer in an obese patient.

2. Using a blend of cutting and coagulation diathermy deepen the incision through fat and fascia onto the sternum, dividing any pectoralis fibres which overlie it.

3. Divide the suprasternal ligament, taking care not to damage the innominate vein. Any bleeding from this area should be controlled with a swab and stopped once the sternum has been opened.

4. Open the linea alba for a few centimetres and divide the xiphisternum with either diathermy or scissors, taking care not to cut into the pericardial cavity.

5. Using the index finger of your right hand, sweep beneath the body of the sternum to free the tissue from its posterior aspect, displacing the pleurae as this is done (Fig. 2.41).

6. Cut the sternum from below with an air-driven vertical saw with a guarded tip, taking care to keep the tip of the saw in contact with the posterior surface of the sternum (Fig. 2.42). Ensure the cut runs up the midline and that the anaesthetist has disconnected the ventilator at this point so that the lungs retreat laterally making it less likely that the pleurae will be opened inadvertently. If this is a repeat operation, an oscillating saw is used as it is less likely to damage underlying structures (the right ventricle is often firmly attached to the sternum).

7. Apply bone wax to the marrow and use diathermy on the cut edges of the periosteum.

8. If cardiopulmonary bypass is intended, this is a good moment to fully heparinize the patient. However, if an internal mammary artery is to be harvested, wait until it has been mobilized.

9. Place folded packs over both edges of the sternum and insert, and slowly open, a retractor.

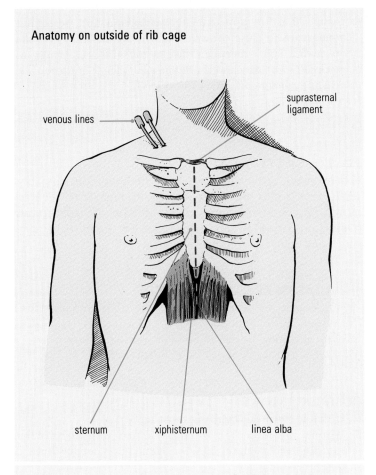

Anatomy on outside of rib cage

venous lines

suprasternal ligament

sternum   xiphisternum   linea alba

Fig. 2.40

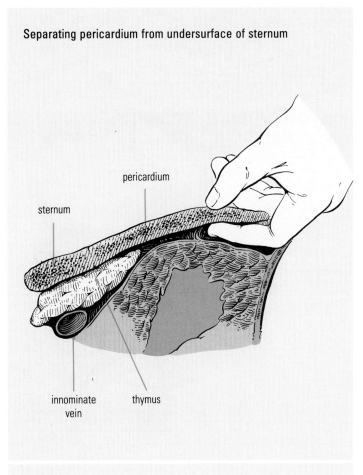

Separating pericardium from undersurface of sternum

sternum

pericardium

innominate vein   thymus

Fig. 2.41

Division of the sternum with a saw

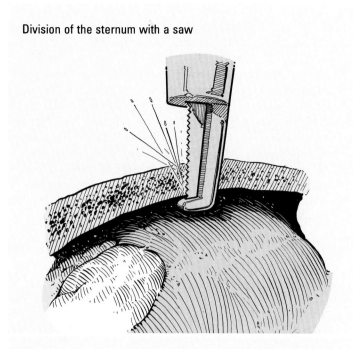

Fig. 2.42

Closure of sternum with wire sutures

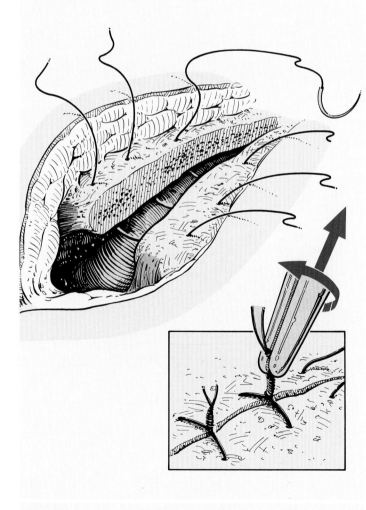

Fig. 2.43

10. To expose the heart, divide the thymus in the midline, either with diathermy or between ties, carefully freeing it from the innominate vein within it. The pleurae are then dissected from the pericardium laterally and the anterior pericardium opened from the origin of the innominate artery to the diaphragm. The incision should be extended laterally at the distal end in a T-shape. Hitch the pericardial edges to the incision in the skin with stout stay sutures. The intended cardiac procedure may now be performed.

Wound closure and dressing

1. At the end of the operation, one pericardial drain is usually placed behind the heart and another behind the sternum. These are brought out at the lower end of the incision through small transverse incisions, and pass through the rectus muscles so that the muscles can be closed in front of them without leaving an epicardial defect. Each is tied in place and an untied mattress suture is left around the emerging drains; these are closed when the drains are removed, usually on the following day.

2. Place six interrupted stainless steel wires through each half of the sternum (Fig. 2.43). Avoid placing them near the cut edge of the sternum which could lead to them cutting out, or around it as this may cause bleeding from intercostal or mammary vessels. Two wires should pass through the manubrium and four through the body of the sternum.

3. Cross and twist the wires tightly around themselves to approximate the sternum. Each wire is then cut approximately 1 cm above the twist and the ends are turned over and buried into the sternum.

4. Using 00 nylon approximate periosteum and pectoralis, taking care to close the space above the sternum and the epicardial space between the rectus muscles. Using an absorbable suture close the fascia (2/0 Vicryl) and then the skin as a subcuticular layer (3/0 Vicryl).

5. Apply a dry gauze dressing.

POSTOPERATIVE CARE

Patients begin to mobilize on the day following the operation when their drains and most monitoring lines have been removed. A continuous intravenous infusion of papaveretum (Omnopon) provides good pain relief for several days, after which oral analgesia will suffice.

SPECIAL OPERATIVE HAZARDS

1. Damage to the heart, especially if there has been previous surgery to the region.
2. Opening into the pleura and damage to the lung.
3. Bleeding from thymus or innominate vein.

COMPLICATIONS

1. Unstable sternum requiring rewiring.
2. Wound infections are often associated with an unstable sternum and require urgent treatment as mediastinitis is potentially fatal.

Use of Cardiopulmonary Bypass

Cardiopulmonary bypass is used for open or closed surgery on the heart, some thoracic aortic procedures, to support the compromised heart for short periods, and to support the heart during massive surgical procedures such as liver transplantation.

The heart–lung machine allows the exclusion of heart and lungs from the circulation so that the heart can be stopped and operated upon without injury to either the heart itself or to other organs which require continuous perfusion.

PREOPERATIVE ASSESSMENT
The choice of bypass circuit depends upon the operation to be performed and any previous cardiac surgery.

RELEVANT ANATOMY
There are three commonly used bypass circuits.
1. Drainage via two pipes, one in each cava, with transfusion back to the aorta (Fig. 2.44). This system allows continued venous drainage as the heart is manipulated to gain access to

the coronary arteries, or if the aorta is opened for aortic valve replacement or the left atrium is opened for mitral valve surgery. If access to the right side of the heart is required (atrial septal defect, tricuspid valve surgery or cardiac transplantation) or if the presence of a patent foramen ovale hinders mitral valve procedures (by allowing blood into the left side of the heart and air into the right) tapes may be passed and tightened around the pipes in each cava to exclude the right atrium from the circuit. During aortic valve surgery where separation of left and right atria will not be critical and in coronary artery surgery where the pattern of disease is such that minimal twisting of the heart will be needed to operate on the vessels, a single venous pipe with end holes in the inferior vena cava and side holes in the right atrium (to take the drainage from the superior vena cava) can be used.
2. Femoral vein to femoral artery bypass is used to support the lower half of the body (including vital organs such as the kidneys) during thoracic aortic procedures (Fig. 2.45).
3. Total bypass can be achieved by the addition of a single

Conventional bypass

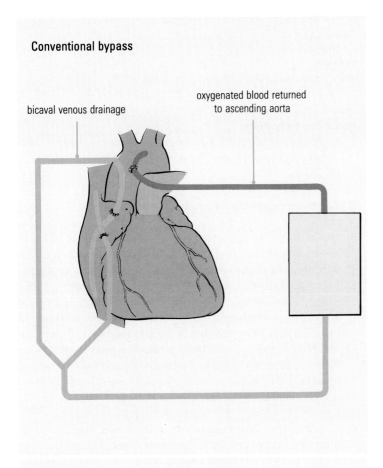

bicaval venous drainage

oxygenated blood returned to ascending aorta

Fig. 2.44

Peripheral bypass

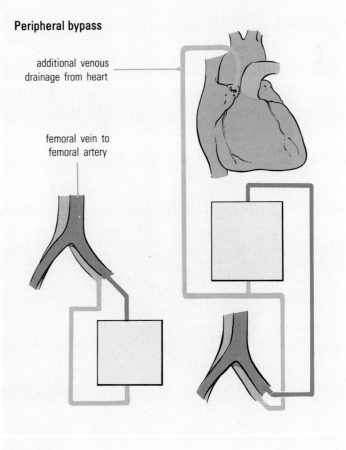

additional venous drainage from heart

femoral vein to femoral artery

Fig. 2.45

Placing 2 concentric purse strings

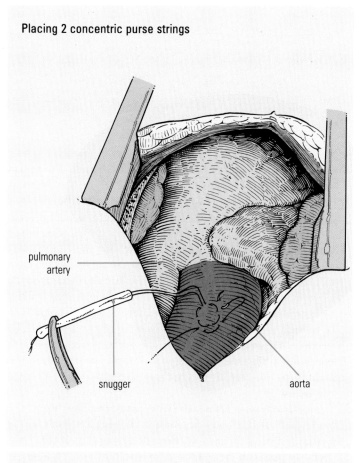

pulmonary
artery

snugger

aorta

Fig. 2.46

Aortotomy in ascending aorta

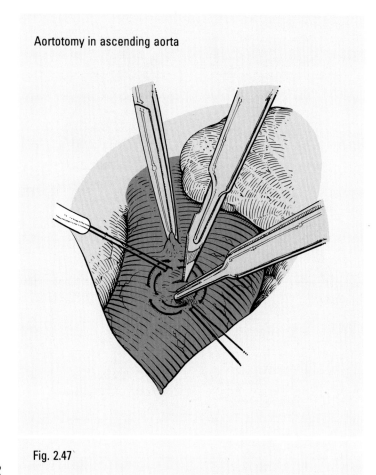

Fig. 2.47

atrial cannula to supplement venous drainage from the femoral vein in femoro–femoral bypass (Fig. 2.45). This arrangement permits surgery on the aortic arch or on the heart in circumstances where aortic cannulation is undesirable or difficult (e.g. in some cases of reoperation). In aortic arch procedures extreme cooling of the patient and short periods of total circulatory arrest with the machine off may be required.

If the aorta is cross-clamped during femoro–femoral bypass it may be desirable to offload the effect of temporarily increased vascular resistance on the heart with a pump-assisted left atrio-femoral bypass or a single shunt from the left ventricular apex to the femoral artery.

The heart–lung bypass machine has a venous reservoir which is primed with crystalloid and receives blood chiefly from the caval pipes, and from pump-assisted drains (e.g. in the pericardium). Blood is pumped from this reservoir and oxygenated with either a membrane oxygenator which allows gas exchange across a silicone membrane, or a bubble oxygenator which bubbles a suitable gas mixture through the blood. The blood is heated or cooled, filtered to remove particulate emboli and infused back into the systemic arterial circulation of the patient, usually via the ascending aorta. Small amounts of air in the venous system are of no consequence whereas air in the arterial side of the circuit can cause an air embolus which may be disastrous (e.g. if it enters the cerebral circulation).

CANNULATION FOR CARDIAC OPERATIONS
Preparation
The patient is placed supine as for a median sternotomy with all monitoring lines inserted (see page 2.28).

Incision
Perform a median sternotomy (see page 2.28).

Operative technique
1. Separate the aorta and the main pulmonary artery by dissection between the two. Some surgeons pass a sling around the aorta.

2. Ask the anaesthetist to heparinize the patient.

3. Insert an 8-mm diameter purse-string suture (consisting of a non-absorbable thread such as 2/0 Ethibond) into the anterior wall of the aorta in the position selected for cannulation according to the procedure to be undertaken. When using this technique on a thick-walled structure like the aorta, the suture must take partial thickness bites of the vessel. Apply a snugger but leave it loose; this will allow the suture to tighten tissue onto a cannula pipe to produce a blood and air-tight seal. A second suture may be placed outside the first and left loose to assist closure of the aorta on completion of the case (Fig. 2.46).

4. Confirm that anticoagulation is adequate, the perfusion lines are ready, and that the mean arterial pressure is no higher than about 75 mmHg, and then open the adventitia of the aorta within the purse-string. Apply a Roberts' clamp to the adventitia of the aorta and ask the assistant to push

this gently in a cephalic direction whilst the aorta is opened within the purse-string using a transverse stab incision with a number 11 blade. Hold the adventitia of the upper margin of this incision with forceps and keep the incision closed by pulling the upper flap down against the upwards pressure from the assistant (Fig. 2.47).

5. Now thrust the aortic cannula into the aorta up to the guard, the level of which was set previously. Arrange for the tip to sit in a central position within the lumen of the aorta and do not let it impinge on the wall of the vessel.

6. While the assistant holds the cannula tighten the purse-string with the snugger and clip it. Tie the snugger and pipe together with a strong tie to retain the pipe securely within the aorta (Fig. 2.48). Clamp the pipe, remove the venting tip from its end and briefly release the clamp to flush out any air.

7. The bypass circuit is passed up to the table as a continuous sash which should be divided at a suitable point along the length of the thinner transfusion tubing. Connect the aortic pipe to the tube and trim the wider venous limb to the desired length at the same time. A controlled release of the clamp on the aortic pipe as it is joined to the transfusion tubing will exclude all air when making the aortic connection.

8. Fix the tubing securely to the edge of the sternotomy.

9. Place non-absorbable (e.g. 2/0 Ethibond) purse strings in the right atrium and attach snuggers. When placing a purse-string suture into flexible tissue like the atrium, envisage the stitch as an anchored tie drawing the cuff of tissue around the pipe (i.e. take small bites on the inside, large ones on the outside). It is usual to place the venous cannulae so that they cross within the atrium, therefore position one purse-string around the atrial appendage (so that a pipe passed into it will lie in the inferior vena cava) and the other on the caudal surface of the atrium (so that its pipe will pass up the superior vena cava). Ensure the tips of the pipes will fit within the orifices of their respective cavae by adjusting the guards on the venous cannulae.

10. Place a vascular clamp across the atrial appendage and amputate its tip with scissors. The surgeon and the assistant hold the resulting hole by grasping opposite sides with forceps. Divide any trabeculae using scissors (Fig. 2.49) and insert the pipe through the atrium into the inferior vena cava as the assistant releases the atrial clamp. A similar technique can be used for the superior vena cava pipe or a stab hole can be made within the purse-string, and dilated to accept the cannula. Once a cannula is in place tighten the purse-string and snugger and tie them together as before.

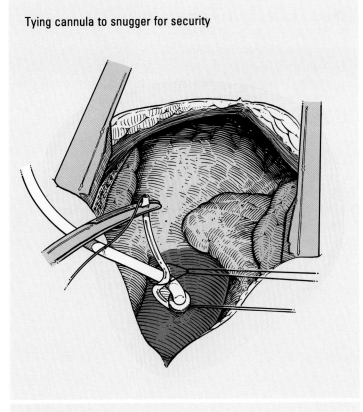

Tying cannula to snugger for security

Fig. 2.48

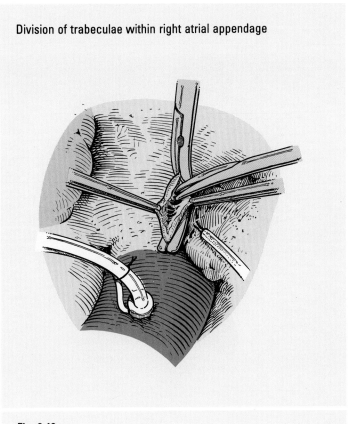

Division of trabeculae within right atrial appendage

Fig. 2.49

11. Fill each venous cannula with blood by lowering its tip, apply a clamp to keep them filled, and join the two via a Y-connector to the venous line to the pump with exclusion of as much air as possible (although there is no risk of air embolus, an airlock should be avoided).

12. Arrange any auxillary circuits required and commence cardiopulmonary bypass.

13. After the operation is completed and bypass has been terminated, remove the venous cannulae. Temporary closure of the atriotomy with the snugger facilitates rapid recannulation if necessary. Otherwise simply tie the purse-strings to close the holes. When heparinization has been reversed with an appropriate dose of protamine and any blood remaining in the pump has been transfused, remove the aortic cannula; this is achieved by the assistant putting a single throw on the outermost of the purse-strings, and tightening it as the surgeon withdraws the pipe after removing the snugger. Now tie the other purse-string and oversew the closure with a non-absorbable (e.g. 4/0 Prolene) suture.

Instillation of cardioplegic solution

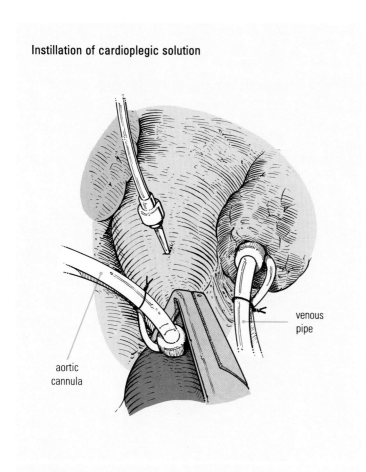

venous pipe

aortic cannula

Fig. 2.50

USING BYPASS

Upon starting cardiopulmonary bypass blood drains away from the heart which thus ceases to eject; the circulation now depends on transfusion of oxygenated blood from the pump. Decompression of the heart to prevent myocardial stretching and damage is important and systemic drainage is supplemented by venting via a cannula placed in a small stab incision in the main pulmonary artery or the apex of the left ventricle.

Blood pressure is controlled during bypass by the use of vasoactive drugs introduced via the pump to manipulate vasoconstriction and by changes in flow rate which nevertheless should remain close to $2.2 \, \mathrm{l \, min^{-1} \, m^{-1}}$ of patient surface area.

Systemic cooling to 28°C is commenced to improve organ preservation and decrease collateral coronary flow. A cross clamp can now be placed across the ascending aorta and the heart stopped in diastole by infusion of a cardioplegic solution (hyperkalaemic and cold, 4°C) into the coronaries either directly or via a cannula in the aortic root (Fig. 2.50). A topical cold circuit over the heart improves myocardial protection. The operation may now proceed.

As the operation draws to a close begin to rewarm the patient, and after open heart procedures de-air the heart by methodical aspiration of the cardiac chambers before removing the aortic cross-clamp to reperfuse the myocardium. The heart usually develops ventricular fibrillation at this point and is defibrillated with a 10–20 J shock directly across the ventricles.

After a suitable period of reperfusion the heart takes over its action and bypass is weaned by gradual reduction of systemic venous drainage so that the heart fills and can eject. Transfusion is simultaneously reduced. Inotropes, chronotropes and vasoactive drugs may be needed at this time to control cardiac power and rate and vascular tone and temporary ventricular pacing may be used to increase rate or overcome heart-block.

SPECIAL OPERATIVE HAZARDS
1. Air and particulate emboli.
2. Ischaemic cardiac damage.
3. Non-specific changes and ischaemic damage to other organs resulting from bypass perfusion (acute renal failure, cerebral changes etc.).
4. Oxygenator failure with overlong usage.

COMPLICATIONS
1. Haemorrhagic risks associated with systemic anticoagulation.
2. Shock lung resulting from endothelial changes on bypass.
3. Platelet consumption, coagulopathies and bleeding.

Surgery for Cardiac Valve Disease

Valve replacement or repair is indicated for haemodynamically significant valvular stenosis or regurgitation and in endocarditis where there is valvular destruction or resistance to antibiotic therapy. Although all four valves are subject to the same pathological processes, surgical interest centres on the mitral and aortic valves since malfunction of these is usually of greater haemodynamic significance than malfunction of those on the right side of the heart.

The surgical options for the treatment of valve disease are replacement, valvotomy (dividing fused commissures) or repair. Sometimes more than one valve requires attention and coronary disease may coexist in which case coronary artery bypass grafting (see page 2.40) may be undertaken at the same time as valve surgery. Occasionally valve surgery is required as part of another procedure (e.g. replacement of the ascending aorta in aortic dissection). With the exception of closed mitral valvotomy, these operations are performed using cardiopulmonary bypass.

PREOPERATIVE ASSESSMENT
1. Echocardiography and cardiac catheterization are used to assess the nature and extent of the valvular disease. Exclude concurrent coronary artery disease with coronary arteriography.
2. Adequately treat bacterial endocarditis to 'sterilize' the valve. Use antibiotics as indicated by blood culture results.
3. Look for and treat septic foci (teeth etc.).
4. Does more than one valve require surgery?
5. If aortic regurgitation is present will this necessitate direct cannulation of the coronary artery ostia to instil the cardioplegic solution?

RELEVANT ANATOMY
The four cardiac valves each guard the outlet from a cardiac chamber and permit the free passage of blood without reflux back into that chamber. The function of the valves is to maintain pressure gradients and ensure unidirectional flow through the heart. Thus the tricuspid valve 'protects' the right atrium, the pulmonary valve the right ventricle, the mitral valve the left atrium and the aortic valve the left ventricle.

The aortic valve is usually tricuspid and its leaflets are semi-lunar in shape. During ventricular diastole the higher pressure in the aortic root pushes the leaflets back towards the ventricle so that their surfaces co-apt to provide a seal (Fig. 2.51a). It is at this phase of the cardiac cycle that coronary perfusion is greatest. In systole the force of blood ejected from the ventricle pushes the leaflets away from each other and opens the valve. The leaflets are attached to the aortic wall at the annulus, a tough fibrous structure which provides a good anchor for sutures. Above the base of each leaflet is a dilatation in the aorta termed an aortic sinus, two of which are sited posteriorly and

one anteriorly, like the valve leaflets. The two main coronary arteries arise from these sinuses, the right from the anterior sinus and the left from the left posterior sinus.

In contrast, the mitral valve is more complex and does more than simply provide an anti-reflux device between two chambers since it also contributes to the power of left ventricular systole, a concept with implications for the value of more conservative valve procedures. The valve is formed of two unequal cusps, the larger lying in an anterior position. The cusps are thicker than those of the aortic valve and contain a few muscle fibres. Like the aortic leaflets they are attached to an annulus. Chordae tendinae run from papillary muscles within the ventricle to the margins of both cusps and also their ventricular surfaces (especially on the smaller posterior cusp). The valve operates as a 'parachute', the papillary muscles contracting in ventricular systole, pulling the cusps towards the atrioventricular orifice and holding blood within the ventricle (Fig. 2.51b). Because the cusps are attached to a strong annulus, this acts as an anchor so that contraction of the papillary muscles also augments the power of ventricular contraction. This effect of the 'mitral apparatus' is considered sufficiently significant for importance

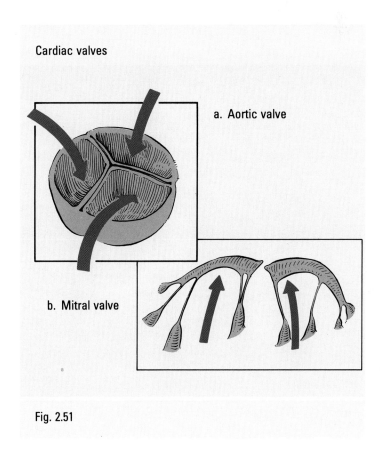

Cardiac valves

a. Aortic valve

b. Mitral valve

Fig. 2.51

to be attached to preserving the attachments of papillary muscles near the annulus by repairing regurgitant valves and even leaving the posterior leaflet in place when replacing the valve.

When conservative surgery is not possible and replacement is needed a variety of prostheses are available. Choice is influenced by age, acceptability of long-term anticoagulation, the presence of other diseases such as chronic renal failure, cost and the surgeon's preference. There are three main types: the human homograft, useful in young patients and those with endocarditis; the xenograft, a porcine valve mounted on a sewing ring (Fig. 2.52) or bovine pericardium affixed to a stent, which are suitable for older patients since the prosthesis is prone to degeneration but does not require long-term anticoagulation; or a variety of mechanical devices such as a captive ball (Fig. 2.53), tilting disc (Fig. 2.54) and bileaflet which suit younger patients since the devices are generally long-lived but carry a

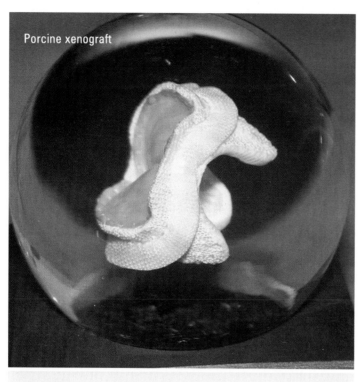

Porcine xenograft

Fig. 2.52

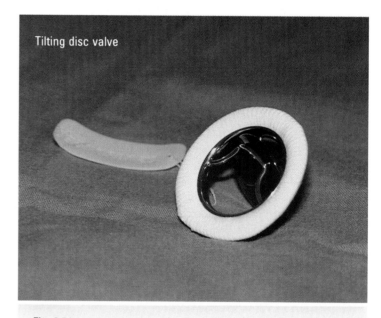

Tilting disc valve

Fig. 2.54

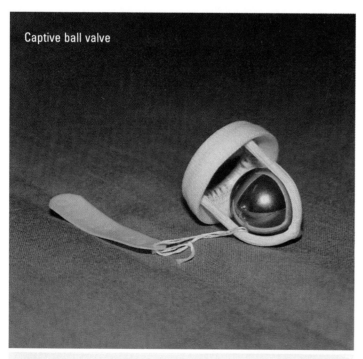

Captive ball valve

Fig. 2.53

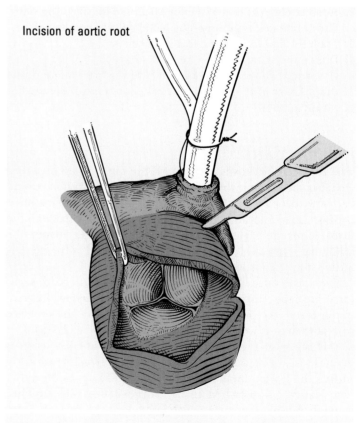

Incision of aortic root

Fig. 2.55

higher risk of thrombosis and embolism and therefore require long-term anticoagulation.

OPERATIONS
Preparation
The patient is draped for a sternotomy, ensuring access to the groin so that femoral cannulation may be performed if needed (this is more likely in revisional surgery). The legs are prepared if coronary artery surgery is anticipated.

Incision
Perform a median sternotomy (see page 2.28).

Operative technique

1. Heparinize the patient and perform routine cannulation for cardiopulmonary bypass (see page 2.32). If mitral surgery is intended two venous cannulae are used to allow the cavae to be snared if this is required, but for aortic surgery a single venous cannula is all that is needed.

2. Commence bypass and begin systemic cooling.

3. Vent the heart with a tube placed through a stab incision in the apex of the left ventricle. During mitral surgery, venting can be performed through the main pulmonary artery.

4. Cross-clamp the aorta, arrest the heart by instillation of cardioplegic solution via a cannula in the aortic root (except where aortic regurgitation necessitates direct cannulation of the coronary ostia) and establish topical cooling.

For aortic valve surgery

5. Access to the aortic valve is via a transverse incision in the ascending aorta which is carried caudally towards the centre of the attachment of the non-coronary cusp of the valve (Fig. 2.55).

6. Inspect the valve and excise it with a knife, scissors and rouengeurs. Care is taken to remove any debris to prevent embolization of this into the systemic or coronary circulations. Wash out the ventricle with cold saline to remove further debris, and remove any calcific deposits from the annulus so that sutures may be easily placed through it and a prosthetic valve can open and close freely. If endocarditis is present, abscess cavities must be opened and drained. It may be appropriate to examine the mitral valve either through the aortic annulus or through the left atrium.

7. Size the annulus with obturators shaped to reproduce the profile of the chosen type of prosthesis and prepare a suitable valve (biological valves need to be washed free of their preservative).

8. Insert a series of individual horizontal mattress sutures around the annulus so as to evert it using non-absorbable material such as 3/0 Ethibond leaving the needles on (Fig. 2.56); five or six sutures per cusp are usually needed (Fig. 2.57).

Sutures placed in annulus

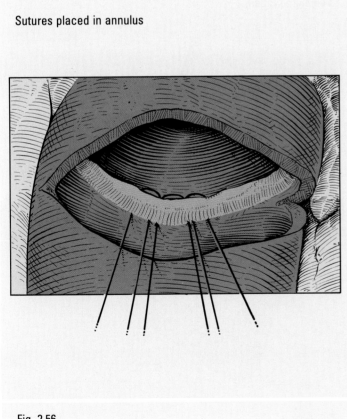

Fig. 2.56

Placement of valve

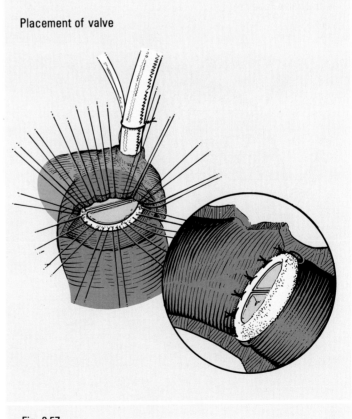

Fig. 2.57

9. Pass the sutures in turn through the sewing ring of the prosthesis and slide it into place within the annulus.

10. Begin systemic rewarming as the sutures are tied in turn and trimmed (see inset to Fig. 2.57). Close the aorta with a continuous non-absorbable suture (e.g. 4/0 Prolene).

For mitral valve surgery

5. Access to the mitral valve is usually through a transverse incision in the left atrium just above the right pulmonary veins (Fig. 2.58, which also shows the next point). On making this incision the unsuspected presence of a patent foramen ovale may lead to airlocking of the venous pipes, in which case snare the cavae.

6. Assess the valve.

7. If a simple commissurotomy is all that is needed, perform this with a knife.

8. Repair of a regurgitant valve may require resection of a quadrangular portion of redundant posterior leaflet (Fig. 2.58) with subsequent repair of the defect (Fig. 2.59). If repair is undertaken, perform an annuloplasty by the insertion of a flexible ring held in place with horizontal mattress sutures, to restore the natural D-shape of the annulus. Repair a ruptured or stretched chorda with a non-absorbable suture. Test any repair by allowing reversal of flow through the left ventricular vent to fill the ventricle with blood.

9. If valve replacement is judged necessary, undertake the procedure in much the same way as for the aortic valve. Preservation of at least some of the chordae and papillary muscles and possibly the whole posterior leaflet is desirable (see earlier in this chapter).

10. Whatever procedure is performed, begin rewarming as the procedure draws to an end and close the atrium with a continuous non-absorbable suture (e.g. 3/0 Prolene).

After surgery on either valve

11. 'De-air' the heart by aspiration from the ventricular apex, aorta, pulmonary veins and left atrium. Hand ventilation of the patient by the anaesthetist forces air and blood through and out of the pulmonary circulation.

12. Remove the cross-clamp and defibrillate the heart after a period of reperfusion. Repeat the 'de-airing' and then close the vent sites with a non-absorbable suture (e.g. 4/0 Prolene).

Mitral valve repair

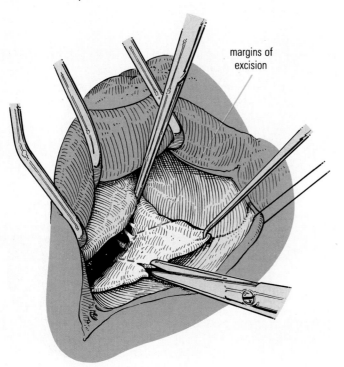

margins of excision

Fig. 2.58

Completed repair

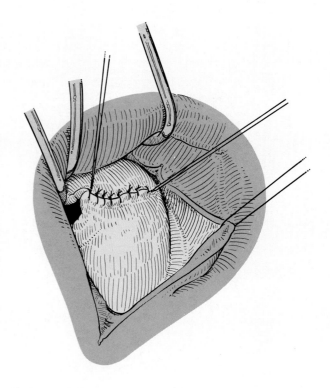

Fig. 2.59

13. Affix temporary pacing wires to the right ventricular muscle. These will be used if heart block appears now or later, or a faster heart rate is desirable.

14. Decannulate, reverse the heparinization with protamine and ensure complete haemostasis.

Wound closure and dressing

Place the drains and close the sternotomy as described previously (see page 2.30).

POSTOPERATIVE CARE

The patients are transferred to the intensive care unit for monitoring for about 18 hours. They are usually extubated if stable and not bleeding after about 4 hours. Drains are removed when drainage of blood has ceased.

A hospital stay of about 8 days after surgery is usual during which time the patient will be anticoagulated with warfarin (temporarily for biological valves, permanently for mechanical valves or where atrial fibrillation has developed).

SPECIAL OPERATIVE HAZARDS
1. Hazards associated with cardiopulmonary bypass.
2. Embolization of valve debris.
3. Discovery of other unsuspected cardiac defects.

COMPLICATIONS
1. Development of paraprosthetic leaks.
2. Intrinsic valve failure, especially with biological valves.
3. Endocarditis and infection of prosthesis.
4. Valve thrombosis or embolus.
5. Bleeding problems from anticoagulation.

Coronary Artery Surgery

Coronary artery surgery is indicated for chronic stable angina resistant to medical therapy, unstable angina, significant left main stem disease, and triple vessel disease which is severe or is associated with a tight left anterior descending lesion or impaired left ventricular function. It is also undertaken as an adjunct to surgery for the complications of infarction (e.g. ventricular septal defect).

Surgery involves the palliative bypassing of blockages and narrowings in the coronary vessels with a conduit from the aorta to a point on the coronary vessel beyond the major disease. Occasionally endarterectomy either with vein patching or grafting is employed but it is probable that many vessels treated in this manner soon re-occlude.

The nature of coronary atheroma lends itself to bypass surgery since it tends to be both proximal and focal although more diffuse patterns are seen, especially in diabetics. More mature atheroma becomes calcified and superadded thrombosis and spasm contribute to the problem.

The most commonly used conduit for surgery is the patient's own vein, harvested at the start of the operation. The long saphenous vein is best since this usually has a uniform diameter with a minimal number of side branches. If this vein has already been removed or is varicose then the short saphenous or the cephalic veins can be considered. The total length of one long saphenous vein is sufficient for three to four grafts. All veins must be reversed so that their valves will permit flow from aorta to distal coronary artery. If vein is in short supply it may be economically used as sequential grafts, adjacent vessels being grafted with a single length of vein (one top end on the aorta, a side-to-side anastomosis to one coronary and an end-to-side anastomosis to another).

It is also possible to use the internal mammary arteries as conduits. The vessel in this case is left attached to its arterial origin so that no proximal anastomosis to the aorta is needed, and the artery is swung down as a pedicle onto the surface of the heart, its tip being anastomosed to the coronary artery. Although it is not always possible to reach all the diseased vessels with either right or left arteries, use of this conduit has the advantage of hugely improved long-term patency rates compared with vein grafts. Intrinsic atheroma in the mammary arteries is a surprisingly rare problem even in elderly patients.

Artificial and preserved biological conduits such as stored bovine mammary artery conduits are almost never used.

PREOPERATIVE ASSESSMENT

1. Examine the legs of the patient to determine the course and quality of the veins, paying particular attention to varicosity, previous surgery which may have compromised or removed the vein and arterial insufficiency which can delay healing.
2. Use an angiogram to determine which vessels require grafting and the quality of left ventricular function. Review the angiogram immediately before operating.

RELEVANT ANATOMY

The long saphenous vein runs up the leg from its commencement at the medial end of the dorsal venous arch anterior to the medial malleolus at the ankle. Its diameter increases progressively as it passes two fingers breadths medial to the posterior border of the tibia, moves a little further posterior at the knee and then gently sweeps up the thigh, pierces the cribriform fascia and terminates at the saphenofemoral junction. It receives tributaries which are more numerous around the knee, making this section less suitable as a conduit.

The mammary artery on each side arises from the inferior surface of the first part of the subclavian artery. The origin is often a little more medial on the right. It arches down across the apex of the lung to run inferiorly on the inner surface of the chest wall just lateral to the border of the sternum. At each intercostal space it gives off two anterior intercostal arteries. The mammary artery terminates at the lower end of the sternum, dividing into superior epigastric and musculophrenic branches. When dissecting the vessel down from the thoracic wall it is important to clip each of these branches to prevent bleeding later. It is also important to carry the dissection right up to the origin of the artery so that the first intercostal branches are divided since if these remain patent a 'steal phenomenon' may develop. The artery, accompanied by two venae comitantes, is covered with fat and pleura and is therefore best displayed after opening the pleura and allowing the lung to fall away from the chest wall, dissection proceeding beneath the elevated sternum.

Relevant anatomy

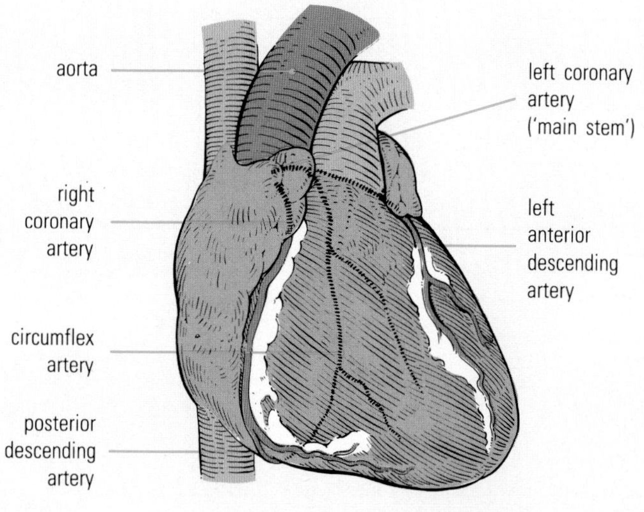

Fig. 2.60

Coronary anatomy suffers from variability in fact and nomenclature but the basic pattern is of two main arteries arising from the aorta within the sinuses of the aortic valve (Fig. 2.60). The right coronary artery passes anteriorly and the left posteriorly around the heart. Each gives off branches, the more major of which pass towards the apex of the heart and are the vessels considered for grafting. Lesser vessels are too small and inaccessible for surgery though their importance, supplying such structures as the conducting system, is not in question.

The left main coronary artery arises from the posterior aortic sinus. It gives off the anterior descending artery which descends to the apex of the heart in the anterior interventricular groove. This vessel provides septal branches to the interventricular septum and diagonal branches to the left ventricular free wall. Both the anterior descending artery and its diagonal branches are important vessels to graft if diseased and suitably placed to accept the left internal mammary artery as a conduit. The left main vessel now passes posteriorly towards the diaphragmatic surface of the heart in the atrioventricular groove where it is known as the circumflex artery. Here, in addition to atrial branches which do not concern the surgeon, it gives off a number of obtuse marginal branches running towards the apex. Some of these are large and if significantly diseased can be grafted, usually with vein.

The right main coronary artery arises from the anterior aortic sinus and passes inferiorly beneath the right atrial appendage in the anterior atrioventricular groove. The main vessel can be grafted here using the right internal mammary artery if the disease is purely proximal. It then gives rise to atrial branches and at the inferior border of the heart the posterior descending artery passes to the apex to anastomose with terminal branches of the anterior descending vessel. Grafting here requires a vein because the anastomosis is too distal for the mammary to reach.

Variations from this pattern are common and coronary vessels can be hard to find if they take an intramuscular course or if they are buried in myocardial fat. In addition, the coronary anatomy as seen by the surgeon differs from textbook descriptions as the heart is anchored within the pericardium and is twisted and manipulated to reveal the vessels. Figs 2.61, 2.62 and 2.63 show the heart in the three positions used to expose the vessels during surgery.

Displaying the coronary arteries 1: anterior descending artery

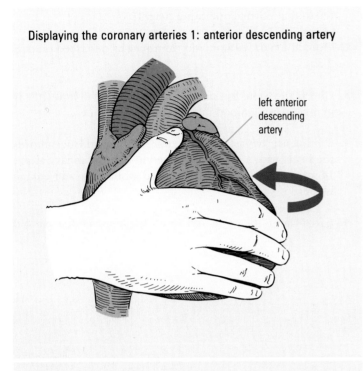

left anterior descending artery

Fig. 2.61

Displaying the coronary arteries 2: obtuse marginal branches

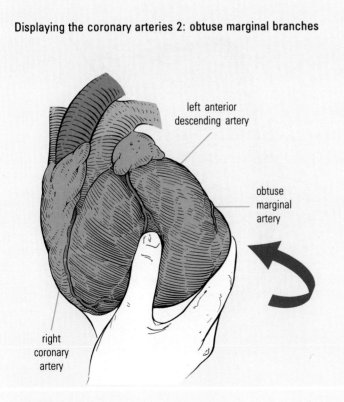

left anterior descending artery

obtuse marginal artery

right coronary artery

Fig. 2.62

Displaying the coronary arteries 3: posterior descending artery

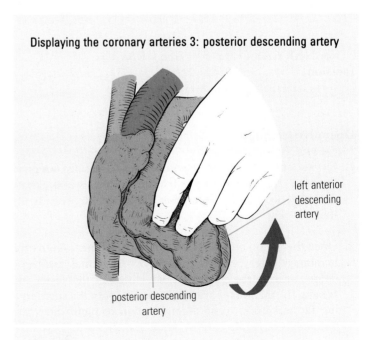

left anterior descending artery

posterior descending artery

Fig. 2.63

2.41

OPERATION
Preparation

One surgeon harvests the long saphenous vein from the chosen leg whilst another performs a median sternotomy as described on page 2.28 and harvests one or both mammary arteries as required.

Prepare the skin and drape the patient so that the chest and both legs are exposed and access to the groins is possible.

HARVESTING THE SAPHENOUS VEIN
Incision

Commence the incision anterior to the medial malleolus just above the ankle with a scalpel.

Operative technique

1. Expose the vein and follow it up the leg using curved Mayo scissors to incise the overlying skin to obtain the length needed.

2. Mobilize the vein with minimal handling, carefully ligating and dividing all tributaries as they are encountered with absorbable ties (e.g. 3/0 Vicryl).

3. Excise the required segment. Cannulate its distal end and pass it to the scrub nurse who will store it in heparinized blood. If the vein appears of poor quality (too narrow or varicose) consider exposing it at the saphenofemoral junction and dissecting downwards or using the vein from the other leg.

4. Ensure careful haemostasis since the patient is about to be anticoagulated.

Wound closure and dressing

Close the leg with a subcutaneous absorbable suture (e.g. 2/0 Vicryl), and the skin with a subcuticular absorbable suture (e.g. 3/0 Vicryl). Apply a bandage.

CORONARY ARTERY BYPASS GRAFTS
Incision

Perform a median sternotomy (see page 2.28).

Operative technique
Harvesting the mammary artery

1. Elevate one side of the sternum with a specially designed retractor, tip the table away from the surgeon and elevate the table so that the operation can proceed beneath the sternum (Fig. 2.64).

2. Open the pleura and allow the lung to fall away. Identify the mammary artery, which runs across the costal cartilages, before incising the pleura on either side of the vessel and freeing the mammary artery as a pedicle with the surrounding fat and fascia using a combination of blunt dissection and diathermy. Clip and divide all branches with 'Ligaclips'.

3. The anaesthetist fully heparinizes the patient.

4. Free the artery to its origin, divide its distal end with a ligature beyond and apply a coronary bulldog clip (Fig. 2.65).

5. Wrap the mammary pedicle in a moist swab and leave it in the chest.

Coronary artery grafting

1. Return the patient and table to their original position (i.e. flat and at normal operating height).

2. Open the pericardium and cannulate as described on page 2.32.

3. Check the vein for quality and any untied branches by gently infusing blood into its cannula.

4. Commence bypass and systemic cooling and decompress the heart with a vent tube placed in the pulmonary artery. Identify the vessels to be grafted while they still contain blood.

5. Cross-clamp the aorta and arrest the heart in diastole with

Mobilization of internal mammary artery

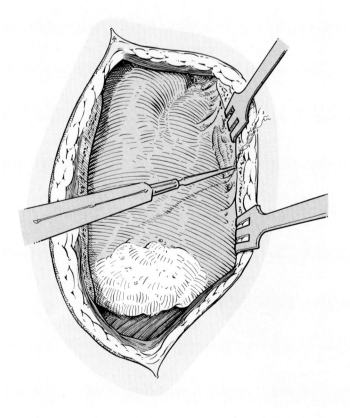

Fig. 2.64

cardioplegic solution instilled into a cannula in the aortic root with simultaneous topical cooling. Establish a continuous topical cooling system.

6. Perform the distal anastomoses of the grafts in turn. The usual pattern is to use the saphenous vein to graft to the right or posterior descending arteries, another segment of saphenous vein to graft the obtuse marginal branches, and the saphenous vein or mammary artery to graft the left anterior descending vessel and its diagonal branches.

7. Pass silastic stays under the chosen vessel for support and open it over 3–4 mm in its midline with a fine or diamond-tipped knife (Fig. 2.66), extending the arteriotomy with fine-angled scissors. Numerous techniques are used for the distal anastomoses, but all involve 6/0 or 7/0 non-absorbable sutures as a continuous running stitch. Figure 2.67 shows one such method which involves bevelling and anchoring the toe and heel of the vein, and running the sutures from each end along each side of the anastomosis and tying them in the middle of each side.

Making an arteriotomy in a coronary artery

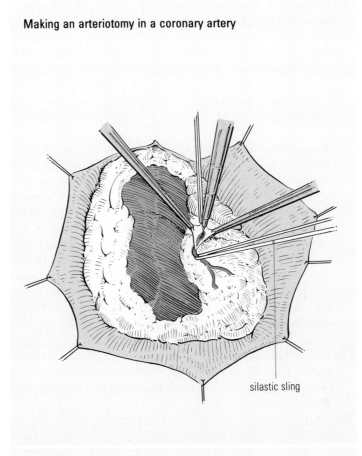

silastic sling

Fig. 2.66

Division of internal mammary artery

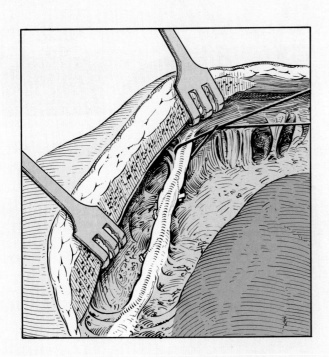

Fig. 2.65

Anastomosis of saphenous vein to coronary artery

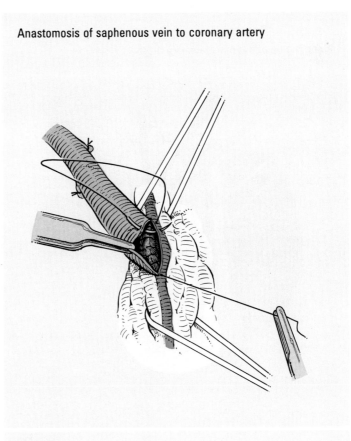

Fig. 2.67

8. Similarly bevel the mammary artery (Fig. 2.68) and anasto-mose it at its tip; even more care is needed with this fragile vessel and the anastomosis is performed with a non-absorbable suture (e.g. 7/0 Prolene). Tack the mammary pedicle to the epicardium (Fig. 2.69), and when the bulldog has been removed from the pedicle rapid flushing of the grafted vessel is seen as this graft is supplied by the heart–lung machine.

9. Begin systemic rewarming. Remove the cross-clamp to partially reperfuse the heart, and anastomose the proximal ends of the vein grafts to the aorta. A side-biting clamp is applied to the aorta and a 4 mm hole cut in it with a punch for each vein graft (Fig. 2.70). Inflate the vein with saline, trim it to the correct length, orientate it so that it lies around the heart with no twists or kinks, and then anasto-mose it end-to-side to the aortotomy with a continuous non-absorbable suture (e.g. 6/0 Prolene) (Fig. 2.71). De-air the graft with a fine needle and remove the clamp to completely revascularize the heart. Completed grafts are seen in Fig. 2.72.

10. Defibrillate the heart, close the vent site with an absorbable suture (e.g. 4/0 Prolene) and wean the patient off bypass (see page 2.34). Decannulation and reversal of anticoagulation follow.

Securing internal mammary artery graft with epicardial suture

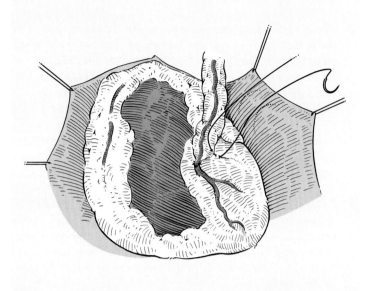

Fig. 2.69

Aortic punch for proximal anastomosis

Preparing tip of internal mammary artery

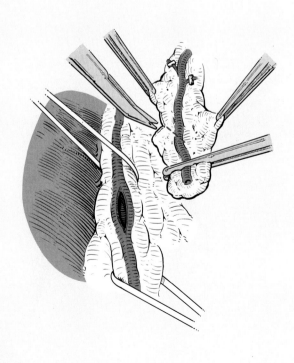

Fig. 2.68

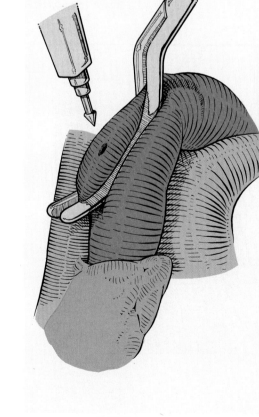

Fig. 2.70

Proximal anastomosis

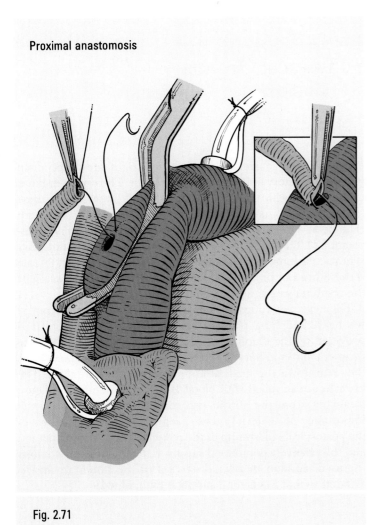

Fig. 2.71

Completed coronary revascularization

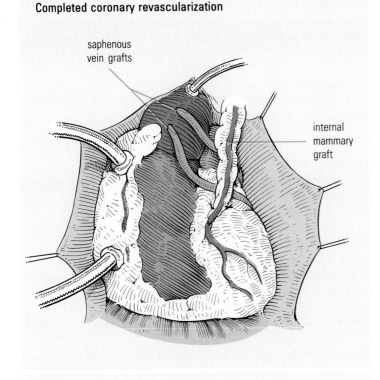

saphenous
vein grafts

internal
mammary
graft

Fig. 2.72

Wound closure and dressing

Place a drain in each of the opened thoracic cavities, one behind the heart and one behind the sternum, and close the chest in the usual way (see page 2.30).

POSTOPERATIVE CARE

The patient is transferred for monitoring and nursing in the intensive therapy ward for about 18 hours, and is extubated when it is clear that he is stable and not bleeding. The drains are removed when the drainage of blood has ceased. Postoperative hospital stay is about 8 days. Low dose aspirin is commenced for its value in maintaining graft patency.

SPECIAL OPERATIVE HAZARDS

1. Problems associated with cardiopulmonary bypass (see page 2.34).
2. Perioperative myocardial infarction.
3. Poor long saphenous vein, in which case consider using the short saphenous or cephalic vein.
4. Persistent bleeding may require re-exploration of the sternotomy.
5. Damage to the saphenous nerve giving an area of anaesthesia on the medial aspect of the foot.
6. Damage to the femoral vein when ligating the saphenofemoral junction.

COMPLICATIONS

1. Blocked grafts due to an embolus or thrombosis secondary to competitive flow or spasm.
2. Recurrent angina as a result of graft occlusion or progression of the native disease.
3. Dysaesthesia of the chest wall after the mammary artery is harvested.
4. Unstable sternum and mediastinitis.
5. Haematoma and infection of leg wound.
6. Sloughing of the leg wound from undermining the skin to expose the saphenous vein.

Transplantation of the Thoracic Organs

Heart, heart and lung, and single or double lung transplantation are practiced. Transplantation of the heart and heart and lungs combined are established parts of the treatment of end-stage failure of these organs. The role of lung transplantation alone is rapidly developing and the indications for this operation are constantly expanding.

Transplantation of the lung alone can often be performed without cardiopulmonary bypass and the donor heart can be given to a second patient. The operation does, however, carry a theoretical increased risk of bronchial anastomotic dehiscence due to poor vascularization of the donor bronchus. This chapter confines itself to the transplantation of the heart and the heart and lungs combined.

RELEVANT ANATOMY

In orthotopic heart transplantation the recipient organ is excised leaving a rim of the left and right atria, the main pulmonary artery and the ascending aorta. The donor organ is excised flush with the pericardium around the atria and these chambers are anastomosed to the stumps of the recipient chambers. The atria are thus enlarged and functionally compromised. This can be improved with caval and pulmonary venous anastomoses. The new heart is denervated and its rate is therefore not under autonomic neural control; on occasions the resultant rate is slow enough to warrant pacing.

The heart and lungs are similarly denervated when removed for heart and lung transplantation, but respiratory effort is provided by the diaphragm which remains innervated by the recipient phrenic nerves. These nerves must be preserved as they run down the mediastinum anterior to each hilum. The bronchi are supplied with blood from the systemic circulation (branches from the aorta); two consequences of this are the importance of achieving good haemostasis in these vessels in the posterior mediastinum of the recipient prior to implantation and the relatively poor blood supply to the tracheal anastomosis (devascularization by over dissection of the donor trachea is avoided so that a collateral supply is maintained).

OPERATIONS

DONOR OPERATIONS

Most organ retrievals are from multi-organ donors. This involves first mobilizing the abdominal organs (e.g. liver and kidneys), and then mobilizing and removing the thoracic organs whilst the now ischaemic abdominal organs are perfused with cold preservation solution *in situ*.

Preparation

The ventilated donor is placed supine and the neck, chest and abdomen are prepared and draped.

Incision

Access for thoracic organ retrieval is via a median sternotomy (see page 2.28).

Operative technique

Heart retrieval

1. Open the pericardium and examine the heart for unsuspected damage or disease.

2. Separate the aorta from the pulmonary artery.

3. Mobilize the superior and inferior venae cavae with sharp dissection and heparinize the donor.

4. Clamp the inferior vena cava and divide the superior vena

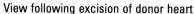

View following excision of donor heart

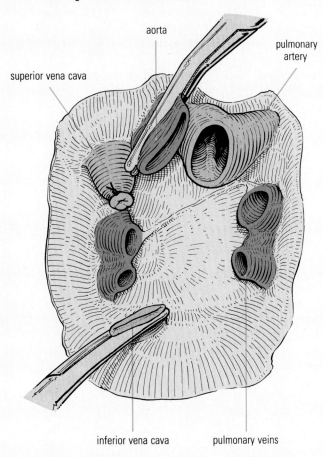

aorta

pulmonary artery

superior vena cava

inferior vena cava   pulmonary veins

Fig. 2.73

cava between two ligatures (well above the sino-auricular node which is preserved) to provide inflow occlusion.

5. Clamp the aorta and commence an infusion of cold cardioplegic solution into a cannula in the aortic root with simultaneous topical cooling to provide rapid electromechanical arrest in diastole.

6. Vent the heart by making an incision in a pulmonary vein and the inferior vena cava.

7. Excise the heart flush with the pericardium and well distal on the aorta and pulmonary arteries (Fig. 2.73).

8. Preserve the heart in its arrested state in cardioplegic solution at 4°C, allowing a total ischaemic time of about 4 hours.

Heart and lung retrieval
1. Inspect the organs carefully.

2. Excise the thymus to reveal the innominate vein, which is divided between ligatures. Also divide the innominate artery.

3. Place a sling around the trachea but do not denude it.

4. Mobilize the cavae and open the pleurae. Expose and divide the azygos vein on the right.

5. Heparinize the donor and insert a cannula into the pulmonary trunk; commence an infusion of epoprostenol (prostacyclin) through this.

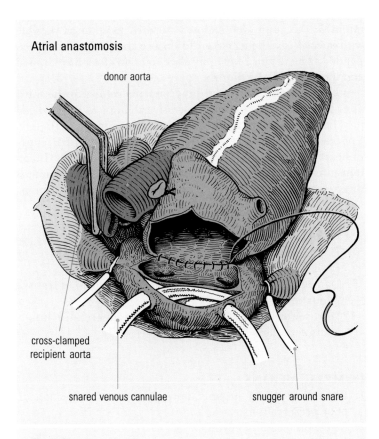

Atrial anastomosis

donor aorta

cross-clamped recipient aorta

snared venous cannulae   snugger around snare

Fig. 2.74

6. Occlude the inflow as described for heart retrieval and cardioplege the heart, venting from the inferior vena cava and the tip of the left atrial appendage on this occasion.

7. As the heart arrests, commence an infusion of cold blood and cystalloid into the pulmonary artery cannula to cool the lungs.

8. Excise the pleurae on each side.

9. Complete the mobilization along the posterior mediastinum by dividing the inferior vena cava and lifting the organs to separate them from the aorta and oesophagus. Take care not to damage the pulmonary hila.

10. Toward the cephalad end of this mobilization divide the ligamentum arteriosum.

11. Ask the anaesthetist to inflate the lungs by hand with air so that no part remains collapsed. The anaesthetist then withdraws the endotracheal tube as the surgeon clamps and divides the trachea so the lungs stay inflated. Dissect down behind the trachea and remove the organs.

12. Staple across the trachea.

13. Store the organs in Ringer's solution at 4°C. The cold pulmonary artery flush evenly distributed as a result of the prostacyclin infusion provides good preservation and early graft function with an ischaemic interval again of up to 4 hours.

RECIPIENT OPERATIONS
Preparation
This is similar to that for cardiopulmonary bypass (see page 2.31).

Incision
Access is via a median sternotomy (see page 2.28).

Operative technique
1. Commence cardiopulmonary bypass and snare the cavae around the venous cannulae so that the heart can be excised. Systemic cooling is to 30°C.

Heart transplantation
2. Cross-clamp the aorta.

3. Open the right atrium and then extend the incision along the septum and across the roof of the left atrium. Divide the aorta and pulmonary trunk and then complete the excision along the free left atrium. The heart is now removed.

4. Examine the donor heart; a patent foramen ovale is closed, the left and right atria are opened and the outflow vessels are trimmed to length.

5. Make the atrial anastomoses with a continuous non-absorbable suture (e.g. Prolene). Suture the left atrium, the inter-

2.47

atrial septum, the septum again, and then right atrium in that order (Fig. 2.74).

6. Anastomose the pulmonary artery and the aorta using continous non-absorbable sutures (e.g. Prolene). Rewarm the patient.

7. Remove the caval snares and de-air the heart. The aortic clamp is then removed and the heart is reperfused. De-airing continues and the heart is defibrillated.

8. After a period of reperfusion recommence ventilation and wean the patient from cardiopulmonary bypass. Temporary pacing wires are attached to right atrium and ventricle.

Heart and lung transplantation

2. Open the pleura and mobilize the hilum of each lung so that the lung may be removed through a window in each pleural sheet; great care is taken to preserve the phrenic and the vagus nerves.

3. If the recipient heart is to be used in a 'domino' operation cardioplege and then remove the heart. Otherwise clamp the aorta and excise the organs.

4. Remove the left and then the right lung after stapling their respective bronchus. The heart is then removed as described in point 3 on Heart transplantation on page 2.47; the left atrial and pulmonary artery remnants play no further part in the operation.

5. Expose the trachea in the posterior mediastinum and minimally mobilize it.

6. Ensure careful haemostasis because the posterior mediastinum will be inaccessible after the operation.

7. Trim the donor and recipient tracheas to the correct length and anastomose them with a continuous non-absorbable suture (e.g. Prolene) (Fig. 2.75). Site the lungs in each thoracic cavity through the window in each pleural sheet.

8. Make the vascular connections; first the aorta and then the right atrium are anastomosed with a continuous non-absorbable suture (e.g. Prolene).

9. Close the holes in the pulmonary artery and the left atrial appendage which were made during the donor procedure. Remove the aortic cross-clamp, de-air the organs as for heart transplantation and then rewarm the patient.

10. Defibrillate the heart and recommence ventilation. After a period of reperfusion wean the patient off the cardiopulmonary bypass. Temporary pacing wires are attached to the heart.

Wound closure and dressing

After decannulation, insert pericardial drains in a heart recipient and pericardial and thoracic drains in a heart and lung recipient. Close and dress the sternotomy (see page 2.30).

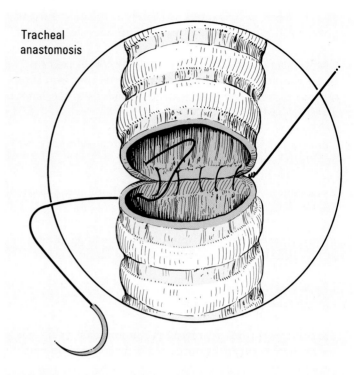

Tracheal anastomosis

Fig. 2.75

POSTOPERATIVE CARE

After receiving a heart the ventilated patient is nursed in isolation. Inotropic support (dopamine), pacing or isoprenaline (to reduce right ventricular afterload) may be needed. Extubation follows the next day.

After transplantation of both the heart and lungs, in the intensive care unit, ventilation is weaned as soon as possible with special care being taken to ensure the lungs remain expanded. The drains remain in place until any leak has stopped and the lungs fill the thoracic space.

Both heart and heart and lung patients return to the ward after 2 or 3 days. Immunosuppressive therapy is commenced just before surgery and continues thereafter indefinitely. Episodes of rejection are confirmed with endomyocardial biopsy in heart transplants and transbronchial biopsy in lungs. Infections are rigorously identified and irradicated. Management is directed at balancing the relative risks of rejection and infection.

SPECIAL OPERATIVE HAZARDS
1. Haemorrhage.
2. Right ventricular overload coming off bypass.
3. Damage to the phrenic nerves in heart and lung transplantation.
4. Devascularization of the trachea in heart and lung transplantation.

COMPLICATIONS
1. Immediate donor organ failure due to poor selection or poor preservation.
2. Rejection (acute or chronic).
3. Infection and other complications of immunosuppression.

3

Breast Surgery

Management of Breast Lumps

PREOPERATIVE ASSESSMENT
1. Decide whether the breast lump is discrete or diffuse.
2. Does the lump undergo cyclical alterations in size and tenderness, suggesting a dysplastic origin?
3. Check for factors that indicate a possible carcinoma. For example, skin changes (e.g. dimpling), nipple changes (e.g. eczema), lymphadenopathy, or a positive family history.
4. Should mammography be performed?
5. Has an attempt been made to aspirate the lump (see later on this page)?
6. Is a preoperative biopsy indicated (see later on this page)?
7. The site of the lump should be marked on the skin with an indelible marker.

RELEVANT ANATOMY
The breast is a glandular organ containing 15–20 radially arranged secretory lobes that are separated by fibrous septa and imbedded in fat (Fig. 3.1). Each lobe drains into a single

Anatomy of glandular tissue of breast

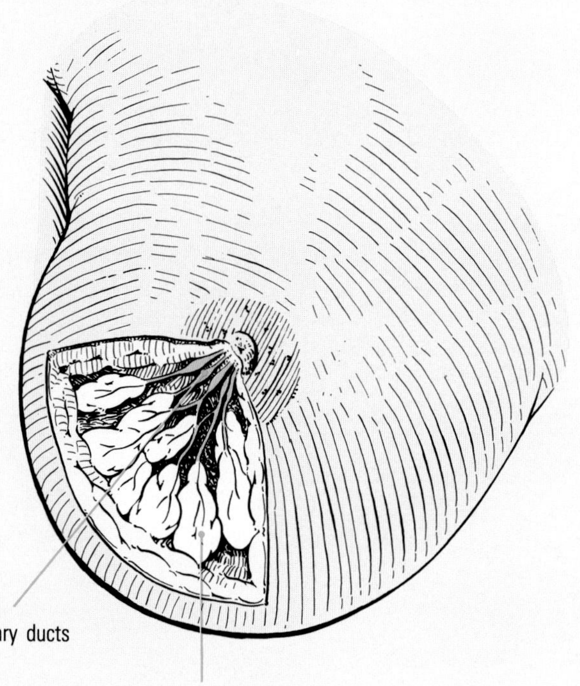

mammary ducts

glandular tissue

Fig. 3.1

3.2

duct which dilates beneath the areola into an ampulla, and then opens onto the surface of the nipple. The breast anatomy is fully covered on page 3.9 in Mastectomy.

Additional supernumerary mammary glands can occur anywhere along the nipple line, which extends from the mid-clavicular line to the groin, and can undergo the same physiological (e.g. lactation) and pathological (e.g. neoplasia) changes as normally sited breast tissue.

OPERATIONS
ASPIRATION OF BREAST CYST
Prior to excision, an attempt to aspirate the breast lump should be made. This is performed without anaesthetic.

Operative technique
1. Hold the lump fixed between the index finger and thumb of the left hand.

2. Cleanse the skin over the lump with an injection swab (70% isopropyl alcohol).

3. Insert a 21G needle into the lump (Fig. 3.2). If it is cystic, the lump is drained to dryness and the fluid is sent for cytology, although the pick-up rate for malignant cells is low. Once the cyst has been aspirated it is important to confirm that a lump no longer exists, and to excise those that recur.

   Cellular aspirate can similarly be obtained from a solid lump; in this case the needle is drawn back and forth through the lump whilst suction is maintained on the syringe and the cells are then spread directly onto a microscope slide.

BREAST BIOPSY
Whilst fine needle aspiration is an excellent method for cytology, with a result available within an hour, it should only be performed in centres that have a pathologist with the necessary expertise to interpret the smears. Otherwise a 'Trucut' biopsy is preferable if a preoperative histological diagnosis is sought.

Operative technique
1. As with cyst aspiration, immobilize the lump between the left index finger and the thumb.

2. Cleanse the skin as before, and inject 1% plain lignocaine into the proposed track of the biopsy needle, from the skin to the lump.

3. With the right hand, push a 'Trucut' needle through the anaesthetized skin and advance it to the lump with the blade shut.

4. Pass the sharp tip of the needle through the lump, with the outer sheath held still (Fig. 3.3); by doing this the sample area rests on the flattened recess of the biopsy needle.

5. Advance the outer sheath through the lump, whilst the inner part is held still; this cuts the biopsy from the tissue lying in the recess (Fig. 3.4).

6. Withdraw the needle, still closed, and then open it to allow retrieval of the biopsy.

7. Apply firm pressure over the biopsy site for a few minutes to stop any bleeding.

BREAST LUMP EXCISION

This should be performed in an operating theatre under general anaesthesia. Before commencing it is essential to confirm that the lump is still present. The patient is placed in a supine position with the ipselateral arm abducted to 90° at the shoulder and supported on an arm board.

Aspiration of breast cyst

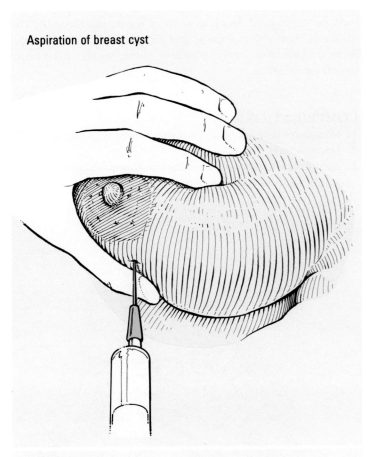

Fig. 3.2

Positioning of 'Trucut' needle for breast biopsy

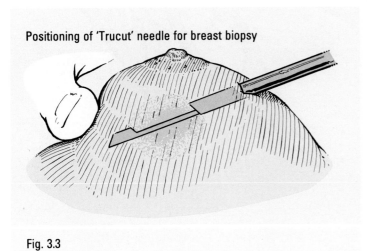

Fig. 3.3

Closure of Trucut device to take biopsy

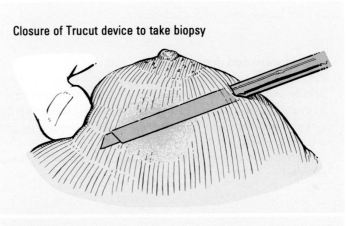

Fig. 3.4

Incision over breast lump

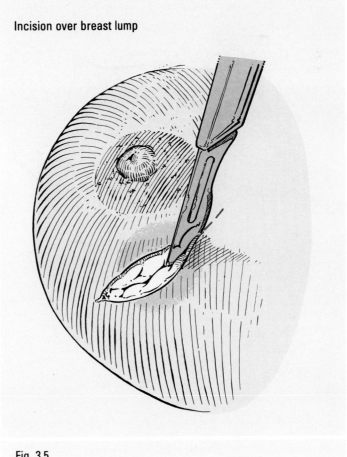

Fig. 3.5

Incision

A circumareolar, circumferential or radial incision is made over the lump (Fig. 3.5). Remember, if the incision is made along Langers lines which run horizontally across the breast, it will heal with the minimum of scarring. However, access must take priority over cosmetic considerations.

Operative technique

1. Deepen the incision and grasp the lump with Allis' or Lane's tissue-holding forceps (Fig. 3.6). The skin edges are then retracted and, whilst traction is applied, the lump is excised with a cuff of normal breast using scissors (Fig. 3.7).

2. Secure haemostasis with diathermy.

Wound closure and dressing

1. Repair the tough breast tissue with 2/0 Vicryl on a cutting needle. Any dead space is drained with a fine suction drain to prevent a haematoma collecting. The fat is closed with 2/0 catgut, and a subcuticular Prolene is used for the skin to give a good cosmetic result.

2. A pressure dressing is unnecessary if a drain has been inserted.

Tissue examination

1. Cut the lump in half with a scalpel. If it is cystic the surrounding breast tissue may harbour an intraduct papilloma or carcinoma which had obstructed the duct. If it is solid the cut surface of a fibroadenoma may bulge and it may appear encapsulated. A cancer often feels gritty, like an unripe pear, and exudes a thin fluid.

2. Place the lump in a labelled container and send it for histological examination.

POSTOPERATIVE CARE

After breast lump excision, the drain is removed once drainage has ceased (this is usually within 24 hours), and the patient can then be discharged home as soon as she is comfortable. The suture is removed at 7 days, and an early follow-up appointment is made to inform the patient of the results of the histological examination.

COMPLICATIONS

1. Mammary fistula can occur if the patient is lactating.
2. Haematoma.
3. Incomplete excision of a carcinoma; this may require further surgery and/or radiotherapy.

Grasping breast lump with Lane's forceps

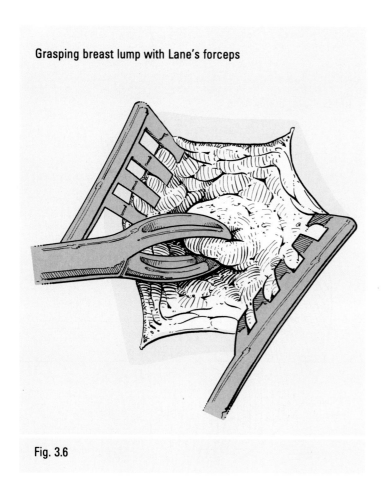

Fig. 3.6

Excision of breast lump

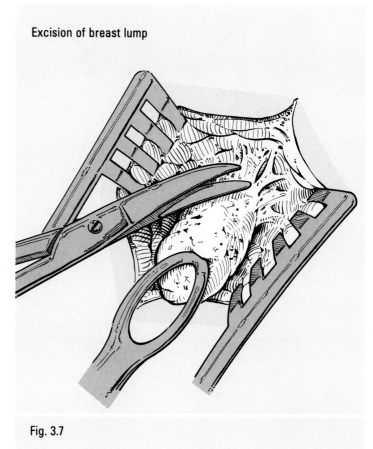

Fig. 3.7

Drainage of Breast Abscess

A breast abscess usually occurs during lactation. When this happens, feeding can continue from the other breast, whilst the affected breast is expressed manually. Alternatively lactation can be suppressed with drugs such as bromocriptine. Mastitis neonatorum occurs in the neonate and is due to an effect of maternal hormones. Occasionally, however, it progresses to suppuration when drainage should be performed urgently to prevent damage to the breast disc and impaired breast development at puberty.

PREOPERATIVE ASSESSMENT

1. Determine whether the infection is purely a cellulitis, in which case it is treated with antibiotics, or whether pus is present and surgical drainage is therefore required.
2. Is lactation to be suppressed?

RELEVANT ANATOMY

This is fully covered on pages 3.2 and 3.9 in Management of Breast Lumps and Mastectomy.

OPERATION
Preparation

Place the patient supine with the ipselateral arm on an arm board, extended at the elbow and abducted to 90° at the shoulder. Abduction beyond 90° stretches the cords of the brachial plexus.

Incision

An incision is made over the point of maximum fluctuance, or over the tenderest point found on a previous examination (Fig. 3.8). It can be either circumareolar for a woman who has completed her family, or radial for a lactating female or one who is likely to have further children; the former leaves a neater scar, while the latter avoids transecting the major ducts.

Operative technique

1. A bacteriology swab or pus sample is taken for culture (Fig. 3.9), and the pus is evacuated from the abscess. To ensure complete drainage any loculi are opened with a finger.

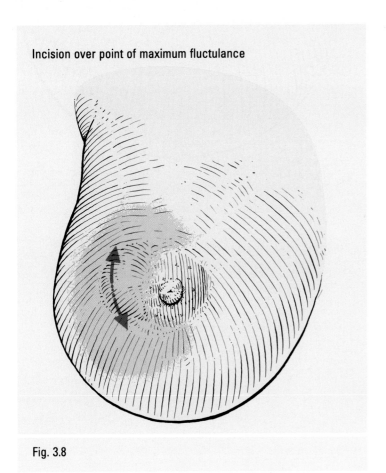

Incision over point of maximum fluctulance

Fig. 3.8

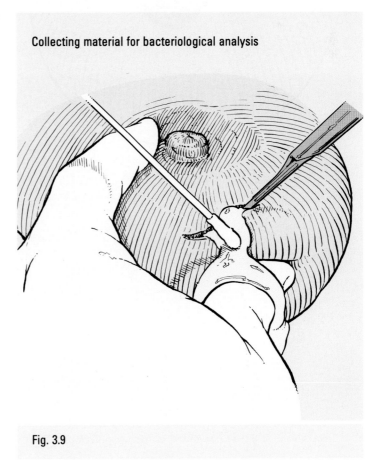

Collecting material for bacteriological analysis

Fig. 3.9

2. The cavity walls are gently curetted with a Volkmann's spoon (Fig. 3.10).

3. In a non-lactating female, or if pus is not found despite adequate exploration, a biopsy of the wall should be taken to exclude an inflammatory carcinoma.

Wound closure and dressing

1. Haemostasis is secured and a ribbon gauze wick, soaked in proflavin cream, is loosely packed into the cavity (Fig. 3.11).

2. An absorbant dressing is applied and the breast supported with strapping.

POSTOPERATIVE CARE

The wick is soaked out in the bath on the following day and the wound redressed daily, keeping the skin edges separated with a small wick of paraffin gauze to allow healing to proceed from the bottom of the cavity. Antibiotics are only indicated if cellulitis is present.

COMPLICATIONS

1. Mammary fistula may follow damage to a major duct during lactation, and will usually close spontaneously if there is no distal obstruction in the duct.

2. A mammary sinus reflects inadequate drainage of an abscess, or follows drainage of an abscess in a breast affected by duct ectasia (or tuberculosis in very rare cases). The tract is defined with methylene blue injection and excised. In cases of tuberculosis, the appropriate chemotherapy is given.

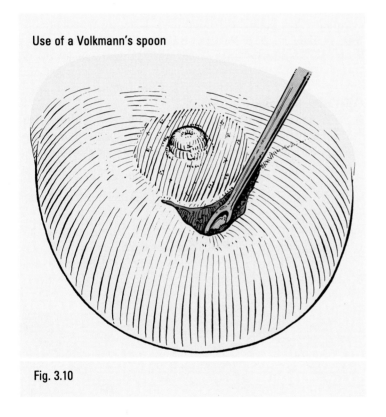

Use of a Volkmann's spoon

Fig. 3.10

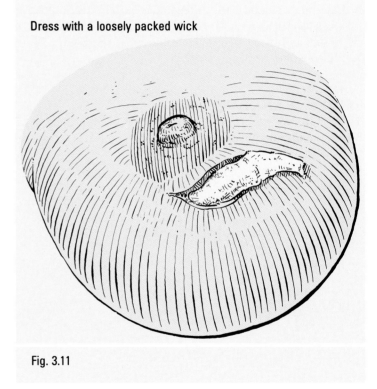

Dress with a loosely packed wick

Fig. 3.11

Microdochectomy

This operation is indicated for patients with a blood-stained discharge from the nipple which derives from a single duct.

PREOPERATIVE ASSESSMENT

1. Discover if pressure on just one point around the areolar elicits a blood-stained discharge; this would indicate that only a single duct is involved. The site is marked on the skin.
2. Ascertain whether there is an associated lump in the breast.
3. Are mammography or a ductogram required to establish the diagnosis?
4. Submit a smear of the discharge for cytology.
5. A bloody discharge from both nipples may occur during pregnancy, but will usually stop spontaneously.

RELEVANT ANATOMY

This is fully covered on pages 3.2 and 3.9 in Management of Breast Lumps and Mastectomy.

An intraduct lesion causes bleeding into a single duct, and this can be expressed by pressure over the ampulla and lobe of the affected duct.

OPERATION
Preparation

The patient is placed in a supine position, and the skin cleansed and draped. After applying pressure to the marked area to elicit discharge from the nipple (Fig. 3.12) a probe is then placed into the duct from which the discharge came (Fig. 3.13).

Incision

A small elliptical incision is made in the nipple, around the affected duct, and extended radially onto the breast for 2–3 cm.

Operative technique

1. The skin edges are gently retracted with skin hooks and the incision is deepened to allow dissection of the duct with scissors.

2. A strong circumferential tie will secure the probe in the duct (Fig. 3.14) or, alternatively, the end of the duct with the probe inside is grasped by an Allis' or Littlewood's tissue-holding forceps.

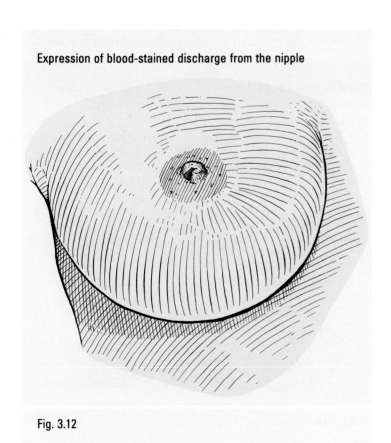

Expression of blood-stained discharge from the nipple

Fig. 3.12

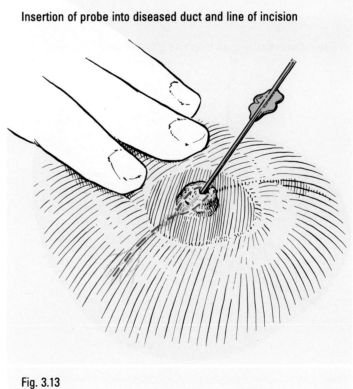

Insertion of probe into diseased duct and line of incision

Fig. 3.13

3. Whilst feeling for the probe, the duct is then further dissected from the surrounding tissue (Fig. 3.15), but not divided. Careful palpatation at this stage may reveal an intraduct lesion.

4. With traction applied to the duct, the secretory tissue is drawn into view, and a generous cuff of the affected lobe is excised *en bloc* with the duct (Fig. 3.16).

Probe secured with ligature

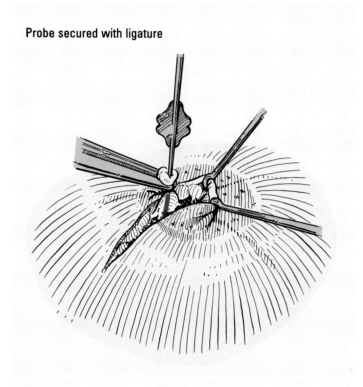

Fig. 3.14

Sharp dissection is used to excise affected duct

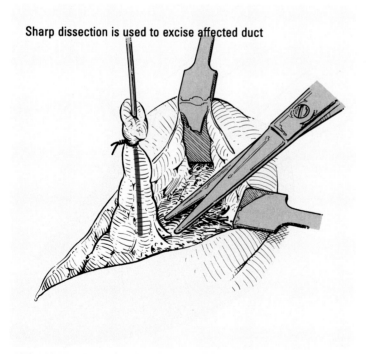

Fig. 3.15

5. Haemostasis is secured.

Wound closure and dressing

1. The breast tissue is repaired with a few interrupted catgut sutures, and a small drain is inserted if there is oozing. The skin is closed with fine interrupted or subcuticular sutures and a dry dressing applied.

2. Opening the excised duct usually reveals the lesion and, whatever the result, the entire specimen is sent for histological examination.

POSTOPERATIVE CARE

If a drain has not been inserted the patient is discharged on the day following surgery. If a drain is present it is removed after 24 hours and the patient discharged on the day after its removal. The sutures remain for a week.

SPECIAL OPERATIVE HAZARDS

1. Excision of the wrong duct. To avoid this it is essential that discharge is elicited from the duct in the theatre, and that the probe is inserted immediately into the duct. Preoperative marking of the position of the affected duct is helpful in localizing it, but the orifices on the summit of the nipple are so close together that this alone is sometimes insufficient. If the discharge cannot be elicited in the theatre, the operation should be postponed. It is wise to prevent anyone, including the patient, from expressing the discharge on the day of the operation.

2. Failure to cannulate the duct, despite it being clearly seen, will require a radial incision to be made from the nipple over the line of the discharging duct, and a wedge of tissue to be excised. Ensure that the tissue under the point which elicits discharge is included. During the dissection the duct may be obvious from its intraduct lesion.

COMPLICATIONS

1. Haematoma due to a wound infection.
2. Mammary duct fistula.
3. Unsuspected invasive intraduct carcinoma; this must be treated on its own merits, with further excisional surgery and/or adjuvant treatment as indicated.

Resected specimen

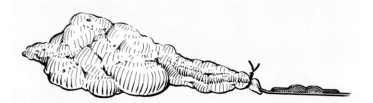

Fig. 3.16

Mastectomy

Many carcinomas of the breast can be removed by local conservative surgery, but centrally placed tumours should be removed by mastectomy, as should large ulcerating lesions and those with extensive skin involvement. Bilateral mastectomy may be indicated for multicentric lobular carcinoma. Axillary lymph node clearance may be facilitated by the division of the pectoralis minor muscle (modified radical mastectomy, after Patey), which originates from the third to fifth ribs and is inserted onto the coracoid process of the scapula.

PREOPERATIVE ASSESSMENT
1. Question whether a mastectomy is the best option for treatment.
2. Preoperative mammography should be used.

3. A histological diagnosis is mandatory prior to embarking upon a mastectomy. This may be performed using a Trucut biopsy, aspiration cytology, or an open biopsy (see pages 3.2 and 3.10); the latter can be carried out under the same anaesthetic as the operation and submitted to frozen section.
4. Are the axillary lymph nodes enlarged?
5. Sympathetic counselling is very important.

RELEVANT ANATOMY
The female breast is a glandular organ, roughly hemispherical in shape, with a pigmented areola at its apex from which the nipple arises centrally. Within the breast, the glandular tissue is imbedded in fat and divided into approximately 15–20 lobes

Anatomy of breast

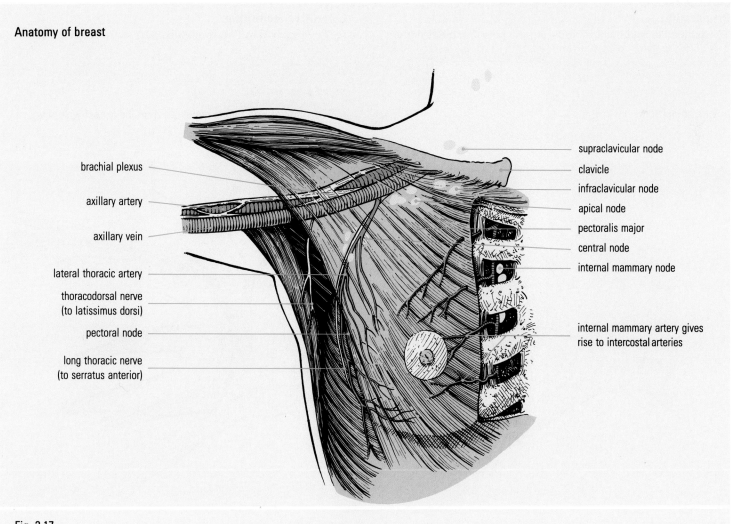

brachial plexus

axillary artery

axillary vein

lateral thoracic artery

thoracodorsal nerve
(to latissimus dorsi)

pectoral node

long thoracic nerve
(to serratus anterior)

supraclavicular node

clavicle

infraclavicular node

apical node

pectoralis major

central node

internal mammary node

internal mammary artery gives
rise to intercostal arteries

Fig. 3.17

each draining into a duct which reaches the skin at the nipple.

The breast is situated in the superficial fascia of the anterior thoracic wall, and despite large variations in the dimensions of the breast, its base has a fairly constant size; overlying the second to sixth ribs, and extending from the lateral border of the sternum to the midaxillary line (Fig. 3.17). The axillary tail extends upward and lateral into the axilla, and is closely related to the nerve supply of latissimus dorsi (the thoraco-dorsal nerve) and serratus anterior (the long thoracic nerve of Bell).

The arterial supply is derived from perforating branches of the internal mammary and intercostal arteries, with large vessels arising from the second and third intercostal spaces, and with an additional supply from the lateral thoracic artery.

Lymphatic drainage is via subareolar and submammary plexuses to nodes along the internal mammary chain medially, and to the pectoral axillary nodes laterally, which drain via the central and apical groups to the supraclavicular and cervical nodes. Seventy-five per cent of the lymphatic drainage from the breast is to the ipselateral axilla. The superior part of the breast drains to the infraclavicular and supraclavicular nodes and thence to the deep cervical nodes. Inferiorly, lymphatic drainage is through the abdominal wall and diaphragm to mediastinal nodes. There is free lymphatic communication across the midline between the two breasts.

OPERATION
Preparation
The patient should be placed in a supine position, tilted slightly away from the surgeon and the ipselateral arm extended at the elbow and abducted on an arm board. If the arm is wrapped after preparation of the skin, its position can be altered during the operation to facilitate dissection of the axilla.

If a biopsy has not been completed, an open biopsy should be performed and the specimen submitted to frozen section. This involves making an incision over and then into the lump, removing a specimen of diseased tissue which is sent fresh for immediate examination. The wound is closed over a swab; ensure that the scrub nurse is aware that you have done this. If the result is malignant, after the wound has been closed all instruments, gloves and drapes should be replaced to prevent implantation of tumour cells into the mastectomy incision. If there is an intraduct or *in situ* carcinoma, a wider excision usually provides adequate treatment.

A permanent marker is used to mark out the skin flaps. These are planned to allow their primary apposition, although this must not be at the expense of adequate clearance of the tumour which should be 5 cm from the tumour margin.

Incision
Make an elliptical incision centred along a line lying transversely across the chest which includes the nipple and areola. This may need to be adjusted according to the site and size of the tumour (Fig. 3.18).

Operative technique
1. The upper skin flap is mobilized by sharp dissection, using a

Line of incision

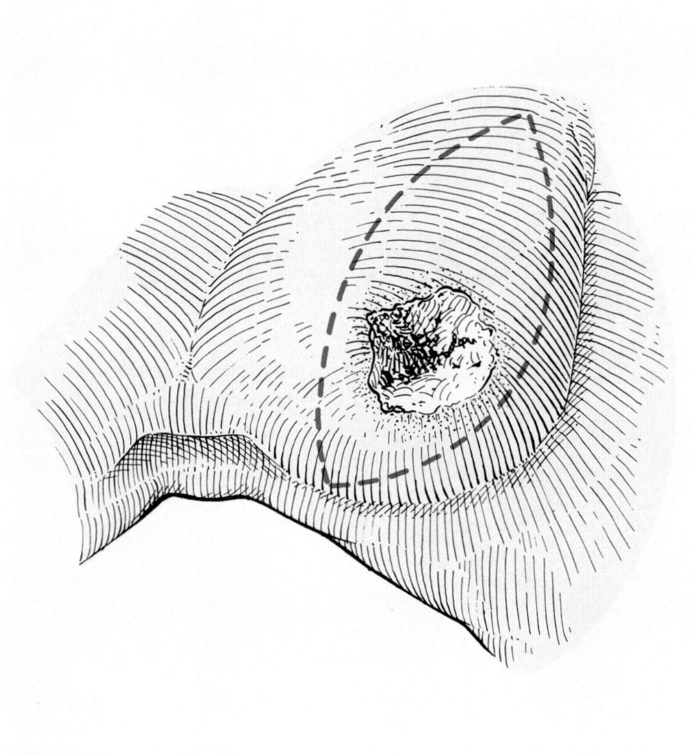

Fig. 3.18

The superior skin flap is mobilized from the breast with sharp dissection

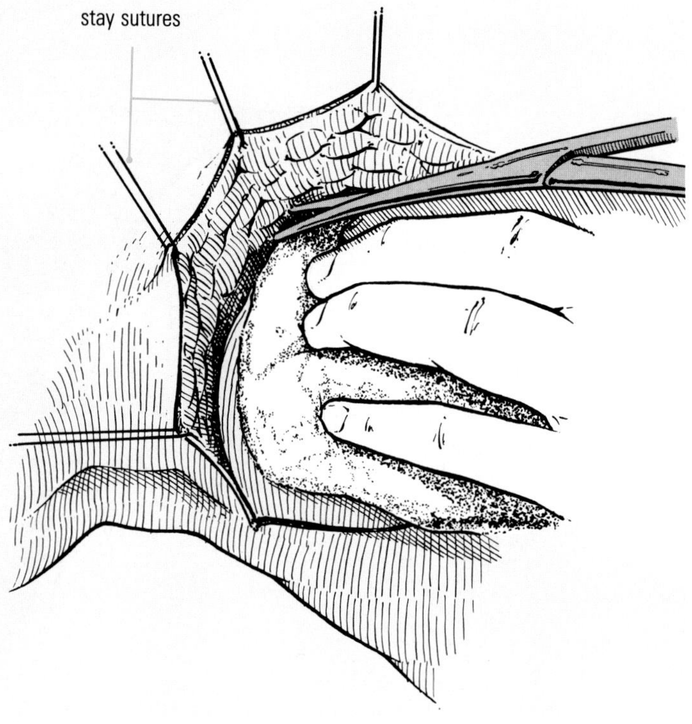

stay sutures

Fig. 3.19

knife or scissors, through the subcutaneous fat in a plane between the skin and the breast tissue until the second intercostal space is reached; sharp straight Mayo scissors are particularly useful for this subcutaneous dissection. The flaps, which should be at least 5 mm thick to prevent devascularization, are held up vertically with stay sutures or tissue forceps (Fig. 3.19). Care must be taken to avoid buttonhole damage to the skin.

2. The lower flap is similarly mobilized until the chest wall is reached, usually at the level of the sixth intercostal space.

3. Starting medially, the breast tissue is now dissected off the anterior thoracic wall, using a mixture of sharp dissection with a knife and blunt dissection with a finger or swab. The breast is lifted and retracted laterally and the large perforating arterial branches are picked up with a clip and ligated (Fig. 3.20). Any muscle which is adherent to the tumour must be excised; it is important not to cut across the tumour. The dissected breast tissue is then placed in a polythene bag that is secured with a ligature to aid in handling and avoid implantation of cancer cells.

4. Laterally, the dissection continues until the axillary tail is reached. This is then mobilized from the overlying skin and underlying musculature. The lower axillary nodes are removed *en bloc*, with ligation of remaining tissues at the apex of the dissection since the contained vessels retract away when divided.

5. With extensive axillary disease the axillary contents are removed up to the level of the axillary vein, and this may be facilitated by division of the pectoralis minor muscle. Care must be taken to avoid the nerve supply to serratus anterior and latissimus dorsi; both are closely applied to the lateral chest wall, which forms the medial border of the axilla (Fig. 3.21). At the apex of the axilla, the axillary vein is encountered before the artery or brachial plexus. This marks the upper limit of the dissection.

6. When removed, a large silk suture placed through the axillary tail will help the pathologists to orientate the specimen; clearly label any separate axillary lymph nodes. Meticulous haemostasis is secured with suture ligation and cautious use of diathermy.

Wound closure
1. Fine suction drains are placed into the axilla and under the superior flap (Fig. 3.22).
2. The skin is closed with interrupted 3/0 nylon sutures, following a rule of halves (Fig. 3.22). Undue tension must be avoided, and if the skin cannot be closed despite mobilization caudally and cranially, a split-skin graft can be applied to the defect (see section on skin grafting).

POSTOPERATIVE CARE
The patient is allowed up the next day. The drains are removed

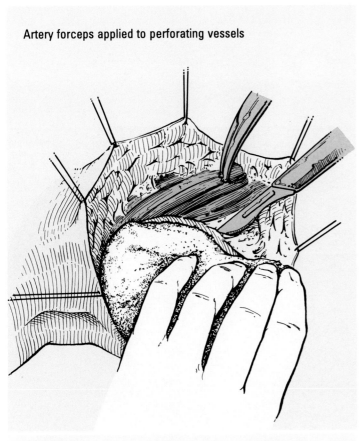

Artery forceps applied to perforating vessels

Fig. 3.20

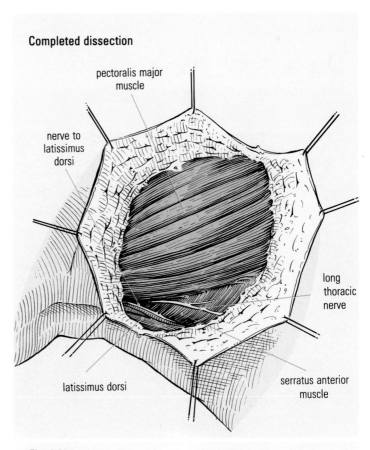

Completed dissection

pectoralis major muscle

nerve to latissimus dorsi

long thoracic nerve

latissimus dorsi

serratus anterior muscle

Fig. 3.21

once they have stopped draining; the sutures remain for 12 days. During the recovery period gentle exercise is encouraged.

By the time the patient is discharged she should be able to raise the ipselateral arm vertically, abduct the arm to 90°, and place that hand on the occiput. Before leaving hospital the patient should be given a foam breast prosthesis (Fig. 3.23), and later supplied with a gel filled prosthesis designed specifically for her (Fig. 3.24). Adjuvant chemotherapy or radiotherapy may be indicated.

Position of suction drains

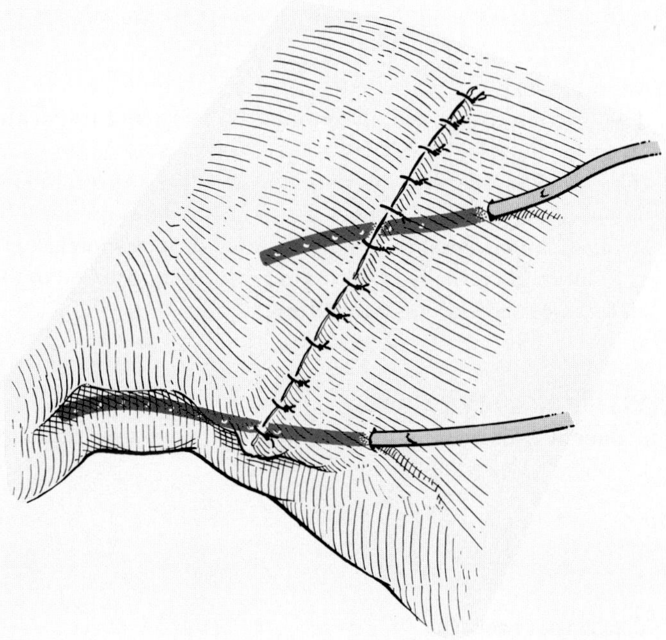

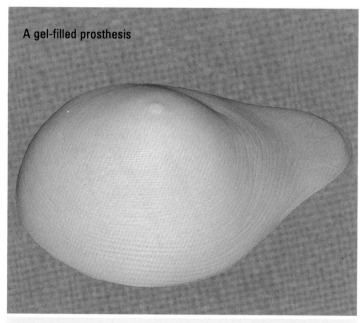

Fig. 3.22

SPECIAL OPERATIVE HAZARDS

1. Ischaemia of the skin flaps occurs if they are cut too thin or the wound is closed under tension.
2. Damage to the axillary vein.
3. Damage to the nerve supply to latissimus dorsi or serratus anterior; the former would cause weakness in extension of the arm, particularly from the flexed position, while the latter results in winging of the scapula.
4. If the axillary contents are removed, the intercostobrachial nerve (T2) is divided causing an area of anaesthesia over the medial aspect of the upper arm.

COMPLICATIONS

1. Haematoma.
2. Seroma under the flaps. This results from either an occluded drain, which should be removed, or when the collection does not discharge down the drain track; aspiration will promote adhesion of the flaps to the underlying chest wall in such cases.
3. A lymphocele of the axilla should only be aspirated if it is tense and uncomfortable; usually it will subside spontaneously.
4. Lymphoedema of the arm occurs particularly in patients who have had an axillary node dissection, lymphatic permeation by a tumour, and loco-regional adjuvant radiotherapy.
5. Local recurrence due to inadequate clearance of the tumour, or tumour cell implantation during surgery.
6. Psychological stigma of disfigurement; the patient may request reconstructive breast surgery, this should not be performed at the time of mastectomy but electively at a later date by a plastic surgeon.

A foam breast prosthesis

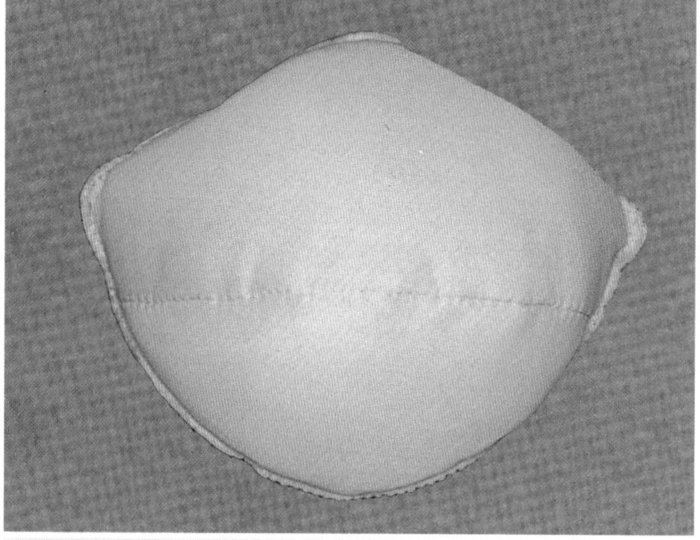

Fig. 3.23

A gel-filled prosthesis

Fig. 3.24

4

Hepatobiliary Surgery
including Spleen and Pancreas

Cholecystectomy

PREOPERATIVE ASSESSMENT

1. Confirm the presence of gall-stones with ultrasound or oral cholecystography.
2. Exclude conditions that mimic gall-stones (e.g. peptic ulcer or hiatus hernia).
3. Encourage the obese to lose weight prior to the operation and smokers to stop.
4. A history of jaundice or abnormal liver function tests indicate that exploration of the common bile duct is likely.
5. Start antithrombotic prophylaxis, and stop females taking oral contraceptives at least 1 month preoperatively.
6. Emergency exploration is required for cases of peritonitis from gangrenous cholecystitis or torsion of the gall bladder.

RELEVANT ANATOMY

The anatomy of the biliary tree and the porta hepatis is variable. Therefore, the normal arrangement will be described first, followed by the more common variations.

The gall bladder comprises a fundus, body and neck. In the presence of gall bladder disease the neck may be dilated; it is then referred to as Hartmann's pouch.

The cystic duct arises from the neck of the gall bladder and passes medially, joining the common hepatic duct to form the common bile duct (CBD). Within the cystic duct lies the spiral valve of Heister which can interfere with the passage of the cholangiography cannula.

The cystic artery arises from the right hepatic artery and

Relevant anatomy

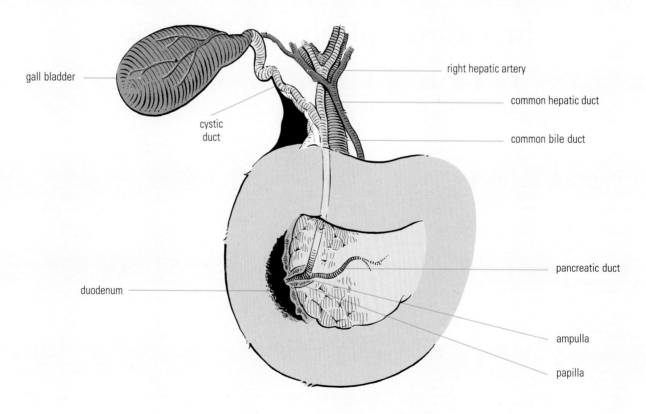

Fig. 4.1

runs above the cystic duct to supply the gall bladder (Fig. 4.1).

A rudimentary fold of mesentery envelopes the gall bladder and attaches it to the liver.

The cystic duct, cystic artery and gall bladder mesentery may vary from the above descriptions in a number of ways:

1. The cystic duct may either join the right hepatic duct or run alongside the common hepatic duct and join it within the head of the pancreas. Sometimes it may be short, and when traction is applied to the gall bladder the CBD may be tented up, mistaken for the cystic duct and inadvertently divided. Small ducts may drain from the liver substance directly into the gall bladder. Very rarely, the cystic duct may join the left hepatic duct or the duodenum directly.

2. The cystic artery may arise from the hepatic artery, or an accessory right hepatic artery which itself arises from the superior mesenteric artery. A tortuous right hepatic artery may be mistaken for the cystic artery and ligated.

3. The gall bladder mesentery may be long and predispose to torsion, or be non-existent (an intra-hepatic gall bladder).

OPERATION
Preparation
Ensure that the patient is placed on a table suitable for taking X-rays, and that the table is tilted 10° to the right to improve operative exposure and to prevent the CBD being superimposed on the spine during cholangiography. The towels are sewn to the skin with silk, since towel clips may obscure the cholangiogram.

Incision
The approach can be by a midline, a right paramedian or a right subcostal (Kocher) incision (see the Introduction) depending on the surgeon's personal preference and previous incisions.

Operative technique
1. Perform a laparotomy (see page 5.2), paying particular attention to the duodenum, caecum and oesophageal hiatus.

2. In difficult cases, break the seal between the liver and the subphrenic space by passing a hand behind the liver and then inserting a wet pack posterior to the liver to lift it forwards.

3. Cholecystectomy can be performed by either the antegrade or retrograde method. The latter approach is advised for difficult cases (e.g. fibrotic gall bladder with dense adhesions, or acutely inflamed gall bladder).

4. Divide any adhesions between the gall bladder and the duodenum or hepatic flexure (Fig. 4.2). The assistant's left hand is then placed over a wet pack covering the stomach and small bowel, with the index and middle finger astride the porta hepatis, and gentle traction is applied to draw the duodenum towards the left iliac fossa.

5. Grasp the fundus of the gall bladder with either a Moynihan clamp or sponge-holding forceps. Apply upward traction and then place a second clamp on Hartmann's pouch.

Division of adhesions between gall bladder and duodenum

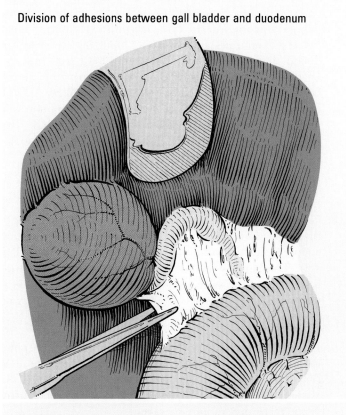

Fig. 4.2

Ligation and division of cystic artery

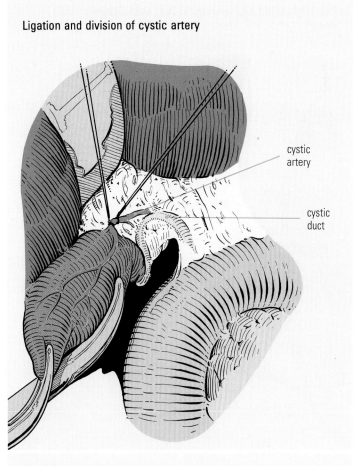

cystic artery

cystic duct

Fig. 4.3

4.3

6. Traction on the gall bladder tents up the cystic duct, exposing its insertion into the common hepatic duct. Divide the peritoneum over the cystic duct with scissors and identify the cystic duct and artery by blunt dissection with a dental roll; the anatomy of this area is variable (see the anatomy section in this chapter) and no structure should be divided until the anatomy has been defined. Having identified the cystic duct, follow it to the common bile duct and ensure that the T-junction is visualized. The anatomy should be confirmed by peroperative cholangiography.

7. Divide the cystic artery between ligatures (Fig. 4.3).

8. Gently palpate the cystic duct and milk back any stones into the gall bladder before ligating the duct distally and placing a loose ligature around the proximal part of the duct (Fig. 4.4). The anterior part of the duct is then opened with scissors, a culture swab of the bile taken and a probe passed down the lumen towards the CBD (Fig. 4.5); this may be difficult because of the spiral valves, or rarely, a stone.

9. Pass a cholangiography cannula (e.g. Stoke on Trent) into the lumen of the cystic duct and secure it with the loose tie (Fig. 4.6). To prevent the introduction of air bubbles in the system, which can be mistaken for stones on the cholangiogram, three precautions are taken:

(i) flush continuously with saline whilst inserting the cannula
(ii) take care when connecting the syringe containing the contrast medium not to introduce air;
(iii) avoid drawing back on the syringe as this may suck air into the CBD through the ampulla.

Insertion of probe into cystic duct

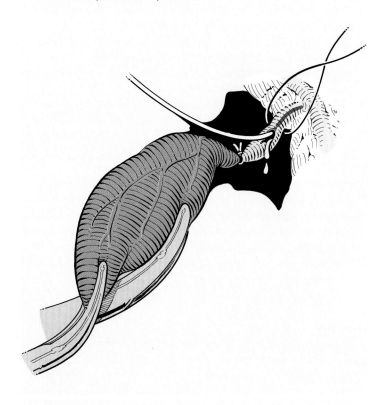

Fig. 4.5

Ligature around proximal cystic duct, with ligation of duct distally

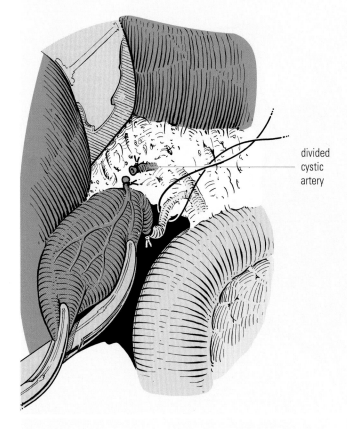

divided cystic artery

Fig. 4.4

Stoke-on-Trent cholangiography cannula

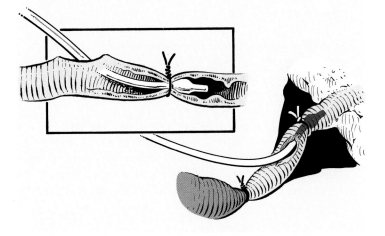

Fig. 4.6

4.4

10. Remove all radio-opaque objects (e.g. swabs and retractors) from the operative field which is covered with a sterile towel. It is usual to take three films after injecting 2, 5 and 8 ml of iodine contrast medium (e.g. 30% Urografin). Ensure co-ordination with the anaesthetist so that there is no ventilatory movement during exposure of the film.

11. Whilst awaiting the X-rays, the surgeon can dissect the gall bladder from the gall bladder fossa by division of the peritoneum which forms the mesentery of the gall bladder (Fig. 4.7). Use diathermy on small vessels in the mesentery and bleeding from the gall bladder bed; the gall bladder should now be attached by the cystic duct alone.

12. Inspect the peroperative cholangiograms (Fig. 4.8) to confirm the perceived anatomy. Important features to look for include:
    (i) no filling defects in the CBD, especially on the early films (as increasing volumes of contrast medium can obscure a small stone);
    (ii) normal calibre of the CBD (<9mm);
    (iii) adequate filling of the hepatic ducts;
    (iv) free flow into the duodenum with tapering of the lumen;
    A concave filling defect is suggestive of a stone. Sometimes contrast medium does not flow into the duodenum although no filling defect is seen. The X-ray should then be repeated with the concurrent administration of 20mg of Buscopan (hyoscine butylbromide) intravenously to relax the sphincter of Oddi.

13. Once a satisfactory peroperative cholangiogram has been obtained, divide the tie securing the cannula, remove the cannula and ligate or transfix the cystic duct with an absorbable suture. The cystic duct is then divided. and the gall bladder removed (Fig. 4.9).

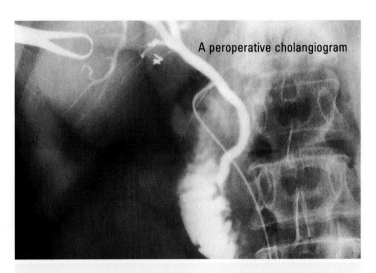

A peroperative cholangiogram

Fig. 4.8

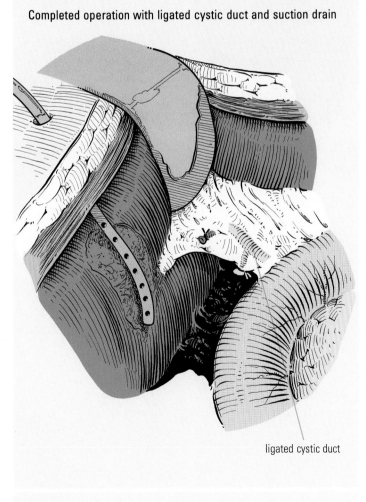

Completed operation with ligated cystic duct and suction drain

ligated cystic duct

Fig. 4.9

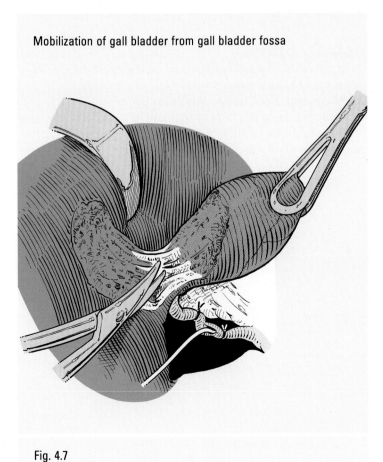

Mobilization of gall bladder from gall bladder fossa

Fig. 4.7

14. In difficult cases, the gall bladder is mobilized fundus first. This retrograde removal makes clarification of the anatomy easier. If the anatomy cannot be defined due to severe inflammation, a Foley catheter is inserted into the fundus of the gall bladder (cholecystotomy), brought out through the skin and placed on drainage to decompress the gall bladder (Fig. 4.10). Formal cholecystectomy is performed 14–21 days later when the inflammation has subsided.

Cholecystostomy with Foley catheter

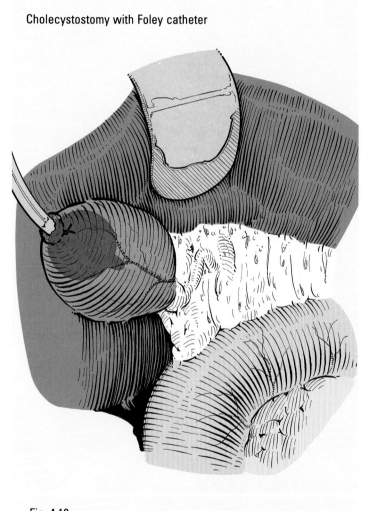

Fig. 4.10

Wound closure

Ensure that haemostasis from the gall bladder bed is secured. A silicone or suction drain is placed to the gall bladder fossa and the abdomen closed with a loop nylon suture and interrupted or subcuticular stitches for the skin.

POSTOPERATIVE CARE

The patient should be given good analgesia without sedation (intercostal blocks) and early chest physiotherapy. Oral fluids can be given from the first postoperative day and the drain is removed if <100 ml of fluid has drained in 24 hours. Occasionally bile may drain, this is usually due to the division of a small biliary radicle in the gall bladder bed or a slipped tie on the cystic duct. If this arises leave the drain *in situ* until the bile leak ceases, or for at least 10 days to form a tract. If there is no distal obstruction the discharge will cease following removal of the drain. The patient is usually allowed home on the fifth postoperative day if there are no complications.

SPECIAL OPERATIVE HAZARDS

1. Damage to the hepatic or common bile ducts most commonly occurs when the surgeon hurries the operation and does not take adequate care to define the anatomy. It can be due either to tenting of the CBD by excessive traction on the gall bladder and mistaking the CBD for the cystic duct, or from blind application of clamps to control bleeding. This should be controlled by packing and applying pressure for 5 minutes. When the pack is removed the bleeding point can be seen and dealt with without damage to surrounding structures.

2. Damage to the hepatic artery.

COMPLICATIONS

1. Haemorrhage from a slipped tie on the cystic duct, or from the gall bladder fossa.

2. Biliary leak (see Postoperative Care).

3. Missed stone in bile duct or remnant of cystic duct which can cause jaundice or cholangitis.

4. Biliary stricture from damage to the biliary tree.

Exploration of the Common Bile Duct
(including transduodenal sphincterotomy and choledochoduodenostomy)

This procedure is indicated for patients known to have stones in the common bile duct (CBD), or who have been shown on peroperative cholangiography to have stones or no flow of contrast medium into the duodenum, despite the administration of Buscopan (hyoscine butylbromide). Peroperative cholangiography is essential to ascertain the anatomy of the biliary system and to demonstrate the number and position of gall-stones.

PREOPERATIVE ASSESSMENT
1. Ensure correct diagnosis and rule out other conditions which cause jaundice (e.g. carcinoma of the head of the pancreas, hepatitis or haemolysis).
2. If the patient is jaundiced correct any clotting abnormalities and ensure a good peroperative diuresis with mannitol to protect renal function.
3. Commence antibiotic prophylaxis.

RELEVANT ANATOMY
The bile canaliculi drain into the bile duct tributaries, which run to the porta hepatis and coalesce to form the right and left hepatic ducts. These join to form the common hepatic duct which runs along the free edge of the lesser omentum. The common hepatic duct is joined by the cystic duct to form the CBD which passes behind the first part of the duodenum and enters the head of the pancreas. The CBD is joined by the pancreatic duct within the pancreas and passes through the wall of the duodenum, opening into it as the papilla of Vater (contrary to popular belief, Vater did not describe an ampulla). Just prior to passing through the wall of the duodenum, the lumen is narrowed by the surrounding smooth muscle sphincter of Oddi (Fig. 4.11). The diameter of the CBD normally has an upper limit of 9–10mm.

The lesser omentum also contains the hepatic artery, medial to the CBD, which divides into right and left branches, and the

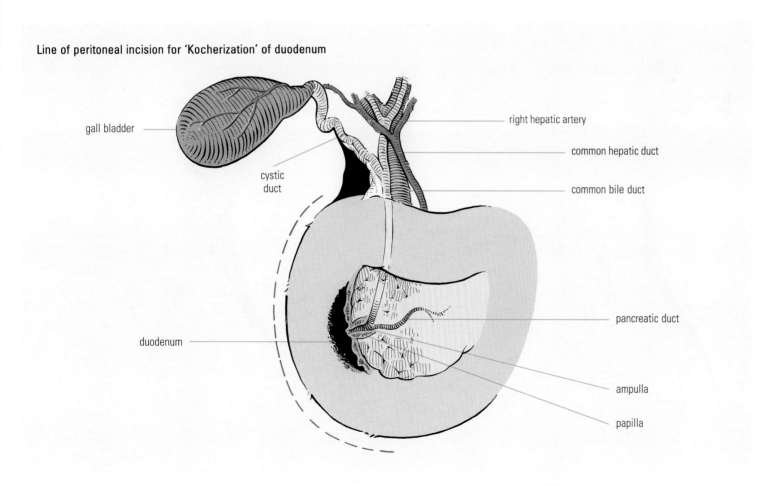

Line of peritoneal incision for 'Kocherization' of duodenum

gall bladder

cystic duct

duodenum

right hepatic artery

common hepatic duct

common bile duct

pancreatic duct

ampulla

papilla

Fig. 4.11

Choledochotomy between stay sutures

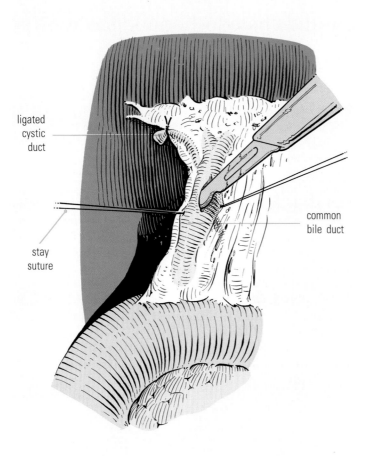

ligated
cystic
duct

stay
suture

common
bile duct

Fig. 4.12

portal vein which lies behind and medial to the CBD.

Anatomical anomalies of the cystic duct are described on page 4.3 in Cholecystectomy. Congenital dilatation of the CBD (choledocal cyst) is rare and may occur in association with distal atresia.

OPERATION
Preparation and incision
This is covered on page 4.3 in Cholecystectomy.

Operative technique
1. Perform a cholecystectomy with peroperative cholangiogram (see page 4.3).

2. Mobilize the duodenum by dividing the peritoneum lateral to the duodenum with scissors ('Kocherization') (Fig. 4.11). Once mobilized the left hand is placed behind the duodenum and the head of the pancreas and CBD palpated.

3. Expose the supraduodenal portion of the CBD by division of its overlying peritoneum and blunt dissection with a

Enlarge choledochotomy with Pott's scissors

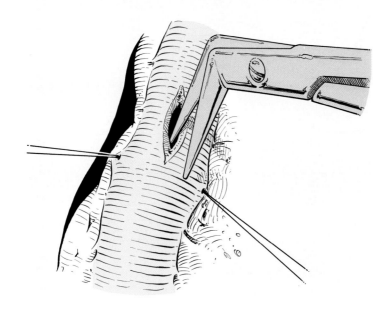

Fig. 4.13

Retrieval of stone with forceps

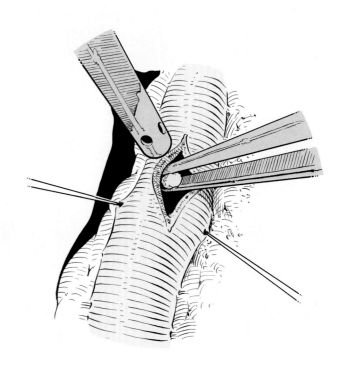

Fig. 4.14

dental roll. A venous plexus (of Saint) surrounds the CBD and this should be carefully diathermized if it is damaged (excessive use of diathermy can cause damage to the CBD).

4. Select a suitable section of the supraduodenal CBD (approximately 2cm long) for exploration. To confirm the anatomy, if there is any uncertainty, aspirate the duct with a 25Fr gauge needle; bile should be withdrawn. Place one stay suture on each side of the CBD to tent it up and open it with a knife (Fig. 4.12). The opening is extended to approximately 2cm with Pott's scissors (Fig. 4.13) and a culture swab of the bile is taken. Occasionally a stone will appear in the opening (Fig. 4.14) and can be lifted out. The stones are usually removed however by either flushing or instrumentation. It is important that stones are not allowed to pass up into the liver during the operation. To prevent this insert a dental pledget with a retaining suture into the proximal duct and place the patient in a head-up position.

5. Insert a 12Fr gauge Jacques catheter into the CBD and flush it rapidly with saline. The catheter is passed both proximally and distally to dislodge debris and calculi; stones commonly lodge at the lower end of the CBD and these are the most difficult to remove.

6. To remove stones by instrumentation, hold Desjardin's forceps in the right hand and pass them into the CBD whilst holding the lower end of the CBD and pancreatic head with the left hand and applying gentle traction downwards. When the stone can be felt against the forceps they are opened and advanced to grasp the stone, which is then extracted (Fig. 4.15).

7. Check that all stones have been removed by using a choledochoscope to visualize the interior of the CBD (Fig. 4.16). Forceps can be attached to this instrument and used to grasp stones while they are being directly viewed. There is also a channel to admit a Fogarty catheter which is passed beyond the stone, the balloon inflated and then the catheter together with the choledochoscope are withdrawn.

8. If a choledochoscope is not available, perform a further cholangiogram having inserted a small Foley catheter into the CBD. After inflating the balloon to keep it in place, inject contrast medium down the catheter and take the X-rays.

9. Pass a series of Bake's dilators with great care along the duct into the duodenum.

Exploration of distal common bile duct with Desjardin's forceps

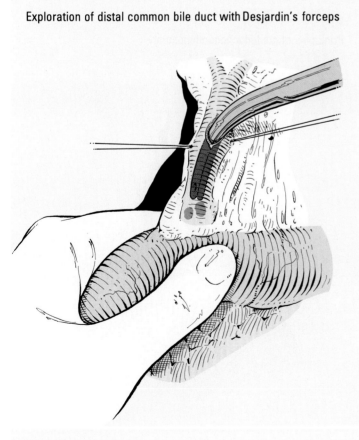

Fig. 4.15

The use of a choledochoscope

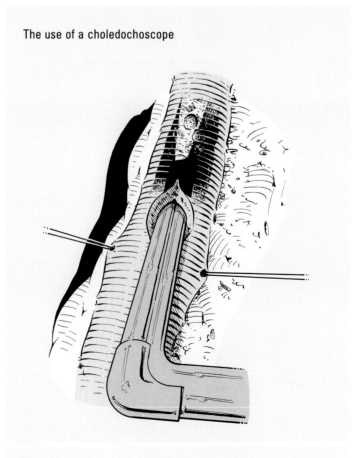

Fig. 4.16

4.9

Insertion of a guttered T-tube

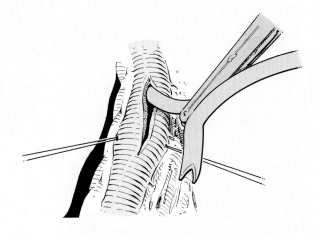

Sphincterotomy of duodenal papilla

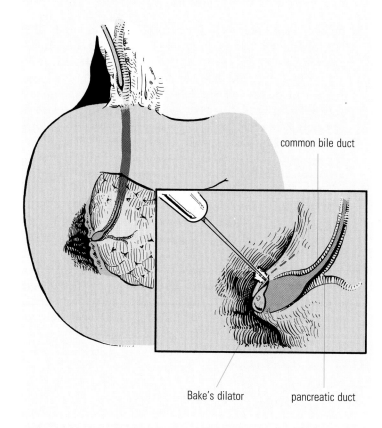

common bile duct

Bake's dilator

pancreatic duct

Fig. 4.19

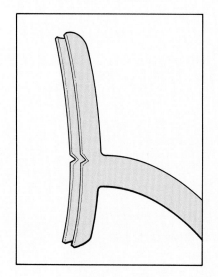

Fig. 4.17

Principles of choledochoduodenostomy

Closure of choledochotomy around T-tube

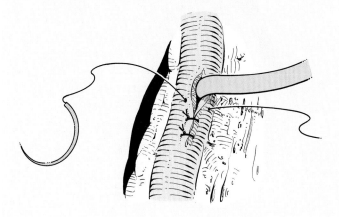

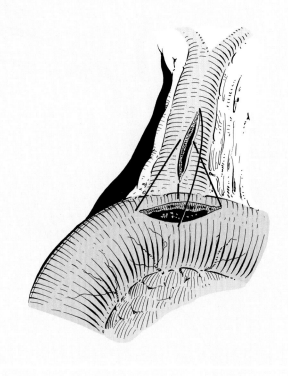

Fig. 4.18

Fig. 4.20

10. Once all the stones have been removed, close the CBD over a 12–16Fr gauge T-tube with interrupted absorbable sutures (e.g. 4/0 catgut) to appose mucosa to mucosa without narrowing the duct (Figs 4.17 and 4.18). Trim the T-tube to form a gutter as shown (inset to Fig. 4.17). Closure is tested for integrity by flushing the T-tube with saline and any leaks closed with further sutures.

11. Ensure haemostasis is secured and place a silicone drain down to the gall bladder fossa.

12. To perform a transduodenal sphincterotomy, pass a Bake's dilator through the choledochotomy down the CBD, and open the second part of the duodenum longitudinally with cutting diathermy.

13. Divide the papilla and underlying lower sphincter superiorly by cutting down onto the olive head of the Bake's dilator for a distance of 1cm with cutting diathermy. This avoids damage to the pancreatic duct and allows the Bake's dilator to pass freely into the duodenum. It is not necessary to insert any stitches into the duodenal mucosa (Fig. 4.19).

14. Close the duodenum longitudinally, not transversely, in two layers with 2/0 Polydioxamone (PDS), ensuring that it is not narrowed.

15. Choledochoduodenostomy is indicated in patients where the CBD obstruction is caused by malignancy, or in elderly patients with impacted stones. It is essential to ensure that the choledochotomy is at least 2.5cm long in order to avoid stenosis, recurrent cholangitis and further stone formation. (Fig. 4.20)

16. Mobilize the duodenum fully to allow the upper aspect of the duodenum to lie against the CBD.

17. Open the duodenum longitudinally and anastomose it to the choledochotomy with interrupted 4/0 PDS so that the final anastomosis is diamond shaped (Fig. 4.21).

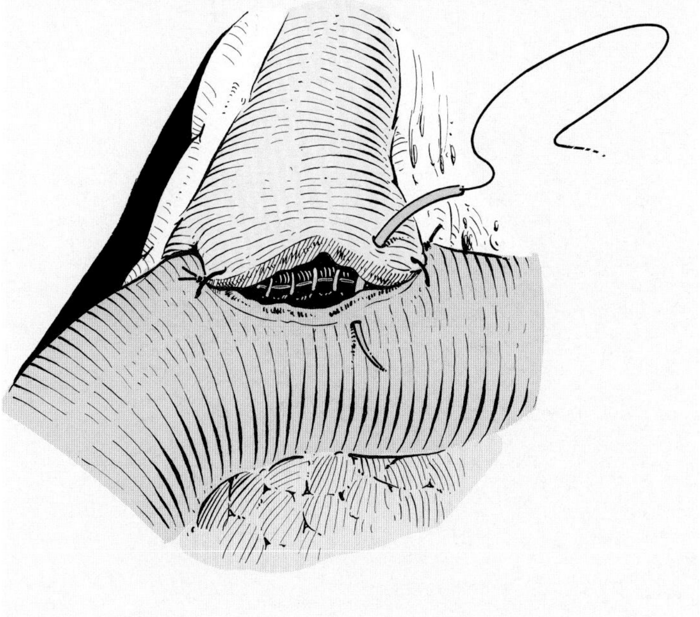

Wound closure

Bring a silicone drain and the T-tube out through separate stab incisions, ensuring that the T-tube leaves by the most direct route as this aids any subsequent instrumentation along the tract. Close the abdomen with continuous loop nylon and the skin with interrupted nylon.

POSTOPERATIVE CARE

Analgesia, physiotherapy and oral fluids are administered as for a cholecystectomy. In the jaundiced patient an adequate urine output must also be maintained. A T-tube cholangiogram is performed after 7–10 days, and if there are no filling defects and free flow into the duodenum, the T-tube is removed on day 10 followed by the silicone drain when drainage has ceased. The patient is then allowed home. Antibiotics are continued if the bile is infected.

SPECIAL OPERATIVE HAZARDS

1. Damage to the biliary tree.
2. Production of a false passage by over zealous instrumentation of the biliary tree. This usually occurs into the retroperitoneal tissues from the distal part of the CBD in a patient with an impacted stone at the lower end of the duct. If it is impossible to remove a stone, transduodenal sphincterotomy or choledochoduodenostomy should be performed.
3. Damage to the hepatic artery or portal vein.

COMPLICATIONS

1. Haemorrhage.
2. Biliary leak either from the incision in the CBD, a slipped tie on the cystic duct, or from the gall bladder fossa. Bile will drain via the silicone drain and the leak will close spontaneously if there is no obstruction of the CBD. Signs of peritonitis are an indication for further surgical exploration.
3. Retained stone seen on the T-tube cholangiogram; this can be dealt with by either ERCP (endoscopic retrograde choledochopancreatography) or by instrumentation along the T-tube tract about 6 weeks postoperatively, the T-tube being left *in situ* until then.
4. Biliary stricture.
5. Cholangitis.
6. Pancreatitis.

Completion of choledochoduodenostomy

Fig. 4.21

Biliary Stricture

Biliary strictures should be dealt with in a specialist unit and only the principles of treatment are outlined in this chapter.

RELEVANT ANATOMY
This is covered on page 4.7 in Exploration of the Common Bile Duct.

OPERATIONS
Resectable short strictures
1. Excise the strictured segment of the bile duct.

2. Mobilize the ends of the resected duct and Kocherize the duodenum until they can be opposed without tension.

3. Perform an end-to-end anastomosis with interrupted Polydioxamone (PDS) sutures over a T-tube, the long arm of which is brought out of the common bile duct below the anastomosis (Figs 4.22 and 4.23).

Resectable long strictures
1. If a primary anastomosis following resection of a stricture cannot be achieved without tension, drain the biliary system into a Roux loop as follows.

2. Divide the jejunum at a convenient point beyond the duodenojejunal flexure and anastomose the proximal cut end of the bowel to the side of the distal segment about 60cm beyond the point of division.

3. Use the distal cut end of the jejunum to re-establish biliary drainage by anastomosing the proximal biliary remnant (usually the common hepatic duct) to the side of the Roux loop just proximal to the cut end; this cut end is oversewn. If there is no common hepatic duct remaining, the divided right and left hepatic ducts can be opposed to the mucosa of the Roux loop using specially designed transhepatic stents which are inserted into the hepatic ducts and brought out through the liver parenchyma (mucosal graft of Smith). Sustained gentle traction on the stents brings about mucosa-

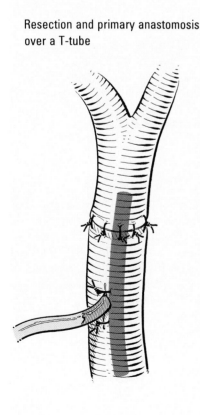

Resection and primary anastomosis over a T-tube

Fig. 4.22

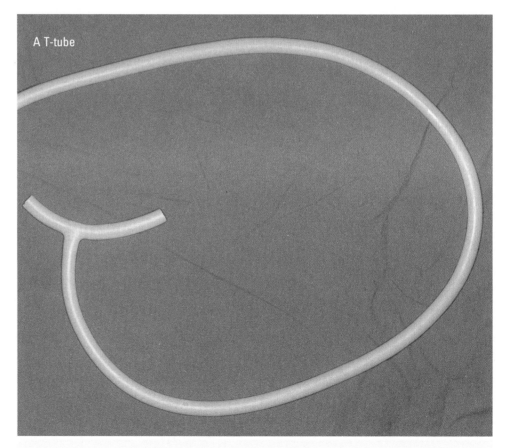

A T-tube

Fig. 4.23

Detail of mucosal graft

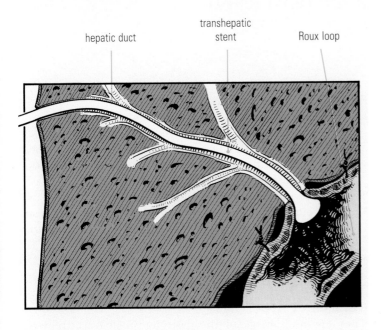

hepatic duct   transhepatic stent   Roux loop

Fig. 4.24

Mucosal graft technique of biliary drainage

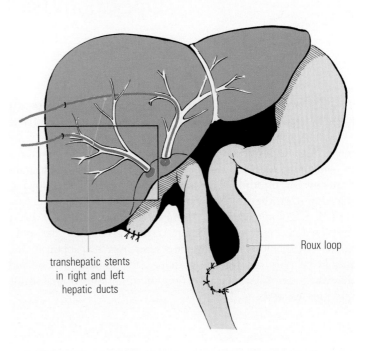

transhepatic stents in right and left hepatic ducts

Roux loop

Fig. 4.25

to-mucosa opposition; no sutures are inserted into the mucosa, but the serosa of the Roux loop is tacked to the undersurface of the liver (Figs 4.24 and 4.25).

Unresectable high strictures

1. These are generally malignant and require a palliative biliary bypass to be fashioned clear of the tumour (Longmire's operation). It is difficult to establish good biliary drainage with this operation.

2. Remove the apex of the left lobe of the liver and find a reasonably sized biliary radicle. A cholangiogram is performed via this radicle to ensure that there is communication between the right and left biliary systems (which is usually the case in obstruction).

3. Suture the end of a Roux loop to the cut edge of the liver (Fig. 4.26) ensuring mucosa-to-mucosa contact. Some surgeons insert an infant feeding tube into the divided biliary radicle, and bring it out further down the Roux loop.

4. If there is no communication between the biliary drainage of the left and right halves of the liver, use a second Roux loop to drain the right side.

Longmire's procedure

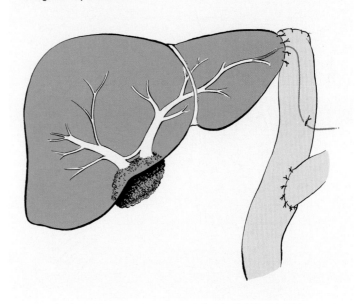

Fig. 4.26

SPECIAL OPERATIVE HAZARDS

1. Failure to find biliary tree.
2. Bleeding from transected liver.

COMPLICATIONS

1. Biliary tract sepsis.
2. Biliary tract stones.
3. Stricture formation.

Operations for Portal Hypertension

The most common indication for surgery in patients with portal hypertension (portal pressure >15cm water) is bleeding from oesophageal varices which has not responded to medical treatment. Although injection sclerotherapy is an effective method of controlling bleeding in most patients, surgery is increasingly required for bleeding from oesophageal ulceration following injection sclerotherapy, gastric varices or bleeding from ectopic sites (e.g. colonic varices). Numerous operations have been described, but nowadays it is important to remember that some of these operations may impede a later liver transplant if this should be required for the patient. Three operations will be described: oesophageal transection, proximal splenorenal shunt and mesocaval shunt.

Oesophageal transection

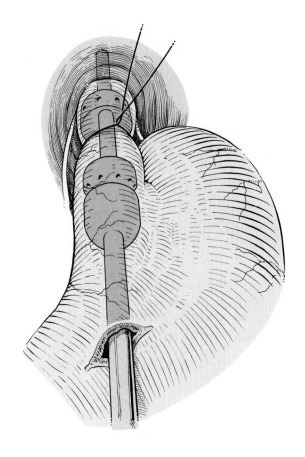

Fig. 4.27

4.14

PREOPERATIVE ASSESSMENT
1. Perform ultrasound, Doppler and angiographic mapping of the portal system anatomy, including if necessary spleno-portography and portal pressure measurements on patients undergoing a shunt operation. Use renal angiography prior to making a splenorenal shunt.
2. Screen serum for hepatitis antigens.
3. Carry out haematological studies (including clotting tests) and give vitamin K, cross-matched blood, fresh frozen plasma and platelets if necessary.
4. Prescribe prophylactic antibiotics.

RELEVANT ANATOMY
The venous drainage of the gastrointestinal tract from the gastro-oesophageal junction to the lower rectum is to the liver via the portal vein. The superior mesenteric vein runs in the root of the mesentery to the right of the superior mesenteric artery. It forms the portal vein by joining the splenic vein which runs from the hilum of the spleen, behind the pancreas, to meet the superior mesenteric vein behind the neck of the pancreas. Caudal to the splenic vein the left renal vein crosses the aorta to drain into the inferior vena cava which lies under the root of the mesentery.

Portal hypertension leads to the development of collaterals between the portal and systemic venous circulations at points where the two meet, clinically the most important site of which is the gastro-oesophageal junction.

OPERATIONS
OESOPHAGEAL TRANSECTION
Although, in theory, oesophageal transection is a simple operation, it can be difficult in those patients who have had chronic injection sclerotherapy since there may be very thickened and haemorrhagic para-oesophageal tissue and a friable oesophagus. It is contra-indicated when there is bleeding from oesophageal ulceration following injection sclerotherapy.

Preparation
Under general anaesthetic the patient is placed supine with slight head-up tilt, and the abdomen and lower chest are cleansed and draped. A nasogastric tube is inserted by the anaesthetist. Ensure that the table is fitted with a crossbar.

Incision
Make a midline incision (see the Introduction). There may be considerable bleeding from the abdominal wall and bleeding points should be cauterized or suture ligated. Insert a self-retaining retractor and retract the sternum upward using the third blade of a Balfour retractor hooked under the crossbar.

Splenorenal shunt

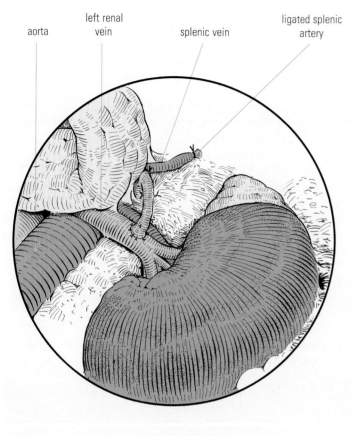

aorta — left renal vein — splenic vein — ligated splenic artery

Fig. 4.28

Operative technique

1. Divide the left triangular ligament so that the left lobe of the liver can be retracted to the right, and then carefully ligate and divide the abnormally thickened serosa which runs across the gastro-oesophageal junction since it will contain numerous collateral vessels. Mobilize the lower 5 cm of the abdominal oesophagus and free the vagal trunks from the oesophageal wall.

2. Make a small longitudinal gastrostomy through the anterior wall of the body of the stomach. Withdraw the nasogastric tube, if it is present, and pass 'sizers' for the anastomotic stapling gun up through the cardia into the oesophagus to determine the largest size of gun that can be used.

3. Pass the appropriately sized gun up into the lower oesophagus and open the anvil. Place a thick silk ligature around the oesophagus just above the oesophagogastric junction (Fig. 4.27) and tie it tightly between the anvil and the staple cartridge of the gun. Care must be taken to avoid incorporating the vagal trunks.

4. Approximate, fire and then unwind and carefully remove the gun. A single complete doughnut of oesophagus which

includes the silk ligature should have been removed by the gun. Close the gastrostomy with two layers of chromic catgut.

5. Inspect the spleen for damage and confirm haemostasis.

Wound closure and dressing
Drainage is not usually necessary. Close the wound with a mass suture technique using monofilament nylon, and interrupted skin sutures. Cover with a waterproof dressing.

PROXIMAL SPLENORENAL SHUNT
Preparation
Under general anaesthesia place the patient supine and cleanse and drape the upper abdomen. Place a small sandbag under the left loin.

Incision
Enter the abdomen through a left subcostal incision (see the Introduction), extended to the right of the midline. Care must be taken to stop all bleeding from blood vessels within the rectus muscle. Ligate and divide the superior epigastric artery and vein.

Operative technique

1. Mobilize the spleen by division of its lateral peritoneal attachments and division and ligation of the short gastric vessels. Divide any attachments to the splenic flexure of the colon (see page 4.28).

2. Dissect out the splenic artery and vein at the hilum of the spleen, and then ligate and divide the artery before dividing the splenic vein between arterial clamps and removing the spleen.

3. Transfix the proximal end of the splenic vein with a silk suture which can be used subsequently to retract the vein whilst it is being mobilized.

4. Mobilize the splenic vein from the tail of the pancreas by ligation and division of the short, friable veins that drain from the pancreas into the splenic vein.

5. Expose the left renal vein lying under the tail of the pancreas and control it with slings. Care must be taken to avoid avulsing the adrenal vein, or a posteriorly sited lumbar vein.

6. Mobilize a sufficient length of the splenic vein to allow an end-to-side splenorenal venous anastomosis to be made without any tension or kinking of the splenic vein.

7. Apply a Satinsky clamp to the side of the renal vein, cut out a segment of the vein wall and make the anastomosis using a continuous non-absorbable suture (e.g. 5/0 Prolene) on the posterior wall and an interrupted non-absorbable suture on the anterior wall (this allows for expansion and contraction of the vein) (Fig. 4.28). Remove the clamps and then measure the fall in portal pressure. This is done by inserting a 21 G needle connected to a pressure transducer into the splenic

4.15

vein and measure the pressure with the anastomosis un-clamped and then clamped.

Wound closure and dressing
Check the position of the nasogastric tube. Drain the area with a large-bore tube drain and close the wound with a mass suture technique using monofilament nylon for all layers, and inter-rupted sutures for the skin. Apply a waterproof dressing.

MESOCAVAL SHUNT
Preparation
Under general anaesthesia place the patient supine and cleanse and drape the entire abdomen.

Incision
Make an upper midline or transverse muscle-cutting incision (see the Introduction) above the umbilicus.

Operative technique
1. Lift the transverse colon, palpate the root of the small bowel mesentery to locate the superior mesenteric artery, and open the peritoneum just to the right of the artery.

Careful dissection through the mesenteric fat will locate the superior mesenteric vein which lies to the right of the artery (Fig. 4.29).

2. Mobilize a length of the vein with some of its branches up to the insertion of the middle colic vein. Slings can be applied around the vein before deciding which segment of this vein will be most suitable for anastomosis to the shunt.

3. Approach the inferior vena cava through the mesentery of the right colon lateral to the superior mesenteric vessels and inferior to the duodenum. If this proves difficult due to a thickened mesentery, the inferior vena cava can be approached by mobilizing the right colon medially and then creating a tunnel through the mesentery for the graft.

4. Perform portal and inferior vena cava pressure measure-ments, if they are not already available, to confirm that there is a sufficient pressure gradient to maintain a shunt.

5. Clean approximately 7 cm of the anterior part of the vena cava so that a Satinsky clamp can be applied and a window of the vein removed.

6. Determine the size of the reinforced Teflon (PTFE, Gore-tex) graft to be used (although in children internal jugular

Exposure of superior mesenteric vein

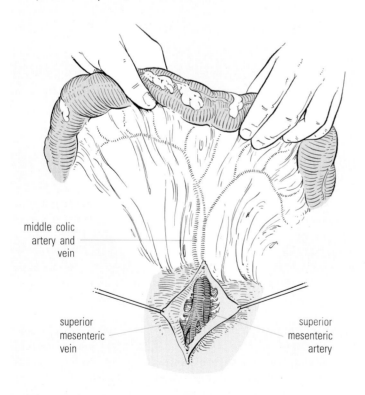

Fig. 4.29

Mesocaval shunt

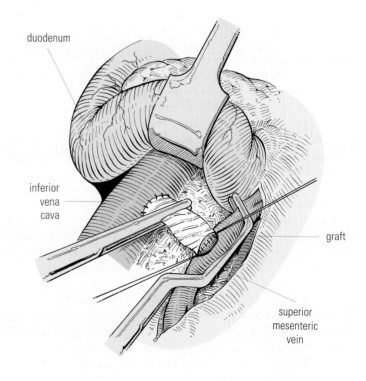

Fig. 4.30

vein is preferred). The size depends on the size of the mesenteric vein, with a 10–14 mm graft being generally used.

7. Remove the reinforced ring at the end of the Teflon graft and anastomose the graft to the vena cava using a continuous 5/0 Teflon or Prolene suture. Fill the graft with heparinized saline, clamp it and then test the anastomosis by releasing the Satinsky clamp.

8. Apply a Satinsky clamp to the appropriate segment of the mesenteric vein, and cut the graft so that it can be anastomosed to the lateral side of the vein and lie without tension or kinking. Remove a small window of vein and again perform the anastomosis with a continuous 5/0 non-absorbable suture; the posterior layer of the anastomosis being performed from the inside of the vein (Fig. 4.30).

9. Once the anastomosis is complete, remove the clamp on the graft and evacuate the air from the graft through its apex with a 21 G needle before removing the clamp on the superior mesenteric vein. The same needle can be used to measure pressures within the graft with and without clamping.

10. Ensure haemostasis has been obtained.

Wound closure and dressing
Close the wound with a mass suture technique using mono-filament nylon for all layers, and interrupted sutures for the skin. Apply a waterproof dressing.

POSTOPERATIVE CARE
Closely monitor the haemodynamic state, hepatic function (including clotting), renal function and the electrolyte balance. Impose a sodium restriction, and ensure the diet following shunt surgery is initially low in protein and gradually increased while being watchful for signs of portosystemic encephalopathy.

SPECIAL OPERATIVE HAZARDS
1. Haemorrhage from raised portal pressure which leads to the vessels becoming distended and easily damaged.
2. Damage to vagal trunks or spleen during oesophageal transection.
3. Damage to the pancreas when performing the spleno-renal shunt.

COMPLICATIONS
1. Intraperitoneal sepsis, hepatic failure from reduced portal flow and recurrent variceal haemorrhage are complications that are liable to occur after all the operations.
2. Anastomotic leakage (rare), anastomotic stricture and oesophageal reflux can occur after oesophageal transection.
3. Transient jaundice (usually disappears within 6 months), portosystemic encephalopathy and shunt thrombosis may follow the shunt operations.

Hepatic Lobectomy

Hepatic resection is indicated for the treatment of some cases of hepatocellular carcinoma, cholangiocarcinoma, solitary liver secondaries, cavernous haemagioma and liver trauma.

PREOPERATIVE ASSESSMENT
1. Exclude extrahepatic metastases.
2. Establish whether the disease is confined to one lobe or segment and decide upon the extent of resection. This may require ultrasound, CT scanning and angiography.

Relevant anatomy

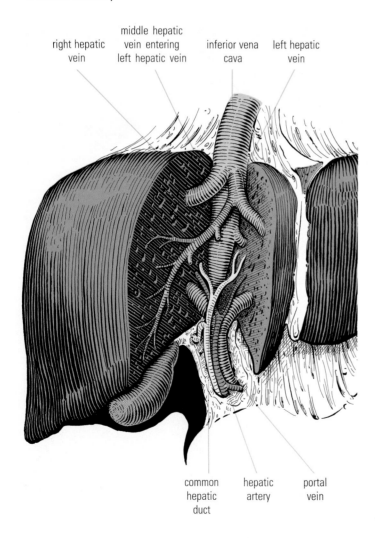

middle hepatic
right hepatic   vein entering   inferior vena   left hepatic
vein   left hepatic vein   cava   vein

common   hepatic   portal
hepatic   artery   vein
duct

Fig. 4.31

4.18

RELEVANT ANATOMY (Fig. 4.31)
Anatomists divide the liver into four lobes: right, left, quadrate and caudate. However, surgically there are only two, the true right and left lobes which are separated by a line passing from the inferior vena cava (IVC) through the gall bladder bed. In addition to wedge excision and resection of the whole of either lobe, the left lateral segment alone can be resected, or a right lobectomy extended to include the medial segment of the left lobe (trisegmentectomy).

Folds of peritoneum pass from the liver to the adjacent diaphragm and lesser curve of the stomach. The left triangular ligament lies ventral to the oesophageal hiatus and runs transversely to meet the falciform ligament and gastrohepatic (lesser) omentum. The right triangular ligament divides into superior and inferior coronary ligaments which encompass the bare area of the liver. The superior coronary ligament passes across the IVC at the diaphragmatic hiatus and joins the left triangular ligament to form the falciform ligament. The ligamentum teres lies in the free edge of the falciform ligament and runs into the umbilical fissure.

The bile ducts, hepatic artery and portal vein each divide into two roughly equal branches at the porta hepatis. Each branch supplies the respective true right or left lobes, with no communication between the two halves, and this marks the point of resection in lobectomy (Fig. 4.31). Following a second bifurcation of the portal triad, each lobe is further divided into two segments. The origin of either hepatic artery may be anomalous; the right may arise from the superior mesenteric artery (17%) or the left may come from the left gastric artery (23%).

Venous drainage is not segmental. The right lobe is drained primarily by the right hepatic vein, the left lateral segment by the left hepatic vein, the middle hepatic vein drains the quadrate lobe and adjacent parts of the right lobe, and the caudate lobe usually has its own separate venous drainage directly into the IVC. The right, middle and left hepatic veins enter the IVC near the upper surface of the liver. The middle vein usually joins the left vein near its termination. Three phrenic veins (left, right and posterior) and several small accessory veins also enter the IVC.

OPERATION
Preparation
The anaesthetized patient is placed supine with adequate venous access for rapid blood replacement should it be necessary. The abdomen and lower chest are prepared and draped.

Incision
Make a midline incision (see the Introduction) as it can be extended laterally on either side to improve access. Rarely, when required, an extension into the chest through the right seventh interspace improves access to the suprahepatic IVC

and diaphragmatic surface of the right lobe. If they are available, table-mounted, self-retaining retractors (e.g. Thompson) provide excellent exposure.

Operative technique

1. Confirm operability by excluding extrahepatic spread or disease in both lobes and determine the extent of resection. Left lateral segmentectomy does not require dissection of the hilum; the line of resection passes just to the left of the umbilical fissure (Fig. 4.32).

2. For left or right lobectomy divide ligaments to the appropriate lobe and identify the entry point of the hepatic vein into the IVC.

3. Dissect the bifurcation of the common hepatic duct, hepatic artery and portal vein at the porta hepatis. The left or right branches, depending on the lobe being removed, are then ligated and divided. In a right hepatic lobectomy the cystic duct is divided (Fig. 4.33). A line of demarcation becomes apparent on the surface of the liver.

4. In trisegmentectomy, following ligation of the right branches the left branches are dissected out and any tributaries divided until the umbilical fissure is reached. The line of resection then passes up the umbilical fissure to the falciform ligament.

5. Clamp, divide and oversew the right or left hepatic vein by retraction of the appropriate lobe (Fig. 4.34). The middle vein is left intact except in trisegmentectomy. It may be

Portal dissection for right hemihepatectomy

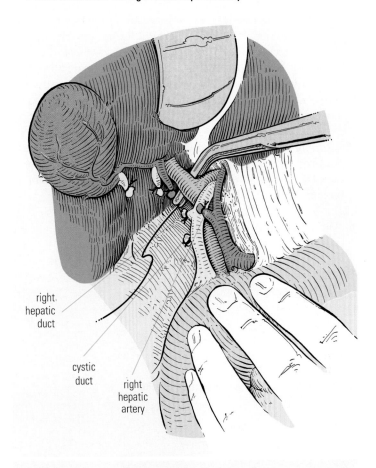

right hepatic duct

cystic duct

right hepatic artery

Fig. 4.33

Large tumour of the left lobe of liver

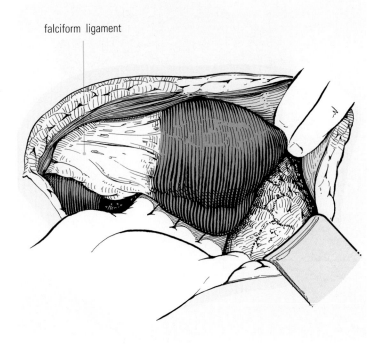

falciform ligament

Fig. 4.32

Control of right hepatic vein

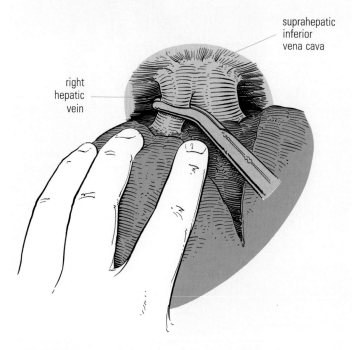

suprahepatic inferior vena cava

right hepatic vein

Fig. 4.34

necessary to divide the liver before the hepatic veins can be isolated.

6. Divide along the line of demarcation, by pinching the parenchyma between the finger and the thumb (the finger-fracture technique). Apply clips to the vessels as they are exposed. Blood loss during left lateral segmentectomy can be reduced by placing a temporary soft clamp across the porta hepatis, or by using a tape and snugger as a tourniquet (Fig. 4.35). Ligate or oversew the clipped vessels.

7. Compress the cut margin with a warm pack for 5 minutes, suture any residual bleeding points, and attempt to oversew the cut edge using vascular sutures threaded through collagen buttons (Fig. 4.36).

8. Drain the cavity with a large-bore silicone drain.

Wound closure
Close the wound with loop nylon.

Appearance following transection of lobe

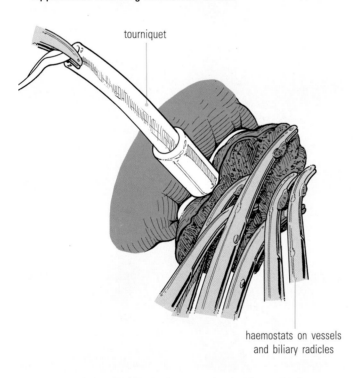

tourniquet

haemostats on vessels
and biliary radicles

Fig. 4.35

POSTOPERATIVE CARE

After major resection the patient is monitored in intensive care, with particular attention given to replacement of blood loss. Fresh frozen plasma and platelets may be required to treat coagulopathy.

Transient derangement of liver function commonly occurs and often large amounts of intravenous albumin need to be administered. If a biliary leak has not occurred the drain is removed around the fifth day.

SPECIAL OPERATIVE HAZARDS

1. The major hazards are haemorrhage and damage to structures at the porta hepatis because of anomalous anatomy.
2. The hepatic veins have almost no extrahepatic course and are easily torn where they enter the IVC.

COMPLICATIONS

1. Haemorrhage is usually from the raw edge of the liver rather than from a slipped tie.
2. Coagulopathy.
3. Jaundice due to impaired bilirubin secretion and clearance by the remaining liver, blood transfusion, and reabsorption of haematoma.
4. Bile leak from a major duct or the cut liver surface.
5. Chest infection.
6. Subphrenic abscess from infected haematoma or bile.

Haemostasis secured with use of sutures and collagen buttons

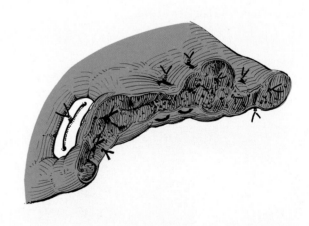

Fig. 4.36

Liver Transplantation

Transplantation of the liver is indicated for the treatment of end-stage chronic liver failure including primary biliary cirrhosis and biliary atresia, acute hepatic failure, inborn errors of the metabolism and some primary liver tumours.

RELEVANT ANATOMY
The liver (Fig. 4.37) lies mainly in the upper right quadrant between the right and left leaves of the peritoneum, which meet at the falciform ligament in front of the liver and follow the ligamentum teres to the porta hepatis where it surrounds the right and left branches of the hepatic artery, portal vein and hepatic ducts (Fig. 4.38). Posteriorly the right and left leaves are separated by the bare area of the liver.

The liver receives its blood supply from the portal vein and hepatic artery, and its venous drainage is via three hepatic veins into the inferior vena cava which is embedded in the posterior surface of the liver. The portal vein, formed by the confluence of the splenic and superior mesenteric veins behind the pancreas, reaches the liver and runs in the free edge of the lesser omentum behind and medial to the bile duct. The hepatic artery lies to the left of the bile duct, and it usually arises as a single trunk from the coeliac artery. However, a replaced or accessory left hepatic artery may arise from the left gastric artery, and the right hepatic artery may form from the superior mesenteric artery and run behind the portal vein to the liver.

OPERATIONS
DONOR HEPATECTOMY
This operation is usually combined with the removal of the kidney and heart or the heart and lungs.

Preparation
The ventilated brain dead donor is placed supine and cleansed and then draped to expose the lower neck, chest and abdomen.

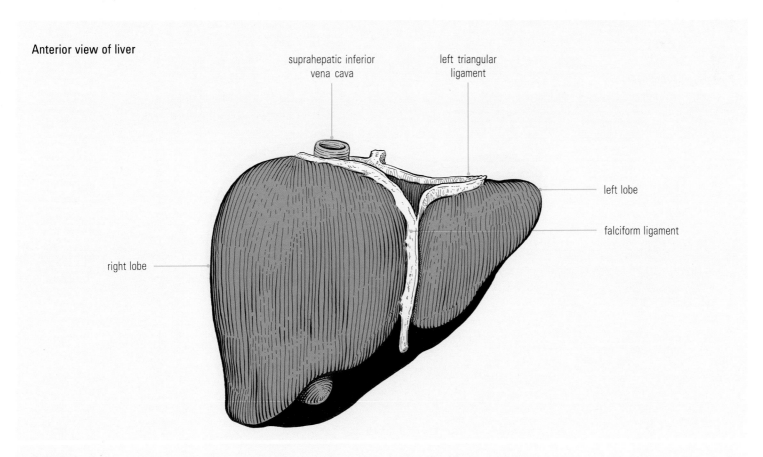

Anterior view of liver

suprahepatic inferior vena cava

left triangular ligament

left lobe

falciform ligament

right lobe

Fig. 4.37

Incision

Make a midline incision from the sternal notch to just above the umbilicus and extend it into each iliac fossa producing an inverted 'Y' shaped incision.

Operative technique

1. Ligate the falciform ligament and divide it back as far as the front of the suprahepatic inferior vena cava.

2. Search for the abdominal arteries supplying the liver; these must be preserved. The structures in the free edge of the lesser omentum are then dissected and the bile duct is divided close to the duodenum.

3. Ligate and divide the gastroduodenal, the splenic and left gastric arteries and identify the coeliac artery. If aberrant arterial anatomy is present, it is dissected out carefully, so that all the arteries can be perfused with an aortic cannula.

4. Ligate and divide any small veins entering the portal vein (e.g. the coronary vein).

5. Mobilize the right side of the colon and small bowel mesentery to allow exposure of the inferior vena cava and abdominal aorta. The inferior vena cava and renal veins are exposed below the liver and are controlled with slings.

6. Divide the peritoneal attachments of the left and right lobes of the liver, including the lesser omentum. Dissection of the bare area is then performed with ligation of the right adrenal vein, freeing the liver and the inferior vena cava from the posterior abdominal wall.

7. Heparinize the patient and insert perfusion cannula into the distal aorta and portal vein via the superior or inferior mesenteric vein.

8. Immediately prior to cardiectomy, cross-clamp the aorta at the diaphragmatic hiatus, and perfuse the liver with preservation fluid through the portal vein and hepatic artery; preservation fluid is a cold solution which prevents cell swelling and minimizes the metabolic rate of the organ. The kidneys are perfused via the aortic cannula. Blood and perfusate run into the pericardial cavity through the divided suprahepatic inferior vena cava which is dissected from the surrounding adherent diaphragm.

9. Once perfusion is complete, divide the portal vein and the inferior vena cava. The arterial supply is removed with a cuff of aorta and the liver is lifted out with its attached segment of inferior vena cava.

10. Oversew the three phrenic veins where they enter the suprahepatic inferior vena cava, and flush the gall bladder and bile duct clean of bile.

Storage of transplant

The liver is packed in cold preservation solution and surrounded with ice to await transplantation.

Posterior view of liver

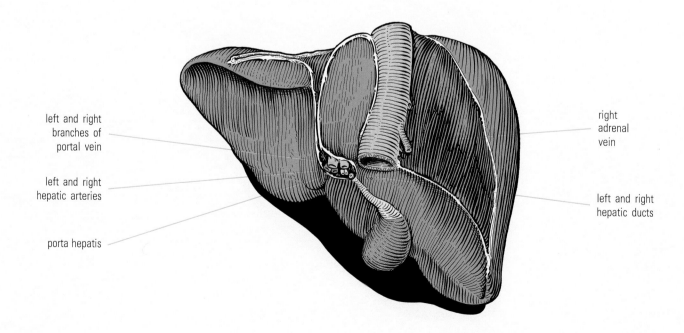

left and right branches of portal vein

left and right hepatic arteries

porta hepatis

right adrenal vein

left and right hepatic ducts

Fig. 4.38

RECIPIENT OPERATION

Incision

Make a 'Mercedes' incision (i.e. a long, curved supraumbilical incision that turns downwards, with a midline limb up to the xiphisternum) (Fig. 4.39).

Operative technique

1. Reflect the two skin flaps upwards, stitch them in position, and then insert a Thompson self-retaining retractor (Fig. 4.40).

2. Expose the vena cava above and below the liver, and divide the peritoneal attachments, ligating the right adrenal vein.

3. Divide the bile duct and control the hepatic artery and portal vein with slings.

4. Divide and ligate the right and left hepatic arteries and clamp and divide the portal vein, and the inferior vena cava above and below the liver.

5. Place the new liver orthotopically in the recipient and then anastomose the suprahepatic inferior vena cava end-to-end with 2/0 Mersilene (Fig. 4.41). The infrahepatic inferior vena cava and the portal vein and anastomosed with 4/0 Prolene and 5/0 Prolene respectively.

6. Before inserting the final stitches of the anastomosis of the infrahepatic inferior vena cava and the portal vein, flush out the preservation fluid from the liver with colloid solution via a cannula in the portal vein; it escapes through the infrahepatic vena cava. The venous anastomoses are then completed, and the venous clamps removed to allow perfusion of the graft with portal blood.

7. Trim the donor coeliac artery and anastomose it to the recipient hepatic artery with non-absorbable sutures (e.g. 6/0 Prolene), usually at the point where the gastroduodenal artery arises.

8. If present, join the superior mesenteric artery with an aberrant right hepatic artery arising from it to the splenic stump of the donor coeliac artery, or interpose the superior mesenteric artery between the donor coeliac and recipient hepatic arteries prior to recipient hepatectomy.

9. The common bile duct can be joined end-to-end to the recipient bile duct, or anastomosed to Hartmann's pouch on the donor gall bladder which is then used as a conduit with an anastomosis being fashioned between the fundus of the gall bladder and the recipient bile duct. A T-tube is used to decompress the biliary anastomosis. If this is no suitable recipient bile duct, such as occurs with sclerosing cholangitis or biliary atresia, biliary drainage is into a Roux loop of jejunum.

Wound closure

Make a thorough check for bleeding prior to closing the wound, and insert several silicone drains.

The Mercedes incision

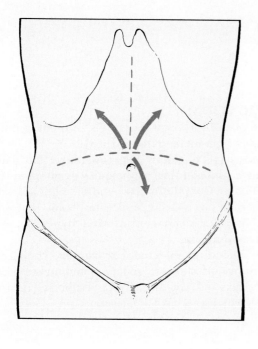

Fig. 4.39

Positioning of Thompson self-retaining retractor

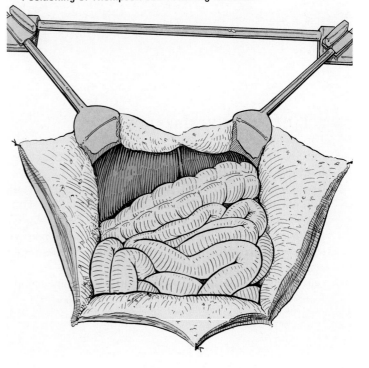

Fig. 4.40

Completed transplantation

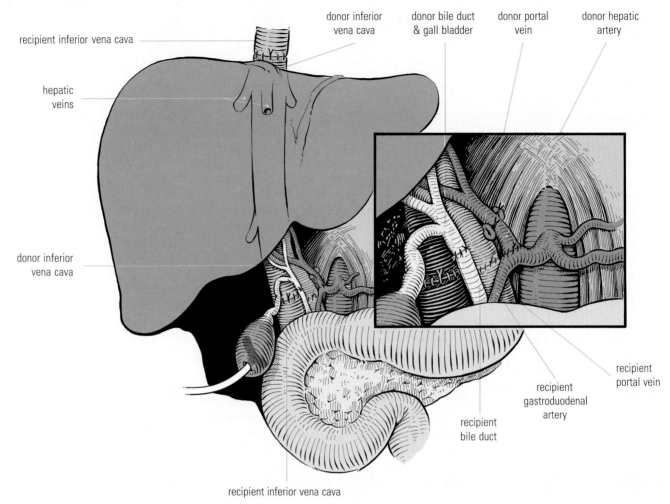

Fig. 4.41

SPECIAL OPERATIVE HAZARDS

1. Portasystemic shunts along the falciform ligament, in the retroperitoneum and in peritoneal adhesions are hazardous and may bleed profusely.
2. The haemodynamic result of cross-clamping the portal vein and inferior vena cava can be life-threatening. For this reason, a trial clamping of the inferior vena cava is performed early in the operation, and if this is poorly tolerated some form of bypass is instituted (e.g. femoral veno-arterial bypass).
3. Cardiac arrest due to cold, acidotic, hyperkalaemic blood from the liver graft entering circulation upon reperfusion.

COMPLICATIONS

1. Primary non-function of the graft is uncommon, but lethal if the patient cannot be retransplanted.
2. Haemorrhage is chiefly a peroperative and early post-operative problem that may require exploration. Bleeding is commonly from the area around the right adrenal gland, but there is rarely a single bleeding point. These patients may have deranged clotting and hypersplenism with thrombocytopenia.
3. Sepsis including infected haematoma, cholangitis and opportunist infections secondary to immunosuppression.
4. Biliary leaks and strictures, graft rejection and recurrence of the original disease may occur later.

Drainage of Subphrenic and Subhepatic Abscess

A collection of pus in one or more of the spaces around the liver may follow an episode of peritonitis, such as follows pancreatitis, perforation due to appendicitis, peptic ulceration or diverticulitis (which may have been silent), or may follow abdominal surgery (especially gastric, biliary, hepatic and colonic), particularly if there has been peritoneal contamination or a residual haematoma. A high index of suspicion should be maintained in patients with persistent swinging pyrexia, leucocytosis and malaise following surgery or peritonitis. The surgical approach employed depends upon the site of the abscess and may be posterolateral or anterior.

PREOPERATIVE ASSESSMENT

1. Radiological imaging is central to the management of subphrenic and subhepatic abscesses. A chest X-ray may show a sympathetic pleural effusion, and ultrasound and CT scanning are equally reliable (75–95%) in making the diagnosis and distinguishing the site. Indium-labelled leucocyte scanning is less accurate for localization.
2. Up to 85% of collections around the liver can be treated successfully by percutaneous drainage under CT or ultrasound guidance, and this has become the treatment of choice regardless of the site and aetiology.
3. Use formal surgical drainage if scanning has been unable to localize the lesion or percutaneous drainage has failed, if there are multiple collections, and for large collections unless a radiologist is confident that he can insert a large-bore drain.
4. Prescribe intravenous broad-spectrum antibiotics in cases with systemic toxicity; base postoperative treatment on the results of culture and sensitivity.
5. Consider parenteral nutrition in severely catabolic patients.

RELEVANT ANATOMY

Collections between the liver and the diaphragm are termed subphrenic, and may be sited anteriorly or posteriorly (Fig. 4.42). The subphrenic spaces are divided into right and left by the falciform ligament. The left space lies over the left lateral segment of the liver and extends over the fundus of the stomach laterally to the gastrosplenic omentum. The right subphrenic space is limited posterolaterally by the anterior leaf of the right coronary ligament.

Collections under the liver are subhepatic. The right subhepatic space lies in the hepatorenal pouch (of Rutherford Morison) between the undersurface of the right lobe of the liver and the right kidney, and is limited on the left by the lesser omentum and the foramen of Winslow.

Extraperitoneal collections are less common and usually occur over the bare area of the liver. They may be secondary to a liver abscess or follow liver resection.

OPERATION
POSTEROLATERAL APPROACH
Preparation

Under a general anaesthetic the patient is placed in the full lateral position, with the table broken at the level of the lower ribs. The side of the chest and the loin are cleansed and draped.

Incision

Make a skin incision along the line of the twelfth rib, from the lateral border of erector spinae to beyond the midaxillary line. Deepen the incision through the subcutaneous tissues, and the latissimus dorsi and underlying muscles, and incise the periosteum of the twelfth rib with diathermy. Using a periosteal elevator free the periosteum from the twelfth rib, from its neck

Relevant anatomy

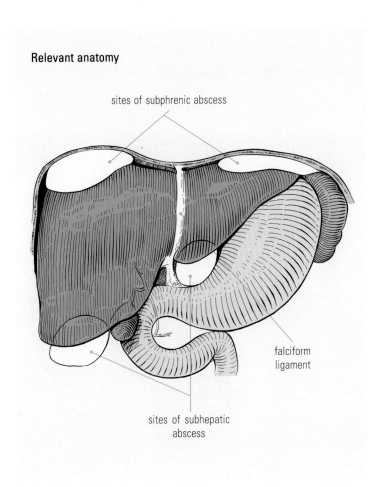

sites of subphrenic abscess

falciform ligament

sites of subhepatic abscess

Fig. 4.42

forward, and excise the rib, dividing it posteriorly with a costa-tome. Incise transversely through the exposed bed of the twelfth rib (Fig. 4.43) dividing the underlying muscles of the eleventh intercostal space anteriorly and the quadratus lumborum muscle posteriorly, together with the attachment of the diaphragm.

Operative technique

1. Insert a self-retaining retractor and slide a hand into the incision with the fingers extended. Feel for the smooth firm outline of the kidney.

2. With the fingers develop a plane outside of Gerota's fascia over the upper pole of the kidney.

3. On the right side, the right lobe of the liver will be easily palpable, and the fingers can be pushed between the dia-phragm and the right lobe of the liver (Fig. 4.44) to enter an extraperitoneal collection and a right posterior subphrenic collection, or below the liver and in front of the kidney to enter a subhepatic abscess.

4. For a posteriorly sited left subphrenic collection develop the plane between the diaphragm above, and spleen and gastric fundus below.

5. Once the abscess has been entered, explore the cavity digitally and break up any loculi. Evacuate the cavity with a sucker having taken a sample of the pus for bacteriology and use swabs, either mounted or loose, to remove debris.

Wound closure and dressing
Insert a wide-bore rubber drain. Close the wound with mono-filament nylon to the muscle, subcutaneous catgut and inter-rupted nylon for the skin. Attach the drain to a collection apparatus and apply an absorbent dressing.

ANTERIOR APPROACH
Preparation
The anaesthetized patient is placed supine with a sandbag under the loin on the side of the abscess. The abdomen is cleansed and draped.

Incision
Make a subcostal incision an inch below and parallel to the costal margin; this should start and finish further laterally than the incision employed for a cholecystectomy (see page 4.2). Divide the abdominal wall musculature with a diathermy point

Incision into bed of twelfth rib

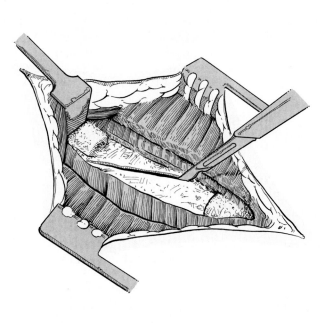

Fig. 4.43

Develop plane between liver and diaphragm

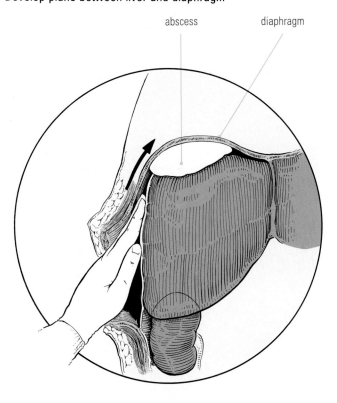

Fig. 4.44

in the line of the skin incision until extraperitoneal fat is reached. The superior epigastric vessels may need to be ligated.

Operative technique
1. Insert a self-retaining retractor and, as with a posterolateral approach, slide a hand with the fingers outstretched into the incision.

2. Feel for the lower border of the liver and enter a subhepatic abscess at this point.

Anterior approach to subphrenic collection

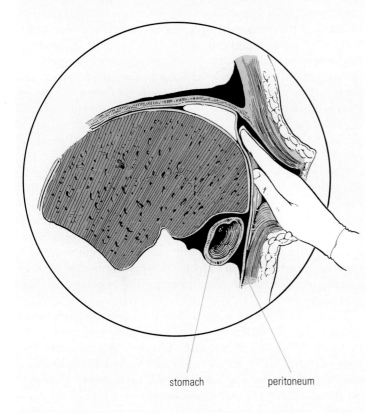

stomach   peritoneum

Fig. 4.45

3. To enter an anteriorly sited subphrenic abscess, develop an extraperitoneal plane with the fingers, sweeping the peritoneum off the inner surface of the abdominal wall muscles and, higher up, the diaphragm (Fig. 4.45).

4. Proceed as described in point 5 of the Posterolateral Approach.

Wound closure and dressing
This is similar to that described for the Posterolateral Approach.

POSTOPERATIVE CARE
Once on the ward, position the patient so as to allow dependent drainage. If this cannot be achieved, consider connecting the drain to a low-pressure suction device. Administer antibiotics until signs of systemic toxicity have resolved. Shorten the drain from the fifth day by about an inch per day. With a long standing abscess, confirm that the cavity has obliterated by injecting contrast medium down the drain prior to its removal. The sutures are removed after 7–10 days.

SPECIAL OPERATIVE HAZARDS
1. Difficulty locating the abscess. The wall of the abscess feels indurated and the tissues nearby will be oedematous. Aspiration with a large needle on a syringe may locate the collection. If the collection is still not apparent, consider laparotomy. It was formerly believed that contamination of the peritoneum with pus was disastrous. In fact with careful peritoneal toilet and modern antibiotics the development of peritonitis is rather uncommon.
2. Opening the pleura. If this has occurred insert an intercostal drain well away from the infection, ask the anaesthetist to inflate the lung, and close the pleura with an absorbable suture. Provided the lung remains fully expanded the drain can be removed the following day.
3. Damage to viscera in the abscess wall (e.g. spleen, liver and stomach).

COMPLICATIONS
1. Fistula formation. If the original cause of the abscess was a fistula (e.g. from the stomach or biliary tract), an external fistula may follow drainage of the abscess. If there is no distal obstruction, such fistulae should heal.
2. Ongoing sepsis may reflect failure to drain the collection adequately, an underlying focus of infection such as osteomyelitis of a rib, or persistance of the cause (e.g. a fistula). The treatment of residual or recurrent pus is drainage.

Splenectomy

Splenectomy is performed as an emergency when trauma has resulted in life-threatening haemorrhage from the spleen. The patient has often suffered multiple injuries in a road traffic accident and a complete assessment of all injuries will be needed. Elective splenectomy is usually performed for a blood dyscrasia (e.g. congenital acholuric jaundice and myelosclerosis), infection by protozoa (e.g. malaria) or parasites (e.g. hydatid), or idiopathic splenomegaly producing thrombocytopenic purpura. A splenectomy may also be needed to either perform an operation (e.g. splenorenal shunt or radical gastrectomy), or if the spleen is damaged accidentally during surgery.

PREOPERATIVE ASSESSMENT
1. Manage the patient for abdominal trauma (see page 8.13).
2. In an elective splenectomy perform a full blood count, including platelets and clotting screen, and make provision to correct any deficit during surgery.

Transverse section at the level of the splenic hilum

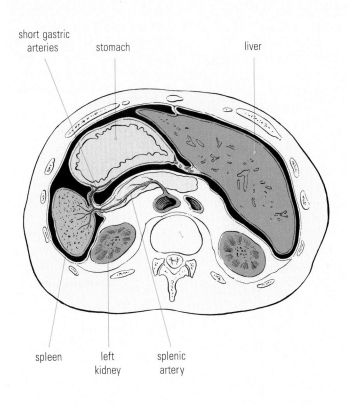

short gastric arteries stomach liver

spleen left kidney splenic artery

Fig. 4.46

3. Give polyvalent anti-pneumococcal vaccine (e.g. Pneumovac) 2 weeks prior to surgery in elective cases.
4. For patients on oral corticosteroids prescribe intravenous hydrocortisone to cover the perioperative period.

RELEVANT ANATOMY
The spleen develops from several 'splenules' within the dorsal mesogastrium and with rotation of the stomach comes to lie below the left hemidiaphragm. In the adult this results in the spleen lying at the left extremity of the lesser sac, anterior to the left kidney and above the splenic flexure of the colon. The two leaves of the dorsal mesogastrium form the gastrosplenic ligament between the greater curve of the stomach and the splenic hilum, and the lienorenal ligament between the splenic hilum and the left kidney (Figs 4.46 and 4.47). The tail of the pancreas lies within the leaves of the lienorenal ligament, alongside the splenic vessels, immediately adjacent to the splenic hilum. The short gastric and gastro-epiploic vessels lie within the gastrosplenic ligament. There is a further fold of peritoneum extending from the hilum towards the lower pole of the spleen, where the left lateral edge of the greater omentum closes off the lesser sac.

The splenic artery is a branch of the coeliac artery and passes along the superior border of the pancreas to the splenic hilum, where it divides into the splenic, short gastric and left gastro-epiploic branches. The splenic vein receives similar tributaries before passing along the superior border of the pancreas, where it receives the inferior mesenteric vein. It then unites with the superior mesenteric vein to form the portal vein. The spleen is a highly vascular organ and if damaged by trauma may bleed profusely.

The close proximity of the tail of the pancreas, the stomach wall and the splenic flexure of the colon make them susceptible to injury during a splenectomy. Accessory spleens develop in approximately one-tenth of individuals in the hilum, the omentum, the pancreas, and rarely in the small bowel mesentery or gonad. These splenuculi are beneficial if the spleen is lost through trauma, but may result in recurrence of the original disease if left behind when splenectomy is performed electively for a blood dyscrasia or idiopathic splenomegaly.

OPERATION
Preparation
The anaesthetized patient is placed supine with a sandbag under the left flank. The abdomen is cleansed and draped.

Incision
In cases of trauma make a midline incision, but an elective splenectomy can be performed through a midline, left paramedian or left subcostal incision (see the Introduction); the

latter is useful if the costal angle is wide. Large spleens can be removed through a generous midline incision because the gastrosplenic and lienorenal ligaments have stretched, creating a mesentery on which the spleen can be manipulated to the midline.

Operative technique

The procedure for an emergency splenectomy and an operation to electively remove a normal sized or moderately enlarged spleen are similar. If, however, the spleen is exceptionally large the method differs and is described separately below. A strong assistant will be required to retract the left side of the wound.

Emergency splenectomy

1. Insert the left hand over the stomach into the left subphrenic space in order to grasp the remnant of the spleen. Remember that when the spleen has ruptured the peritoneal cavity will be full of blood, so this initial part of the operation is performed 'blind'.

2. Lifting the remnant upwards and medially, slit the peritoneum of the outer leaf of the lienorenal ligament upwards and downwards using a long pair of scissors (Fig. 4.48). This will allow the splenic remnant to be lifted further upwards and medially into the wound, bringing the pancreatic tail and splenic flexure of the colon with it.

Relevant anatomy

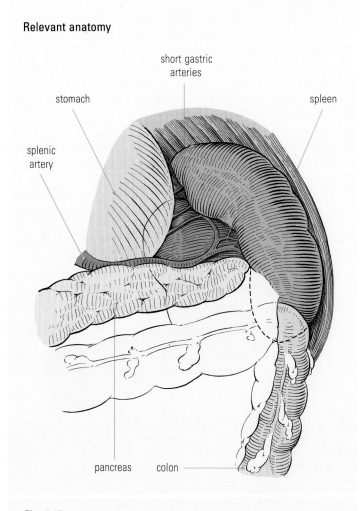

Fig. 4.47

Division of lienorenal ligament

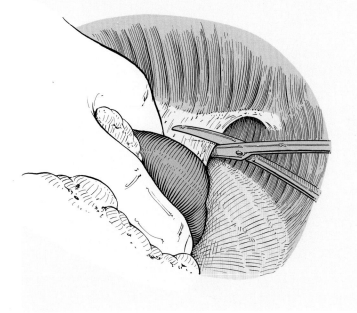

Fig. 4.48

Occlusion of vessels at splenic hilum

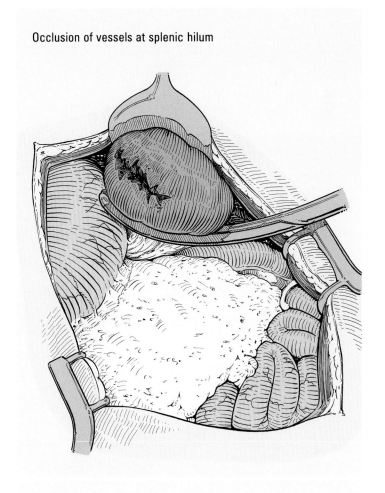

Fig. 4.49

3. Place a soft Crafoord clamp gently across the splenic hilum to control haemorrhage, and insert a large pack into the splenic fossa to prevent the spleen falling back (Fig. 4.49).

4. Clamp, divide and ligate the short gastric vessels carefully, taking care not to damage the fundus and greater curvaïre of the stomach, before clamping, dividing and ligating the attachments of the spleen to the greater omentum and colon in similar fashion.

5. Rotate the spleen to allow inspection of the posterior aspect of its pedicle (Fig. 4.50). Identify the splenic vessels at the hilum, and divide and doubly ligate them with strong, non-absorbable ties, taking care not to damage the tail of the pancreas (Fig. 4.51).

6. Clear the peritoneal cavity of blood and perform a careful laparotomy to exclude damage to any other intra-abdominal organ.

7. Inspect the operative area for residual bleeding sites.

8. In an attempt to preserve some splenic function, dice up some of the removed spleen and wrap it in the greater omentum where it may grow and function as an autograft.

Elective splenectomy

If the spleen is normal size or only moderately enlarged, proceed as for an emergency splenectomy, with two differences. There is no need to apply a vascular clamp to the splenic hilum prior to dissecting and ligating the vessels, and do not attempt to autograft the splenic tissue. With a massively enlarged spleen it is wise to ligate the splenic artery prior to mobilization. This is performed as follows.

1. Lift the spleen, which will be obscuring the operative field, gently to allow access to the gastrocolic omentum.

2. Open the lesser sac through the gastrocolic omentum by clipping, cutting and ligating the gastro-epiploic vessels. Alternatively, open the lesser omentum.

3. Identify the pancreas on the posterior abdominal wall with the splenic artery lying along its superior edge. Incise the peritoneum overlying the vessel and carefully isolate a segment of the vessel as near to the tail of the pancreas as possible.

4. Use an aneurysm needle to pass a strong non-absorbable ligature around the splenic artery (Fig. 4.52) and ligate it in continuity.

Inspection of pedicle from behind

Completed operation

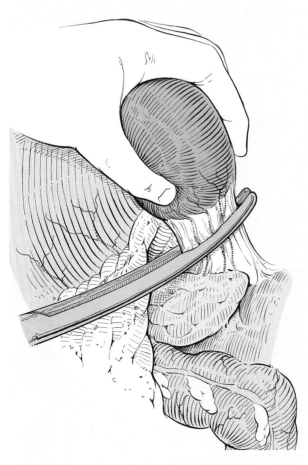

Fig. 4.50

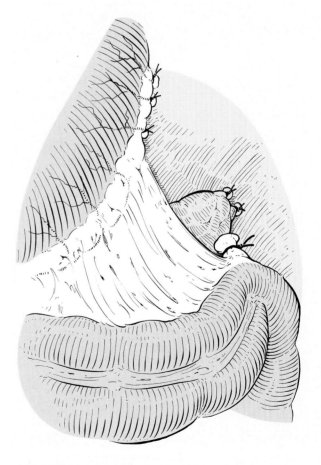

Fig. 4.51

4.30

5. Mobilize the spleen as previously described, dividing the short gastric vessels, gastro-epiploic vessels and omental attachments between clips prior to removal, taking care not to damage adjacent organs.

Wound closure and dressing

Insert a large silicone drain to the splenic fossa and check the position of the nasogastric tube. Close the wound with monofilament nylon, and the skin with interrupted stitches or a subcuticular suture. Apply a waterproof dressing.

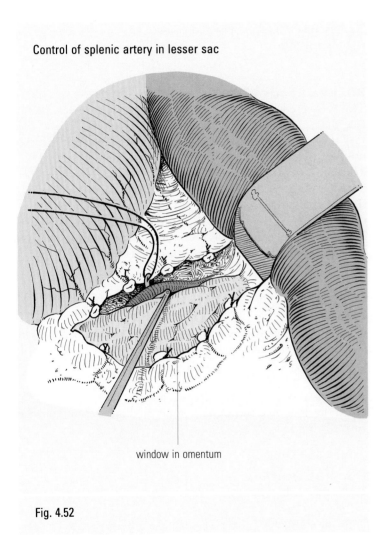

Control of splenic artery in lesser sac

window in omentum

Fig. 4.52

POSTOPERATIVE CARE

The nasogastric tube must remain until gastric emptying recovers. Check the serum amylase level on the first postoperative day to ensure that the tail of the pancreas has not been damaged. The drain can be removed after 48 hours if there has been less than 50 ml drainage in the previous 24 hours. If drainage is excessive perform an amylase estimation on the drain fluid and if it is very high keep the drain in until drainage ceases.

The platelet count is checked daily and although the risks of venous thrombosis are not greatly increased by reactive thrombocytosis it is our policy to prescribe antiplatelet agents (e.g. aspirin or dipyridamole) if the count exceeds 1000×10^9 per litre.

Following splenectomy the risk of infection with capsulated organisms, particularly pneumococcus, is increased. In patients undergoing emergency splenectomy give antipneumococcal vaccine (e.g. Pneumovac), although it is less effective if given postoperatively. It is our policy to prescribe prophylactic oral penicillin V for 2 years in children and 1 year in adults (over 21).

If an autograft has been performed it is possible to tell whether or not it is functioning by examining a blood film after 1 year.

SPECIAL OPERATIVE HAZARDS
1. Damage to the tail of the pancreas. This may lead to an abscess, which must be drained, or a fistula (see Postoperative Care).
2. Damage to the fundus of the stomach which may follow hurried attempts to clamp and tie the short gastric vessels and may also lead to abscess or fistula formation.
3. Damage to the splenic flexure of the colon.

COMPLICATIONS
1. Pancreatic or gastric fistula.
2. Thrombo-embolism.
3. Sepsis, including overwhelming postsplenectomy infection (OPSI).
4. Recurrence of haematological disease following failure to remove a splenunculus.

Triple Bypass

With the exception of true periampullary tumours, where radical resection may offer the prospect of long-term survival, carcinoma of the head of the pancreas is now generally considered incurable, and management directed towards adequate palliation. Patients who present only with obstructive jaundice can usually be treated by stenting of the common bile duct either endoscopically or percutaneously. When these techniques fail, or when duodenal obstruction is present, operative bypass may be indicated. If this operation is undertaken, both the duodenum and bile duct should be bypassed, otherwise a subsequent obstruction is likely to occur.

PREOPERATIVE ASSESSMENT
1. Confirm the diagnosis and extent of the disease using CT scanning. Widespread intraperitoneal or metastatic disease is a contra-indication to surgery.
2. Use a barium meal to visualize duodenal obstruction, and ERCP or percutaneous cholangiography in cases with jaundice.
3. Correct fluid and electrolyte disturbances.
4. Perform gastric lavage in cases with duodenal obstruction.

5. Correct prolonged prothrombin time in jaundiced patients with vitamin K, and fresh frozen plasma if necessary.
6. Encourage preoperative and peroperative diuresis using intravenous fluids and 200 ml of 10% mannitol, and monitor the urine output via a urethral catheter.
7. Prescribe broad-spectrum intravenous antibiotics to be given at induction.

RELEVANT ANATOMY
This is covered on page 4.7 in the Exploration of the Common Bile Duct.

If the gall bladder is distended and not diseased it may be used for the biliary bypass, but it must be remembered that the drainage is only as wide as the cystic duct and, if the cystic duct has a low insertion into the common bile duct, subsequent extension of the carcinoma may result in recurrent jaundice. For these reasons, if the hepatic duct is dilated and readily accessible or if the gall bladder has been removed previously, a bypass to the common hepatic duct is to be preferred.

OPERATION
Preparation
The patient is placed supine, the whole abdomen is cleansed and draped, and a nasogastric tube is inserted.

Incision
Open the abdomen through an upper midline incision (see the Introduction).

Operative technique
1. Perform a laparotomy.

2. After confirming the diagnosis take a biopsy from omental or peritoneal deposits, if present, or transduodenally from the head of the pancreas using a 'Trucut' needle.

3. Perform a gastrojejunostomy using the most proximal loop of jejunum and make an antecolic anastomosis to avoid invasion by a local extension of the cancer. An 8-cm stoma using two layers of continuous absorbable suture (e.g. Vicryl or Polydioxamone) is satisfactory (see details on gastroenterostomy, page 5.35).

4. Choose a proximal loop of jejunum for the biliary bypass, and perform an entero-enterostomy to divert jejunal content away from the biliary tree. This stoma should be 5–6 cm in diameter, and is carried out in a similar way to the gastro-jejunostomy, using non-crushing clamps and two layers of continuous absorbable sutures (Figs 4.53 and 4.54). In addi-

Fashioning of entero-enterostomy

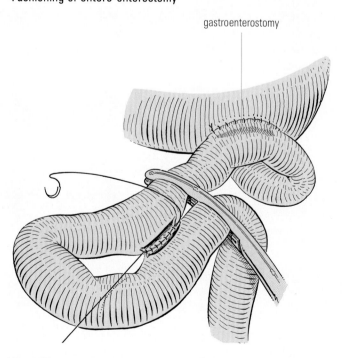

gastroenterostomy

Fig. 4.53

4.32

tion, partially occlude the afferent loop with sutures beyond the enteroenterostomy to discourage contamination of the biliary tree (Fig. 4.55). These procedures should be done before the biliary anastomosis because access becomes more difficult after this point. Alternatively a less bulky Roux loop may be constructed (see page 4.12).

5. If the gall bladder is to be used for the bypass, decompress it using a trocar and suction cannula to allow application of a non-crushing clamp, and make a 2-cm incision (Fig. 4.56). If the common hepatic duct is to be used, make a 2-cm longitudinal incision between stay sutures (Fig. 4.57). A sample of bile is sent for culture.

Incision into gall bladder

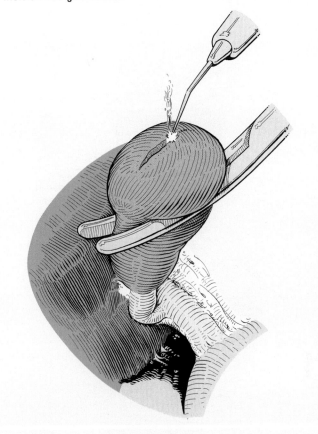

Fig. 4.56

Completion of entero-enterostomy

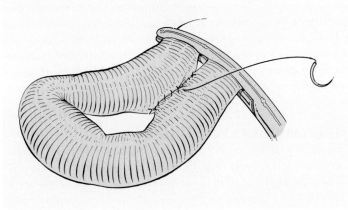

Fig. 4.54

Sutures to partially occlude afferent loop

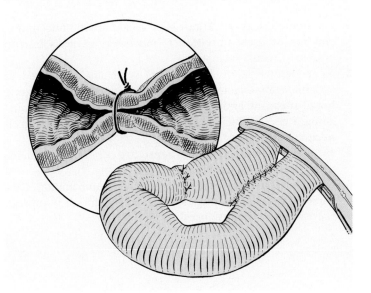

Fig. 4.55

Choledochotomy in common hepatic duct

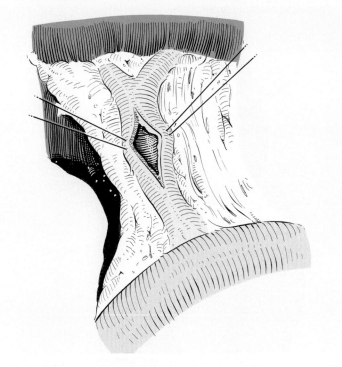

Fig. 4.57

Posterior suture line of cholecystojejunostomy

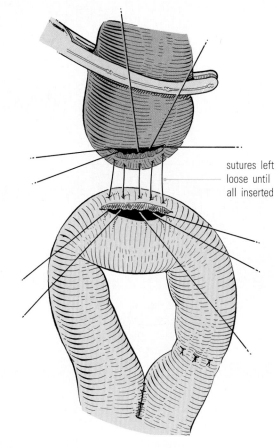

sutures left
loose until
all inserted

Fig. 4.58

Completed posterior layer

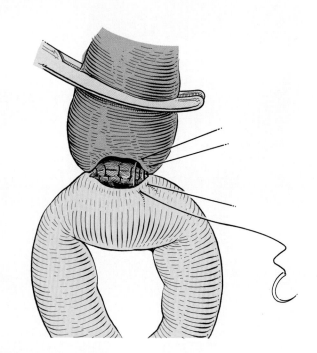

Fig. 4.59

6. Open the apex of the jejunal loop using diathermy and fashion the biliary anastomosis with a single layer of interrupted absorbable sutures (e.g. 3/0 Polydioxamone) spaced 3–4mm apart, placing all the sutures in the posterior wall before tying them as this improves access (Figs 4.58 and 4.59). Perform an anastomosis between the loop and common hepatic duct in an identical fashion to a choledochoduodenostomy (see page 4.10). The knots in the anastomosis of posterior wall thus lie in the lumen, and those for the anterior layer on the outside.

Wound closure and dressing

Insert a suction drain in the subhepatic space. Perform a mass closure using continuous monofilament nylon and close the skin with interrupted nylon sutures. Apply a dry dressing.

POSTOPERATIVE CARE

Nasogastric drainage and intravenous fluids are continued until the postoperative ileus subsides, usually on the second or third postoperative day, when the drain can also be removed unless it is draining bile. Broad-spectrum antibiotics should be continued for 48 hours and the urine output is carefully observed during the postoperative period. Skin sutures should not be removed before the twelfth day.

SPECIAL OPERATIVE HAZARD

Inability to drain the common hepatic duct due to spread of tumour to the porta hepatis. More complicated methods of drainage can be used in these instances, such as a Longmire's (see page 4.13) operation, but it is often more appropriate to either pass a stent or do nothing.

COMPLICATIONS

1. Haemorrhage in the jaundiced patient, especially from the gastric anastomosis. This can be avoided if the twin clamps are removed before the anterior wall of the anastomosis is completed so that bleeding points may be observed and controlled.
2. Anastomotic leakage. Minor biliary leaks are not uncommon and not of great importance; more serious leaks lead to abscess or fistula formation.
3. Renal failure from 'hepatorenal syndrome' is related to systemic endotoxaemia. This can be reduced by continuing broad-spectrum antibiotics for at least 48 hours, and encouraging a good urine output with intravenous fluids and, if necessary, diuretics.
4. Intra-abdominal and wound sepsis are common in patients with jaundice and malignant disease.
5. Ulceration at the gastrojejunal stoma is uncommon after triple bypass, but prophylaxis with an H_2 blocker is appropriate in these circumstances.

Surgery for Pancreatic Pseudocyst

A pancreatic pseudocyst is a collection of serous fluid in relation to the pancreas following acute pancreatitis. The most common site is the lesser sac as a result of blockage of the gastro-epiploic foramen by inflammatory adhesions, but pseudocysts may occur anywhere adjacent to, or sometimes within, the pancreas. If pancreatography is performed, most pseudocysts will be found to have a connection with the pancreatic ductal system. Routine ultrasound or CT scanning will detect pseudocysts in up to 30% of patients with acute pancreatitis, but most pseudocysts will resolve spontaneously, and clinically significant pseudocysts form in only about 5% of cases. It follows that intervention is not indicated unless there is a clinical reason. This may be persisting pancreatic inflammation with hyperamylasaemia, palpable abdominal swelling which may compress the stomach and cause vomiting, or occasionally infection or haemorrhage into the cyst. If possible, surgical intervention should be avoided until the pseudocyst is at least 6 weeks old, by which time the wall will usually be fibrotic enough to hold sutures. Percutaneous aspiration may be carried out earlier under ultrasound or CT control, but recurrence is frequent, and pancreatic fistulae

may occasionally result. Surgery at this stage should be restricted to external drainage.

PREOPERATIVE ASSESSMENT
1. Visualize the configuration of the pseudocyst with CT scanning.
2. Use ultrasound or CT to look for gall-stones as the cause of the pancreatitis. If present, cholecystectomy may be performed at the same operation.
3. Correct electrolyte and serum calcium disturbances in cases with persisting pancreatitis.
4. Perform endoscopic retrograde pancreatography if there is any suspicion of malignant disease of the pancreas or obstruction of the main duct.

RELEVANT ANATOMY
The majority of pseudocysts occupy the lesser sac and are retrogastric, displacing the stomach anteriorly (Fig. 4.60). How-

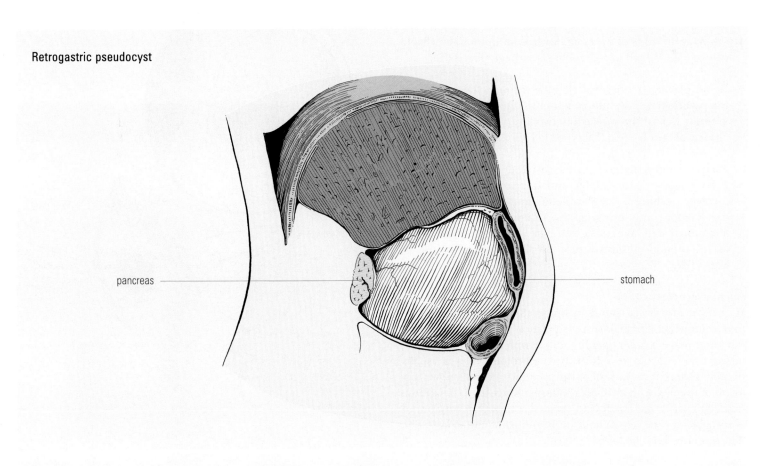

Retrogastric pseudocyst

pancreas

stomach

Fig. 4.60

ever, some lie more inferiorly, bulging into the transverse mesocolon (Fig. 4.61).

OPERATION
Preparation
The patient is placed supine, and the whole abdomen cleansed and draped. A nasogastric tube is passed because gastric emptying is often impaired. A single intravenous dose of broad-spectrum antibiotics is given at induction.

Incision
Make an upper midline incision (see the Introduction). Confirm the position of the pseudocyst and perform a thorough laparotomy with special attention to the gall bladder as a possible cause of the pancreatitis.

Operative technique
Retrogastric pseudocyst (Fig. 4.60)
1. Perform a gastrostomy using cutting diathermy to open the anterior wall of the stomach between stay sutures.

2. Confirm the position of the pseudocyst by aspirating through the posterior wall of the stomach with a needle.

3. Incise the posterior wall and the adherent pseudocyst wall with cutting diathermy and suck out the contents of the pseudocyst, breaking down any loculi in the cavity with a finger. Ensure that the opening between the stomach and the cyst is at least 3 cm in diameter.

4. Oversew the edge of the stoma with a continuous absorbable suture (e.g. Vicryl) to control haemorrhage (Fig. 4.62).

5. Avoid placing the nasogastric tube through the stoma into the pseudocyst (it should be left in the stomach). Repair the anterior wall of the stomach in two layers with a continuous absorbable suture (e.g. Vicryl or Polydioxamone).

6. Rodney Smith's method of transgastric drainage with a large Foley catheter is a simpler and quicker alternative. This involves pushing a Foley catheter into the cavity, inflating the balloon, and bringing the catheter out through the abdominal wall. When the catheter is later removed it will leave a pseudocyst-gastrostomy into the stomach (see inset to Fig. 4.62).

Inferior pseudocyst
If the pseudocyst is found to bulge through the transverse mesocolon (Fig. 4.61) confirm its position using needle aspiration, and make a 3-cm opening into it with cutting diathermy, taking care to avoid vessels in the mesocolon which is usually densely adherent to the wall of the pseudocyst. Break down any loculi in the cyst with a finger, fashion a Roux loop of jejunum (see page 4.12) and stitch it to the cyst wall with a continuous absorbable suture (e.g. Vicryl or Polydioxamone) (Fig. 4.63). The loop need not be long.

Pseudocyst related to head or tail of pancreas
Those at the head may be drained into the duodenum by a

4.36

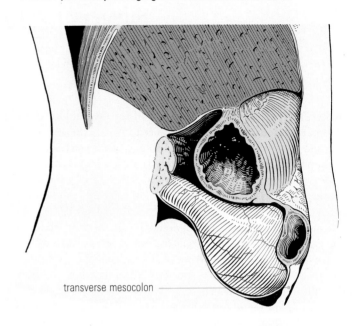

Inferior pseudocyst bulging into transverse mesocolon

transverse mesocolon

Fig. 4.61

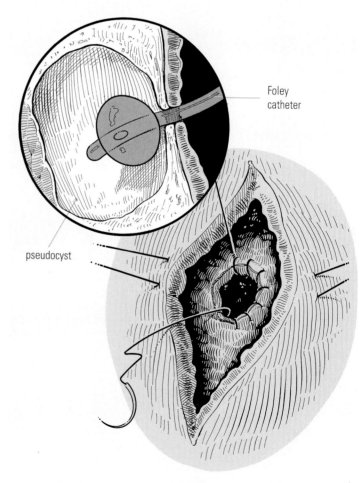

Posterior cystogastrostomy

Foley catheter

pseudocyst

Fig. 4.62

cystduodenostomy, and those related to the tail of the pancreas are best managed by distal pancreatectomy with a splenectomy.

7. If the patient has suffered from gall-stone pancreatitis perform a cholecystectomy (see page 4.2).

8. Check for haemostasis.

Wound closure and dressing

Close the wound by a mass closure technique with a monofilament suture, and interrupted nylon sutures for the skin. Apply a dry dressing.

POSTOPERATIVE CARE

The serum amylase should be measured postoperatively as acute pancreatitis may occasionally flare up following surgery. If the serum amylase is less than three times the upper limit of the normal range, the nasogastric tube may be removed on the second day and oral fluids commenced. The skin sutures are removed on the tenth day.

SPECIAL OPERATIVE HAZARDS

1. Haemorrhage from the pseudocyst wall or inflamed wall of the stomach during cystogastrostomy may be quite brisk. Continuous sutures are used for the anastomosis to control this.
2. Damage to the middle colic vessels during infracolic Roux loop drainage, which is avoided if the mesocolon is carefully inspected and the opening made where the pseudocyst appears to point. If the transverse colon is devascularized it should be exteriorized if pancreatitis is still active, and re-anastomosis carried out at a later date.
3. Cutting out of sutures in the pseudocyst wall increases the risk of pancreatic ascites. If this occurs the anastomosis should be abandoned, and external drainage carried out.

COMPLICATIONS

1. Acute pancreatitis is managed conservatively in the usual way, and generally settles rapidly if the pseudocyst has been adequately drained.

2. Haemorrhage from the suture lines or from the vessels in the wall of the pseudocyst as it collapses. This may be profuse requiring reoperation for control.
3. Pancreatic ascites due to leakage of cyst contents can be detected by comparing amylase levels in peritoneal aspirate and serum. Reoperation and external drainage are required.
4. External pancreatic fistulae can be controlled and managed conservatively with a view to internal drainage later if spontaneous closure does not occur.
5. Recurrent pseudocyst formation is due either to inadequate stoma size, or to failure to break down loculi within the pseudocyst.

Drainage of inferior pseudocyst

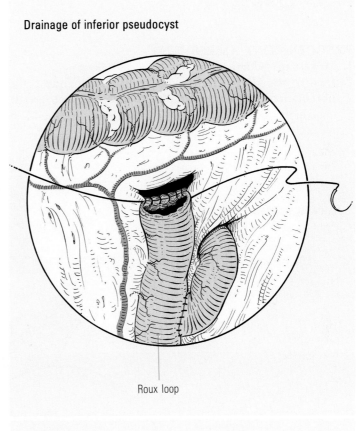

Roux loop

Fig. 4.63

Whipple's Operation or Pancreaticoduodenectomy

This operation is indicated for curative resection of malignancies of the duodenum, ampulla of Vater, lower bile duct and occasionally pancreatic head. In addition, it is occasionally indicated in cases of trauma. It is not, however, an appropriate operation for palliation of malignancy, and it should be noted that the 5-year survival rate for even carefully selected cases of malignancy is very low.

PREOPERATIVE ASSESSMENT
1. Correct any deranged clotting in the jaundiced patient.
2. Ensure the diagnosis is confirmed using endoscopy, percutaneous cholangiography, endoscopic retrograde cholangiopancreatography and endoscopic ultrasound as necessary.

3. Ensure adequate diuresis is maintained during the operative period.
4. Prescribe peroperative and postoperative antibiotics.

RELEVANT ANATOMY
Lying within the concavity of the duodenum, the head of the pancreas rests in the right paravertebral gutter. It is retroperitoneal, lying under the attachment of the transverse mesocolon, crossing the inferior vena cava and renal veins, and extending to the left as the neck of the pancreas which overlies the superior mesenteric vein and portal vein. The uncinate process of the pancreas extends to the left from the inferior part of the head and is crossed by the superior mesenteric vessels. Exocrine secretions drain from the head and neck of the pancreas into

Relevant anatomy

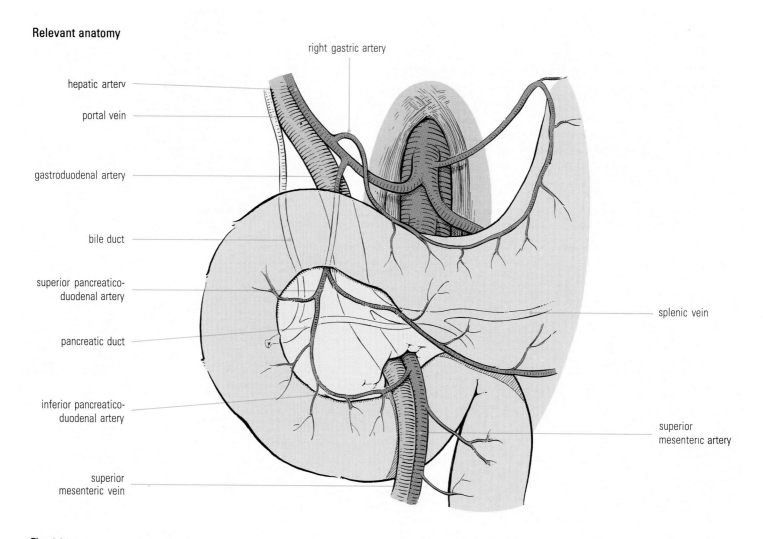

Fig. 4.64

the main pancreatic duct (the duct of Wirsung). This duct is joined by the common bile duct and enters the duodenum at the papilla. The uncinate process drains into a smaller accessory pancreatic duct, the duct of Santorini, which opens more proximally into the duodenum.

The head of the pancreas is supplied with blood by the superior (from gastroduodenal) and inferior (from superior mesenteric) pancreaticoduodenal arteries (Fig. 4.64). The rest of the pancreas receives blood from branches arising from the splenic artery, a branch of the coeliac artery.

The distal stomach is usually resected in Whipple's operation. The blood supply to the antrum and pylorus of the stomach is from branches of the hepatic artery, with the right gastric artery running along the lesser curvature and the right gastro-epiploic artery running along the greater curvature, from where the greater omentum arises.

The distal extent of the duodenum is marked by the ligament of Treitz. At this point the retroperitoneal duodenum becomes the intraperitoneal jejunum.

OPERATION
Preparation
Place the patient supine, and clean and drape the abdomen.

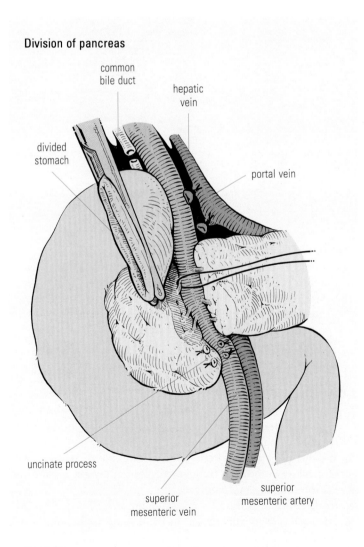

Division of pancreas

common bile duct

hepatic vein

divided stomach

portal vein

uncinate process

superior mesenteric vein

superior mesenteric artery

Fig. 4.65

Incision
Make a midline incision (see the Introduction).

Operative technique

1. Make a very careful assessment of resectability and if there are no obvious liver, lymph node or peritoneal metastases, pinch the finger and thumb together behind the neck of the pancreas to ensure that there is no invasion of the portal or superior mesenteric vein. The resected specimen will include the distal stomach, distal bile duct, pancreatic head and uncinate process, duodenum and proximal jejunum.

2. Mobilize the duodenum using Kocher's manoeuvre (i.e. by division of the peritoneum along its lateral side, see page 4.6), and then lift the head of the pancreas off the inferior vena cava.

3. Divide the lesser and greater omenta up to the wall of the stomach, ligating the gastric and gastro-epiploic arteries.

4. Dissect the hepatic artery before ligating and dividing the gastroduodenal and right gastric arteries.

5. Transect the stomach. Some surgeons prefer to preserve the pylorus and right gastric artery by dividing the first part of the duodenum to prevent postgastrectomy symptoms such as dumping.

6. Divide the supraduodenal common bile duct.

7. Lift the transverse colon up and mobilize the distal duodenum.

8. Divide the small bowel at a convenient point in the proximal jejunum. The origin of the middle colic artery marks the position of the superior mesenteric artery. Pass a blunt dissector between the portal vein and the pancreas to protect the vein and divide the neck of the pancreas with a knife. Carefully ligate any branches entering the right side of the portal vein and duodenum; these are thin walled and easily torn (Fig. 4.65).

9. Dissect the superior mesenteric vessels from the uncinate process, with ligation and division of the inferior pancreaticoduodenal artery. The specimen is now free (Fig. 4.66).

10. Bring the cut end of the jejunum through the transverse mesocolon and anastomose it to the cut end of the bile duct, end-to-side, with 5/0 absorbable sutures. The cut end of the jejunum is oversewn.

11. Fashion a gastroenterostomy between the antimesenteric border of the jejunum and the cut end of the stomach (or the transected duodenum in a pylorus-preserving procedure) with two layers of a continuous 2/0 or 3/0 absorbable suture. A small enterotomy is made distal to this and the mucosa of the pancreatic duct is sutured to the mucosa of the jejunum over an infant feeding tube. Suture the capsule of the pancreas to the wall of the jejunum to immobilize this anastomosis and prevent leakage of pancreatic juice.

Resected specimen

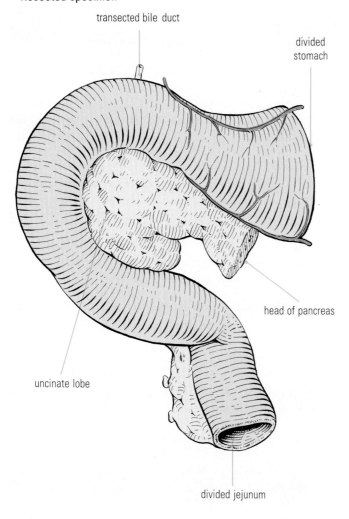

Fig. 4.66

Completed pancreaticoduodenectomy

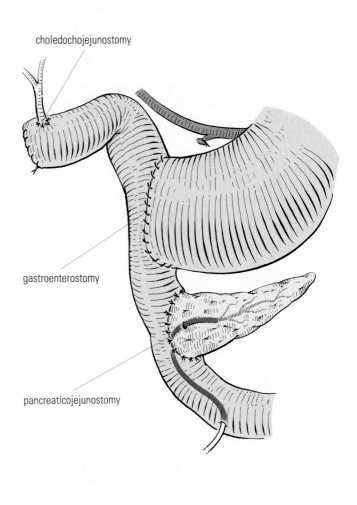

Fig. 4.67

12. Bring the infant feeding tube through the bowel wall approximately 15 cm further downstream (Fig. 4.67) and secure it with a catgut purse-string suture.

Wound closure and dressing

Insert a large silicone drain and close the wound with a loop nylon suture, and interrupted nylon for the skin. A dry dressing is applied.

POSTOPERATIVE CARE

The patient is generally nursed in an intensive care unit for the first 24–48 hours, and transfused as required. Postoperative antibiotics are given. Intravenous fluids and nasogastric drainage continue until gut motility returns. The drain is removed after 2–3 days unless there is evidence of pancreatic or biliary drainage, in which case it must remain for at least 10 days. The infant feeding tube remains for 14 days and should drain clear pancreatic juice during this period.

SPECIAL OPERATIVE HAZARDS

1. Damage to the portal vein, hepatic artery or superior mesenteric vessels.

2. Peroperative bleeding is frequently a sustained ooze rather than a single bleeding point and can be difficult to control. Apply pressure with swabs for 5–10 minutes in such cases.

COMPLICATIONS

1. Anastomotic leakage can occur from any of the three anastomoses, particularly the pancreatic, leading to abscess or fistula formation.

2. Wound infection and cholangitis. The bile of patients with obstructive jaundice is frequently colonized by gut organisms.

3. Postoperative pancreatitis.

4. Recurrence of tumour is not uncommon.

5. Postgastrectomy diarrhoea and dumping if the stomach is resected.

6. Stomal ulceration at the gastroenterostomy.

7. Malabsorption or diabetes due to pancreatic insufficiency.

Laparoscopic cholecystectomy

Laparoscopic surgery is enjoying popularity, with laparoscopic cholecystectomy being the most commonly performed general surgical procedure. Other laparoscopic procedures are possible, including appendicectomy, cervical sympathectomy, selective vagotomy, and perforated duodenal ulcer repair, in addition to its gynaecological indications. Laparoscopic cholecystectomy has popularized the use of laser energy as a dissecting tool. The most appropriate lasers at present are the NdYAG and the JTP532, both of which utilize a contact probe heated by the laser energy. However a laser is not necessary for this operation, and is considered dangerous by some who prefer to use diathermy alone. The use of a laser does require more equipment and personnel in the operating theatre.

PREOPERATIVE ASSESSMENT

1. Gross obesity and intra-abdominal adhesions are relative contra-indications to any laparoscopic surgery.
2. Confirm the diagnosis of gallbladder pathology and exclude other possible causes of symptoms such as peptic ulcer disease.
3. Acute cholecystitis, acute pancreatitis and jaundice are contra-indications. A history of common duct stones (e.g. jaundice, pancreatitis) should be sought, and their presence excluded pre-operatively by ultrasound, intravenous cholangiography or ERCP. If stones are present a pre-operative papillotomy and stone extraction is performed, or if facilities for ERCP are not available an open operation and exploration of the common bile duct is indicated.
4. The surgeon must be equipped to cope with possible complications, such as injury to portal vein, hepatic artery and bile duct, and instruments should be available for immediate conversion to an open procedure.

RELEVANT ANATOMY

The anatomy of the gall bladder is discussed on page 4.2. It is particularly important to be aware of possible anatomical anomalies such as a short cystic duct or an early bifurcation of the hepatic artery.

OPERATION

Preparation

Catheterize the patient and insert a nasogastric tube; both of these are removed at the end of the operation. Positioned supine, with the abdomen cleansed and draped, place the patient in the Trendelenberg (head down) position while the Veress needle (Fig. 4.68) is introduced, and then in the reverse Trendelenberg (head up) position for the dissection. Figure 4.69 shows a suggested layout of equipment.

Incision

A 1cm transverse subumbilical skin incision is made and the Veress insufflation needle introduced into the peritoneal cavity, angled towards the pelvis clear of the great vessels. Three to 4 litres of CO_2 are introduced before the Veress needle is removed and replaced by a 10mm trochar and cannula.

Three further incisions are made (see Fig. 4.70) under direct vision through the laparoscope.

Operative technique

1. Perform a laparoscopic survey of the entire abdomen to exclude coincident or alternative pathology. Identify the structures making up Calot's triangle as in the open operation. A peanut swab on a grasping forceps is a useful instrument for this blunt dissection.

2. Clip the cystic artery and proximal cystic duct with ligaclips. Perform a cholangiogram by introducing a catheter into the cystic duct to verify the anatomy and to look for common duct stones. Introduce the cholangiogram catheter into the abdomen either through a separate stab incision or within the specially-designed Olsen cholangiogram catheter.

3. Divide the cystic duct and artery and dissect the gall bladder from the liver by a combination of blunt dissection and cautery.

Veress needle

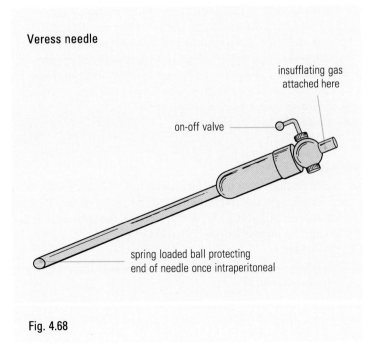

insufflating gas attached here

on-off valve

spring loaded ball protecting end of needle once intraperitoneal

Fig. 4.68

Suggested layout of equipment

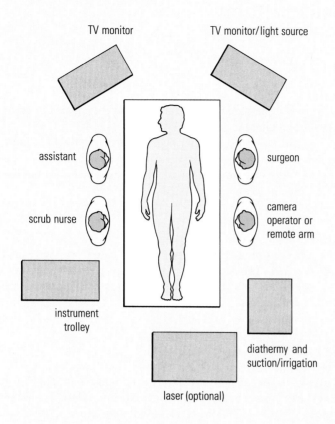

Fig. 4.69

Veress insufflation needle introduced into peritoneal cavity

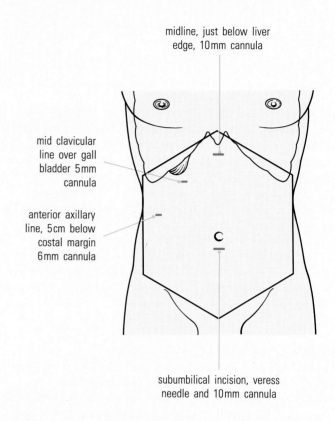

Fig. 4.70

4. Once free, check the liver bed for haemostasis and remove the gall bladder through the sub-umbilical portal. If a large stone is present the sub-umbilical incision may need extending laterally.

5. Exsufflate the abdomen by removing the instruments and opening the trumpet valves on the cannulae. Withdraw the cannulae.

Wound closure and dressing
Close the incisions with clips. If the subumbilical portal has been extended the fascia should first be opposed using a suture on a J-needle.

POSTOPERATIVE CARE
The patient is usually well enough to be fully mobile and eating the following day, and may be allowed home. Clips may be removed and replaced with paper skin closure. The patient should be back to work within two weeks.

SPECIAL OPERATIVE HAZARDS
1. Injury to the bowel or great vessels during insufflation.
2. Carbon dioxide retention due to absorption of intraperitoneal CO_2. End tidal CO_2 monitoring by the anaesthetist will enable accurate ventilatory compensation.
3. Accidental perforation of the gall bladder makes extraction difficult. Perforations are best secured when made, to prevent scattering calculi throughout the abdomen.
4. Damage to common bile duct, portal vein, or hepatic artery; failure to recognize abnormal anatomical variants.
5. Inability to complete the operation.
6. Common duct stones.

COMPLICATIONS
1. Right shoulder tip pain is common in the first 24 hours due to diaphragmatic irritation. It can be reduced by releasing all the insufflated CO_2 at the end of the procedure and asking the anaesthetist to expand the lungs.
2. Bile leakage.
3. Bleeding from gall bladder bed, a slipped ligature clip or iatrogenic injury.

5

Gastrointestinal Surgery

Laparotomy

Modern imaging techniques and laparoscopy have reduced the need for diagnostic laparotomy. However, the ability to assess an abdomen carefully and thoroughly is essential in certain circumstances, particularly abdominal trauma, laparotomy for undiagnosed abdominal pain, and in the staging of tumours. It is useful experience for the trainee to perform a complete laparotomy as frequently as possible in order to obtain a feel for normal variations, and to develop a systematic routine for the examination of the entire abdominal cavity. Thorough laparotomy is inadvisable in cases of localized abdominal sepsis, with the possible exception of perforated tumours, because it may disseminate infection. The order of examination is a matter of personal preference; one technique is described below and shown in Fig. 5.1. The essential feature is that nothing should be overlooked and most of the assessment is by palpation requiring 'educated' surgical hands.

PREOPERATIVE ASSESSMENT
1. This is largely determined by the nature of the problem, but in all cases the patient must be suitably prepared for surgery with adequate resuscitation and correction of haematological and biochemical abnormalities.
2. Any investigations which might have a bearing on the problem must be available in the theatre and relevant X-rays displayed.

RELEVANT ANATOMY
The abdominal cavity extends from the level of the nipples to the gluteal crease and even the most sensitive examining hand can only get a limited amount of information preoperatively.

The laparotomy provides the opportunity to examine the most inaccessible reaches of the peritoneal cavity. The amount of information obtained is proportional to the time and care taken during surgical exploration.

OPERATION
Preparation
The anaesthetized patient is generally positioned supine, although in the presence of pelvic pathology the Lloyd-Davies position may be more appropriate. The patient is cleansed and draped to expose the abdomen, and the chest in cases of trauma.

Incision
Abdominal incisions are covered in the Introduction. Routine laparotomy rarely alters management. The length and siting of the incision should be governed by the nature of the operation being performed rather than to allow ideal conditions for thorough assessment of the entire abdominal contents. When a full assessment is needed, a midline incision is usually employed because it can be extended to expose any of the four quadrants of the abdomen. It has the additional advantages of speed in access when dealing with abdominal trauma, and sound wound closure. In young children a transverse incision sited just above the umbilicus provides good exposure and heals well.

Operative technique
1. It is logical to start by examining the small bowel because once this has been eviscerated, visibility is improved for the remainder of the examination. Therefore, deliver the omentum and transverse colon into the wound and ask the assistant to hold them upwards (Fig. 5.2). Starting at the duodenojejunal flexure, inspect the paraduodenal fossa and examine the entire small bowel. Palpate the root of the

Sequence of examination

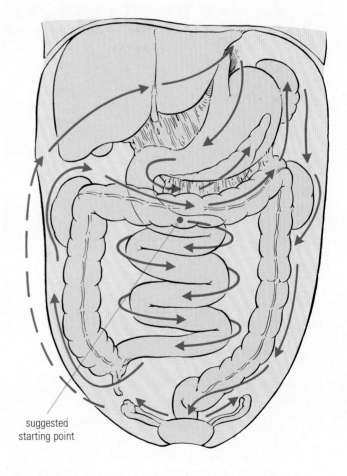

suggested
starting point

Fig. 5.1

mesentery, paravertebral retroperitoneum, aorta and mesenteric vessels, and displace the small bowel to the left of the wound. Inspect the blood vessels in the mesentery.

2. Retract the abdominal incision to the right, allowing visualization and palpation of the caecum, appendix, ascending colon, hepatic flexure and right kidney. Examine the transverse colon carefully, then displace the small bowel to the right and retract the incision to the left.

3. Examine the splenic flexure of the colon and spleen; particular care is needed here because if adhesions are present the capsule of the spleen is easily torn. Pass a hand over the spleen to palpate the left hemidiaphragm, subphrenic space, and assess the size and condition of the spleen. In deep-chested or obese patients it is easy to miss a small carcinoma of the splenic flexure of the colon.

4. Palpate the left kidney, descending colon, sigmoid colon and rectum in turn. The hand is then turned over to palpate the rectovesical or recto-uterine pouch and the pelvic contents. Having completed the examination of the infracolic compartment, return the small bowel and transverse colon to the abdomen.

5. Insert a Morris or Deaver retractor into the upper end of the incision and lift it upwards. Pass the hand to the side of the falciform ligament, and palpate the left lobe of the liver between finger and thumb (Fig. 5.3). The assistant retracts the right costal margin to allow bimanual palpation of the right lobe of the liver and palpation of the right subphrenic and subhepatic spaces (Fig. 5.4).

Palpation of liver

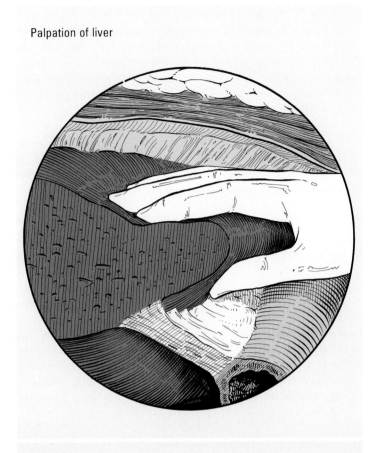

·Fig. 5.3

Lift transverse colon to examine infra-colic compartment

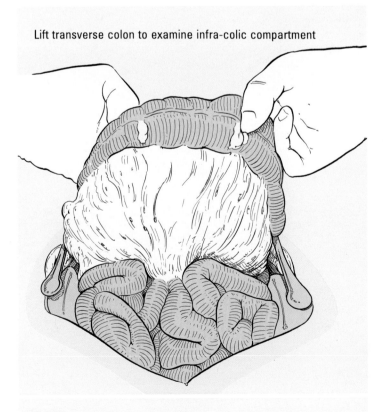

Fig. 5.2

Retract right costal margin to examine right lobe of liver

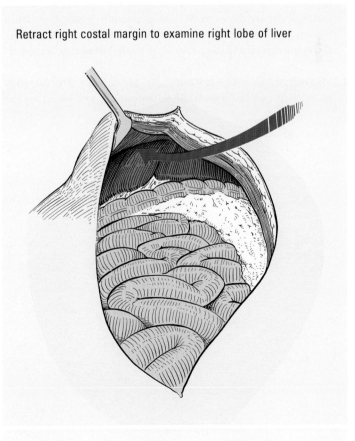

Fig. 5.4

5.3

6. Assess the oesophageal hiatus with the index finger, and then pass the hand down over the fundus and body of the stomach. Using the examining hand, stretch out the stomach to look for puckering of the serosal surface that might indicate an ulcer or small tumour, and examine the upper part of the aorta and body and tail of the pancreas by palpation through the lesser omentum.

7. The assistant draws the stomach to the left and displaces the transverse colon inferiorly to expose the pylorus and first part of the duodenum. Feel the head of the pancreas in the concavity of the duodenum.

8. Palpate the common bile duct, hepatic artery and portal vein through the foramen of Winslow, and examine the gall bladder for stones; an anomalous hepatic arterial supply is common.

Additional manoeuvres

1. For a full assessment of the first and second parts of the duodenum, head of the pancreas and distal common bile duct, mobilize the duodenum by incising the peritoneum between the duodenum and inferior vena cava. Insert a finger behind the duodenum, which is then lifted forwards (Kocher's manoeuvre).

2. If access to the lesser sac, posterior wall of the stomach and pancreas is required, divide the avascular portion of the transverse mesocolon or the gastrocolic omentum.

3. Exposure of the kidney, ureter and iliac vessels is obtained by mobilizing the ascending colon, or descending colon and the spleen, by division of the peritoneum along its antimesenteric border. When combined with Kocher's manoeuvre, the inferior vena cava and the right kidney are exposed.

4. During staging laparotomy for Hodgkin's disease (less frequently indicated with the advent of CT scanning), or for exposure of the great vessels below the duodenum, displace the small bowel to the right, and divide the peritoneum in the midline, avoiding injury to the mesenteric vessels.

5. For a full assessment of the right hemidiaphragm and bare area of the liver, together with access to the suprahepatic inferior vena cava, incise the right triangular ligament and upper leaf of the coronary ligament.

Wound closure and dressing

Close the wound with monofilament nylon and the skin by the method of choice. No drain is required for an exploratory laparotomy alone. A waterproof dressing is applied.

POSTOPERATIVE CARE

This will be largely determined by the operation which has been undertaken. If there has been no additional procedure, a nasogastric tube is advisable until any ileus from handling the bowel has subsided. Fluids and diet are then reintroduced. Skin sutures are removed after 8–10 days.

SPECIAL OPERATIVE HAZARDS
1. Poor siting of the incision.
2. Failure to assess the entire abdominal cavity, particularly if there are multiple adhesions.
3. Damage to the capsule of the spleen which usually responds to packing. Rarely, a splenectomy may be needed.

COMPLICATIONS
1. Paralytic ileus.
2. Wound problems, such as haematoma, infection and dehiscence.

Nissen Fundoplication

This operation is indicated for a minority of cases of reflux oesophagitis associated with a sliding hiatus hernia, in which there are either intractable symptoms of gastro-oesophageal reflux or complications of gastro-oesophageal reflux (e.g. stricture formation with or without aspiration pneumonitis, ulceration and haemorrhage). The aim of the operation is to restore a length of intra-abdominal oesophagus and create a valvular wrap around it using the fundus of the stomach.

The operation can be performed through the chest or abdomen according to the surgeon's preference, but the latter route is advised for cases where other intra-abdominal pathology such as gall-stones requires assessment.

PREOPERATIVE ASSESSMENT

1. Other causes of dyspepsia (e.g. peptic ulceration and gall-stones) must first be excluded. If doubts exist about the diagnosis, oesophageal manometry and pH monitoring are useful in addition to endoscopy and routine radiology.
2. Warn the patient of 'gas bloat' (see Complications later in this chapter) and the inability to vomit following the operation.
3. Reflux oesophagitis can lead to stricture formation. Any associated stricture must be treated on its own merits. Once other causes, especially malignancy, have been excluded the stricture can be endoscopically dilated.

RELEVANT ANATOMY

The oesophagus passes through the diaphragm at the level of the tenth thoracic vertebra (Fig. 5.5). The oesophageal hiatus is more vertical than horizontal and the fibres of the right crus of the diaphragm loop around the oesophagus at this level; the action of this muscular loop, together with the effect of intra-abdominal pressure on the intra-abdominal oesophagus and the weak intrinsic cardiac sphincter all act to prevent reflux of food, acid and bile from the stomach. In a sliding hiatus hernia, the gastro-oesophageal junction slides up into the chest through the hiatus, leaving the cardiac sphincter alone to prevent gastro-oesophageal reflux. Gastro-oesophageal reflux can occur without a hiatus hernia and reflux need not accompany a hiatus hernia.

The normal intra-abdominal oesophagus is approximately 1 cm long, and on its surface lie the anterior and posterior vagal trunks. It is enveloped between two leaves of peritoneum which fuse on its right as the uppermost part of the lesser omentum and on its left as the upper extremity of the greater omentum; both omenta are firmly attached to the diaphragm. Lying in front of the gastro-oesophageal junction is the lateral segment of the left lobe of the liver; this is attached to the diaphragm by the left triangular ligament.

The oesophagus enters the stomach at the cardiac orifice. The fundus of the stomach is that part which extends above the level of the cardiac orifice and which is in contact with the left hemidiaphragm. It is closely related to the spleen, being attached by two folds of peritoneum called the gastrosplenic omentum which contains the short gastric arteries (vasa brevia); these arise from the splenic artery (Fig. 5.6).

OPERATION
ABDOMINAL APPROACH
Preparation

The patient is placed supine on the operating table and a crossbar inserted into the table to allow the third blade of a Balfour retractor to be hooked under it, to provide sternal retraction. A wide-bore, for example 40 Fr, orogastric tube is passed by the anaesthetist to prevent undue narrowing of the lower oesophagus when performing the fundoplication. The skin is cleansed and drapes are applied to expose the lower chest and upper abdomen.

Incision

The abdomen is entered through an upper midline incision, starting at the level of the xiphisternum (see the Introduction).

Peritoneal attachments at hiatus

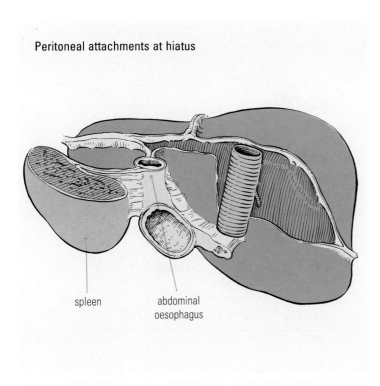

spleen   abdominal
          oesophagus

Fig. 5.5

Operative technique

1. Following a thorough laparotomy, expose the gastro-oesophageal junction by division of the left triangular ligament (Fig. 5.7). This allows the lateral segment of the left lobe of the liver to be gently retracted forward and to the right.

2. Gentle traction on the upper part of the stomach reduces the hiatus hernia. Divide the peritoneum over the front of the abdominal oesophagus and mobilize the lower oesophagus, taking care not to damage the vagi.

3. Extend this incision to the upper part of the lesser omentum. Avoid damage to an accessory left hepatic artery arising from the left gastric artery; this occurs in 23% of patients.

4. Mobilize the fundus of the stomach by division of its peritoneal attachment to the diaphragm; ligation and division of the upper short gastric arteries may be necessary (Fig. 5.8).

5. With the fingers of the right hand, push the anterior wall of the fundus of the stomach behind the oesophagus to the patient's right and grasp it with a Babcock's forceps (Fig. 5.9).

6. Insert non-absorbable sutures (e.g. 00 silk) into the gastric fundus to the right of the oesophagus, through the anterior wall of the oesophagus and into the upper stomach to the left of the oesophagus, thus wrapping the fundus around the lower oesophagus (Fig. 5.10). Generally only three or four sutures are required.

Anatomy of the cardia

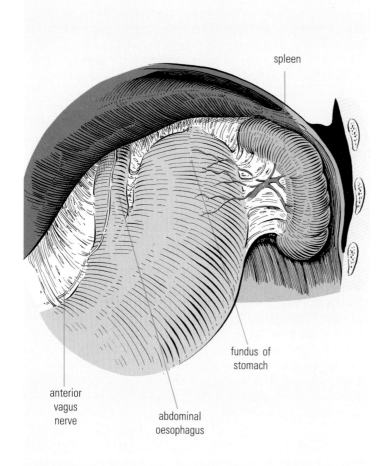

Fig. 5.6

Division of left triangular ligament to expose abdominal oesophagus and hiatus

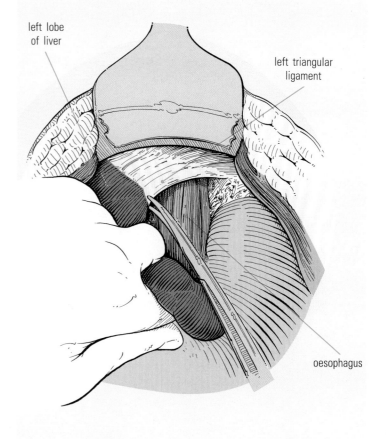

Fig. 5.7

Incision of peritoneum over oesophagus and division of short gastric vessels

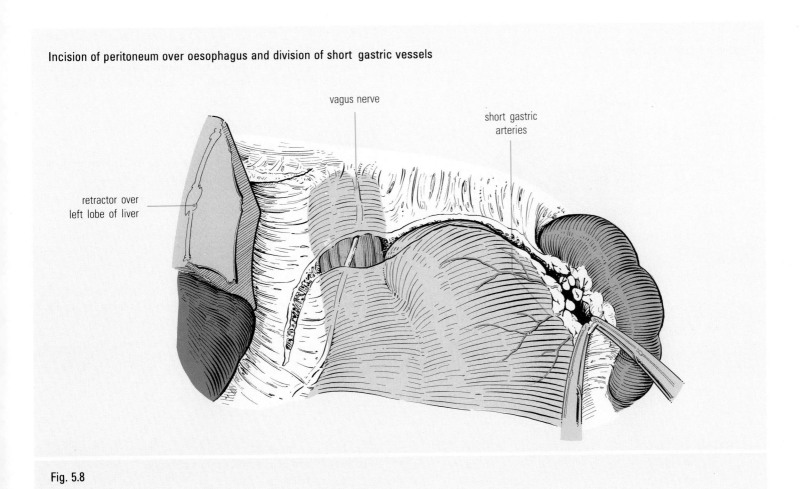

vagus nerve

short gastric arteries

retractor over left lobe of liver

Fig. 5.8

Wrapping fundus around the oesophagus

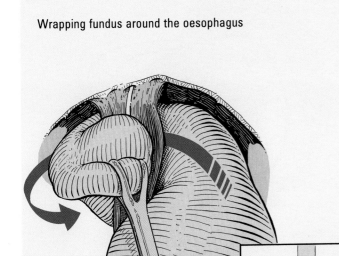

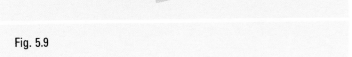

Fig. 5.9

Completion of fundoplication

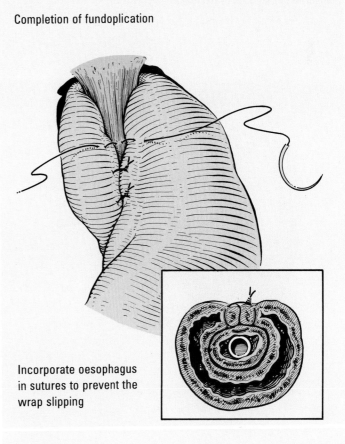

Incorporate oesophagus in sutures to prevent the wrap slipping

Fig. 5.10

Posterior repair of hiatus

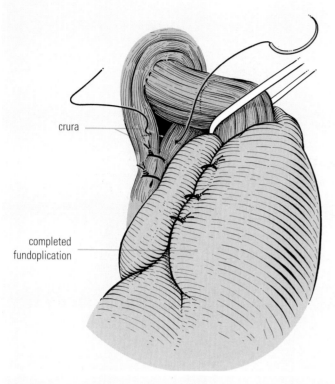

crura

completed
fundoplication

Fig. 5.11

Insertion of sutures to narrow hiatus

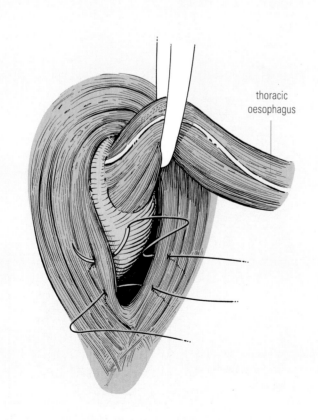

thoracic
oesophagus

Fig. 5.12

7. With gentle traction on a sling placed around the oesophagus, the margins of the hiatus are defined posteriorly
and the two crura opposed with interrupted non-absorbable
sutures (Fig. 5.11). The resulting hiatus should be snug but
not tight.

Wound closure and dressing
1. Check that there is no bleeding from the spleen and close
the wound. A drain is not necessary.
2. Replace the wide-bore tube with a standard nasogastric tube.
A dry dressing is applied.

THORACIC APPROACH
Preparation
The patient is anaesthetized and then intubated with a double-
lumen endotracheal tube and placed in the full lateral position.

Fixation of fundoplication to margin of hiatus

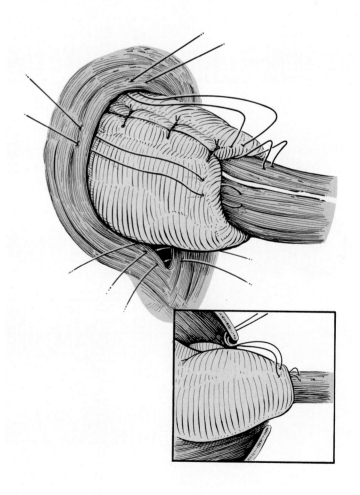

Fig. 5.13

Incision

Perform a left posterolateral thoracotomy (see page 2.20) above the seventh rib.

Operative technique

1. Open the pleura and ask the anaesthetist to deflate the left lung. The inferior pulmonary ligament is divided as far as the inferior pulmonary vein and the lung retracted upward and anteriorly.

2. Divide the parietal pleura over the lower third of the oesophagus and mobilize this segment, passing a linen tape around it. A nasogastric tube helps identification of the oesophagus and can now be withdrawn. Throughout the operation care is taken to preserve the vagus nerves which are clearly felt as cord like structures beneath the fingers, and are often visible.

3. Continue the mobilization caudally, separating the oesophagus and hiatus hernia from the crura of the diaphragm. This is achieved by dividing the condensation of connective tissue between the oesophagus and diaphragm (phreno-oesophageal ligament) and opening the basal pleura and peritoneum in order that a finger may be passed into the abdomen and swept completely around the gastro-oesophageal junction.

4. Deliver the gastric fundus into the chest and ligate the upper short gastric vessels. Reduce the stomach into the abdomen (see Fig. 5.12).

5. Define the crura and insert three non-absorbable sutures (e.g. Ethibond) between them posteriorly. These are left un-tied at this stage, but are later tied to repair the hiatus so that it will just admit two fingers (Fig. 5.12).

6. Draw the stomach into the chest, clear the fat pad from the gastro-oesophageal junction, and ask the anaesthetist to introduce a size 50 or 55 Hurst–Maloney bougie to prevent undue narrowing of the lumen of the oesophagus.

7. Wrap the fundus of the stomach 360° around the lower 3–4 cm of oesophagus from behind and secure it with three non-absorbable sutures (e.g. Ethibond), passed from one side of the fundus to the other via the encircled oesophagus. Withdraw the bougie.

8. Insert two or three non-absorbable sutures horizontally through oesophagus, fundus and crus so that when tightened the wrap is reduced into the abdomen (Fig. 5.13).

9. Tie the crural sutures, which were inserted earlier, to narrow the hiatus (Fig. 5.14).

Wound closure and dressing

Insert a chest drain, reinflate the left lung and close the chest.

POSTOPERATIVE CARE

The nasogastric tube should remain in place until gastric motility

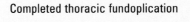

Completed thoracic fundoplication

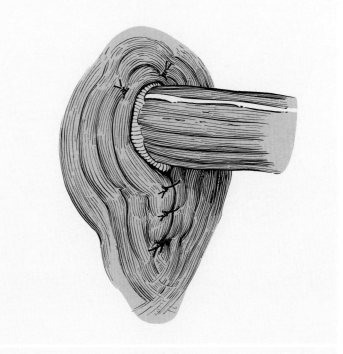

Fig. 5.14

returns; oral fluids can then be reintroduced. The skin sutures are removed after 8 days. Following the thoracic approach, the chest drain is removed on the first postoperative day unless there is an air leak from the lung.

SPECIAL OPERATIVE HAZARDS

1. Damage to the spleen. This may be treated by conservative measures, but generally a splenectomy is necessary.
2. Damage to the vagi can cause functional gastric outlet obstruction, requiring a pyloroplasty or gastroenterostomy.
3. Inability to bring the gastro-oesophageal junction into the abdomen. This is usually due to scarring and consequent shortening of the oesophagus. There are two alternatives to overcome this problem:
   (i) perform a Nissen fundoplication in the left chest;
   (ii) create a 'neo-oesophagus' by performing a Collis gastroplasty with a linear stapler (Fig. 5.15).
4. A tight peptic stricture which cannot be dilated, even when operated under direct vision. In such cases a Thal fundic patch can be performed by incising the stricture in the line of the oesophagus and suturing the fundus of the stomach to the margins of the incision. Then a fundoplication is performed.

COMPLICATIONS

1. 'Gas bloat' is a term used to describe the unpleasant gaseous

Principles of gastroplasty

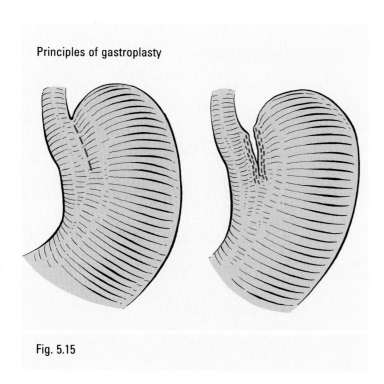

Fig. 5.15

distention experienced by some patients following a fundo-plication. It occurs particularly after fizzy drinks, which should be avoided. The valvular wrap created by this operation cannot relax and consequently the patient frequently cannot belch or vomit.

2. Dysphagia is usually transient and due to oedema around the lower oesophagus. However, in cases where a wide oro-gastric tube is not inserted at the start of the operation, the wrap can be made too tight in which case the dysphagia will not be transient.

Oesophagogastrectomy

This operation is indicated for the treatment of carcinoma of the distal oesophagus and gastro-oesophageal junction. With any further involvement of the stomach a total gastrectomy should be considered, or an Ivor–Lewis oesophagectomy if the involvement is more proximal.

PREOPERATIVE ASSESSMENT
1. Establish the diagnosis and extent of the disease with a barium meal, endoscopy with biopsy, chest X-ray, liver ultrasound and CT scanning.
2. Malnourished patients may benefit from preoperative parenteral nutrition.
3. In patients with poor respiratory function, particularly with aspiration from oesophageal obstruction, consider a procedure which does not require a thoracotomy (e.g. a purely abdominal or an abdominocervical approach).
4. Arrange a preoperative visit to the intensive care unit.

RELEVANT ANATOMY
This is covered on pages 2.11 and 5.23 in Oesophagectomy and Partial Gastrectomy.

After the operation the gastric remnant will rely on the right gastric and right gastro-epiploic arteries (both derived from the hepatic artery) for its blood supply.

OPERATION
Preparation
The anaesthetized patient is intubated and ventilated with a double-lumen endotracheal tube (to allow selective deflation of the left lung), and positioned for a thoraco-abdominal incision (see page 5.30).

Incision
Make an oblique, left-sided abdominal incision and, having confirmed resectability, extend it as a left thoraco-abdominal incision as described on page 5.30.

Operative technique
1. With the left lung drawn upwards, divide the inferior pulmonary ligament using scissors.

2. Divide the diaphragm radially down to the hiatus and insert stay sutures at intervals to allow retraction of the diaphragm and reopposition afterwards. If the tumour is adherent to the margins of the hiatus plan to remove this *en bloc*.

3. Open the pleura overlying the thoracic aorta with scissors and free the thoracic oesophagus from the aorta, coagula-

ting or ligating any small arteries running into the oesophagus directly from the aorta. Mobilize the oesophagus, keeping with it as much surrounding lymphatic and connective tissue as possible, to allow transection at least 5 cm above the upper extremity of the tumour; this may require mobilization up to the level of the aortic arch. Free the peritoneal attachments at the hiatus, excising any muscle adherent to the tumour *en bloc*, and divide the left triangular ligament if it will improve access (Fig. 5.16).

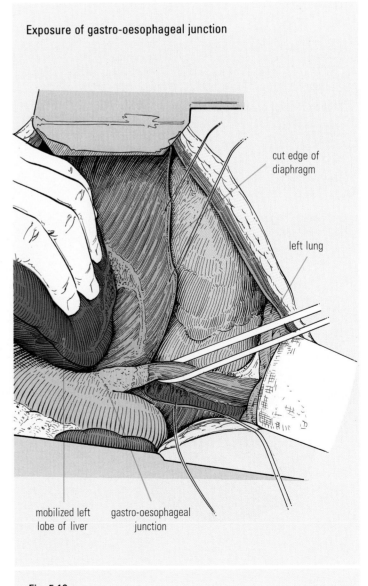

Exposure of gastro-oesophageal junction

cut edge of diaphragm

left lung

mobilized left lobe of liver

gastro-oesophageal junction

Fig. 5.16

4. Enter the lesser sac by dividing the gastrocolic omentum between ligatures and divide any adhesions between the stomach and pancreas. Keeping well clear of the stomach so as to preserve the gastro-epiploic arcade, work up to the fundus, dividing the short gastric arteries and left gastro-epiploic arteries close to their origin (Fig. 5.17).

5. Fully mobilize (Kocherize) the duodenum. Divide the lesser omentum close to the stomach, with ligation and division of any aberrant arterial input to the left lobe of the liver from the left gastric artery, and expose the origin of the left gastric artery from the coeliac artery just above the upper border of the pancreas. With the stomach lifted forwards doubly ligate and divide the left gastric artery at its origin; this is often more easily performed from the left, working

behind the stomach. Dissect the vessel free as it crosses the floor of the lesser sac with its surrounding lymphatic tissue until the upper stomach and lower oesophagus are completely free (Fig. 5.18).

6. Divide the thoracic oesophagus at the selected site and transect the stomach obliquely just below a crushing clamp below the cardia, with a non-crushing clamp across the stomach. The left gastric pedicle with its attached lymphatics forms part of the specimen. Check that the mobilized stomach can comfortably reach the cut end of the oesophagus. If it will not, divide the greater and lesser omenta further but ensure that the right gastric and gastro-epiploic arteries are not damaged.

Mobilization of greater curvature and fundus

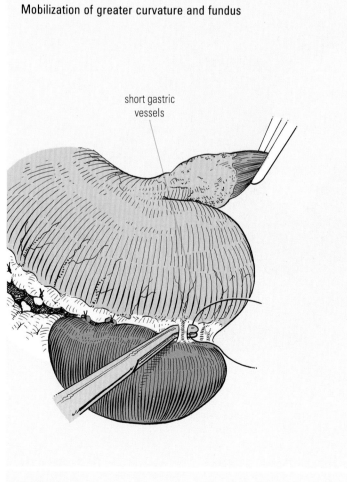

short gastric vessels

Fig. 5.17

Completed mobilization

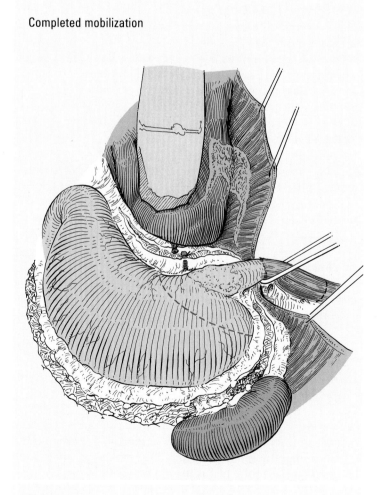

Fig. 5.18

7. Close the lesser curve defect completely with either two layers of continuous absorbable sutures, such as Vicryl or Polydioxamone (Fig. 5.19), or a linear stapling device.

8. Using diathermy make an incision in the anterior wall of the fundus of the stomach to match in size the cut end of the oesophagus and fashion an anastomosis between them using either one or two concentric layers of interrupted sutures (Fig. 5.20). It is easiest to insert all the posterior layer of sutures first, then tie them with the knots on the inside. Include the oesophageal mucosa in each stitch as it tends to retract, and if a second layer is used umbricate the outer layer of the anastomosis in an ink-well fashion (see the inset on Fig. 5.20). Alternatively, this anastomosis can be made with a stapling device, introduced through a pyloroplasty incision in the stomach in a similar fashion to that described for total gastrectomy (see page 5.31). If stapling devices are used to both close the stomach and for the anastomosis, it is important not to leave a narrow potentially devascularized area between these two staple lines; the anastomosis must either include part of the staple line or be well separated from it.

Closure of cardia

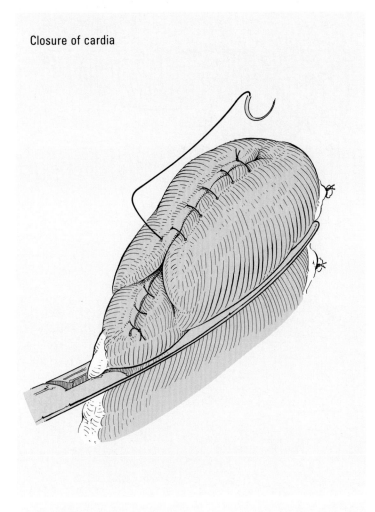

Hand sewn oesophagogastric anastomosis

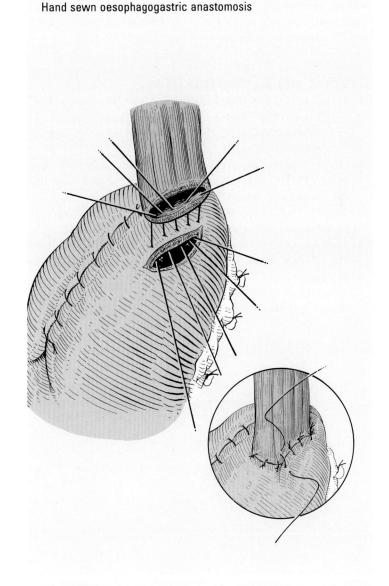

Fig. 5.19

Fig. 5.20

9. Perform a pyloromyotomy with diathermy (Fig. 5.21) or a pyloroplasty (see page 5.21) since the vagi will have been divided.

10. Ensure haemostasis, particularly around the spleen, and check the position of a nasogastric tube which is passed through the anastomosis.

Wound closure and dressing
Insert apical and basal chest drains and close and dress the thoraco-abdominal wound as described on page 5.33

POSTOPERATIVE CARE
The patient is nursed in an intensive care unit for the first 24–48 hours and electively ventilated overnight. Good analgesia without respiratory depression can be achieved by administering opiates via a thoracic epidural cannula. The patient is kept nil-by-mouth with a nasogastric tube until the sixth day, when a Gastrografin (meglumine diatrizoate) swallow is performed to visualize the anastomosis. During this period parenteral nutrition is administered. If the anastomosis is intact the nasogastric tube is removed and oral fluids are reintroduced. The apical drain is removed if the lung is fully expanded after 24–48 hours, and if there is no air leak. The basal drain remains until the seventh day. Sutures are removed after 8–10 days.

SPECIAL OPERATIVE HAZARDS
1. Disseminated tumour, in which case palliative resection might be justified particularly for cases with dysphagia. If not, consider bypassing the tumour with a loop of bowel, or palliative intubation.
2. There may be an accessory left hepatic artery, which generally arises from the left gastric artery and must be sacrificed if present.
3. Damage to the spleen, which requires a splenectomy if this does not respond to packing with moist swabs.
4. Damage to the inferior pulmonary vein when dividing the inferior pulmonary ligament.
5. Damage to the thoracic duct leading to a chylous effusion or ascites. If noted at the time of surgery, ligate the duct with a non-absorbable tie.

COMPLICATIONS
1. Anastomotic leakage should be treated conservatively with a nasogastric tube and parenteral nutrition until radiologically healed.
2. Anastomotic strictures may be benign or malignant and are treated by dilatation or palliative intubation.
3. Chest infection. Physiotherapy should be used in all patients after extubation.
4. Post-thoracotomy pain.

Pyloromyotomy

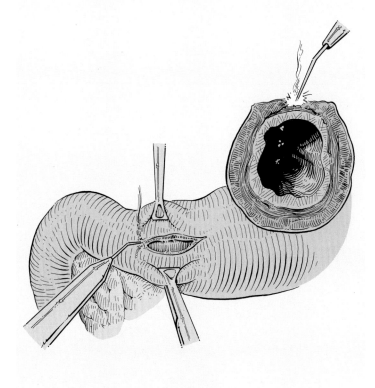

Fig. 5.21

Highly selective vagotomy (parietal cell vagotomy) is an acid reducing operation for patients with duodenal ulceration refractory to adequate medical therapy. This procedure aims to denervate the gastric parietal cells whilst preserving the hepatic, coeliac and antral branches of the vagus nerves. Intact antral innervation ensures adequate gastric emptying, obviating the need for a gastric drainage procedure. This operation carries a lower morbidity than truncal vagotomy and drainage (see page 5.18), but there is concern about the increasing long-term recurrence rate. Highly selective vagotomy is contra-indicated in obese patients because of the technical difficulties. It is generally considered that this procedure is too time-consuming to be appropriate as part of an emergency operation for complications of duodenal ulceration (e.g. bleeding).

PREOPERATIVE ASSESSMENT

1. Confirm the presence of persistent or recurrent duodenal ulceration using endoscopy or a barium meal.

2. Exclude pyloric stenosis as this is usually considered a contra-indication to highly selective vagotomy, although there are techniques of duodenal dilation and duodenoplasty.

3. Exclude, if suspected, a gastrinoma by the fasting serum gastrin estimation method, and duodenal Crohn's disease by biopsy.

RELEVANT ANATOMY (Fig. 5.22)

The anterior vagus nerve lies on the anterior surface of the abdominal oesophagus, and the posterior vagus lies behind and to the right of the oesophagus. Both give rise to multiple small branches which run onto the stomach. The vagal trunks also give rise to the hepatic and coeliac branches, and continue adjacent to the lesser curve of the stomach as the anterior and posterior nerves of Latarjet; these supply multiple secretory branches to the stomach, each accompanied by branches of the left and right gastric vessels. The nerves of Latarjet give off a leash of branches to the gastric antrum, and the watershed

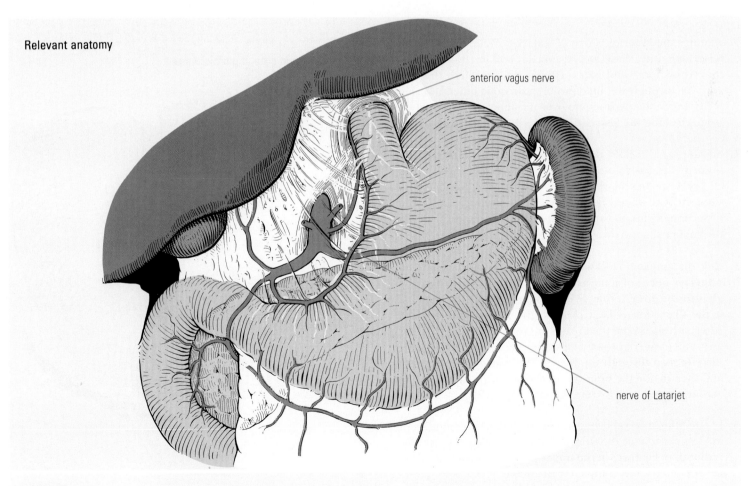

Relevant anatomy

anterior vagus nerve

nerve of Latarjet

Fig. 5.22

between these motor branches and the secretory branches to the body of the stomach is usually clearly seen at the proximal extremity of the 'crows's foot', 5–6cm proximal to the pylorus.

OPERATION
Preparation
The patient is placed supine, and the mid and upper abdomen and lower chest is cleansed and draped. A crossbar is fitted to the table. A nasogastric tube is passed, and a single dose of broad-spectrum intravenous antibiotics are given at induction.

Incision
Make an upper midline incision (see the Introduction) and carry it up into the notch between the xiphoid and costal margin to achieve the best exposure of the oesophageal hiatus. Insert a self-retaining retractor and retract the sternum with the third blade of a Balfour retractor, hooked under the crossbar.

Operative technique
1. Confirm the diagnosis of chronic duodenal ulceration, assess the gastric outlet using a finger and thumb (Fig. 5.23) and perform a thorough laparotomy.

2. Open the lesser sac by opening the gastrocolic omentum, taking care to preserve the gastro-epiploic arcade. Free adhesions between the posterior wall of the stomach and pancreas and check that there is no unsuspected gastric ulcer.

3. Identify the anterior nerve of Latarjet. Make a hole in the lesser omentum close to the stomach wall just to the left of the 'crow's foot', and pass a rubber sling through this hole and out through the hole in the gastrocolic omentum (Fig. 5.24). Incise the peritoneum over the anterior surface of the stomach along the lesser curve.

4. Starting at the hole in the lesser omentum and working towards the gastro-oesophageal junction, ligate and divide all the branches of the anterior nerve of Latarjet to the stomach with their accompanying vessels (Fig. 5.25). The dissection begins no further than 6cm from the pylorus. Use the rubber sling to draw the nerve of Latarjet taut.

5. Roll the stomach clockwise to expose the branches of the posterior nerve of Latarjet (Fig. 5.26). It is not necessary to identify the posterior nerve itself, as it should not be damaged if the dissection is kept close to the wall of the stomach. Alternatively, rotate the greater curve of the stomach superiorly and to the right so the posterior nerve of Latarjet can be directly seen through the hole in the gastrocolic omentum, and then divide the branches of the posterior vagus and the accompanying vessels from behind (Fig. 5.27).

6. Ligate and divide the remaining neurovascular bundles on the lesser curve of the stomach; it may be easier to use clips rather than ligatures in the upper part of the dissection. The lesser curve is thus completely denuded.

7. Incise the serosa over the gastro-oesophageal junction from

5.16

Digital assessment of gastric outlet

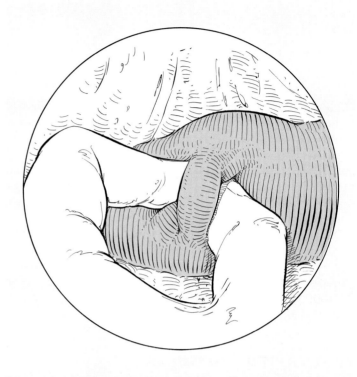

Fig. 5.23

Sling passed around gastric antrum

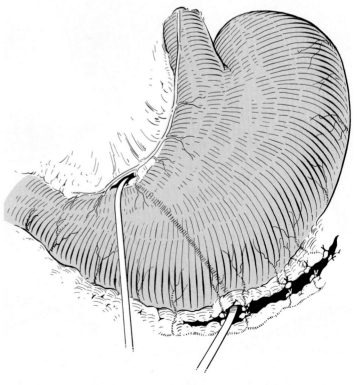

Fig. 5.24

Division of branches of anterior nerve of Latarjet

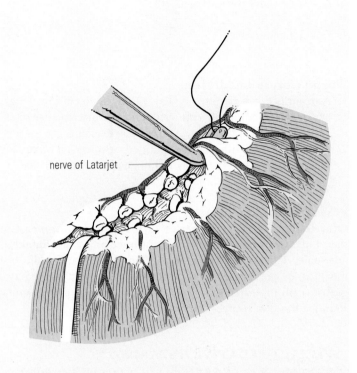

nerve of Latarjet

Fig. 5.25

the lesser curve to the oesophagogastric angle, dividing all the branches of the anterior vagus nerve to the upper stomach. Carefully preserve the vagal trunk itself and retract it to the right. It is useful to place a sling around the oesophagus to draw it downwards at this stage, taking care to exclude the posterior vagal trunk from the sling (Fig. 5.28).

8. Meticulously clear the lower 6 cm of the oesophagus circumferentially of all vagal fibres running down from above (Fig.

Posterior trunk approached through the lesser sac

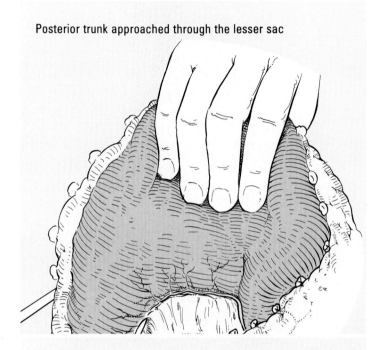

Fig. 5.27

Division of posterior branches

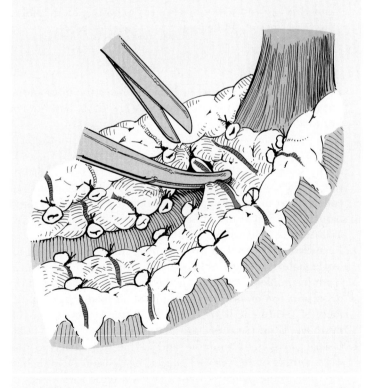

Fig. 5.26

Dissection extended over gastro-oesophageal junction

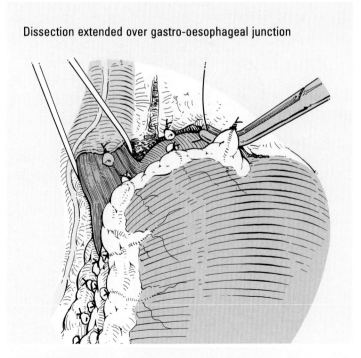

Fig. 5.28

Lower 6 cm of oesophagus cleared

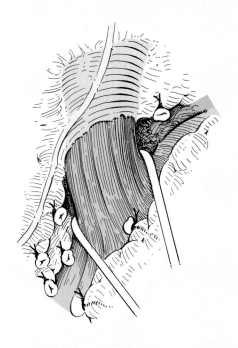

Fig. 5.29

Posterior vagus completely freed from lower oesophagus

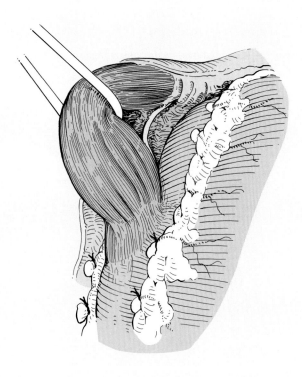

Fig. 5.30

5.18

5.29); some traction on the oesophageal sling may be necessary to obtain adequate exposure. From this level down, completely separate the back of the oesophagus from the posterior vagal trunk (Fig. 5.30).

9. Check haemostasis.

Wound closure and dressing
1. A drain is not generally needed. Close the wound by a mass closure technique with a monofilament suture, and use interrupted nylon for the skin. Apply a dry dressing.
2. The nasogastric tube can be retained or removed according to preference; it is probably not needed postoperatively.

POSTOPERATIVE CARE
Oral fluids may be commenced on the first postoperative day, but intravenous fluids are continued until oral intake is adequate. To confirm parietal cell denervation an insulin test meal can be performed, observing the acid output in the nasogastric aspirate in response to insulin-induced hypoglycaemia. Remove the skin sutures on the eighth day.

SPECIAL OPERATIVE HAZARDS
1. Tearing of the spleen due to traction on the stomach during dissection. Small tears may be repaired, but more extensive damage will necessitate splenectomy.
2. Division of the vagal trunk. If this is recognized intra-operatively a pyloroplasty is advisable, otherwise gastric stasis is likely to follow.
3. Bleeding from a vessel which retracts between the leaves of the lesser omentum. Great care must be taken to avoid damage to the nerve of Latarjet so the blind application of clips must be avoided. If bleeding persists despite sustained pressure the vessel requires exposure by incising the peritoneum and ligation.

COMPLICATIONS
1. Dysphagia due to oedema or haematoma of the distal oesophagus. This usually settles within a few days, and always within a month.
2. Lesser curve necrosis is a rare but serious complication which leads to leakage of gastric content due to necrosis of the wall of the stomach in the region of the incisura. It is probably due to inclusion of part of the gastric wall in ligatures. If conservative management with nasogastric suction and antibiotics does not bring about rapid resolution, laparotomy and suture repair will be necessary.
3. Recurrent duodenal or pyloric ulceration may be due to inadequate vagotomy. This is not uncommon, and results from incomplete clearance of the lower oesophagus and/or dissection commenced too far proximal to the pylorus. If medical treatment is unsuccessful, truncal vagotomy and drainage or autrectomy are necessary.
4. Gastric stasis is uncommon, and is due to damage to the vagal trunks or nerves of Latarjet, or division of branches too close to the pylorus. Many cases will settle with a period of intravenous fluids and nasogastric suction, but some will require reoperation and a drainage procedure.

Truncal Vagotomy and Pyloroplasty

The aim of truncal vagotomy is to reduce the gastric acid secretion of patients with peptic ulceration of the duodenum which is resistant to medical therapy. Delayed gastric emptying is a frequent result of truncal vagotomy, and a drainage procedure is therefore necessary. The drainage operation described here is pyloroplasty, but alternatively the pylorus may be bypassed by a gastrojejunostomy (see page 5.35), and this is appropriate in cases of severe pyloric scarring or stenosis. Highly selective vagotomy (see page 5.15) obviates the need for a drainage procedure by preserving the innervation of the gastric antrum, but is more time-consuming, difficult in obese patients, and results in a higher ulcer recurrence rate. Truncal vagotomy and pyloroplasty is also the procedure of choice when surgery is required for a bleeding duodenal ulcer (see page 5.41).

PREOPERATIVE ASSESSMENT
1. Confirm the presence of persistent or recurrent duodenal ulceration by endoscopy or a barium meal.
2. Exclude, if suspected, a gastrinoma causing Zollinger–Ellison syndrome by fasting serum gastrin estimation. Crohn's disease of the duodenum is very rare.

RELEVANT ANATOMY
The left triangular ligament of the liver often overlies the oesophageal hiatus, and the oesophagus is firmly attached to the diaphragm by a fold of reflected peritoneum (the phreno-oesophageal ligament).

The distribution of the vagal trunks is quite variable. The posterior vagal trunk is usually single and lies behind the oesophagus a little to the right, either closely applied to the oesophagus or in the soft tissues more posteriorly. The anterior vagus has often divided into two or more branches before entering the abdomen, and these run down the anterior surface of the oesophagus onto the stomach, the largest usually lying somewhat to the left. Small blood vessels frequently accompany the nerve trunks.

The pylorus is identified by the prepyloric vein crossing it anteriorly, and confirmed by palpating the pyloric sphincter between the finger and thumb.

OPERATION
Preparation
The patient is placed supine on the operating table and a crossbar attached. The mid and upper abdomen and lower chest are cleansed and draped and a 16 Fr nasogastric tube is passed.

Incision
Make an upper midline incision (see the Introduction) and carry it up into the notch between the xiphoid and costal margin in order to achieve adequate exposure of the oesophageal hiatus.

Operative technique
1. Insert a self-retaining retractor and retract the sternum with the third blade of a Balfour retractor hooked under the crossbar. Confirm the diagnosis of chronic duodenal ulceration and perform a thorough laparotomy.
2. Divide the left triangular ligament with scissors and reflect the left lobe of the liver to the patient's right (see Fig. 5.7 on page 5.6).
3. Confirm the position of the nasogastric tube and, with the fingers of the left hand on either side of the tube, mobilize the phreno-oesophageal ligament with scissors whilst grasping it with Roberts' forceps (Fig. 5.31) and push the perito-

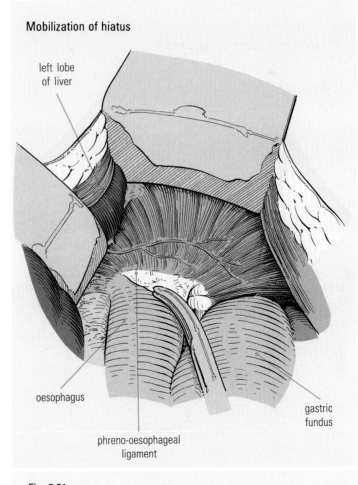

Mobilization of hiatus

left lobe of liver

oesophagus

phreno-oesophageal ligament

gastric fundus

Fig. 5.31

neal reflection on the anterior surface of the oesophagus superiorly using a pledget.

4. Gently mobilize the oesophagus using the fingers, and pass a soft rubber sling or a length of Paul's tubing around it (see Fig. 5.32).

5. With traction on the sling, pass the fingers of the right hand behind the oesophagus. If the posterior vagal trunk is in the sling it will be felt as a tight band behind the oesophagus. If it is not, it will be found posteriorly, usually in the sulcus between the vertebral column and the aorta. Push the posterior vagus forward on the tip of the right middle finger to the right of the oesophagus (Fig. 5.32).

6. Grasp the posterior vagus with three pairs of Roberts' forceps and divide the trunk above and below the middle pair (Fig. 5.33). Ligate or use diathermy on the upper and lower cut ends, and send the excised segment for histological analysis. Look for a second posterior trunk and, if present, deal with it in the same way.

7. Lift the anterior vagus nerve with a nerve hook (Fig. 5.34), excise a segment in a similar manner to the posterior vagus nerve; the segment is also sent for histological analysis. Search carefully for multiple anterior nerves which are felt

Division of posterior vagus nerve

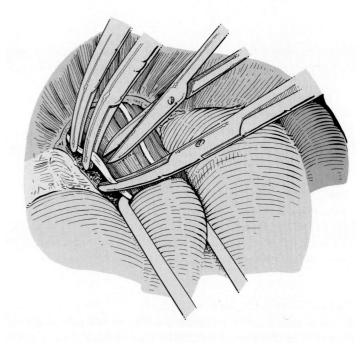

Fig. 5.33

Visualization of posterior vagus nerve

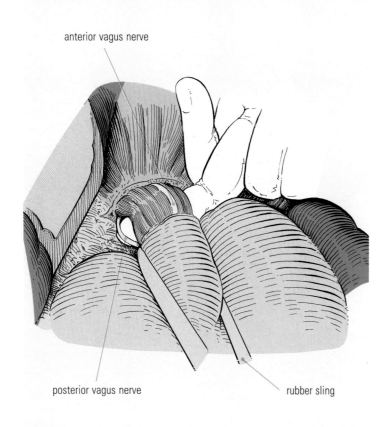

anterior vagus nerve

posterior vagus nerve

rubber sling

Fig. 5.32

Lifting anterior vagus nerve free from oesophagus

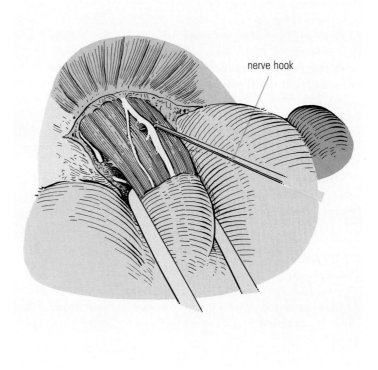

nerve hook

Fig. 5.34

Incision for Heineke–Mikulicz pyloroplasty

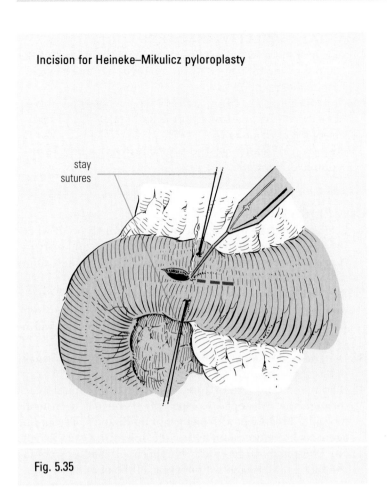

Fig. 5.35

as cord-like structures on the surface of the oesophagus. Lift these smaller nerves from the oesophagus with a nerve hook and diathermize and divide them.

8. Steady the pylorus with superior and inferior stay sutures and perform a pyloroplasty. This is made easier if the duodenum is mobilized (Kocherized) by division of the peritoneum along its lateral side. Two techniques of pyloroplasty are described in this chapter:

For a Heineke–Mikulicz pyloroplasty
9. Open the pylorus longitudinally for 3–4cm using a cutting diathermy point (Fig. 5.35).

10. With traction applied to the stay sutures, bring the proximal and distal ends of the incision into apposition and close the incision transversely in two layers; an over-and-over, inner continuous layer (Fig. 5.36) and an outer layer of interrupted seromuscular (Lembert) stitches using an absorbable suture (e.g. 2/0 Vicryl) (Fig. 5.37).

For a Finney pyloroplasty
9. Prior to opening the stomach, oppose the adjacent walls of the antrum and descending duodenum with a continuous seromuscular stitch, although some surgeon's consider this step unnecessary (Fig. 5.38). Make a curved, inverted U-

Inner all-coats layer

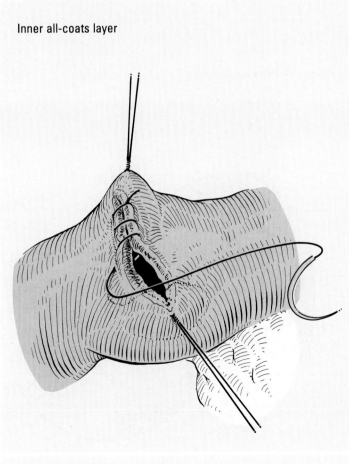

Fig. 5.36

Interrupted seromuscular outer layer

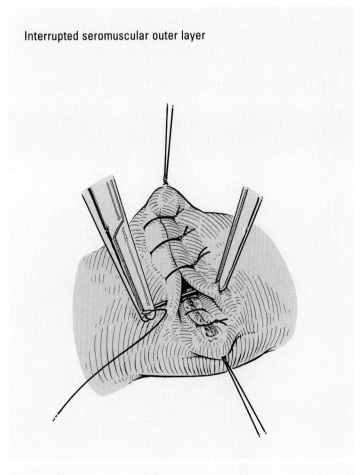

Fig. 5.37

shaped gastroduodenotomy with cutting diathermy from the gastric antrum to the descending duodenum (see Fig. 5.38).

10. Starting at the apex of the 'U', sew the cut edges of the stomach and descending duodenum together with a continuous over-and-over suture until the ends of the gastroduodenotomy are reached. Complete the anterior layer with an over-and-over suture inverting the mucosa with each stitch and bury it with a layer of interrupted seromuscular Lembert stitches (Fig. 5.39).

11. Check the completed pyloroplasty to ensure that it is widely patent by invaginating the thumb and index finger through the lumen. Also check the hiatus for haemostasis and adjust the position of the nasogastric tube so that it lies in the gastric antrum.

Wound closure and dressing
The use of a drain is a matter of personal preference. Close the wound by a mass closure technique with a monofilament suture, and use interrupted nylon sutures for the skin. Apply a dry dressing.

POSTOPERATIVE CARE
Intravenous fluids and nasogastric suction are continued until gastric emptying is established, usually on the second or third postoperative day. The drain, if used, is removed after 2–3 days and the skin sutures after 8–10 days.

SPECIAL OPERATIVE HAZARDS
1. Tearing the spleen due to traction on the stomach during vagotomy. Small tears may be repaired, but more extensive damage will necessitate splenectomy.
2. Perforation of the oesophagus during mobilization; this is usually due to inadequate mobilization of the phreno-oesophageal ligament.
3. Failure to identify all the vagal nerves, leading to incomplete vagotomy.

COMPLICATIONS
1. Leakage from the pyloroplasty may occasionally occur where sutures have cut out in the presence of oedema and scarring. If gross scarring or oedema is present, a gastroenterostomy is a wiser choice of drainage procedure.
2. Delayed gastric emptying. If this is due to postoperative oedema it will settle with a few days of nasogastric suction. If the pyloroplasty is too narrow, surgical revision will be necessary.
3. Diarrhoea is due to rapid gastric emptying, and usually settles spontaneously.
4. Bilious vomiting results from reflux of bile into the stomach through the pyloroplasty, especially if this has been made too wide. Treatment with metoclopramide and a bile-binding agent such as aluminium hydroxide or hydrotalcite will help. No revisional surgery for diarrhoea or bilious vomiting should be undertaken within a year of the operation.
5. Recurrent ulceration is usually due to incomplete vagotomy. This may heal with H$_2$ blockers, but revisional surgery with revagotomy or partial gastrectomy may be necessary.

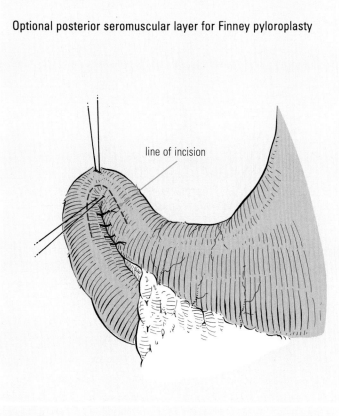

Optional posterior seromuscular layer for Finney pyloroplasty

line of incision

Fig. 5.38

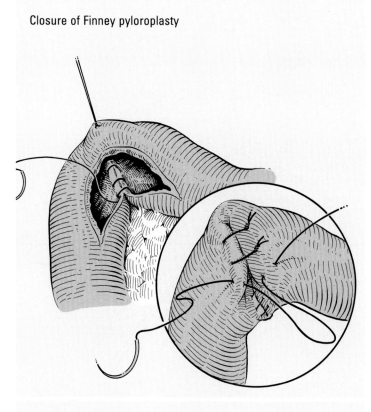

Closure of Finney pyloroplasty

Fig. 5.39

Partial Gastrectomy

There are two principle indications for this procedure. The first is benign peptic ulceration in which there has been either failure of medical treatment, or complications such as perforation or haemorrhage; particularly if vagotomy and drainage is inappropriate or has been performed previously. The second is either a benign (e.g. leiomyoma) or malignant lesion of the distal two-thirds of the stomach. In cases of malignancy, as much lymphatic tissue as possible is resected with the specimen and the vessels ligated close to their origins.

Following resection of the distal stomach, reconstruction can be performed by either fashioning a new lesser curve and creating a gastroduodenal anastomosis (Billroth I) or by anastomosis of the gastric remnant to a loop of jejunum, with closure of the duodenal stump (Billroth II or Pólya gastrectomy).

PREOPERATIVE ASSESSMENT

1. Adequate resuscitation prior to surgery is essential for patients with either haemorrhage or perforation.
2. Preoperative endoscopy should be performed in cases of haemorrhage to establish the site of bleeding and to biopsy a gastric ulcer.

RELEVANT ANATOMY

The stomach lies in the epigastrium and left hypochondrium, and forms part of the anterior wall of the lesser sac (Fig. 5.40). It comprises four regions: the fundus (the region above the cardiac orifice) which is closely related to the spleen; the body which is separated from the pancreas by the lesser sac; the

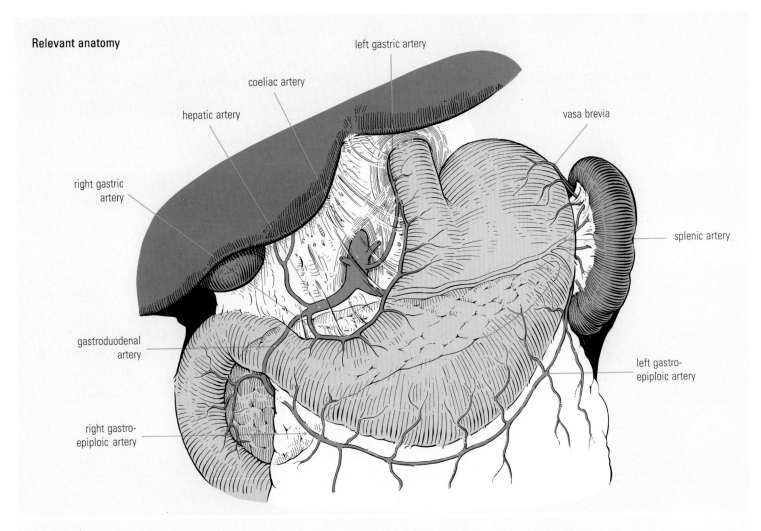

Relevant anatomy

Fig. 5.40

antrum which is the propulsive distal portion of the stomach; and the pylorus, which is the muscular valve controlling gastric emptying into the duodenum, the first part of which is intra-peritoneal and overlies the common bile duct.

The two leaves of peritoneum forming the lesser omentum extend from the liver to the lesser curvature of the stomach, where they then separate to enclose the stomach and fuse once again along the greater curvature of the stomach to form the greater omentum. This overlies and is adherent to the transverse colon and mesocolon.

The stomach derives its blood supply from the coeliac axis as follows.

1. The left gastric artery arises directly from the coeliac axis and runs across the floor of the lesser sac towards the oeso-phageal hiatus. It then passes between the leaves of the lesser omentum and runs along the lesser curvature to anastomose with the right gastric artery.
2. The right gastric artery arises from the hepatic artery and similarly runs between the leaves of the lesser omentum.
3. The gastroduodenal artery, a branch of the hepatic artery, runs behind the first part of the duodenum and gives rise to the right gastro-epiploic artery which passes from the pylorus along the greater curvature towards the fundus to meet the left gastro-epiploic artery. It gives off gastric branches to the

stomach and epiploic arteries to the greater omentum.
4. The left gastro-epiploic artery arises from the splenic artery and similarly runs between the leaves of the greater omentum towards the pylorus.
5. The vasa brevia, or short gastric arteries, of which there are five or six, arise from the splenic artery and run in the gastrosplenic omentum to reach the fundus of the stomach. The lymphatic drainage of the stomach follows the arterial supply and drains to the pre-aortic nodes around the coeliac axis. Venous blood drains into the splenic and portal veins.

OPERATION
Preparation
The operation is performed under general anaesthesia with a nasogastric tube introduced by the anaesthetist. A crossbar suitable for a sternal retractor is fixed to the table. The patient is placed supine, the skin is prepared and drapes are placed.

Incision
Make a midline abdominal incision (see the Introduction).

Develop plane between greater omentum and transverse mesocolon

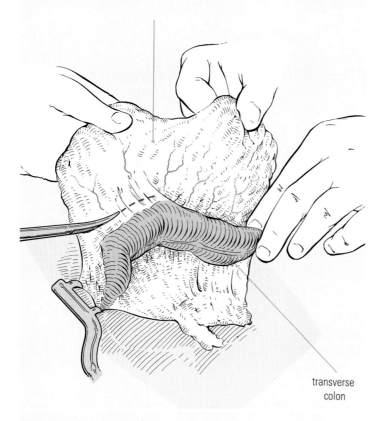

transverse colon

Fig. 5.41

Division of right gastric artery

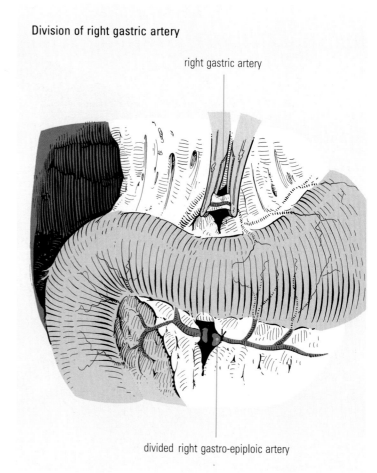

right gastric artery

divided right gastro-epiploic artery

Fig. 5.42

Operative technique

1. Perform a laparotomy and insert a self-retaining retractor. In cases of haemorrhage the bleeding site must be located and haemostasis secured (see page 5.41 in Management of Gastroduodenal Bleeding).

2. Commence mobilization of the stomach. In benign conditions, divide the gastrocolic omentum with ligation and division of the gastro-epiploic vessels to gain access to the lesser sac. In cases of malignancy, lift the omentum up and dissect it off the transverse colon and mesocolon (Fig. 5.41) in the so-called bloodless plane, taking care to identify and avoid the middle colic artery which runs in the transverse mesocolon close to the pylorus.

3. Divide any adhesions in the lesser sac between the pancreas and the stomach.

4. If present, a posterior gastric ulcer eroding into the pancreas should be pinched off leaving the excluded ulcer base stuck to the pancreas. The resulting hole in the stomach must be closed to prevent contamination.

5. Mobilization of the greater curvature is completed by ligation and division of the lower short gastric vessels, the left gastro-epiploic artery and also the right gastro-epiploic pedicle, which is divided below the duodenum (see Fig. 5.42).

6. Divide the right gastric pedicle on the lesser curvature (Fig. 5.42).

7. Divide and ligate the lesser omentum from the pylorus proximally until the left gastric pedicle is reached. This is then doubly ligated and divided, with care being taken to preserve an aberrant left hepatic artery if it is present.

8. Place a crushing clamp just distal to the pylorus and a soft clamp across the duodenum before dividing the duodenum between the two clamps (Fig. 5.43).

To perform a gastroduodenal anastomosis

9. Ensure that the nasogastric tube is withdrawn into the fundus and place a long non-crushing clamp across the stomach from the greater curvature for a distance that will be suitable to anastomose to the duodenal stump. Apply a crushing clamp alongside and distal to it and divide the stomach between the clamps.

10. Apply a second pair of clamps at an angle to the first pair from the apex of the previous incision to the lesser curvature ensuring that the ulcer will be included in the resected specimen. Divide the remaining stomach (Fig. 5.44) and remove the resected specimen.

11. Fashion a new lesser curve by suturing over-and-over the upper non-crushing clamp with a 2/0 absorbable suture

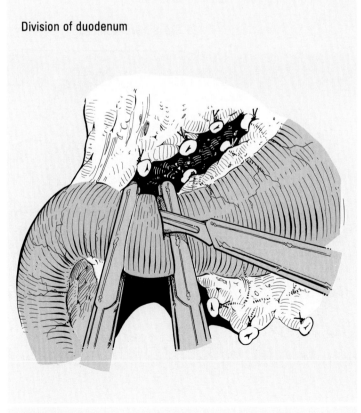

Division of duodenum

Fig. 5.43

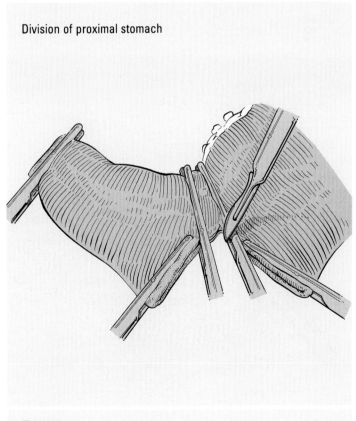

Division of proximal stomach

Fig. 5.44

(Fig. 5.45). Tighten the sutures after removing the clamp and bury the suture line with a continuous seromuscular stitch (Fig. 5.46).

12. The gastroduodenal anastomosis should be performed in two layers, with an inner all-coats layer and an outer seromuscular suture (Fig. 5.47). The weakest point of the anastomosis is at the Y-junction formed with the newly fashioned lesser curve. This should be reinforced with a horizontal mattress suture (Fig. 5.47, inset).

Gastroduodenal anastomosis

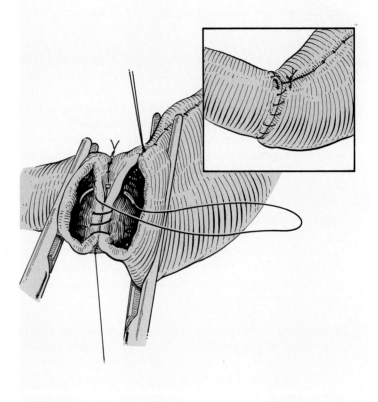

Fig. 5.47

Creation of new lesser curvature

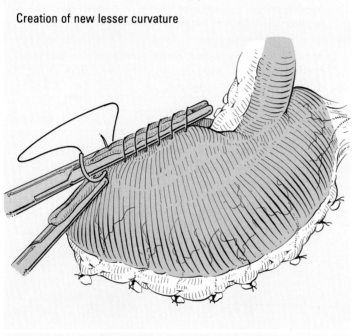

Fig. 5.45

Two-layer closure of lesser curve

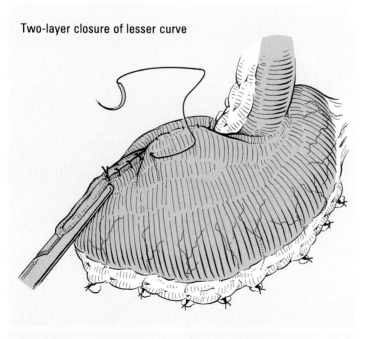

Fig. 5.46

Use of stapling device to close duodenum

Hand-sewn technique

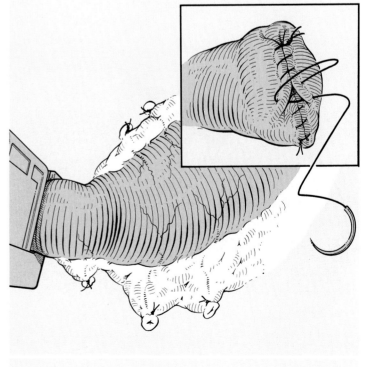

Fig. 5.48

To perform a gastrojejunal anastomosis

9. Close the duodenal stump by inserting an over-and-over, continuous absorbable suture which is drawn tight as the clamp is eased off. Insert a second layer of continuous, or interrupted sutures to invert the previous suture line (see inset to Fig. 5.48). Alternatively a linear stapler may be used to close the duodenum prior to dividing it (Fig. 5.48).

10. Choose the level of resection of the stomach, aiming to remove the distal two-thirds in peptic ulceration and at least a 5 cm margin with a malignancy. Place a non-crushing clamp across the stomach, 2 cm proximal to the chosen level of resection.

11. Bring a loop of proximal jejunum, taken from as close to the duodenojejunal flexure as possible, in front of or through the transverse mesocolon to the left of the middle colic artery and place it in an isoperistalsic position (afferent end to the greater curve) (Fig. 5.49). The afferent loop should be kept short.

12. Pull the stomach remnant over to the left and allow it to hang over the costal margin. Place a non-crushing clamp across the jejunal loop, or alternatively use a pair of interlocking Lane's twin gastroenterostomy clamps, and insert a posterior continuous 2/0 absorbable seromuscular suture to unite the jejunum to the stomach beyond the clamp.

13. Place crushing clamps across the stomach from the lesser and greater curves and open the posterior wall of the stomach remnant with diathermy (Fig. 5.50).

14. Using a diathermy point, open the jejunum adjacent to the gastric stoma with a longitudinal incision which should match the divided stomach (see Fig. 5.51).

15. Anastomose the adjacent edges of the gastric and jejunal incisions with an over-and-over, all-layer, continuous absorbable suture (Fig. 5.51) to complete the posterior wall of the anastomosis.

Partially dividing stomach

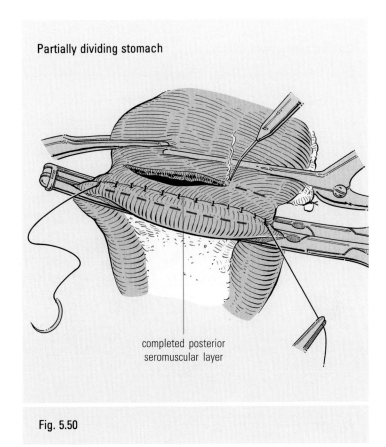

completed posterior seromuscular layer

Fig. 5.50

Positioning twin clamp for gastrojejunal anastomosis

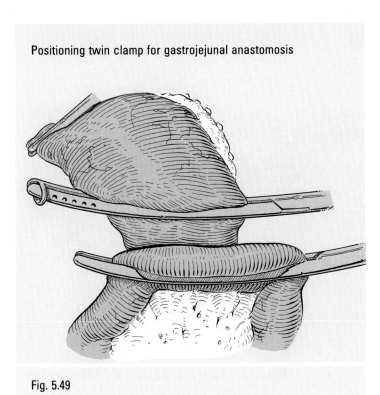

Fig. 5.49

Completing posterior layer of anastomosis

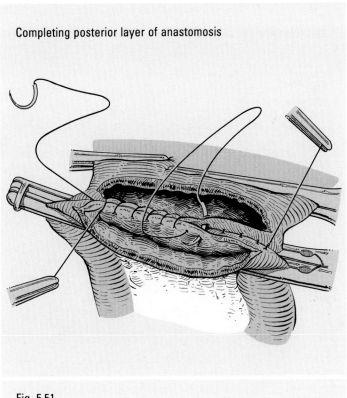

Fig. 5.51

16. Now remove the stomach remnant by division of the anterior stomach wall with diathermy (Fig. 5.52) and continue the all-layers suture around the incision to complete the

inner layer of the anastomosis. An over-and-over stitch should be used to ensure haemostatic closure (Fig. 5.53). Remove the clamps.

17. Complete the anterior seromuscular layer (Fig. 5.54) and check the stoma for adequate patency by invaginating a finger and thumb through the anastomosis.

18. If a partial width stoma is preferred to reduce bile reflux into the stomach, a Hofmeister valve can be fashioned, reducing the stoma length to around 5 cm. This is achieved by resecting the stomach remnant with cutting diathermy after completion of the posterior serosal layer. Fashion the valve by suturing together the anterior and posterior cut edges of the stomach from the lesser curve towards the greater curve until 5 cm of gastric stoma remains. Then open the jejunum over this length and complete the anastomosis as above including the valve segment in the anterior seromuscular layer (Fig. 5.55).

Wound closure and dressing

Place a drain and close the abdomen with loop nylon and interrupted skin sutures. Apply a dry dressing.

POSTOPERATIVE CARE

The patient should be managed with intravenous fluids and nasogastric tube on free drainage. Once bowel sounds have returned and the drainage from the nasogastric tube has diminished, oral intake can be increased and the nasogastric tube can be removed.

Dividing anterior wall of stomach

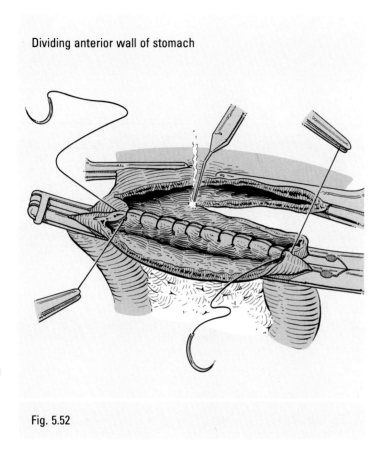

Fig. 5.52

All coats suture of anterior wall

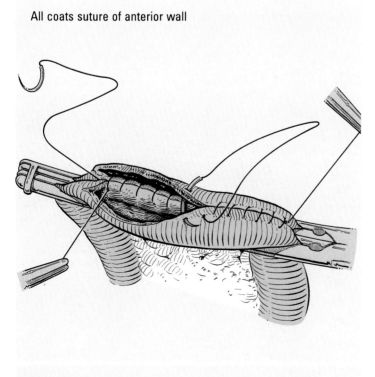

Fig. 5.53

Completion of gastrojejunal anastomosis

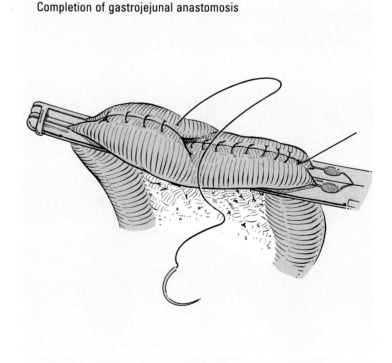

Fig. 5.54

The drain should be left for 24–48 hours unless, in a Billroth II gastrectomy, the closure of the duodenal stump was difficult, in which case the drain is left for 10 days until a tract has formed.

SPECIAL OPERATIVE HAZARDS

1. The common bile duct may be damaged when mobilizing the first part of the duodenum. It should be repaired around a T-tube in these circumstances.
2. Damage to the middle colic artery in the transverse mesocolon, which can lead to ischaemia of the colon and necessitate resection.
3. With an ulcer high on the lesser curve, Pauchet's procedure can be employed in which a tongue of lesser curve (including the ulcer) is taken prior to making a new lesser curve. With a high ulcer that is not on the lesser curve, the stomach can be rotated to allow the ulcer to be resected as though it was on the lesser curve (Tanner's rotation). Alternatively the ulcer can be locally excised and the defect closed prior to distal gastrectomy.
4. It may be impossible to close the duodenal stump securely. In such cases the stump is closed around a 30 Fr Foley catheter which is brought out through the anterior abdominal wall and removed on the fourteenth post-operative day. By this time a tract will have formed, creating a controlled fistula which should close spontaneously.
5. Occasionally when a large posterior duodenal ulcer is present, full mobilization of the duodenum is not possible. Nissen's method of closure can then be performed by suturing the anterior edge of the duodenum to the lateral edge of the ulcer crater, thus excluding the ulcer from the gastrointestinal tract.
6. Damage to the spleen when mobilizing the stomach.

COMPLICATIONS

1. Haemorrhage can occur either from an inadequately under-run artery in the base of the ulcer or from the cut edges of stomach and small bowel particularly if a continuous haemo-static over-and-over stitch is not used. Haemorrhage may also result from a splenic tear that was overlooked.
2. Leakage may occur from either the duodenal stump or from the anastomosis. If there are no signs of peritonitis and drainage is satisfactory, parenteral nutrition should be instituted and the patient placed 'nil-by-mouth'. If there are signs of peritonitis, laparotomy should be performed and the leak repaired if it is from the anastomosis. If it is from the duodenal stump, the stump should be closed around a large Foley catheter (see Special Operative Hazards).

3. Postgastrectomy complications may occur as follows:
   (i) Vasomotor dumping; if symptoms do not settle with medical treatment, various operative techniques are available to interpose a loop of jejunum between the stomach and the duodenum, either isoperistalsic or anti-peristalsic to slow down gastric emptying.
   (ii) Late dumping; the patient is advised to eat small amounts of food frequently.
   (iii) Small stomach and dumping; several procedures have been described to form a reservoir (e.g. the Poth pouch and the Hunt–Lawrence pouch).
   (iv) Reflux gastritis; this is best treated by a Roux-en-Y diversion.
4. The risk of gastric malignancy in the stomach remnant is increased.
5. Anaemia from iron or B_{12} deficiency.

Hofmeister valve

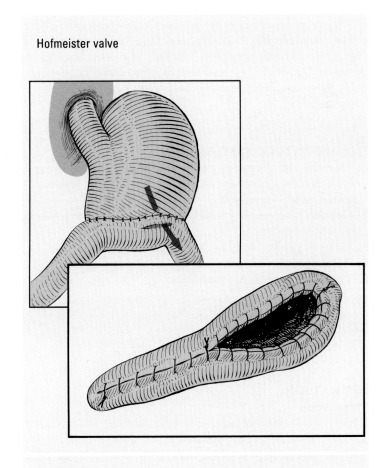

Fig. 5.55

Total Gastrectomy for Gastric Malignancy

To offer a potential cure from gastric cancer, radical resection of the stomach and its surrounding lymph nodes is indicated in selected patients with gastric malignancy. Continuity is restored by oesophagojejunal anastomosis. The extent of the lymph-adenectomy forms the basis by which radical gastrectomy is classified as R1, R2 or R3 types. An R1 resection includes the immediate lymph nodes along the stomach wall, an R2 resection (described below) also includes the nodes around the splenic hilum and along the coeliac artery and its branches, and in an R3 resection the nodes from the porta hepatis, the front of the aorta, behind the head of the pancreas and in the base of the mesentery and transverse mesocolon are also removed. There remains some debate as to whether a more radical operation is necessarily going to benefit the patient. The operation can be performed through a long midline incision, but in large individuals a thoraco-abdominal approach gives better access to the lower oesophagus.

PREOPERATIVE ASSESSMENT
1. Establish the diagnosis and extent of the disease using a barium meal, endoscopy with biopsy, chest X-ray, liver ultrasound and CT scanning.
2. Consider preoperative total parenteral nutrition in severely wasted patients.
3. Perform gastric lavage in cases of gastric obstruction.
4. Arrange for an intensive care bed postoperatively.
5. Prescribe prophylactic antibiotics.

RELEVANT ANATOMY
This is covered on page 5.23 in Partial Gastrectomy.

OPERATION
Preparation
If a thoraco-abdominal incision is to be used, the anaesthetized patient is intubated and ventilated with a double-lumen endotracheal tube to allow selective deflation of the left lung. They are supported on the operating table on their right side but tilted backward to lie midway between a full lateral and semi-lateral position. The left leg is flexed at the knee and the hip and right leg extended with a pillow between the knees. The left arm is bandaged to a support in the position shown in Fig. 5.56.

For an abdominal approach the patient is placed supine.

Incision
If a thoraco-abdominal approach is to be used, make an oblique abdominal incision from the midline to the costal margin. Divide the underlying muscles in the line of the skin incision with cutting diathermy, ligate and divide the superior epigastric vessels which lie deep to the rectus abdominus muscle and open

the peritoneum. After a preliminary laparotomy to confirm suitability for resection, extend the skin incision laterally along the line of the eighth or ninth rib to the lateral border of erector spinae, and deepen it onto the rib with cutting diathermy. Incise the periosteum and strip it upwards and off the upper border of the rib as far as its neck using a periosteal elevator. Excise a 2–3 cm portion of the rib posteriorly with a costatome, and the costal cartilage anteriorly where it crosses the relevant interspace with a knife. Open the pleura, insert a Finochietto retractor, and crank the retractor open. The diaphragm is then divided radially down to the oesophageal hiatus after stay sutures have been inserted at intervals to allow its accurate reopposition afterwards (see Fig. 5.16). If the tumour is adherent to the margins of the hiatus plan to remove this *en bloc*.

For an abdominal approach make a long midline incision (see the Introduction) with division of the xiphisternum.

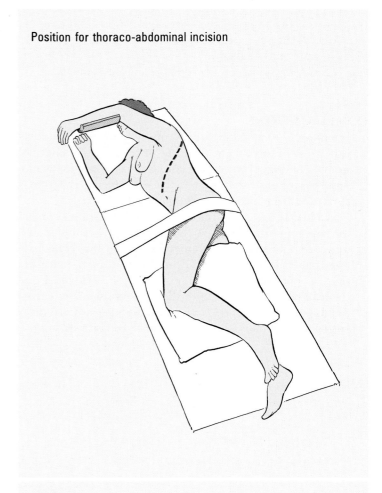

Position for thoraco-abdominal incision

Fig. 5.56

Operative technique

1. Divide the left triangular ligament and the peritoneum over the gastro-oesophageal junction with scissors as for a truncal vagotomy (see page 5.19).

2. Divide and free the oesophagus from the margins of the diaphragmatic hiatus unless tumour is adherent.

3. Mobilize the lower oesophagus and place a sling around it; division of the vagi will provide extra length. If a thoraco-abdominal approach is used the thoracic oesophagus can be more easily mobilized after division of the inferior pulmonary ligament and upward retraction of the left lung.

4. Divide the peritoneal attachments of the spleen to the diaphragm and posterior abdominal wall with scissors and draw the spleen and attached fundus of the stomach medially, lifting the tail of the pancreas forward.

5. Divide the peritoneal fold attaching the splenic flexure to the spleen; this often contains a blood vessel which requires ligation or diathermy. Lift up the omentum and with scissors develop the bloodless plane between it and the transverse mesocolon from the hepatic to the splenic flexure so that it remains attached only to the stomach.

6. Mobilize the duodenum by division of the lateral reflection of peritoneum, and continue to incise the peritoneum as it crosses the bile duct and hepatic artery to become the lesser omentum. Keep close to the liver and continue until the cardio-oesophageal junction is reached (see Fig. 5.57), sacrificing an accessory left hepatic artery arising from the left gastric artery if present. This completes the division of the peritoneal attachment of the stomach.

7. Divide the right gastric and right gastro-epiploic arteries close to their origin from the hepatic and gastroduodenal arteries above and below the pylorus respectively (Fig. 5.57). Clamp and divide the first part of the duodenum and close the distal end, using either a linear stapling device or two layers of sutures with an inner continuous and an outer interrupted or continuous layer, as for a Pólya gastrectomy (see page 5.27).

8. Lift the spleen forward and dissect the pancreas free from its posterior attachments until the coeliac artery is reached. Dissect out and divide the splenic and left gastric arteries. Clear the coeliac artery of surrounding lymphatic tissue keeping this tissue with the specimen.

9. Ligate and divide the splenic vein and divide the pancreas

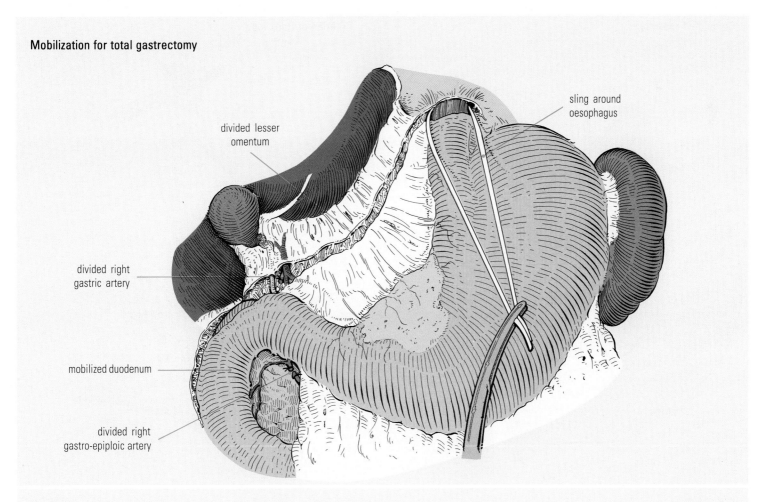

Mobilization for total gastrectomy

divided lesser omentum

sling around oesophagus

divided right gastric artery

mobilized duodenum

divided right gastro-epiploic artery

Fig. 5.57

just to the left of the aorta with a knife. Secure haemostasis from any bleeding points with fine sutures or diathermy. Carefully transfix the cut end of the pancreatic duct and oversew the cut end of the gland with non-absorbable sutures (Fig. 5.58).

10. Place a right-angled non-crushing clamp across the oesophagus and divide it distally above the gastro-oesophageal junction, ensuring at least 5 cm clearance from the tumour margin, and remove the specimen. When completed the oesophagojejunal anastomosis should lie within the abdomen.

11. To fashion the Roux loop, take a mobile loop of jejunum just distal to the duodenojejunal flexure and holding it by the apex of the loop, divide the proximal bowel at the base of the loop between non-crushing clamps, and partially divide its mesentery with ligation of its contained blood vessels so that the cut end of the loop will reach the cut end of the oesophagus.

12. Make a hole in the transverse mesocolon and take the

jejunum through this hole and up to the hiatus (Fig. 5.59). The oesophagojejunal anastomosis is now fashioned, either by suturing or stapling. To suture the anastomosis, make a hole in the antimesenteric border of the bowel with diathermy to match the lumen of the oesophagus, 3–4 cm from the cut end of the jejunal loop. Oversew the cut end of the jejunum with two layers of an absorbable suture such as Vicryl. Fashion the oesophagojejunal anastomosis with a single layer of interrupted non-absorbable sutures; if preferred, this suture line can be buried with a second layer of interrupted sutures (Fig. 5.60), picking up the diaphragm with a couple of these to keep the anastomosis in the abdomen. There must be good vascularity and no tension on this anastomosis.

To staple the oesophagojejunal anastomosis insert a purse-string suture into the distal end of the oesophagus and introduce a circular stapling gun into the cut end of the jejunal loop with the upper stapling head removed. Push the central post of the device through the antimesenteric wall of the bowel 3–4 cm from the end, screw on the upper stapling head and slide the end of the oesophagus over it (see the inset on Fig. 5.60), tightening the purse

Completed resection

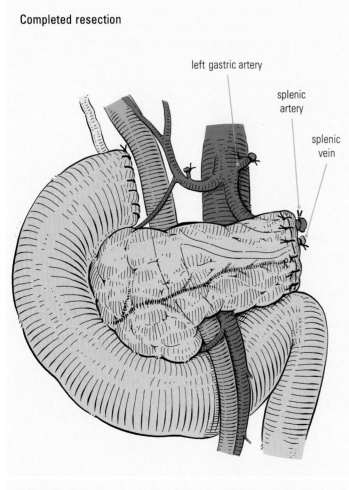

Fig. 5.58

Creation of Roux loop

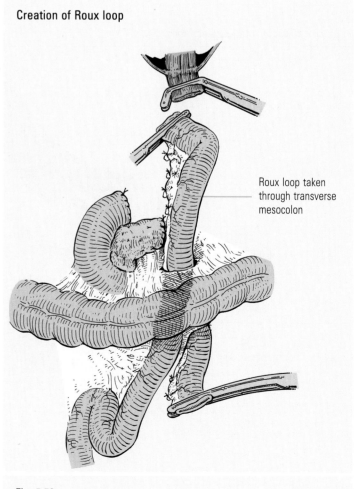

Fig. 5.59

Oesophagojejunal anastomosis

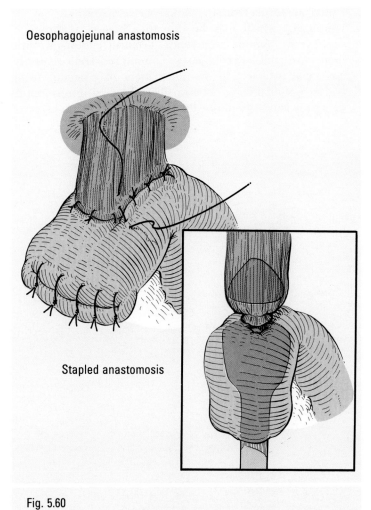

Stapled anastomosis

Fig. 5.60

Completed reconstruction

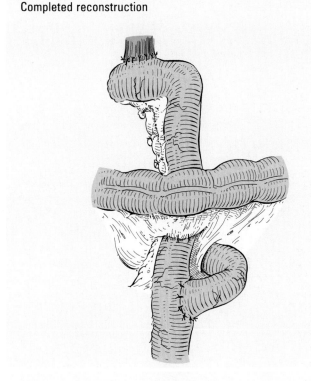

Fig. 5.61

string. Screw up the stapling gun, fire it, and unscrew and remove the gun before closing the open end of the jejunum either with a linear stapler or by suturing in two layers.

Suture the jejunum to the edges of the opening in the mesocolon.

13. Perform an end-to-side anastomosis between the divided proximal jejunum and a conveniently sited enterotomy in one or two layers according to preference. Use catgut sutures to close any holes in the mesentery through which a loop of bowel could herniate (Fig. 5.61).

14. Ask the anaesthetist to pass a nasogastric tube which should be positioned in the efferent limb of the jejunum.

Wound closure and dressing

Insert abdominal drains to the anastomosis and duodenal stump. For a thoraco-abdominal approach insert chest drains into the left pleural space and repair the diaphragm with interrupted non-absorbable sutures using the stay sutures to realign the cut edges. Leave the last few sutures untied until the chest is closed and tie them from below. Insert a rib approximator and close the chest as for a thoracotomy (see page 2.23). The abdomen is closed with monofilament nylon and the skin with sutures or staples. Suture the drains in position, place a silk purse string around each chest drain, and connect to an underwater seal. Dress the wound with a light non-occlusive dressing.

POSTOPERATIVE CARE

If facilities are available the patient should be ventilated until the following day and nursed in an intensive care or high dependency unit. Give parenteral nutrition.

If the lung is fully expanded and when there is minimal drainage, the chest drains are removed and the surrounding purse-strings tied. The nasogastric tube should remain for 6 days and the patient kept strictly nil-by-mouth during this period. On the sixth day a barium or Gastrografin (meglumine diatrizoate) swallow is performed and if there is no anastomotic leakage the nasogastric tube is removed and the patient is allowed to drink and then eat. Skin sutures or staples are removed after 8–10 days. The patient should be encouraged to eat normally. Long-term, vitamin B_{12} injections will be required each month.

SPECIAL OPERATIVE HAZARDS

1. Unresectability. If at the preliminary laparotomy there is local invasion, it may be possible to extend the resection margins (e.g. to include the transverse colon and mesocolon) to allow *en bloc* excision of the tumour. If local extension is unresectable (e.g. involvement of the superior mesenteric vessels) or if there is distant spread (e.g. peritoneal seedings or multiple liver metastases), it may be more appropriate to perform a simpler palliative operation such as a gastroenterostomy or partial gastrectomy, although a total gastrectomy can give good palliation.
2. Damage to to the bile duct.
3. Damage to the hepatic artery.
4. Damage to the middle colic artery, which may compromise the blood supply of the colon.

COMPLICATIONS

1. Major leakage from the oesophagojejunal anastomosis is often fatal from mediastinitis. Most leaks, however, are minor and only demonstrated radiologically. Continue parenteral nutrition in such cases and keep nil-by-mouth until healing is radiologically confirmed.
2. Leakage from the duodenal stump.
3. Pancreatic fistula from the pancreatic remnant.
4. Dysphagia, which may be due to a benign anastomotic stricture or tumour recurrence. Perform endoscopy with biopsy to establish the diagnosis. Tumour recurrence is rarely amenable to resection but the patient may benefit from endoscopic dilation or occasionally endoscopic intubation. A benign stricture should be dilated.

Gastroenterostomy

A gastroenterostomy is performed to bypass an obstruction to the gastric outlet or duodenum by such causes as carcinoma of the distal stomach or pancreatic head (see page 4.32 in Triple Bypass) and pyloric stenosis following scarring from duodenal ulceration. It can be combined with a truncal vagotomy as an alternative to pyloroplasty (see page 5.19).

Whilst popular for many years, the posterior retrocolic gastroenterostomy (where the small bowel is taken through the transverse mesocolon and anastomosed to the posterior wall of the stomach) offers little advantage over the simpler anterior anastomosis. An anterior gastroenterostomy is described below.

PREOPERATIVE ASSESSMENT
1. Confirm the diagnosis using a barium meal and/or endoscopy with biopsy.
2. Correct fluid and electrolyte disturbances.
3. Perform a gastric lavage with a wide-bore tube if there is food residue in their stomach.
4. Prescribe prophylactic antibiotics.

RELEVANT ANATOMY
The greater omentum is attached to the greater curvature of the stomach and sweeps down over the transverse mesocolon and colon. The jejunum arises under the root of the transverse mesocolon at the duodenojejunal flexure. To perform a gastroenterostomy a proximal loop of jejunum is selected which will comfortably reach the anterior surface of the body/antrum of the stomach, lying in front of the transverse colon, mesocolon and omentum.

OPERATION
Preparation
Place the patient supine and cleanse and drape the abdomen.

Incision
Enter the abdomen through a midline or right paramedian incision (see the Introduction). The former is preferable if a truncal vagotomy is anticipated.

Operative technique
1. Perform a thorough laparotomy. In cases of benign ulceration perform a truncal vagotomy because of the high incidence of stomal ulceration if acid secretion is allowed to continue (see page 5.19). For patients with gastric malignancy assess the position and extent of the tumour, the regional lymphatics and the liver; the best palliation in gastric cancer (and the only chance of a cure) comes from resection, although this may be inappropriate in elderly

unfit patients. In patients with tumours of the pancreatic head, gastroenterostomy is combined with a biliary diversion (see page 4.32).

2. Confirm the position of the nasogastric tube and aspirate the stomach contents before the stomach is opened.

3. Select the site for the anastomosis on the anterior wall of the stomach; this should be placed distally (in the antrum if possible) to allow the anastomosis to be dependant, although in cases of malignancy it is essential to adjust the site in order to prevent malignant involvement and early obstruction of the stoma.

4. Pick up the anterior wall of the stomach with two pairs of Babcock's tissue forceps placed at either end of the proposed site for the stoma. Identify the duodenojejunal flexure under the transverse mesocolon and follow it to the first loop of proximal jejunum which is similarly picked up with Babcock's forceps and laid alongside the stomach (Fig. 5.62), in front of the transverse colon. Ensure that the

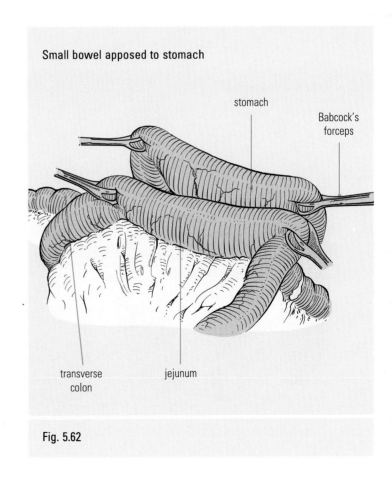

Small bowel apposed to stomach

stomach

Babcock's forceps

transverse colon

jejunum

Fig. 5.62

small bowel lies without tension with the proximal end of the loop on the greater curvature side of the stomach (i.e. isoperistaltic rather than antiperistaltic).

5. Ask the anaesthetist to withdraw the nasogastric tube if necessary (to avoid it being picked up by the clamp), before applying a Lane's gastroenterostomy twin-clamp to the

Posterior seromuscular layer

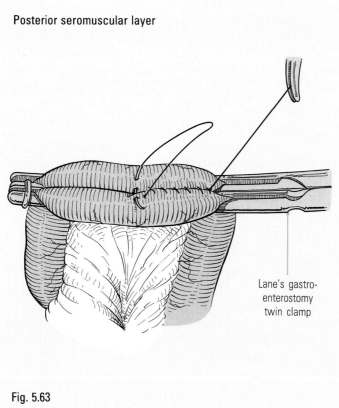

Lane's gastro-enterostomy twin clamp

Fig. 5.63

Posterior all-coats over-and-over stitch

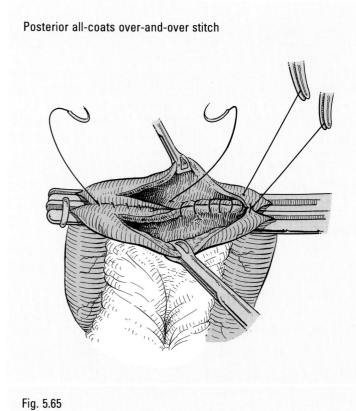

Fig. 5.65

Gastrotomy and enterotomy

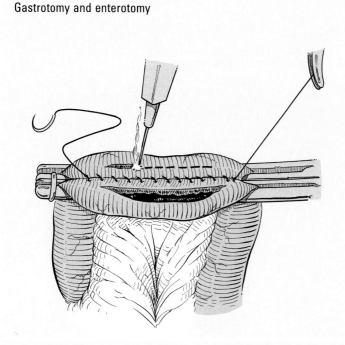

Fig. 5.64

Anterior all-coats layer

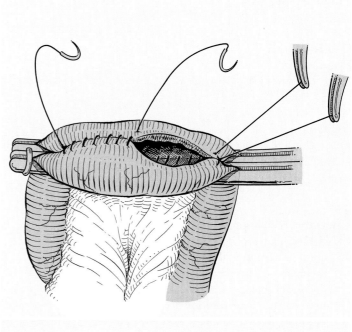

Fig. 5.66

stomach and small bowel and interlocking the two halves of the clamp (see Fig. 5.63). Close the clamp firmly to prevent venous congestion and bleeding.

6. Remove the Babcock's forceps and insert a running seromuscular suture (e.g. 2/0 Polydioxamone) between the stomach and bowel (Fig. 5.63). In cases of benign disease aim to make the stoma 5–6cm long, but for a malignancy it should be longer (up to 10cm). Cut the proximal end of this seromuscular stitch long and mark it with a clip, then lock the suture at the distal end and place a clip onto the needle; this will be used later for the anterior seromuscular layer.

7. Using cutting diathermy, open the stomach and antimesenteric border of the bowel about 0.75cm from the seromuscular stitch, along a length which is 1cm shorter than the seromuscular suture at each end (Fig. 5.64). Insert an all-coats, over-and-over, absorbable continuous suture (e.g. 2/0 Polydioxamone) to complete the posterior layer of the anastomosis (Fig. 5.65). The proximal end is left long and clipped with an artery forceps. Continue this suture around as the anterior layer (Fig. 5.66) until the starting point is reached, when the suture is tied to its clipped proximal end. A Connell stitch will allow the edges to invert, but is not haemostatic and for this reason not recommended.

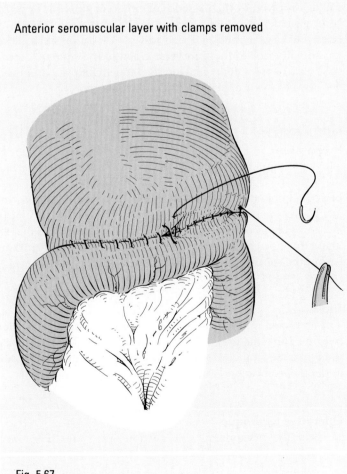

Anterior seromuscular layer with clamps removed

Fig. 5.67

8. Remove the clamps and then complete the anastomosis by coming back using the first suture to complete the anterior seromuscular layer (Fig. 5.67).

9. Confirm the patency of the stoma by invaginating the thumb and index finger through the anastomosis.

10. Ensure that the bowel lies without kinks, and draw the transverse colon to the right to check that it is not dragging down on the anastomosis.

Wound closure and dressing

Insert a silicone drain, check the position of the nasogastric tube, and close the abdomen with monofilament nylon and interrupted skin sutures. Apply a waterproof wound dressing.

POSTOPERATIVE CARE

The patient is nursed with a nasogastric tube and intravenous fluids until the stomach starts to empty. This may take several days and if slow, regular metoclopramide may help; if persistent a barium meal is advisable. The drain is removed after 48 hours unless drainage is excessive, or there is ascites in which case it should remain longer. Sutures are removed after 8–10 days.

SPECIAL OPERATIVE HAZARDS
1. Extensive gastric malignancy, in which case a palliative total gastrectomy may be appropriate in occasional cases. Alternatively, consider anatomosing a jejunal loop onto the upper body or fundus of the stomach, with or without exclusion of the tumour.
2. Difficulty in bringing the stomach and jejunum together without tension. This may require opening the gastrocolic omentum and performing a retrocolic posterior gastroenterostomy, bringing the jejunum through the mesocolon to the left of the middle colic vessels and anastomosing it to the posterior wall of the stomach. Oppose the edges of the defect in the mesocolon to the anastomosis to prevent an internal hernia.

COMPLICATIONS
1. Haemorrhage, which is usually from the gastric side of the anastomosis. If the bleeding is into the lumen of the gut it may not be apparent at operation since it only starts when the clamps are released, by which time the lumen is not visible. It occasionally requires exploration.
2. Leakage, possibly as a result of tension on the anastomosis.
3. Sepsis, either as a wound infection or an intra-abdominal abscess.
4. Recurrent obstruction. Early obstruction follows oedema around the stoma or kinking, but later is probably due to progression of a malignancy. Reduce the risk by making the stoma as wide as is practical and well clear of the tumour in cases of malignancy.
5. Stomal ulceration, which can be prevented by a vagotomy in cases of peptic ulceration, or H_2 blockers.
6. Pancreatitis due to afferent loop obstruction.

Perforated Peptic Ulcer

Improved medical management of peptic ulceration has reduced the incidence of perforation, although this remains a common cause of peritonitis. In the majority of cases surgery is advisable, but in very unfit patients, conservative treatment with antibiotics, intravenous fluids and nasogastric aspiration can be employed.

PREOPERATIVE ASSESSMENT

1. Ensure that there is adequate resuscitation with intravenous fluids and antibiotics.
2. A history of chronic dyspepsia, previous peptic ulceration or perforation whilst on H_2 blockers indicates that it may be advisable to perform a definitive anti-ulcer procedure rather than simple closure of the perforation, provided that the patient is fit and that there is little peritoneal contamination (see pages 5.19 and 5.23).
3. A history of previous peptic ulcer surgery may indicate a perforated stomal ulcer (e.g. after a Pólya gastrectomy or gastroenterostomy). Again a definitive anti-ulcer procedure may be advisable.

Perforation on anterior wall of first part of duodenum

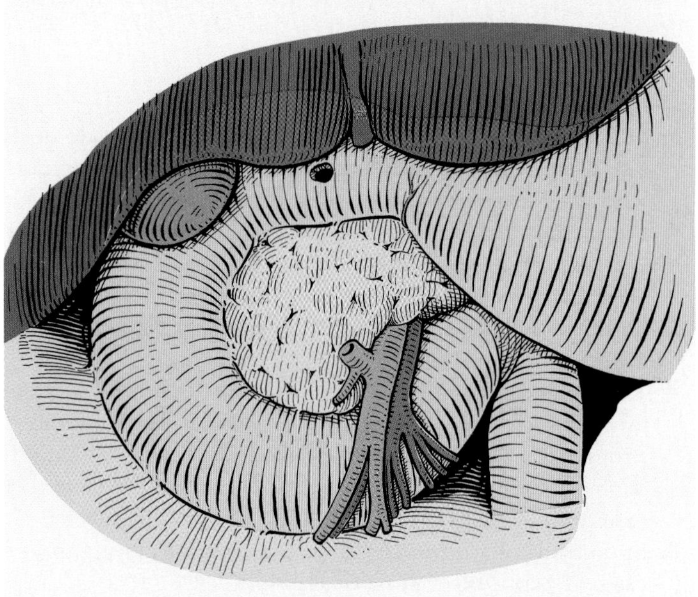

Fig. 5.68

5.38

4. The safest procedure, particularly when either the patient is unfit or the surgeon is inexperienced in gastroduodenal surgery, or both, is simple closure of the perforation with postoperative medical treatment to heal the ulcer.

RELEVANT ANATOMY

The majority of perforations are through the anterior wall of the first part of the duodenum; this is easily located just below the lower border of the liver, immediately to the right of the midline. The first part of the duodenum (2.5 cm long) is suspended in continuity with the stomach from the liver by the lesser omentum, the duodenum becoming retroperitoneal in its second part. The position of the pylorus at the junction of the stomach and duodenum is shown by the presence of the prepyloric vein (Mayo's vein), a prominent vessel that crosses the anterior gastric surface immediately proximal to the pylorus. The prominent circular muscle of the pylorus is easy to feel.

In the case of a perforated gastric ulcer, access may be required to the anterior and posterior aspects of the stomach; for the relevant anatomy of this see page 5.23 in Partial Gastrectomy.

In the case of a perforated stomal ulcer, the usual anatomy will be distorted by the presence of either an antecolic or retrocolic gastroenterostomy. An antecolic gastroenterostomy is relatively easy to find as there will be a loop of small bowel passing anterior to the transverse colon to the stoma. A retrocolic gastroenterostomy may not be immediately apparent as it lies deep to the transverse colon and omentum.

OPERATION

Preparation

The operation is performed under general anaesthesia and the anaesthetist inserts a nasogastric tube. The patient is then placed supine and the skin prepared from the nipples to the groin; this degree of preparation is important as the initial incision may have to be extended (e.g. to expose oesophageal hiatus for a vagotomy). Suction should be ready and working before the start of the operation.

Incision

The abdomen is usually opened with an upper midline incision (see the Introduction). When the peritoneum is first opened there may be a puff of escaping gas which should be odourless in peptic perforation.

Operative technique

1. Clear the peritoneum with suction and swabs. Peritoneal fluid from a gastroduodenal perforation is characteristic, containing food residue and bile; it is not purulent or faeculent with a recent perforation.

2. Perform a laparotomy (see page 5.2) to identify the site of the perforation. The commonest site is the anterior wall of the first part of the duodenum (Fig. 5.69) and such a site can usually be treated by simple closure.

3. Pack off the area around the duodenum with moistened abdominal packs.

4. Pick up the pylorus between the finger and thumb (Fig. 5.69) or with Babcock's forceps, and insert a series of full thickness sutures of a heavy, slowly absorbable material (e.g. 00 Vicryl) in a line transversely across the duodenum spanning the area of the ulcer (Fig. 5.70); leave them untied with artery forceps attached until they are all inserted. Between three and five sutures will be required depending upon the size of the ulcer.

5. Tie the sutures to close the ulcer, taking care to avoid over-tightening as they will cut out. The ends are left long (Fig. 5.71).

Insertion of closure sutures transversely across perforation

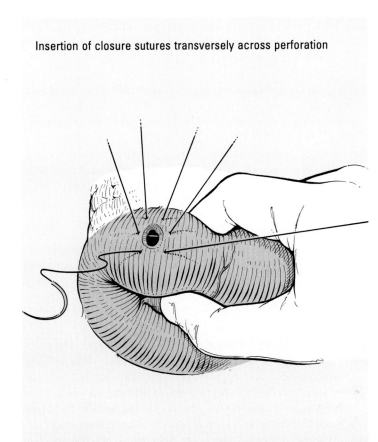

Fig. 5.70

Perforated duodenal ulcer

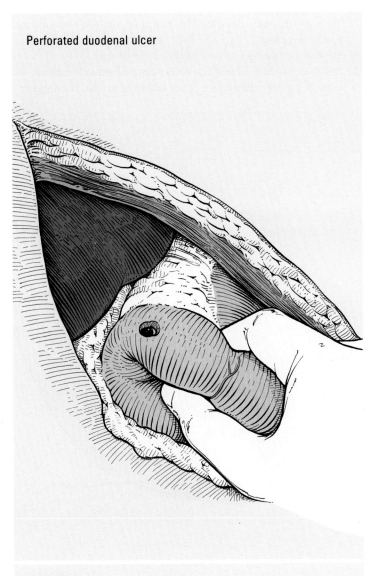

Fig. 5.69

Sutures tied to close perforation

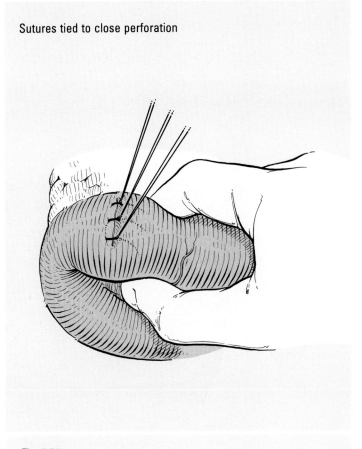

Fig. 5.71

6. Find a piece of greater omentum that will easily reach to the site of perforation and thread a tongue of this omentum over the line of sutures (Fig. 5.72).

7. With the omentum covering the repair, secure it in position by gently tying the sutures over it (Fig. 5.73). Avoid over-tightening the sutures which will strangulate the omentum.

8. Thoroughly wash out the peritoneal cavity with warm sterile saline, removing all visible solid debris, particularly from the subphrenic and hepatorenal spaces, and the pelvis.

Wound closure and dressing
1. Place a large silicone drain into the subhepatic space.
2. Close the incision with a mass closure technique using loop nylon and the skin with interrupted sutures. Apply a wound dressing.

POSTOPERATIVE CARE
This involves good analgesia without excessive sedation (e.g. intercostal blocks) and regular chest physiotherapy. The naso-gastric tube is removed and oral fluids introduced when flatus has been passed. Antibiotics should be prescribed for a full 5 days unless there is minimal peritoneal contamination. The drain can be removed when less than 50 ml per day of clear serous fluid is drained, provided that the patient is afebrile.

Postoperative medical therapy involves use of an H_2 antago-nist to heal the ulcer. Outpatient follow-up is essential after 6 weeks, as up to 25% of patients will have further complications from an acute ulcer, and up to 80% from a chronic ulcer (see below).

SPECIAL OPERATIVE HAZARDS
1. If no perforation site is evident on initial laparotomy, expose the posterior surface of the stomach in the lesser sac (see additional manoeuvres on page 5.4).
2. If access to the duodenum is poor, perform Kocher's manoeuvre to mobilize it (see page 5.4).
3. If the duodenal ulcer is too large and/or the tissues are too friable to perform a simple closure, a partial gastrec-tomy may be required (see page 5.23).
4. A perforated gastric ulcer needs careful assessment. A proportion (8%) will be malignant and gastric ulcers are more likely to reperforate after simple closure. There-fore, if the expertise is available, a resection is advisable (either partial gastrectomy or ulcer excision with a vago-tomy). If it is not available it is reasonable to perform simple closure but biopsies must be taken from all four quadrants of the ulcer and medical therapy started.

COMPLICATIONS
1. Intraperitoneal abscess, for instance, in the subphrenic space or pelvis.
2. Persistence or recurrence of ulcer symptoms.
3. Leakage from oversewn perforation and reperforation.
4. Gastric outlet obstruction from scarring of the duodenum.

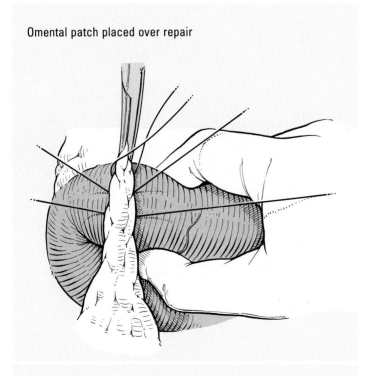

Omental patch placed over repair

Fig. 5.72

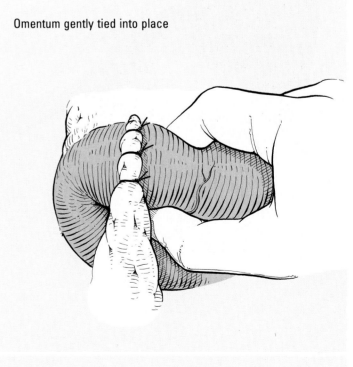

Omentum gently tied into place

Fig. 5.73

Management of Gastroduodenal Bleeding

Gastrointestinal haemorrhage is potentially life threatening and failure to respond to medical management (i.e. recurrent or continuing bleeding) is an indication for urgent surgery. As patients over 60 years of age do not tolerate blood loss well the threshold to operate should be lower in these cases.

It is important to establish the site of the bleeding early in the patient's management. Endoscopy is the most accurate method for locating the source of an upper gastrointestinal bleed, and if active bleeding or clot is seen in an ulcer early surgery should be strongly considered. Endoscopy also allows biopsy of gastric ulcers which may be malignant and, in selected cases, permits the local injection of adrenaline solution to help control bleeding. In the majority of cases bleeding is due to mucosal ulceration (benign and malignant), gastric erosions and, less often, bleeding from varices; the latter is considered elsewhere (see page 4.14).

PREOPERATIVE ASSESSMENT
1. Ensure adequate resuscitation with blood transfusion. The patient should have a urinary catheter and a central venous line for venous access and pressure monitoring. A nasogastric tube can rarely cope with a significant gastrointestinal bleed.
2. Wherever possible establish the diagnosis preoperatively with endoscopy. Look for stigmata of chronic liver disease which might suggest oesophageal varices.
3. In patients who have undergone massive blood transfusion, correct clotting abnormalities with intravenous calcium (to reverse citrate toxicity), fresh frozen plasma and platelet transfusion.
4. Give broad-spectrum prophylactic antibiotics.

RELEVANT ANATOMY
This is covered on page 5.19 in Truncal Vagotomy and Pyloroplasty and page 5.23 in Partial Gastrectomy.

OPERATION
Preparation
The patient is placed supine and the entire abdomen is cleansed and draped. A crossbar will allow the insertion of a sternal retractor for access to the hiatus to perform a vagotomy if this is required.

Incision
Enter the abdomen through a midline incision (see the Introduction).

Operative technique
1. Locate and confirm the cause of bleeding, such as a gastric or duodenal ulcer, and look for splenomegaly and other evidence of portal hypertension. The bowel may appear blue and distended from the contained blood.

2. Perform Kocher's manoeuvre to mobilize the duodenum (see page 4.7). If the bleeding is known to be coming from the duodenum, make a pyloroplasty-type incision from the distal stomach across the pylorus into the proximal duodenum, having picked up the wall with Babcock's forceps or stay sutures (Fig. 5.74). Locate a bleeding duodenal ulcer which is usually on the posterior wall.

3. If the site of bleeding is unknown or in the stomach, pick up the antrum of the stomach with two pairs of Babcock's forceps and using cutting diathermy make a gastrotomy incision, 8–10cm long, in the anterior wall of the stomach

Opening of the pylorus

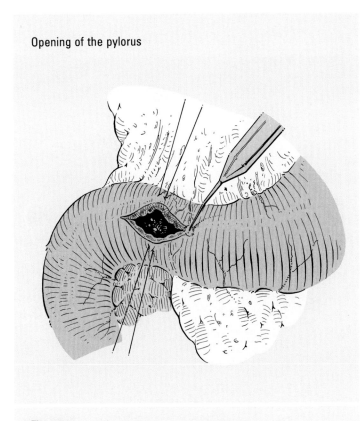

Fig. 5.74

(Fig. 5.75). Avoid extending the incision across the pylorus into the duodenum at this stage since it will make a subsequent partial gastrectomy more difficult. Evacuate the blood clot with a sucker and locate a bleeding gastric ulcer or bleeding erosions if present. If the site was unknown and is still not apparent, blood may be seen welling up from the proximal stomach or from the duodenum. If the bleeding is coming from higher up insert a narrow-bladed Deaver retractor into the lumen of the stomach to allow visualization of the fundus and cardia; this may require the gastrotomy to be extended. The mucosa can then be brought into view by digitally invaginating it into the gastrotomy (Fig. 5.77). Examine the entire lining of the stomach. If the blood is coming from distally, extend the gastrotomy incision across the pylorus into the first part of the duodenum.

4. Establish temporary control of a bleeding ulcer with digital pressure for 5 minutes. If unexpected bleeding varices are found consider either inserting a James', Linton or Sengstaken tube or, if the surgeon has sufficient experience and the patient's condition is reasonable, perform suture ligation of the varices, or oesophageal transection shunt or a shunt (see page 4.14).

5. A spurting vessel such as the gastroduodenal artery or a bleeding point will usually be visible in the base of the ulcer; underrun the vessel or bleeding point with interrupted non-absorbable sutures such as 00 linen or silk in a figure-of-8 fashion (Fig. 5.77), placing the sutures under the vessel on either side of the bleeding point. Avoid biting too deeply

into the posterior wall of the duodenum where the bile duct can be damaged and do not overtighten the stitch or it will cut out of the friable ulcer. Ensure complete haemostasis before proceeding; it is now necessary to perform a definitive operation to prevent rebleeding.

6. For a duodenal ulcer perform a vagotomy and pyloroplasty (see page 5.19). With an extensive gastroduodenotomy perform a Finney-type pyloroplasty, and if, in an obese patient the vagi are inaccessible, a Pólya-type partial gastrectomy should be performed (see page 5.27).

For a bleeding gastric ulcer perform a partial gastrectomy to include the ulcer; vagotomy and pyloroplasty carries a higher risk of rebleeding and an unsuspected malignant gastric ulcer will be allowed to remain. The rim of an eroding posterior ulcer, once underrun, should be pinched off the pancreas, leaving its base excluded from the gut lumen. If the ulcer is high up in the stomach, rotate the stomach so that the ulcer comes to lie on the lesser curvature and then excise and oversew the lesser curve and fashion a gastroduodenal anastomosis (Billroth I, see page 5.25). Erosions can be treated by underrunning alone but if extensive perform a vagotomy with pyloroplasty (see page 5.19) or, preferably, a gastrectomy (see page 5.23). Ensure any bleeding points in the remaining proximal gastric remnant are carefully underrun.

A bleeding carcinoma can be resected by whatever operation would have been chosen if the case were elective. Alternatively bleeding can be controlled with sutures if resection is inappropriate.

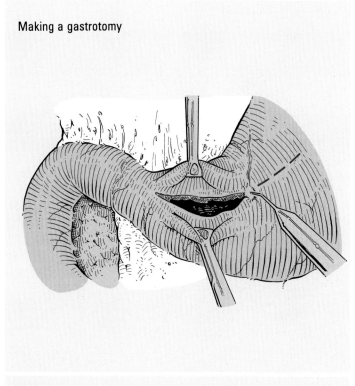

Making a gastrotomy

Fig. 5.75

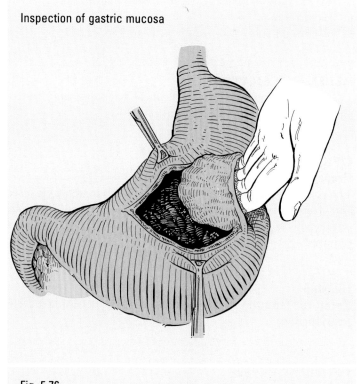

Inspection of gastric mucosa

Fig. 5.76

Wound closure and dressing

Ask the anaesthetist to insert a nasogastric tube and check its position in the stomach. Insert a drain and close the wound with monofilament nylon and the skin with interrupted sutures. Apply a waterproof dressing.

POSTOPERATIVE CARE

Careful correction and maintenance of fluid and electrolyte balance is most important, with under- and over-transfusion both being potential hazards. The need for ongoing monitoring and in some cases postoperative ventilation often demands that these patients are managed in an intensive care unit after the operation. Carefully observe the patient for bleeding but remember that some melaena is inevitable. The nasogastric tube is allowed to drain but should not be aspirated; continue intravenous fluids and nasogastric drainage until bowel sounds return and flatus is passed. If doubt exists regarding completeness of vagotomy prescribe H_2 antagonists or omeprazole until the histology of the vagi is available. Remove the drain after 48 hours if there is no significant drainage. Sutures can be removed after 8–10 days.

SPECIAL OPERATIVE HAZARDS

1. Damage to the bile duct; the retroduodenal portion of the bile duct is vulnerable if sutures are hurriedly inserted to underrun a bleeding gastroduodenal artery. If a duodenal ulcer has caused much distortion of the tissues open the supraduodenal portion of the bile duct and insert a rubber Jacques catheter to aid its identification. Close the duct over a T-tube.
2. No gastroduodenal cause found for the bleeding, in which case perform a complete small bowel laparotomy and carefully examine the pancreas, gall bladder and bile duct, and the aorta where it is crossed by the fourth part of the duodenum. If the site is still not apparent and the bleeding has stopped, close the abdomen.

COMPLICATIONS

See also the complications on page 5.19 in Truncal Vagotomy and Pyloroplasty, and page 5.23 in Partial Gastrectomy.

1. Rebleeding, which may be from a gastric suture line or from the original bleeding site. If it persists, despite H_2 antagonists and correction of any clotting abnormalities, elect to re-operate, reopening the anterior gastric suture line and securing haemostasis.
2. Discovery of an unsuspected gastric cancer following partial gastrectomy. In a young fit patient, or if the excision margins appear to be involved with tumour, consider electively performing a more radical resection.
3. Incomplete vagotomy, in which case continue H_2 antagonists rather than considering another operation.
4. Leakage from a suture line or duodenal stump.

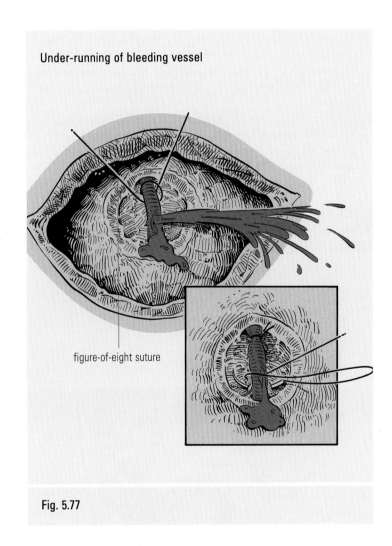

Under-running of bleeding vessel

figure-of-eight suture

Fig. 5.77

Ramstedt's Pyloromyotomy

This idiopathic condition occurs in neonates at around 4 weeks of age. It is more common in first born male infants and there is a familial tendency towards it.

PREOPERATIVE ASSESSMENT
1. To confirm the diagnosis, the hypertrophied pyloric muscle is palpated during a 'test feed' with glucose water; this may be followed by projectile vomiting. On rare occasions confirmation may require the use of ultrasonography or barium studies.
2. Correct any dehydration and acid-base disturbances.
3. Empty the stomach by nasogastric aspiration, combined with gastric lavage to remove milk curd and, if present, barium from the stomach.

RELEVANT ANATOMY
While the pylorus lies midway between the umbilicus and the xiphoid in the adult, in the infant it is slightly more caudal and overlapped by the inferior margin of the liver. The more mobile pylorus in the neonate can be delivered through an abdominal incision without difficulty.

OPERATION
Preparation
The anaesthetist should be skilled and experienced in paediatric anaesthesia, and care should be taken to ensure that heat loss is minimized by placing the baby on a heated mattress. The skin is prepared and drapes placed. At the cephalic end it is useful to use a clear, sterile, plastic sheet spread over a wire cage so that the patient's head remains visible, while the abdomen is covered by a transparent adhesive drape.

Incision
1. Incise the skin with a transverse incision in the right upper quadrant, above the palpable liver edge and extend it towards the midline for 2.5 cm (Fig. 5.78).

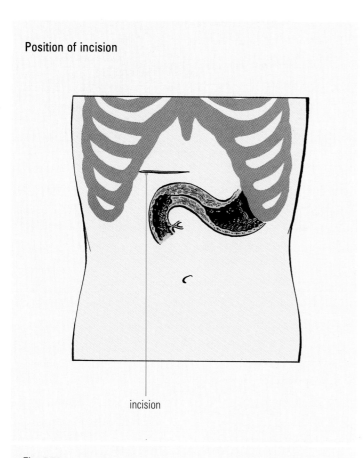

Position of incision

incision

Fig. 5.78

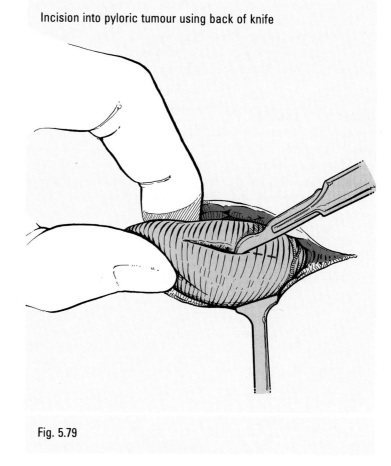

Incision into pyloric tumour using back of knife

Fig. 5.79

2. Enter the peritoneal cavity by dividing the right rectus abdominus muscle and the peritoneum in the line of the skin incision, paying meticulous attention to haemostasis.

Operative technique
1. Gently retract the liver upwards and grasp the gastric antrum, this is then delivered into the wound followed by the thickened pylorus which can be held with a pair of Denis Browne forceps.

2. Using the back of a scalpel blade make a longitudinal incision through an avascular portion of the serosa along the length of the hypertrophied segment (Fig. 5.79), extending onto the antrium.

3. Introduce a Denis Browne spreader or small artery forceps into this incision and open them transversely to split the hypertrophied muscle down to the mucosa, which then bulges into the incision (Figs 5.80 and 5.81). Check that all the muscle fibres are divided.

4. Ensure that the mucosa has not been opened by squeezing air from the stomach into the duodenum; a leak in the mucosa can be detected by a tell-tale bubble and should be repaired with 4/0 catgut. Slight oozing from the pyloro-myotomy is usually due to venous engorgement and will stop when the pylorus is returned to the abdomen. Avoid using diathermy on the mucosa.

Wound closure
1. Close the abdomen in two layers, first the peritoneum with the posterior rectus sheath and then the anterior rectus sheath, using a slowly absorbable 3/0 suture such as Poly-dioxamone (PDS).
2. Close the skin with 3/0 subcuticular stitches.

POSTOPERATIVE CARE
Oral feeding with an electrolyte/dextrose solution ($10\,ml\,kg^{-1}$ body weight) is commenced 4 hours postoperatively and given every 2 hours for the subsequent 12 hours. If tolerated, half strength milk ($15\,ml\,kg^{-1}$ body weight) is given 2-hourly, converting to full strength after 6 hours with normal feeding being resumed within 24 hours. If vomiting occurs, return to the previous phase of the regime. The patient can be discharged home when tolerating feeds, this usually occurs by day 2–3.

SPECIAL OPERATIVE HAZARDS
1. Opening the mucosa; this is most likely to occur at the duodenal fornix.
2. Incorrect diagnosis.

COMPLICATIONS
1. Unrecognized mucosal perforation can be avoided by checking for air leaks (see above).

2. Postoperative vomiting is rarely due to inadequate myotomy, and is usually due to gastro-oesophageal reflux which can be reduced by nursing the baby in a chair inclined at 60° to the horizontal.

Principle of pyloromyotomy

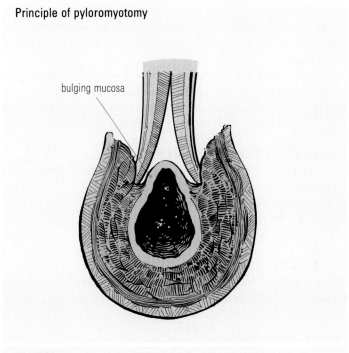

bulging mucosa

Fig. 5.80

Opening the tumour with Denis Browne spreader

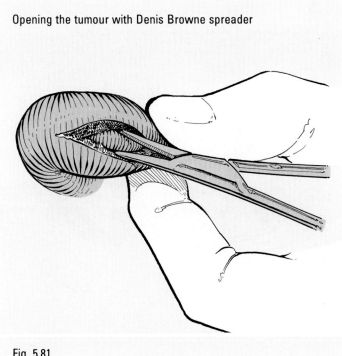

Fig. 5.81

Laparotomy for Adhesions

After abdominal surgery, blood and inflammatory exudate in the peritoneal cavity can become organized to form fibrous adhesions, which is one of the commonest causes of small bowel obstruction.

A laparotomy is indicated if conservative treatment fails, if there are recurrent obstructive symptoms, or if there are signs of ischaemic bowel as indicated by signs of toxicity or peritonitis.

PREOPERATIVE ASSESSMENT
1. Rehydrate and resuscitate the patient with intravenous fluids.
2. Correct any electrolyte or acid/base disorders.
3. Initiate nasogastric aspiration.

RELEVANT ANATOMY
The small bowel loops usually lie in the infracolic compartment of the abdomen and in the pelvis. They receive their blood supply via the mesentery from branches of the superior mesenteric artery.

Adhesions can affect any or all of the small bowel, binding the loops to each other and to the abdominal wall, particularly to the back of wounds and to sites of previous sepsis.

A volvulus around a band compromises the blood supply to the bowel and if vascular occlusion is complete it will lead to gangrene and perforation.

OPERATION
Preparation
Under general anaesthesia, place the patient supine on the operating table. Expose, cleanse, and drape the entire abdomen.

Incision
Either reopen the old scar and extend the incision to allow good exposure or make a fresh midline incision (see the Introduction). The fresh incision is frequently a 'false economy' since the bowel which is adherent to the old incision will have to be encountered and dealt with at some point, and better access is afforded by the old incision. Very careful dissection is needed at this stage since bowel may be adherent to the scar. It is safest to begin the incision on fresh tissue, just beyond the end of the old incision. Enter the peritoneal cavity initially at this point, and dissect the bowel off the inside of the scar before reopening it.

Operative technique
1. Separate loops of bowel by a combination of sharp and blunt dissection to clear the wound edges (Fig. 5.82).

2. Insert a self-retaining retractor, or apply Kocher's tissue-holding forceps to the deeper layers of the wound edge and have an assistant lift them vertically.

3. Separate the adhesions using gentle traction and sharp dissection (Fig. 5.83). If the seromuscular coat is divided during the mobilization of the bowel, repair it with a 2/0 continuous catgut stitch. Continue until the whole length of the small bowel is mobilized.

4. Decompress the small bowel by milking the contents into the stomach, from where they are aspirated via the nasogastric tube.

5. Resect any loops of bowel that have been rendered ischaemic by obstructive bands or have been damaged during mobilization (see page 5.50 in Small Bowel Resection).

6. Adhesions are likely to reform and may cause further small

Adhesons between bowel loops and abdominal wall

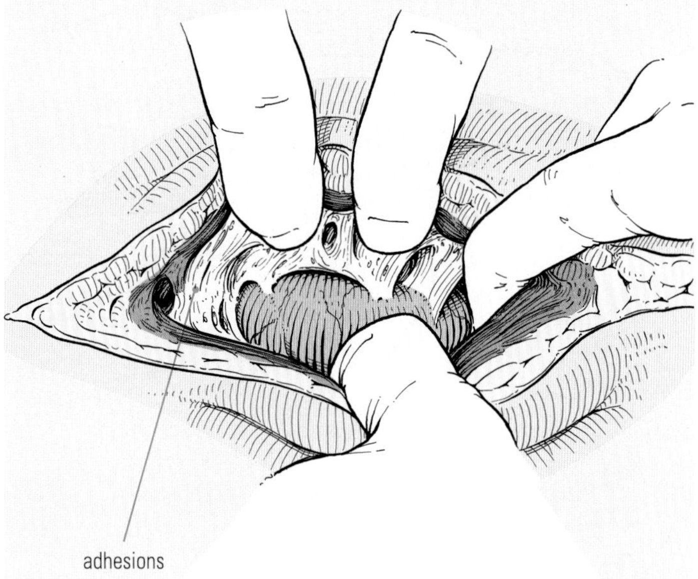

adhesions

Fig. 5.82

Divide adhesions with sharp dissection

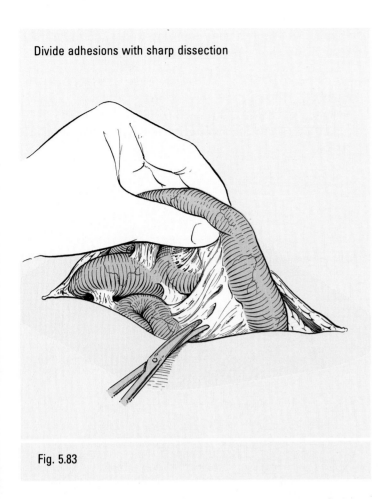

Fig. 5.83

bowel obstruction. A number of procedures are described to reduce the risks of subsequent obstruction and these procedures have the common objective of tethering the bowel loops in a concertina form. Insertion of a Jones' tube is one way to achieve this goal (Fig. 5.84). The tube is a 3 m long, 18 Fr gauge balloon catheter with side holes in the distal half to allow decompression of the bowel. The tube is inserted just beyond the duodenojejunal flexure and passed to the caecum. It acts as an internal splint, so that when adhesions reform they do so with the bowel positioned in gentle loops without sharp kinks.

7. To insert the Jones' tube, make a stab incision in the anterior abdominal wall to the left of the wound at a point overlying the duodenojejunal flexure. Pull the Jones' tube through the abdominal wall with Roberts' forceps (Fig. 5.85).

8. Make a small enterotomy near the duodenojejunal flexure with a knife and place a catgut purse-string suture around it. Insert the Jones' tube through the enterotomy and inflate the balloon with 5 ml of saline. Tie the purse-string loosely around the tube.

Jones' tube

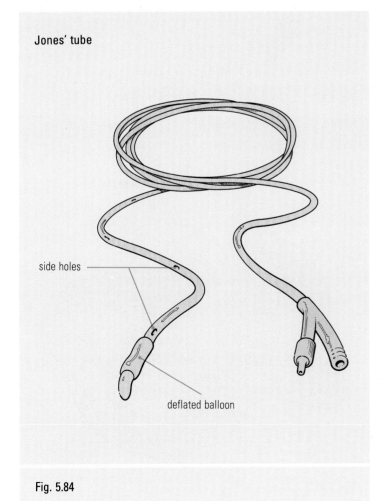

side holes

deflated balloon

Fig. 5.84

Introduce Jones' tube through anterior abdominal wall

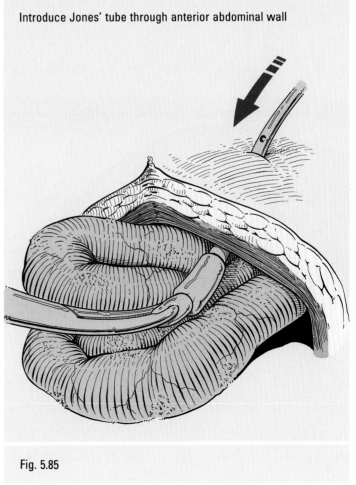

Fig. 5.85

9. Milk the tip of the Jones' tube along the small bowel distally by applying gentle traction on the balloon (Fig. 5.86). When the balloon reaches the ileocaecal valve, deflate it, pass the tip into the caecum (Fig. 5.87) and then reinflate the balloon with 10 ml of saline, to retain it beyond the ileocaecal valve.

10. Insert a second purse-string stitch around the enterotomy site which is tightened and then tacked to the abdominal wall close to the point of entry of the Jones' tube to prevent intra-abdominal leakage of small bowel contents when the Jones' tube is removed.

11. Lay the small bowel in gentle curves (Fig. 5.88) and cover it with the greater omentum.

Wound closure and dressing
The wound is closed with a monofilament nylon and interrupted skin stitches, and the Jones' tube secured to this skin at the exit site. A light dressing is applied.

POSTOPERATIVE CARE
Nasogastric aspiration and intravenous fluid replacement should be continued until bowel function returns. Adequate postoperative analgesia is essential because the patient may suffer intestinal colic from the Jones' tube.

The Jones' tube should be allowed to drain freely initially, but it is spigotted when bowel function returns with twice-daily flushing with saline to prevent the tube from blocking. Remove the tube after 14 days; this can be done on the ward with analgesia supplemented if necessary with an oxygen/nitrous

oxide mixture. Apply a gauze dressing to the enterotomy site until the fistula closes spontaneously.

SPECIAL OPERATIVE HAZARDS
Damage to the bowel whilst opening the abdomen and dividing the adhesions. Any damaged bowel is either repaired or resected.

Balloon retains tip in the caecum

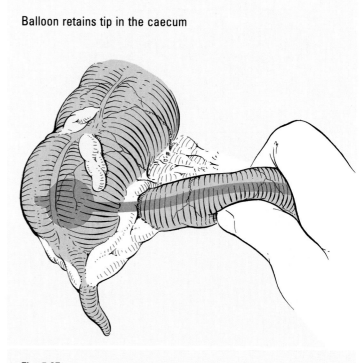

Fig. 5.87

With the balloon inflated, milk the Jones' tube along the bowel

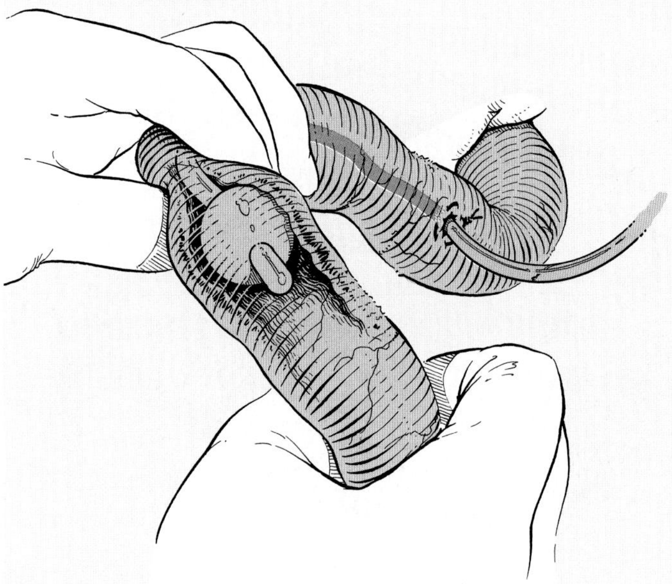

Lay out bowel in orderly fashion with gentle curves

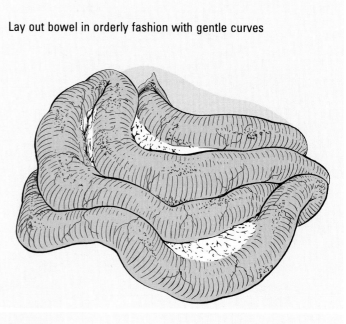

Fig. 5.86

Fig. 5.88

Noble's plication of the small intestine

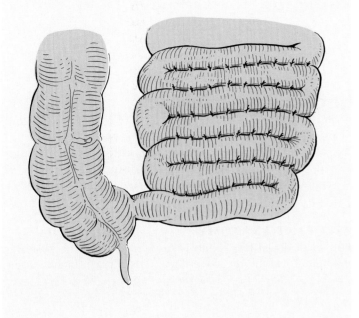

Fig. 5.89

COMPLICATIONS

1. Recurrence of bowel obstruction.
2. Leakage from the site of the Jones' tube.

ALTERNATIVE METHODS OF BOWEL PLICATION

An alternative to Jones' intubation is Noble's plication. Once the small bowel has been freed from adhesions, it is sutured together with interrupted seromuscular sutures (e.g. 3/0 catgut) so that the plicated bowel lies in regular folds (Fig. 5.89). The procedure is very time-consuming and carries the risk of small intestinal fistula formation. As with Jones' intubation, it reduces but does not completely prevent recurrent small bowel obstruction.

A second alternative is to pass non-absorbable sutures through the mesentery to prevent sharp angulation of the bowel. This carries the risk of bleeding as the result of damage to a mesenteric vessel and again does not guarantee the obstruction will not occur again.

Small Bowel Resection

Small bowel resection is indicated for: cases of obstruction where the bowel is judged to be non-viable once the cause of the obstruction is released; irreducible small bowel intussusception; ischaemia secondary to arterial embolus; traumatic damage; a Meckel's diverticulum causing symptoms, such as intussusception and bleeding; strictures, as occur for example in Crohn's disease; and tumours of the small bowel. Primary small bowel tumours, both benign (e.g. hamartoma and lipoma) and malignant (e.g. lymphoma, adenocarcinoma and carcinoid), are uncommon but a loop of small bowel is frequently adherent to large bowel tumours and needs to be resected.

PREOPERATIVE ASSESSMENT
1. Barium follow-through in cases of Crohn's disease and primary small bowel tumours.
2. Nasogastric aspiration, rehydration with intravenous fluids and correction of any electrolyte disturbance in cases of small bowel obstruction.

RELEVANT ANATOMY
The small bowel (Fig. 5.90) is suspended from the posterior abdominal wall by the mesentery. It has a rich blood supply

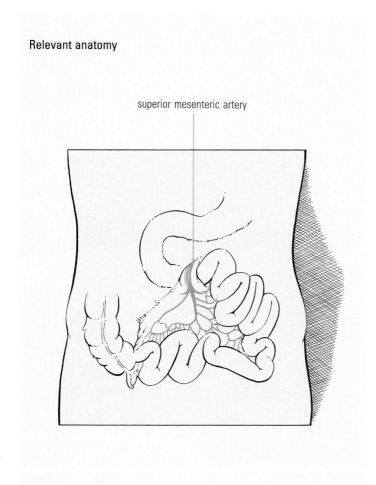

Relevant anatomy

superior mesenteric artery

Fig. 5.90

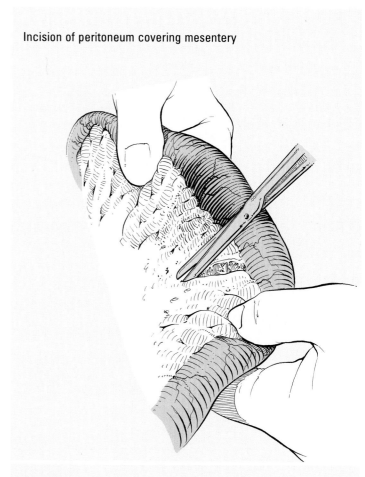

Incision of peritoneum covering mesentery

Fig. 5.91

Division of mesenteric vessels

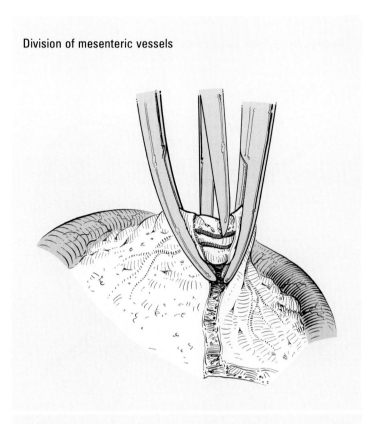

Fig. 5.92

Ligation of mesenteric vessels

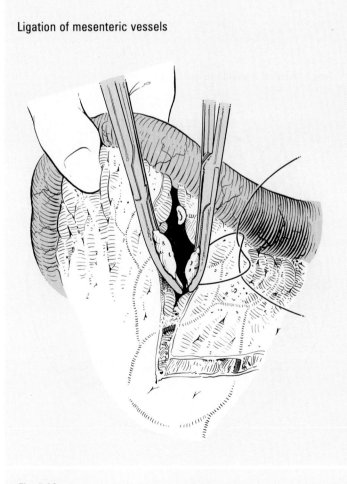

Fig. 5.93

from branches of the superior mesenteric artery, which pierce the mesenteric border of the bowel wall. Venous drainage is to the superior mesenteric vein and thence to the portal vein and the liver. The lymphatic vessels run with the arteries and drain into pre-aortic nodes around the origin of the superior mesenteric artery. The small bowel is intraperitoneal throughout its length. Approximately 60 cm proximal to the ileocaecal valve, a diverticulum (Meckel's) arises from the antimesenteric border in approximately 2% of the population.

Since the small bowel lies free in the peritoneal cavity and is freely mobile, it is prone to kinking, compression and obstruction by adhesions, which can be either congenital or acquired (e.g. after previous surgery or sepsis). Its mobility also allows it to enter the sac of an abdominal wall hernia, putting it at risk of ischaemic damage by pressure at the neck of the hernia (strangulation), which is generally the narrowest point.

OPERATION
Preparation
Place the patient supine, and cleanse and drape in the usual manner. Ask the anaesthetist to pass a nasogastric tube.

Incision
Make a midline incision, unless there is a conveniently sited previous incision which can be reopened. In cases of strangulated external hernia, an incision will have been made to approach it. If it is found that a resection is necessary, either extend this incision (e.g. through the posterior wall of the inguinal canal) if it is possible, or make a separate laparotomy incision.

Operative technique
1. Perform a thorough laparotomy (see page 5.2).

2. In cases of obstruction, locate the cause and deal with it, for example by dividing an obstructing fibrous band.

3. Carefully inspect both the segment of small bowel requiring resection and also the remaining bowel, and choose the resection margins. In cases of malignancy, a 5 cm margin should be taken on each side. This is not necessary in benign disease, such as ischaemia and Crohn's disease, where the amount resected is kept to a minimum, ensuring however that the margins are viable and healthy.

4. Using scissors divide the peritoneum covering one side of the mesentery between the margins of resection (Fig. 5.91). In benign disease keep close to the bowel wall, but for malignant disease, take a generous V-shaped wedge of mesentery with the bowel segment to remove the local lymphatic tissue which runs with the arteries.

5. With scissors, divide the mesentery between clips along the line of this incision (Fig. 5.92). By shining a light through the mesentery from behind the vessels can be seen more clearly. Ligate the vessels with absorbable (e.g. 00 Vicryl) ties (Fig. 5.93). Take as little fat and connective tissue with the vessel as possible since when tied, the vessels may slip back into the mesentery and bleed.

6. Clear the mesentery up to the bowel wall (Fig. 5.94) and apply crushing clamps to the bowel immediately beyond the point of section. Then, after the bowel contents have been milked from the intervening segment, apply soft (non-crushing) clamps proximal and distal to the crushing clamps (Fig. 5.94).

7. Using a knife divide the bowel flush with the crushing clamp (Fig. 5.95).

8. Anastomose the two cut ends in one or two layers (see the Introduction) according to preference.

9. Close the defect in the mesentery with a continuous 00 chromic catgut stitch on a round-bodied needle (Fig. 5.96). Only the peritoneum covering the mesentery should be picked up with this stitch to avoid damaging the blood supply to the anastomosis (Fig. 5.97). Alternatively leave the ties ligating the vessels long and tie them together in pairs to close the hole in the mesentery.

10. Lay the omentum around the anastomosis.

Wound closure and dressing

Drainage is not usually necessary. Close the wound with loop nylon, catgut and 00 nylon for the skin.

POSTOPERATIVE CARE

Nasogastric aspiration and intravenous fluids should be continued until gut motility returns, as indicated by decreasing volumes of aspirate, normal bowel sounds and the passage of flatus.

SPECIAL OPERATIVE HAZARDS

1. Damage to the main trunk of the superior mesenteric artery can only occur if the dissection extends too deep into the root of the mesentery. If must be repaired.
2. Gross disparity between the sizes of the cut ends. This can occur with long-standing obstruction, in which case either perform an end-to-side anastomosis or divide the narrower bowel obliquely.
3. With extensive adhesions and obstruction, consider either a Noble's plication or insertion of a Jones' tube (see page 5.46).
4. Extensive infarction and difficulty in deciding where the bowel becomes viable. This is seen in cases of superior mesenteric artery thrombosis and embolus of the main trunk. It may be necessary to resect what is definitely non-viable and either exteriorize the ends or anastomose and perform a second-look laparotomy 24 hours later.

COMPLICATIONS

1. Anastomotic leakage will lead to either an abscess, fistula, or both. The rich blood supply to the small bowel makes this uncommon, but it is particularly seen in cases of Crohn's disease and in irradiated bowel. A fistula may close spontaneously if the patient is kept nil-by-mouth and fed intravenously; an abscess needs to be drained.

Application of intestinal clamps

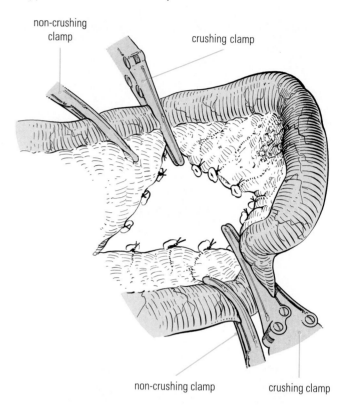

non-crushing clamp

crushing clamp

non-crushing clamp

crushing clamp

Fig. 5.94

Divide bowel flush with crushing clamp

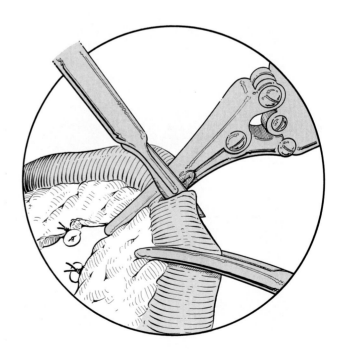

Fig. 5.95

2. Stricture formation; because of the fluid nature of the small bowel content, this has to be quite severe to cause symptoms. It generally requires resection if symptomatic.
3. 'Short gut syndrome', in which massive small bowel resection will lead to malabsorption and intractable diarrhoea. It can be managed with either an enteral elemental diet or parenteral nutrition. Surgical reversal of a segment of the bowel can be performed to slow down intestinal transit.

Closure of mesentery with running peritoneal suture

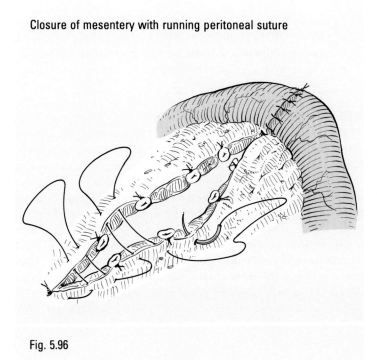

Fig. 5.96

Closure of mesentery with suture drawn tight

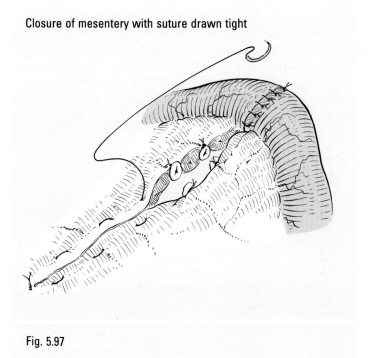

Fig. 5.97

An intussusception is an invagination, or telescoping, of the proximal bowel into the distal bowel. Intussusception in adults should be treated as a symptom of an underlying condition and the precipitating condition should be sought. Idiopathic intussusception occurs in infants around the time of weaning and is attributed to enlargement of Peyer's patches, due either to a change in gut flora or to a viral infection.

PREOPERATIVE ASSESSMENT

1. Intussusception may cause a strangulation obstruction and hence must be treated with urgency.
2. In a child, careful digital examination should distinguish a rectal prolapse, where the rectal mucosa is continuous with skin from the apex of an intussusception presenting at the anus.
3. Circumoral pigmentation suggests Peutz–Jeghers syndrome which may present with multiple intussusceptions from small bowel hamartomas.

4. In the infant, a diagnostic barium enema may achieve reduction of the intussusception by hydrostatic pressure. Operative reduction is indicated if hydrostatic reduction fails, or if there are features suggesting perforation.

RELEVANT ANATOMY

At the apex of the invaginating bowel, or intussusceptum, there is usually a lesion which is proud of the mucosa such as a polyp, hamartoma, an inverted Meckel's diverticulum or a carcinoma (Fig. 5.98). This is pulled distally by peristalsis, drawing the bowel along with it. The inner (entering) tube and middle (returning) tube of bowel form the intussusceptum, while the outer shelter is known as the intussuscipiens.

The intussusception is almost always antegrade, single, and usually involves terminal ileum as the intussusceptum, with colon forming the intussuscipiens. This three-walled segment of bowel is usually easily palpable along the line of the colon.

Intussusception due to polyp

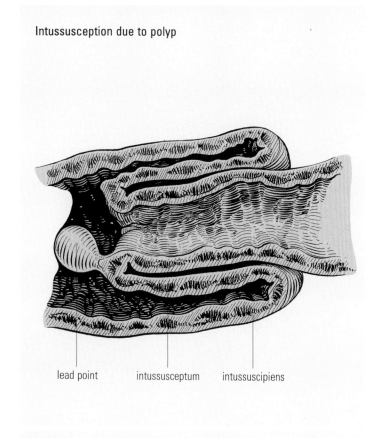

lead point   intussusceptum   intussuscipiens

Fig. 5.98

Reduce from distal end

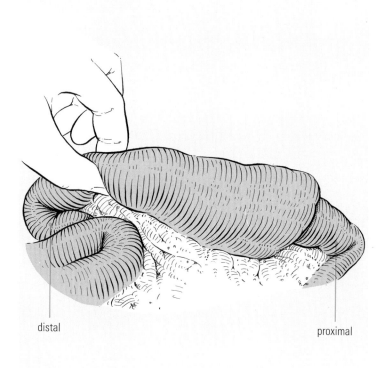

distal   proximal

Fig. 5.99

OPERATION
Preparation
The patient should be adequately resuscitated before surgery and have a nasogastric tube. The abdomen is cleansed and draped in the normal way.

Incision
A midline laparotomy incision is most suitable in the adult, but a transverse or high gridiron incision is better in the infant.

Operative technique
1. Locate the intussusception and attempt to reduce it by gently squeezing the distal bowel over the apex, trying to milk the proximal bowel back (Figs 5.99 and 5.100), rather like squeezing toothpaste from a tube. The intussusceptum may be friable and should not be pulled out proximally.

2. Once the bowel has been fully reduced, palpate it for any intraluminal lesions which may have acted as the apex. If there is any doubt an enterotomy should be made and the lumen assessed directly.

3. If there is no lesion present, as is common in the infant, the bowel can be left as postoperative adhesions make the likelihood of recurrent intussusception very low.

4. If there is a lesion present, excise it as appropriate. Hence a Meckel's diverticulum is resected, and a neoplasm requires the appropriate bowel resection (e.g. a right hemicolectomy) together with a laparotomy. An enterotomy and polypectomy are performed for a simple polyp.

5. If the intussusception cannot be reduced or it is of dubious viability once reduced, resect the bowel.

6. In cases of Peutz–Jeghers syndrome, multiple intussusceptions may be present and all should be reduced. Remove the hamartomatous polyps which are responsible for the intussusceptions through a minimum number of enterotomies by intraluminal resection.

Wound closure and dressing
The abdomen is closed in routine fashion with loop nylon and nylon skin sutures in the adult. For an infant, slowly absorbable sutures such as PDS should be used for the deeper layers. A dry dressing is applied.

POSTOPERATIVE CARE
After simple reduction, oral fluids can be introduced after 24–48 hours. If the bowel has been opened or resected, the management will be similar to that described for small bowel resection on page 5.52.

SPECIAL OPERATIVE HAZARDS
Damage to the intussusceptum with perforation by traction on the proximal bowel.

COMPLICATIONS
Recurrence is rare, providing an underlying cause has not been overlooked.

Technique of reduction

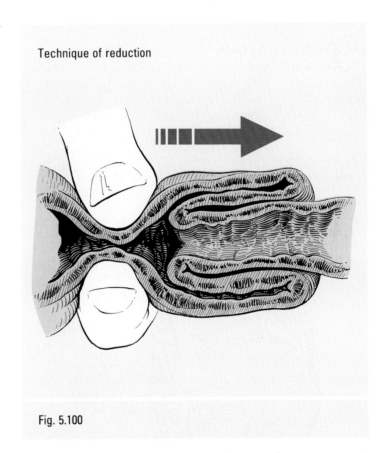

Fig. 5.100

Appendicectomy

PREOPERATIVE ASSESSMENT

1. Exclude an intrascrotal pathology (e.g. testicular torsion) and infection or calculus disease of the renal tract which can mimic appendicitis.
2. Perform a rectal examination in the presence of urinary symptoms to exclude a pelvic appendix lying in contact with the bladder.
3. The very young and very old have a low tolerance to peritonitis and immediate exploration is recommended if the history is suggestive.
4. If the history is not conclusive in a young woman with pelvic pain, laparoscopy may be more appropriate.
5. Give a metronidazole suppository.

RELEVANT ANATOMY

The vermiform appendix arises from the posteromedial wall of the caecum, 2 cm below the end of the ileum (Fig. 5.101). Its base is located deep to a point one-third of the distance between the right anterior superior iliac spine and the umbilicus (McBurney's point). The position of the caecum should be verified in the anaesthetized patient prior to making an incision, as pregnancy and arrested caecal descent result in a more cranial position in the right upper quadrant. Malrotation places the appendix in the left iliac fossa (Fig. 5.102).

The appendix varies from 2 to 20 cm in length, and arises where the three taeniae coli converge on the caecum; this provides a valuable guide to its position. As the appendix is relatively free it may point in any direction, but it usually lies in a pelvic or retrocaecal position. Occasionally, subcaecal and paracaecal positions may cause diagnostic and surgical difficulties. The mesoappendix carries the appendicular artery, which is a terminal branch of the ileocolic artery, which lies in its free border.

The overlying abdominal wall consists of skin, subcutaneous connective tissue, Scarpa's fascia and deep connective tissue. Beneath lie, in order, the external oblique aponeurosis running obliquely, parallel to the inguinal ligament to become the rectus sheath; the internal oblique muscle running upward and medial with its fibres at right angles to those of the external oblique; the transversus abdominis muscle running horizontally across the abdomen and the transversalis fascia and extraperitoneal fat which covers the parietal peritoneum overlying the caecum. The ilio-inguinal nerve and accompanying vessels pass through the abdominal muscles to lie on the internal oblique muscles close to McBurney's point.

OPERATION

Preparation

Under general anaesthesia the patient is placed supine, the abdomen is cleaned and drapes are applied to expose the right lower quadrant. Ensure that the proposed incision can be extended medially or laterally should it become necessary.

Incision

A skin crease (Lanz) or a gridiron oblique incision is centred over McBurney's point and extended laterally to within a finger's breadth of the anterior superior iliac spine (Fig. 5.103). The Lanz incision provides a more cosmetic scar, but the gridiron affords better and swifter access. It is also extended more easily.

Operative technique

1. Incise the fat and fascia to reveal the external oblique aponeurosis (Fig. 5.104), which is opened with a knife and then scissors in the line of its fibres for the full length of the wound.

Relevant anatomy

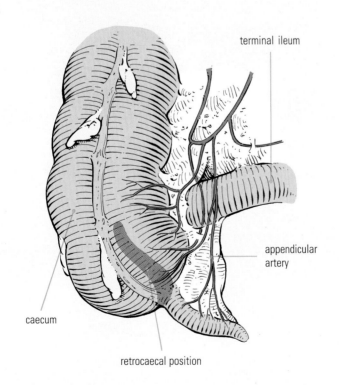

terminal ileum

appendicular artery

caecum

retrocaecal position

Fig. 5.101

2. Split the internal oblique and transversus abdominus muscles between their fibres. This is started with the points of a pair of Mayo scissors that are opened at right angles to the fibres (Fig. 5.105), and enlarged with the finger.

Possible sites for appendix

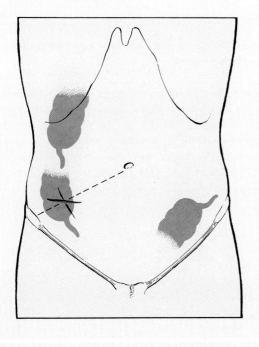

Fig. 5.102

Incision of external oblique aponeurosis

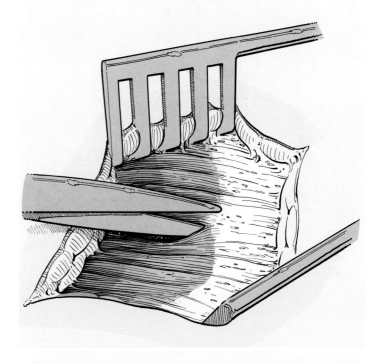

Fig. 5.104

Skin incision

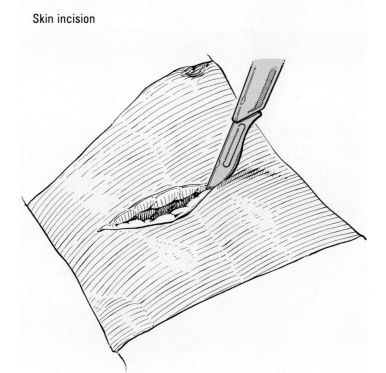

Fig. 5.103

Separating fibres of internal oblique and transversus abdominis muscles

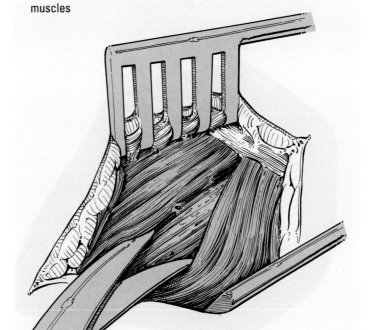

Fig. 5.105

5.57

Tenting up and opening the peritoneum

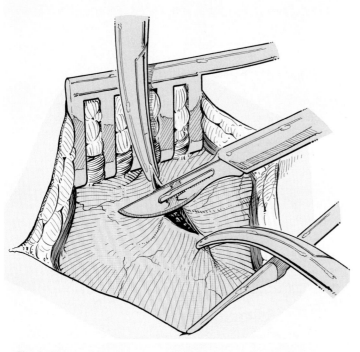

Fig. 5.106

3. Sweep aside the preperitoneal fat and tent the peritoneum between two artery forceps, before incising it with a scalpel (Fig. 5.106) and enlarging the incision transversely using scissors. A foul smell or the presence of pus at this stage indicates advanced appendicitis.

4. If greater exposure is required, incise the rectus sheath and retract the rectus muscle medially, or divide the muscles laterally in the line of the skin incision.

5. After locating the appendix by pursuing the caecal taeniae distally, take a swab of any free fluid present for bacteriological assessment.

6. Deliver the appendix, together with the caecum, into the wound and hold it with a Babcock tissue forceps. Alternatively, an artery forceps may be placed on the distal mesoappendix. If the appendix is reluctant to appear, it can sometimes be swept into the wound with the surgeon's right index finger; this procedure may be facilitated by

Clamping the appendicular artery in the mesoappendix

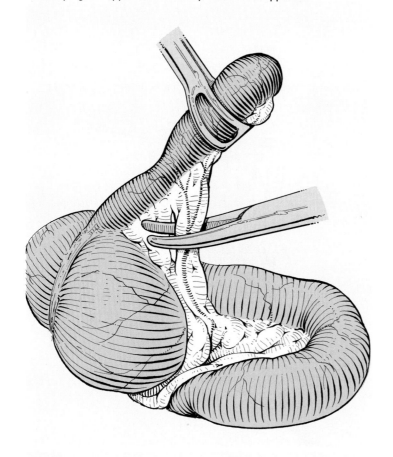

Fig. 5.107

Crushing the appendix stump

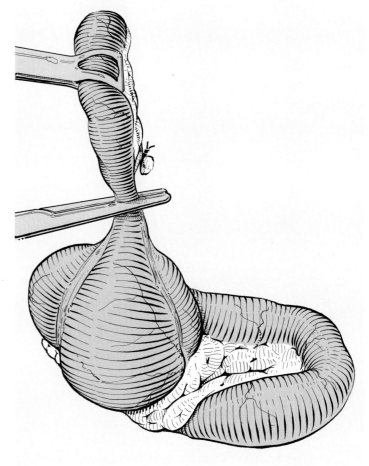

Fig. 5.108

gentle traction on the caecum which is held with a small gauge swab in the left hand.

7. Divide the mesoappendix with the contained appendicular artery between artery forceps (Fig. 5.107) and ligate it with 2/0 chromic catgut ligatures.

8. Using the Babcock forceps, hold the appendix up and crush its base with heavy artery forceps, e.g. Spencer Wells (Fig. 5.108). The artery forceps is then opened, moved up the appendix and closed again.

9. Tie a strong 00 catgut ligature around the base of the appendix where it was crushed, leaving a cuff of about 3 mm between the heavy artery forceps and the tie (Fig. 5.109).

10. Place a small artery forceps adjacent to the knot of the stump tie, and cut the ends.

11. Divide the appendix with a scalpel blade by running it along the underside of the forceps (Fig. 5.110).

12. Insert a purse-string suture around the stump using 2/0 chromic catgut, picking up the seromuscular wall of the caecum. The stump is then invaginated into the caecum using the artery forceps and the purse string is tied (Fig. 5.111).

13. Check the ligated mesoappendix for haemostasis.

14. In cases with perforation aspirate any collection of pus with a sucker and ensure that all particulate matter is removed.

Wound closure and dressing
1. Close the peritoneum with a continuous catgut suture (Fig. 5.112).

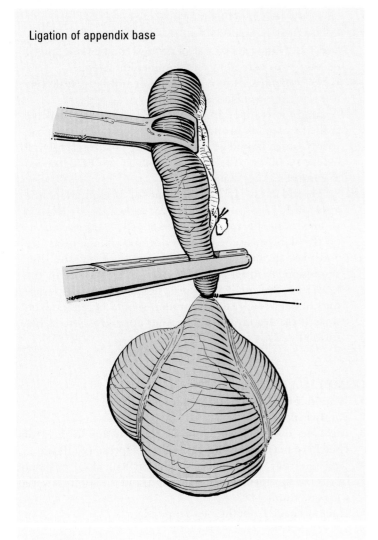

Ligation of appendix base

Fig. 5.109

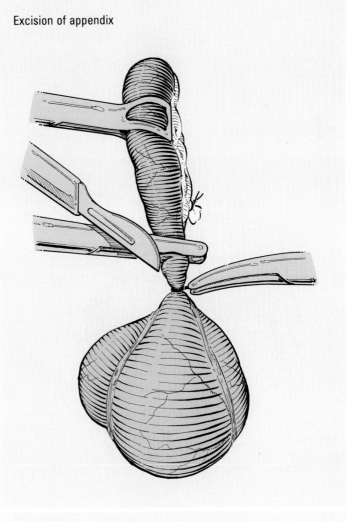

Excision of appendix

Fig. 5.110

Purse-string technique for burial of appendix stump

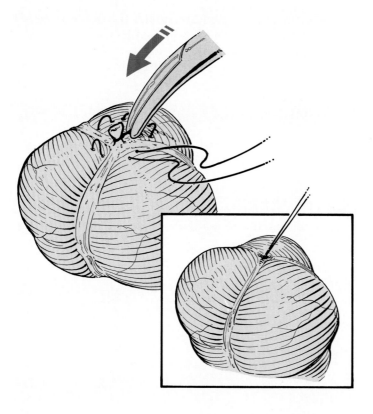

Fig. 5.111

Closure of peritoneum

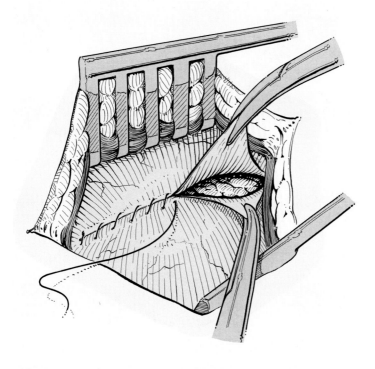

Fig. 5.112

2. Close each of the remaining layers with interrupted chromic catgut.
3. Use interrupted nylon sutures to close the skin. If the wound has been contaminated, either a corrugated wound drain is inserted into the wound or the skin closure may be deferred with delayed primary suturing 3 to 5 days later.

POSTOPERATIVE CARE
Metronidazole is continued for two doses to reduce the incidence of wound infection. Oral fluids can usually be started the following morning, and the patient should be eating and fully mobile by the third postoperative day.

SPECIAL OPERATIVE HAZARDS
1. Poor access, which can be improved by converting the muscle-splitting incision into a muscle-cutting incision by dividing the internal oblique laterally and the rectus sheath medially.
2. Incorrect diagnosis. A normal appendix should be removed and a search made for alternative pathology; the small bowel mesentery should be inspected for mesenteric adenitis, the bowel for Crohn's ileitis and a Meckel's diverticulum, and the female pelvis should be examined for ovarian cysts or tubal pathology. A swab on sponge-holding forceps should be passed into the pelvis to discover whether free blood or pus is present.
3. Retrocaecal appendix, in which case the caecum is mobilized by dividing its lateral peritoneal attachment and, if necessary, by extending the skin incision laterally.
4. If the appendix cannot be found, it will be revealed by following the taeniae coli caudally.
5. A gangrenous appendix base. To avoid the risk of leakage from the caecum through the gangrenous portion a purse string suture should be inserted in the healthy caecal wall before mobilizing the appendix, which can be tightened to control leakage if it occurs.
6. Appendix mass. If, by the time of presentation, the appendicitis has progressed to an inflammatory mass, it should be initially treated conservatively. Mark its contour on the skin surface to observe for any change in its size and plan an interval appendicectomy 2–3 months after resolution. If there is worsening pain or the size of the mass increases, or if signs of systemic toxicity or peritonitis develop, surgical exploration should be undertaken since these are indications that an appendix abscess has formed.

COMPLICATIONS
1. Wound infection and intra-abdominal abscess.
2. Paralytic ileus.
3. Incorrect diagnosis, for example serositis due to pus from elsewhere may be misinterpreted as the primary infection.
4. Leakage from the appendix stump; difficult closures should be oversewn with catgut and drained, and the stump covered with omentum.
5. Haemorrhage from the mesoappendix.

Right Hemicolectomy and Extended Right Hemicolectomy

The most frequent indications for right hemicolectomy are malignant disease of the caecum and ascending colon, Crohn's disease and angiodysplasia.

PREOPERATIVE ASSESSMENT

1. The diagnosis must be confirmed and synchronous pathology in the rest of the colon excluded by barium enema or colonoscopy, with or without biopsy.
2. In cases of malignancy, chest X-ray, liver scanning, liver function tests and assays for tumour markers (e.g. carcinoembryonic antigen) should be carried out.
3. If the patient has angiodysplasia, carry out angiography and red cell scanning.
4. Commence antibiotic cover, and prophylaxis for deep vein thrombosis.
5. Ensure adequate fluid replacement and correct any electrolyte disturbances in the presence of an intestinal obstruction.

RELEVANT ANATOMY

The right side of the colon extends from the caecum to the hepatic flexure (Fig. 5.113); the terminal ileum opens into the medial wall of the large intestine at the junction of the caecum and ascending colon. The caecum is covered on three sides by peritoneum, its posterior aspect is applied to the posterior abdominal wall. The appendix arises from the lower pole of the caecum.

The ascending colon, which is 15–18 cm long, runs from the caecum to the hepatic flexure. Lateral to the ascending colon is the right paracolic gutter, and medially is the right infracolic compartment. The ascending colon turns medially at the hepatic flexure to become the transverse colon.

The right side of the colon and its blood supply overlie the right ureter, genitofemoral nerve and the right gonadal vessels. The hepatic flexure overlies the lower pole of the right kidney, and may be covered by the inferior surface of the liver. The second part of the duodenum is medially related to the hepatic flexure. The transverse colon hangs down in the peritoneal cavity, and within its concavity lies the greater curvature of the stomach; the gastrocolic omentum stretches between the two and continues as the greater omentum below the transverse colon.

The blood supply to the right side of the colon comes from arteries which arise from the right side of the superior mesenteric artery. This runs in the root of the small bowel mesentery,

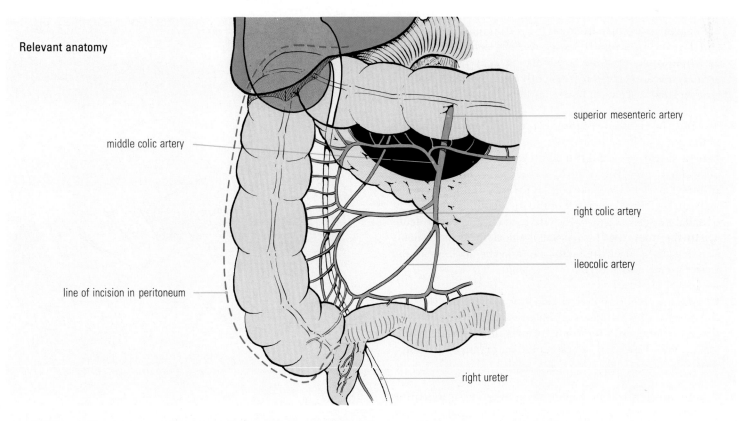

Relevant anatomy

middle colic artery

line of incision in peritoneum

superior mesenteric artery

right colic artery

ileocolic artery

right ureter

Fig. 5.113

gives rise to the middle and right colic arteries, and the ileocolic artery. The right colic and ileocolic arteries run to the right, beneath the peritoneum on the posterior abdominal wall. The middle colic artery runs in the transverse mesocolon. Each vessel divides into ascending and descending branches close to the bowel wall, which form a single marginal artery (of Drummond); this runs from the caecum to the rectum, being supplied on the left side by the branches of the inferior mesenteric artery. Venous drainage follows the arterial supply, with the veins draining into the superior mesenteric vein, and from there to the liver via the portal vein.

The lymphatic drainage is to epicolic nodes lying on the mesenteric border of the bowel wall, and then through paracolic nodes located along the arterial trunks to pre-aortic nodes around the origin of the superior mesenteric artery. Malignancies of this region of the bowel are spread through these pathways.

OPERATIONS
RIGHT HEMICOLECTOMY
Incision

1. Place the patient supine and enter the abdomen through a midline, transverse or right paramedian incision (see the Introduction) according to preference or any previous incisions.

2. Occasionally, a caecal carcinoma may present as appendicitis and is discovered during the operation. In such cases, extend the gridiron incision obliquely as a muscle-cutting incision to allow adequate access.

Operative technique

1. In cases of malignancy, confirm the site of the lesion and assess its mobility. Perform a thorough laparotomy (see page 5.2), paying particular attention to the draining lymph nodes and the liver. In Crohn's disease, carefully examine the entire gastrointestinal tract for evidence of active disease. For angiodysplasia, the colon frequently looks normal although an abnormal vascular pattern may be apparent.

2. Mobilize the right side of the colon by division of the peritoneum on its lateral side from the terminal ileum to the hepatic flexure (Fig. 5.113). Lift the colon off the posterior abdominal wall and swing it towards the midline on its primitive mesentery. Take care to identify and preserve the right ureter, the second part of the duodenum and the right gonadal vessels (Fig. 5.114). The caecum and distal ileum are further mobilized by dividing the peritoneal attachments between the root of the mesentery and the abdominal wall under the ileocaecal region.

3. Choose the level of bowel section; for malignant disease of the caecum which appears curable resect 30 cm of the distal ileum, together with the colon as far as the proximal transverse colon. Resection can be more conservative for benign disease.

4. Divide the gastrocolic omentum and greater omentum between clips up to the point chosen for sectioning of the colon.

Right paracolic gutter

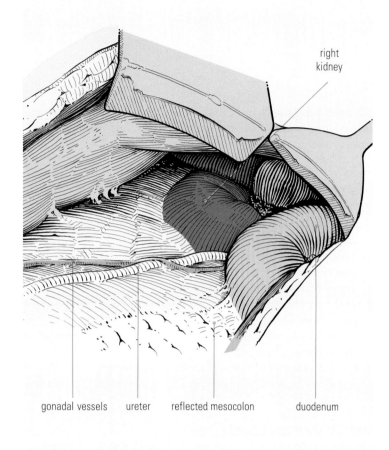

right kidney

gonadal vessels   ureter   reflected mesocolon   duodenum

Fig. 5.114

Identification of vessels

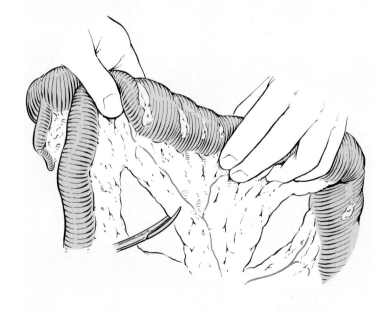

Fig. 5.115

Ligation and division of blood vessels

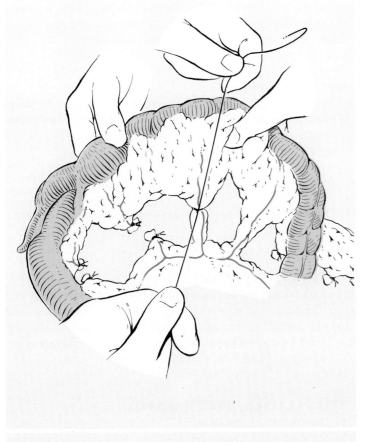

Fig. 5.116

5. If the mesentery is held up to the light, the vessels running in it can be clearly seen, provided there is not too much fat. The intervening mesentery is relatively avascular and can be divided with scissors (Fig. 5.115). Ligate and divide the ileo-colic and right colic arteries, and the right branch of the middle colic artery (Fig. 5.116). In cases of malignancy, divide the vessels close to their origin from the superior mesenteric or middle colic artery in order to remove as much lymphatic tissue as possible. In benign disorders, divide the mesentery close to the bowel wall.

6. Once the mesentery and omentum have been divided, exclude the bowel from the operative field with large acri-flavine-soaked swabs and apply crushing clamps to the bowel at the site chosen for resection. Apply non-crushing clamps to the bowel on either side of the specimen 5 cm from the crushing clamps, having milked any bowel contents out of the intervening segment (Fig. 5.117). Ensure the clamps are applied firmly or venous engorgement will occur. Using a knife, divide the bowel flush with the crushing clamp so that this clamp remains with the specimen.

7. Hold the bowel lumen open with Babcock's tissue-holding forceps (Fig. 5.118) and dab it clean with aqueous iodine-soaked dental swabs; coagulate any bleeding points with diathermy or fine catgut ligatures. Unite the bowel ends in

Bowel clamps applied

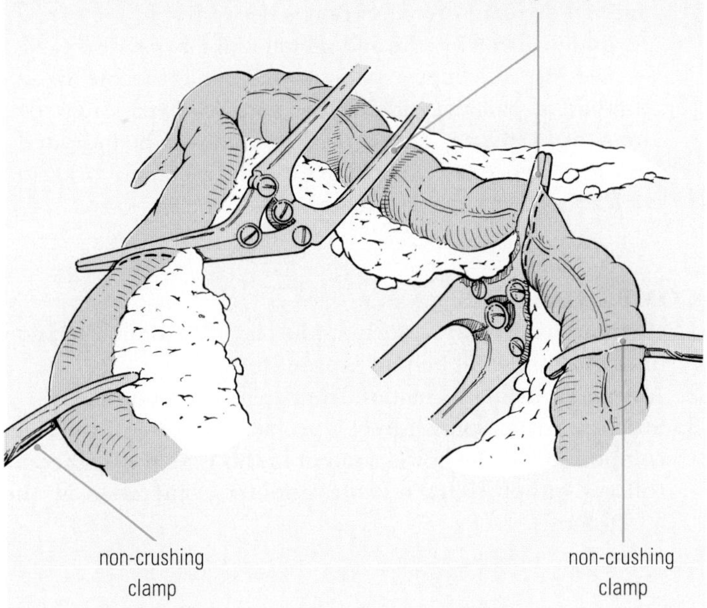

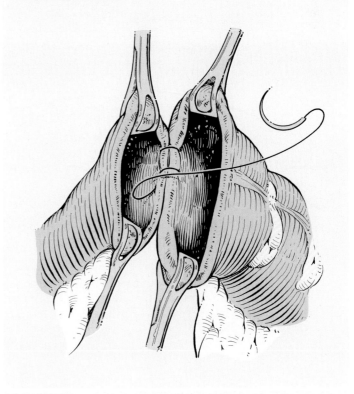

crushing clamps

non-crushing clamp

non-crushing clamp

Fig. 5.117

Ileocolic anastomosis

Fig. 5.118

one or two layers (see the Introduction) according to preference. Any disparity in size between the ileum and colon can be overcome by a more oblique division of the ileum, resecting more tissue from the antimesenteric border so as not to compromise the blood supply, or by performing an end-to-side or side-to-end anastomosis and oversewing the other end with two layers of absorbable sutures. On completion, remove the non-crushing clamps and discard the acriflavine-soaked swabs. Suture the cut edge of the mesocolon to the cut edge of mesentery with 2/0 catgut in order to avoid leaving a hole through which bowel could herniate (Fig. 5.119). Pick up only the peritoneum with the suture, as there is a risk of damage to the blood supply of the anastomosis if vessels running in the edge of mesentery or mesocolon are sutured.

8. Make a careful check for haemostasis, and wrap the remaining omentum around the anastomosis.

Wound closure and dressing

Place a silicone drain in the right paracolic gutter. Close the wound with loop nylon; if a midline incision was made it is closed in one layer, if the incision was paramedian or transverse, close in two layers. Use catgut to the fascia and 2/0 nylon for the skin.

Closure of defect in mesentery

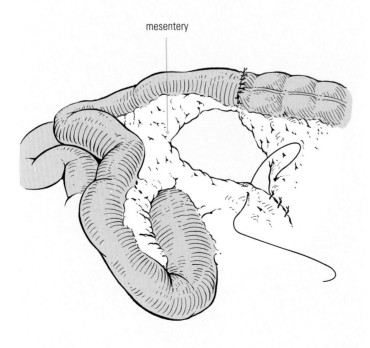

mesentery

EXTENDED RIGHT HEMICOLECTOMY

Lesions of the transverse colon, splenic flexure, and even the descending colon can be treated by extended right hemicolectomy; this prevents a colo-colic anastomosis with its more precarious blood supply, and can be safely performed in unprepared bowel (e.g. in the presence of obstruction).

Operative technique

1. In addition to the mobilization as described above, the transverse colon and splenic flexure are mobilized with ligation and division of the middle colic artery and if need be the upper left colic vessels.

2. Anastomose the ileum to the descending colon.

3. Oppose the mesentery and mesocolon in front of the proximal jejunum.

POSTOPERATIVE CARE

A nasogastric tube is left *in situ* until gastric emptying recovers. Oral fluids should be increased as bowel sounds return and flatus is passed. Prophylactic antibiotics are usually continued for 24–48 hours and the drain is removed when drainage is less than 100 ml per day. The skin sutures remain for 8–10 days.

SPECIAL OPERATIVE HAZARDS
1. Damage to the duodenum.
2. Damage to the right ureter.
3. Damage to the middle colic artery in a right hemicolectomy, which may compromise the blood supply to the anastomosis and the remaining colon.
4. Damage to the superior mesenteric artery.
5. Occluded inferior mesenteric artery in patients undergoing extended right hemicolectomy. In such cases the descending and sigmoid colon rely on the marginal artery and superior mesenteric artery for their blood supply and a more extensive resection is necessary.
6. A tumour involving the abdominal wall may be resectable *en bloc*. In an elderly patient with an incurable fixed tumour, a pallative side-to-side ileocolic bypass may be more appropriate. This procedure may also be indicated in the presence of obstruction in an unfit patient, prior to definitive operative treatment.

COMPLICATIONS
1. Haemorrhage from a poorly applied ligature; double ligation of large vessels will help to prevent this.
2. Abscess or fistula formation from an anastomotic leak.
3. Stricture formation is rarely a problem because of the fluid composition of the bowel content in this region. It generally follows either ischaemia or tumour recurrence at the anastomosis.

Fig. 5.119

Sigmoid Colectomy

Segmental resection of the sigmoid colon is performed for cases of limited diverticular disease, sigmoid volvulus, benign colonic polyps not amenable to endoscopic removal and some cases of carcinoma of the sigmoid colon. Cases of carcinoma frequently require a more radical resection, but this is not appropriate in all cases, for example in the presence of liver metastases.

PREOPERATIVE ASSESSMENT
1. Confirm the diagnosis with barium enema and/or colonoscopy with biopsy.
2. Prepare the bowel and administer prophylactic antibiotics.
3. Ascertain whether a restorative operation is safe. In the emergency situation such as obstruction, perforation or with abscess formation, exteriorization of the proximal end may be preferable as a temporary measure (see page 6.36).

RELEVANT ANATOMY
For a full description see page 6.22 in Abdominoperineal Excision of the Rectum.

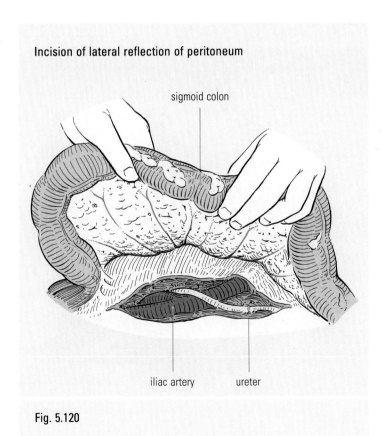

Incision of lateral reflection of peritoneum

sigmoid colon

iliac artery   ureter

Fig. 5.120

OPERATION
Preparation
Under a general anaesthetic the patient is catheterized and placed in Lloyd–Davies position (see page 6.49). This allows the distal bowel to be washed out prior to anastomosis and, if necessary, a stapling device can be inserted through the anus.

Incision
Enter the abdomen through a lower midline or left paramedian incision (see the Introduction).

Operative technique
1. Perform a thorough laparotomy. If the operation is for diverticulitis the rectum is spared from the disease, but the proximal limit of severe disease must be confirmed.

2. With the patient in a head-down tilt, pack the small bowel away into the upper abdomen with a large damp abdominal swab.

3. Frequently there are some fibrous adhesions between the sigmoid colon and the parietal peritoneum in the left iliac fossa. These are divided, followed by the peritoneum over the lateral side of the sigmoid mesocolon (Fig. 5.120). Free the sigmoid colon from any adherent viscus such as bladder or small bowel, repairing any defect that this creates.

4. Extend the peritoneal incision down into the pelvis alongside the upper rectum, while the sigmoid loop is retracted to the patient's right by the assistant. Identify and preserve the left ureter as it crosses the bifurcation of the common iliac artery.

5. Draw the colon to the left and similarly divide the peritoneum on the other side of the sigmoid mesocolon (Fig. 5.121); a finger is insinuated under the inferior mesenteric vessels in the root of the mesocolon. Identify and lift up the inferior mesenteric artery and vein, and continue the dissection in the plane behind these vessels down as far as the upper rectum. Unlike an anterior resection, the lateral ligaments of the rectum are not divided.

6. Select the proximal level of bowel section which is usually at the junction of the descending and sigmoid colon. The distal level of resection is also selected, generally in the upper rectum.

7. Locate the sigmoid arteries which can be seen in the mesocolon, and decide whether one or more of the sigmoid vessels is to be preserved, or if the proximal bowel is to rely on the lower left colic artery for its blood supply. Ligate

5.65

Incision of peritoneum on medial side of root of mesocolon

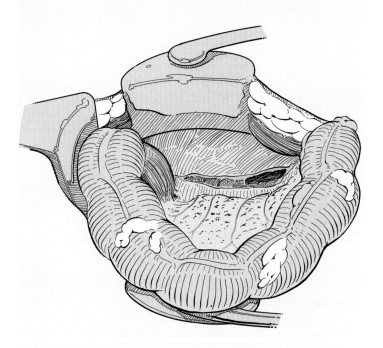

Fig. 5.121

Fully mobilized sigmoid colon

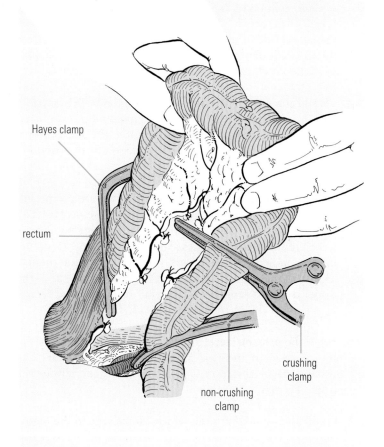

Hayes clamp

rectum

non-crushing
clamp

crushing
clamp

Fig. 5.122

and divide the inferior mesenteric vessels beyond the lowest branch to be preserved and divide the mesocolon between clips up to the point of proximal bowel section. Distally the mesorectum is divided between clips and ligated up to the bowel wall at the level of proposed transection.

8. Apply a Hayes clamp to the upper rectum, and crushing and non-crushing clamps to the proximal bowel as shown in Fig. 5.122. The distal bowel beyond the Hayes clamp is washed out with saline using a wide bore tube introduced through the anus, and sucked dry via a proctoscope. Support the distal bowel with Babcock's forceps and divide it flush with the underside of the Hayes clamp (Fig. 5.123). Insert stay sutures into each corner of the distal bowel.

9. Divide the proximal colon between the clamps and anastomose the bowel end-to-end with either one or two layers of sutures according to preference (a single layer anastomosis is shown in Figs 5.124 and 5.125). It is generally unnecessary to use a stapling device since the anastomosis is at the level of sacral promontory and therefore easily hand-sewn. To ensure the anastomosis is lying without tension, the lateral peritoneum alongside the descending colon can be divided and, if necessary, the splenic flexure is mobilized by division of the peritoneal attachment between the colon and the spleen (Fig. 5.126). This must be done with sharp dissection; if done bluntly the splenic capsule will tear and bleed. There is frequently a moderate sized vessel in the peritoneal reflection which is ligated or cauterized.

10. Test the anastomosis to ensure that it is watertight. This is performed by inflating the rectum with air via a sigmoido-

Division of distal bowel

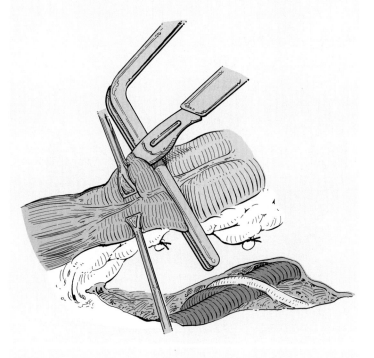

Fig. 5.123

Posterior layer of single-layer anastomosis completed

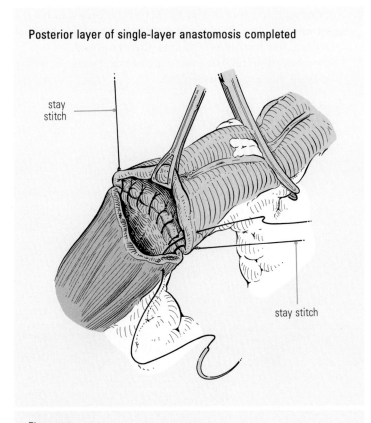

stay stitch

stay stitch

Fig. 5.124

scope while the pelvis is full of sterile saline and the proximal non-crushing clamp is still applied. Additional sutures are inserted if required.

Wound closure and dressing
Insert a silicone drain and close the wound with loop nylon and interrupted skin sutures. Apply a waterproof dressing.

POSTOPERATIVE CARE
The patient returns to the ward with a nasogastric tube and an intravenous drip. The nasogastric tube is removed and oral fluids are reintroduced as bowel function recovers. A further 24 hours of intravenous antibiotics are given. The drain remains for 7 days, and the urinary catheter is removed when the patient is mobile. Sutures are removed on the eighth day.

SPECIAL OPERATIVE HAZARDS
1. Damage to the ureter.
2. Damage to the hypogastric nerves as they cross the pelvic brim; this causes retrograde ejaculation in the male but is of little consequence in the female.

Completed anastomosis

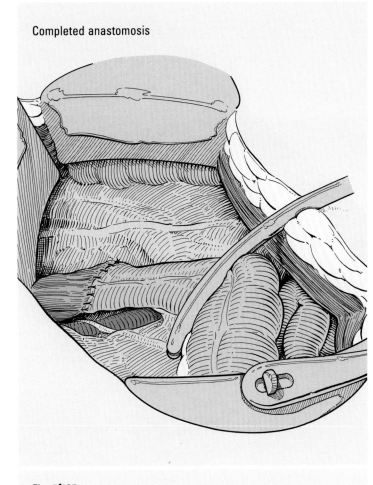

Fig. 5.125

Further mobilization of left colon

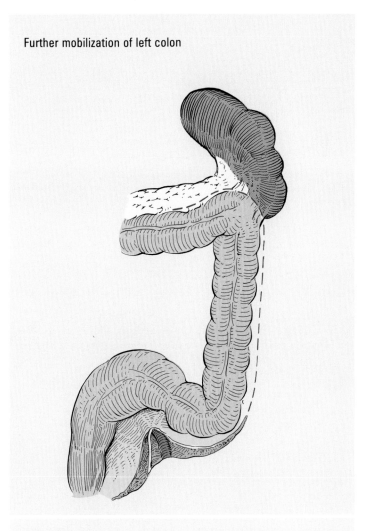

Fig. 5.126

5.67

COMPLICATIONS

1. Anastomotic leakage and fistula formation; these are unlikely if there is no tension on the anastomosis. A fistula can be treated conservatively but if a leak leads to a generalized peritonitis, a laparotomy and defunctioning colostomy is required.

2. Anastomotic stricture is also likely to follow tension on the anastomosis. This can sometimes be treated by peranal dilatation, but further resection is often required.

3. Recurrence of original disease (e.g. diverticulitis in persisting diverticuli in the proximal colon).

Proctocolectomy and Ileostomy

Proctocolectomy (removal of the colon, rectum and anus) with an ileostomy is performed for familial adenomatous polyposis, ulcerative colitis, colonic Crohn's disease and for patients with multiple large bowel carcinomas. A total colectomy with conservation of the rectum can be performed with ileorectal anastomosis for familial adenomatous polyposis or as the first stage of a restorative proctocolectomy (see page 6.49).

PREOPERATIVE ASSESSMENT

1. Perform a barium enema and colonoscopy with biopsy to confirm the diagnosis and assess the extent of disease.
2. Consider performing a sphincter-saving procedure. A restorative proctocolectomy (see page 6.49 in Park's Pouch) is suitable for selected patients with ulcerative colitis and familial adenomatous polyposis.
3. Patients with ulcerative colitis requiring emergency surgery are best treated by total colectomy, closing off or exteriorizing but preserving the rectal stump. Proctocolectomy in these patients carries a higher morbidity and prevents a restorative pouch operation being performed at a later date.
4. Explain to the patient that they are to have a permanent ileostomy. Arrange for counselling from a specialist stoma nurse who will mark the site of the stoma with an indelible marker pen.
5. Perform full bowel preparation and prescribe prophylactic antibiotics such as penicillin, gentamicin and metronidazole.

RELEVANT ANATOMY
This is fully covered on pages 5.62 and 6.22.

OPERATION
ABDOMINAL OPERATION
Preparation
Under general anaesthetic, which is often accompanied by an epidural, a urinary catheter is inserted and the patient is placed in Lloyd-Davies position (see page 6.49), with a sandbag under the buttocks. In the male, use adhesive tape to secure the scrotum to the thigh on one side to prevent it getting in the way of the perineum. For both sexes insert a 00 silk purse-string suture into the skin around the anus close to the anal verge to occlude the lumen, and cleanse and drape the entire abdomen and perineum, keeping the proposed site for the ileostomy exposed.

Incision
The abdomen is entered through a midline or long left paramedian incision (see the Introduction). In a female patient the uterus can be retracted by suturing it up to the lower end of the wound.

Operative technique
1. Perform a thorough laparotomy. In cases of familial adenomatous polyposis look for malignant change and in inflammatory bowel disease examine for evidence of small bowel involvement. Insert a self-retaining retractor. The technique for mobilization of the colon is fully covered in the chapters on colonic resection and summarized below.

2. Mobilize the caecum and right side of the colon as far as the hepatic flexure by division of the peritoneum along its lateral side (see page 5.63). Draw the colon medially and identify and preserve the duodenum, gonadal vessels and right ureter.

3. Incise the peritoneum covering the mesentery with scissors and identify and divide between ligatures the right colic and ileocolic arteries. The vessels can be divided quite close to the bowel wall rather than flush with the superior mesenteric artery in cases of benign disease.

4. Decide on the point of bowel section in the terminal ileum and divide the mesentery up to this point; the vessels are more easily seen if the mesentery is transilluminated. It is essential to ensure a good vascular supply to the stoma, but important to avoid leaving too much bulky mesentery around the distal ileum as this will interfere with the creation of the spout ileostomy later.

5. Apply a set of three de Martell clamps to the bowel at the proposed point of section and divide the bowel having removed the middle clamp (Fig. 5.127).

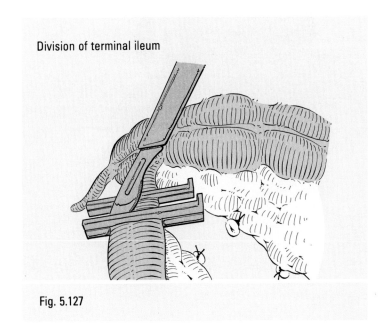

Division of terminal ileum

Fig. 5.127

6. With an assistant lifting the greater omentum upwards, draw the transverse colon caudally and using scissors dissect in the bloodless plane between omentum and transverse mesocolon and preserve the omentum.

7. Divide any adhesions between the sigmoid colon and parietal peritoneum, and using scissors mobilize the left side of the colon by dividing the lateral peritoneal reflection upwards from the pelvic brim towards the splenic flexure. Draw the colon medially and identify and preserve the left ureter and gonadal vessels.

8. Mobilize the splenic flexure by division of the fold of peritoneum between the spleen and colon with scissors whilst gently drawing both the proximal (transverse) and distal (descending) colon downwards with the other hand (Fig. 5.128). This fold often contains a blood vessel which is coagulated with diathermy or ligated. Avoid excessive traction to the colon which can strip the splenic capsule causing the spleen to bleed.

9. Divide and ligate the middle colic, upper and lower left colic and sigmoid vessels close to the bowel wall, dividing the intervening mesocolon. For convenience the mobilized bowel can now be placed into a sterile polythene bag.

10. With an assistant between the patient's legs displaying the

3 point fixation with mucocutaneous sutures

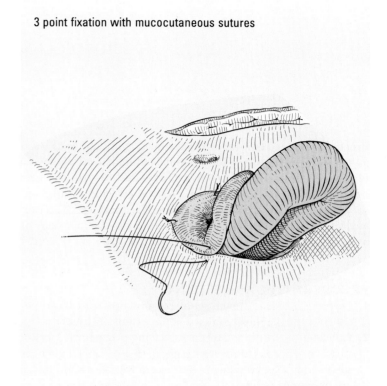

Fig. 5.129

Mobilization of splenic flexure

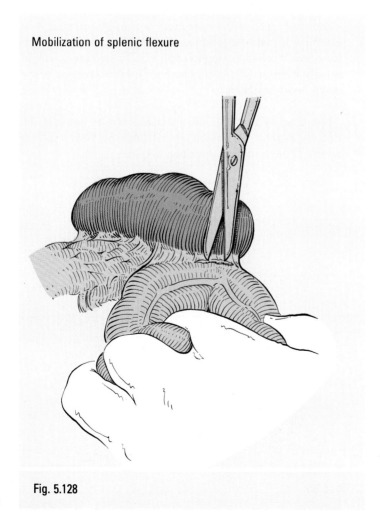

Fig. 5.128

Evertion of spout

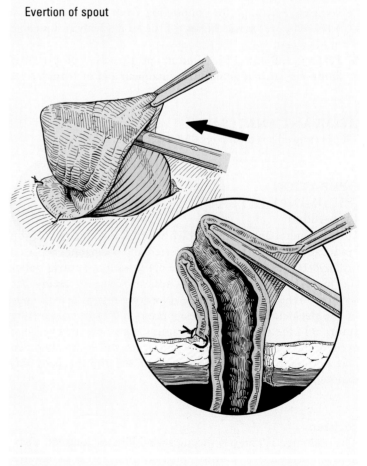

Fig. 5.130

rectum by downward traction on a St Mark's retractor, incise the pelvic peritoneum along each side of the rectum and continue these two incisions across the front of the rectum to meet each other. Keep both ureters in sight, placing a sling around them if necessary.

11. With the rectum drawn forward, divide the inferior mesenteric vessels at the pelvic brim, and the posterior fascial attachments of the rectum to the sacrum. Keep close to the rectum, ligating or diathermizing any vessels as they are encountered.

12. Mobilize the rectum anteriorly from the seminal vesicles and prostate in the male and from the uterus and cervix in the female.

13. With traction up and to the left, clamp (using Lloyd-Davies clamps), divide and ligate the right lateral ligament and its enclosed middle rectal artery close to the bowel wall. Repeat this for the left side. The remainder of the mobilization will have been performed from below (see later in this chapter) and the entire large bowel can now be removed from the patient.

14. Close the pelvic peritoneum with a running 00 catgut stitch.

15. Grasp the centre of the proposed stoma site with Lane's tissue-holding forceps and, whilst tenting it up, excise a disc of skin with a knife. Similarly excise a disc of underlying fat and incise the anterior rectus sheath in cruciate fashion with a knife. Insinuate two fingers between the fibres of the rectus abdominis muscle and either create an extraperitoneal tunnel to the original incision in the peritoneum lateral to the right side of the colon (for an extraperitoneal ileostomy), or open the posterior rectus sheath and peritoneum at this point with scissors (for an intraperitoneal ileostomy).

16. Bring the terminal ileum to the surface by feeding the de Martell clamp through the tunnel or the posterior rectus sheath and allow 8–10cm of ileum to protrude.

17. For an intraperitoneal ileostomy secure the ileum to the peritoneum and close off the lateral space with catgut to prevent parastomal and lateral space herniae (see page 6.30).

Abdominal wound closure and dressing
Insert a silicone drain, close the wound with loop nylon and use interrupted sutures or staples for the skin. Apply a waterproof dressing to the wound. Once the wound is covered create the spout ileostomy as described below.

Formation of ileostomy
1. Secure the ileostomy to the anterior rectus sheath with a few non-absorbable sutures.

2. Cut the ileum flush with the undersurface of the clamp and insert three mucocutaneous sutures at the 3, 9 and 12 o'clock positions using 00 chromic catgut mounted on a cutting needle as shown in Fig. 5.129.

3. Using a pair of non-toothed forceps (e.g. Canadian pattern) inserted at the 6 o'clock position, gently push the ileum through the stoma from within so as to evert the ileum (Fig. 5.130). Insert interrupted circumferential chromic catgut sutures, picking up the skin, the deep serosal surface of the ileum and the cut end of the ileum (Fig. 5.131).

4. Apply a transparent ileostomy appliance.

PERINEAL OPERATION
In the presence of rectal malignancy or severe sepsis such as may occur in Crohn's disease, proceed as for Abdominoperineal Excision of the Rectum (see page 6.27). Widespread sepsis with ulceration and fistula formation may make closure of the wound unsafe and it should be packed and allowed to heal by secondary intention. In other cases an intersphincteric dissection of the rectum is used as described below.

Preparation
This has been described for the Abdominal Operation.

Incision
By careful palpation a groove can be felt around the anus between the internal and external sphincters. Make a circular

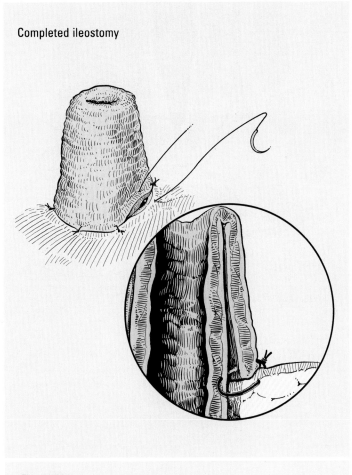

Completed ileostomy

Fig. 5.131

incision over this groove and identify the lower borders of the internal and external sphincters. The intersphincteric plane lies between them.

Operative technique

1. Grasp the anus with a Lane's tissue holding forceps, insert a self-retaining retractor and using sharp dissection with scissors develop the intersphincteric plane (Fig. 5.132). Injection of dilute adrenaline solution (1:300,000) will aid identification of the plane.

2. Posteriorly and laterally stay in this plane until the abdominal dissection is reached. Anteriorly, as the dissection proceeds, divide the anterior fibres of the external sphincter to enter the plane behind the prostate in the male and behind the vagina in the female to meet the abdominal operator.

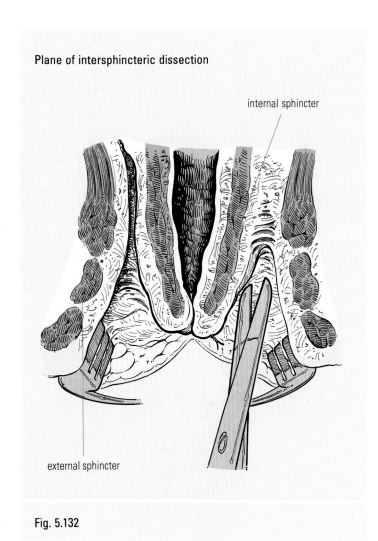

Plane of intersphincteric dissection

internal sphincter

external sphincter

Fig. 5.132

3. Once the large bowel has been withdrawn ensure haemostasis.

Perineal wound closure and dressing

Insert a fine suction drain, oppose the external sphincters with interrupted absorbable sutures (e.g. Vicryl), and close the skin with a subcuticular suture. Cover with a gauze pad and T-bandage.

POSTOPERATIVE CARE

Maintain nasogastric aspiration and intravenous fluids until gas and fluid appear in the ileostomy bag, then reintroduce fluids and food. Continue to use the epidural catheter for analgesia for the first 2–3 days. Remove the drain when drainage has ceased, usually after 2–3 days, and take out the catheter when the patient is mobile. Remove the sutures after 8 days.

SPECIAL OPERATIVE HAZARDS

1. Damage to the ureters when mobilizing the colon.
2. Damage to the spleen when mobilizing the splenic flexure. In which case, pack the area for 10 minutes with warm packs to control bleeding; haemostatic gauze (e.g. oxidized cellulose) may also help. It is uncommon to have to resort to splenectomy to control the bleeding.
3. Bleeding from the pelvic dissection, which also will generally stop if packed.

COMPLICATIONS

1. Ischaemia, retraction, or stenosis of the ileostomy usually reflects that the ileostomy was created under tension.
2. Ileostomy prolapse which may necessitate revision.
3. Pelvic floor herniation.
4. Parastomal and lateral space herniation are usually complications of an intraperitoneal ileostomy and may require surgery and resiting of the stoma.
5. Impotence in males from damage to the hypogastric nerves, which should not occur if the surgeon keeps in the right plane, close to the rectal wall.
6. Failure of the perineal wound to heal with sinus formation. This is usually a feature of Crohn's disease; any sepsis must be drained, excising the coccyx if need be, and cavities saucerized and allowed to heal by secondary intention. Ensure that no foreign material (including non-absorbable sutures) remains. In selected cases a gracilis or gluteal flap can be raised and used to pack the defect.
7. Dehydration and salt depletion following high output from the ileostomy. When bowel function returns postoperatively the output is often high initially and treated by adequate intravenous hydration. Later, if the problem persists, prescribe codeine phosphate or loperamide.
8. Recurrence of Crohn's disease in the small bowel.

Transverse Loop Colostomy

A loop colostomy defunctions the distal colon and rectum and is intended as a temporary measure either to relieve a distal obstruction prior to a definitive procedure, or to allow a distal anastomosis to heal. In some circumstances it may be performed as a palliative procedure and remain permanently.

PREOPERATIVE ASSESSMENT
1. Forewarn the patient undergoing a distal colonic resection that a temporary colostomy may be necessary.
2. A stoma therapist should mark the position of the colostomy on the patient's abdomen preoperatively, either in the right upper quadrant or right iliac fossa for a transverse loop colostomy or in the left iliac fossa for a sigmoid loop colostomy.

RELEVANT ANATOMY
A loop colostomy is usually placed in the proximal transverse colon, although it can be sited in the sigmoid colon. The colon and upper rectum receive blood from the superior and inferior mesenteric arteries, with major branches feeding the marginal artery along its length (Fig. 5.133). A proportion of patients do not have an inferior mesenteric artery blood supply. This is either because it has been ligated flush to the aorta during resections of the left colon and rectum, or because, in many elderly patients, the vessel is no longer patent. The left colon is then supplied by the marginal vessel extending from the left branch of the middle colic artery. To avoid impeding this blood supply a transverse loop colostomy is formed to the right of the middle colic artery.

OPERATION
Preparation
The patient is either placed supine, or in the Lloyd-Davies position if a low colonic anastomosis has been performed.

Incision
Make a midline or left paramedian incision in the abdomen (see the Introduction). A separate transverse incision will be required for the colostomy after the colon has been mobilized.

Operative technique
1. Identify the transverse colon and middle colic vessels, and select and manipulate a point to the right of these vessels to

Relevant anatomy

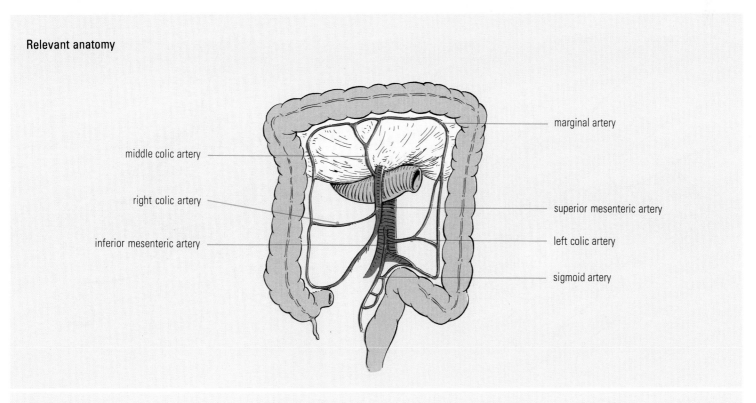

Fig. 5.133

ensure the colon can lie without tension at the intended site.

2. If the transverse colon is to be used, clear the omentum from a short length, and open the mesocolon adjacent to the serosa to allow the passage of a glass rod which is attached to a rubber colostomy tube (Fig. 5.134). Avoid the marginal artery if possible.

3. Make a transverse skin incision 5 cm long at the site marked for the colostomy. If no site is marked, it should be on the right side, midway from umbilicus to costal margin or, if the transverse colon can be brought down, a right iliac fossa colostomy is more manageable. In either case it should not be in the line of skin creases or near the laparotomy incision.

4. Deepen the transverse skin incision through the connective tissue and anterior and posterior rectus sheaths, dividing the lateral half of rectus abdominis.

5. Open the peritoneum and draw the loop of bowel through by traction on the rubber tube so it lies without tension or twisting on the abdominal wall (Fig. 5.135).

6. Having closed and dressed the laparotomy wound, open the colon longitudinally using a 3 cm linear incision along one of the taeniae; a transverse or cruciate incision may be used with a dilated obstructed colon. Start the incision with a scalpel, since if the bowel has been obstructed diathermy may ignite the intraluminal gases.

Bowel drawn through abdominal wall

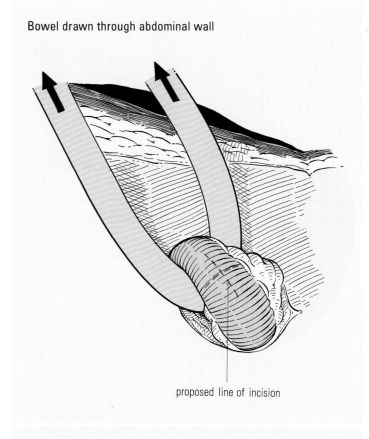

proposed line of incision

Fig. 5.135

Glass rod passed through mesocolon

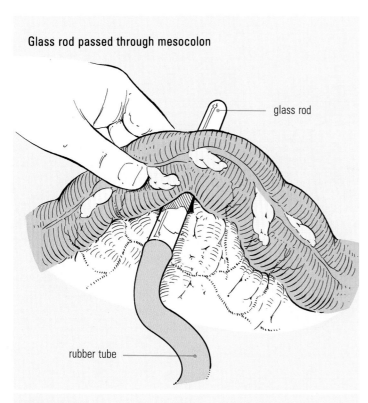

glass rod

rubber tube

Fig. 5.134

Mucocutaneous sutures to secure colostomy

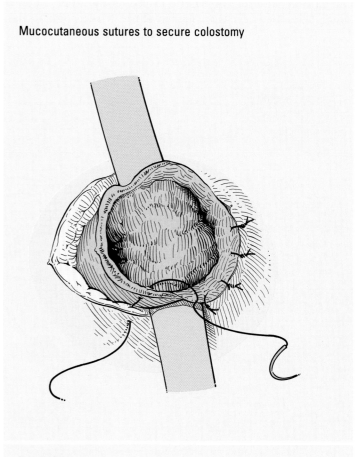

Fig. 5.136

Completed loop colostomy

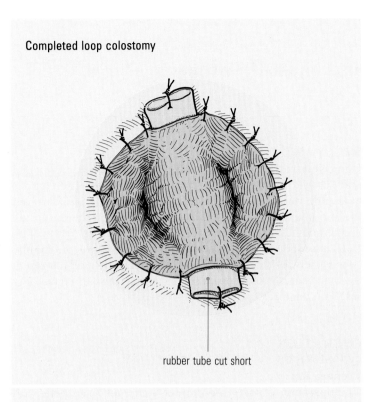

rubber tube cut short

Fig. 5.137

Bag applied

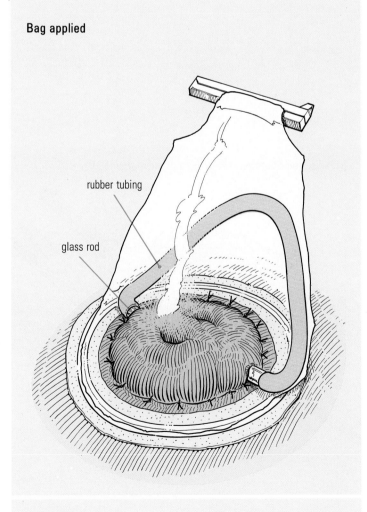

rubber tubing

glass rod

Fig. 5.138

7. Suture the full thickness of the edge of the colon wall to the skin edge using interrupted 2/0 chromic catgut on a cutting needle (Fig. 5.136), ensuring mucocutaneous apposition.

8. Insert a finger down both proximal and distal lumina to ensure patency.

9. Cut off surplus rubber tube and secure it to the skin, transfixing it with 2/0 silk sutures (Fig. 5.137). Alternatively thread the glass rod back under the colon, keeping its ends linked with the rubber tube (Fig. 5.138).

10. Spray the surrounding skin with tincture of benzoin and fit a colostomy bag.

POSTOPERATIVE CARE
Nurse the patient with a nasogastric tube and intravenous fluids until wind is seen in the bag. Remove the colostomy bridge on the tenth day. Once distal contrast X-ray studies have proved patency and no leaks close the loop colostomy at any time (see page 5.77). A delay of 4 to 6 weeks reduces oedema and facilitates the procedure.

SPECIAL OPERATIVE HAZARDS
1. Damage to the left branch of the middle colic artery impairs the blood supply to the distal colon and any anastomosis.
2. Ischaemia of the colostomy due to tension or twisting.

COMPLICATIONS
1. Colostomy retraction as a result of tension on the loop can be avoided by adequate mobilization.
2. Parastomal hernia.
3. Colostomy prolapse.

Closure of Loop Colostomy (and Ileostomy)

Once the requirement for a loop colostomy has passed (e.g. an anastomosis has healed), the colostomy can be closed and the distal bowel put back into intestinal circuit.

PREOPERATIVE ASSESSMENT

1. A distal loop barium enema and/or endoscopic examination (sigmoidoscopy or colonoscopy) are required prior to closure. This will confirm that the colon distal to the colostomy is healthy and that any anastomosis has healed.
2. Preparation of both the proximal and distal colon is required, using both an oral purgative and a distal loop wash-out with saline.

RELEVANT ANATOMY

The colon as the result of a loop colostomy has been opened and sutured to the skin, most commonly in the right upper quadrant. Both the proximal and the distal colon pass through the abdominal wall, where the serosa becomes adherent to the abdominal wall muscles and connective tissue (Fig. 5.139). The transverse loop is placed to the right-hand side of the middle colic vessels, so that, should the marginal artery be damaged, the blood supply to the distal colon is not compromised (see Fig. 5.133 on page 5.73).

OPERATION
CLOSURE OF A LOOP COLOSTOMY
Preparation

The operation is performed under a general anaesthetic with muscle relaxation. The patient is placed supine and the colostomy bag is removed.

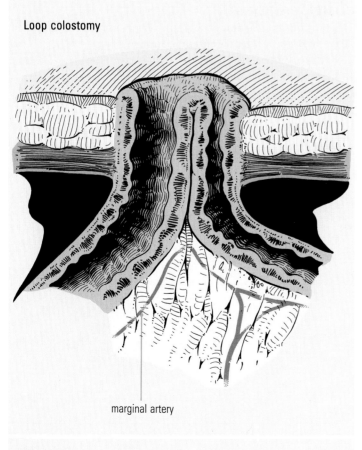

Loop colostomy

marginal artery

Fig. 5.139

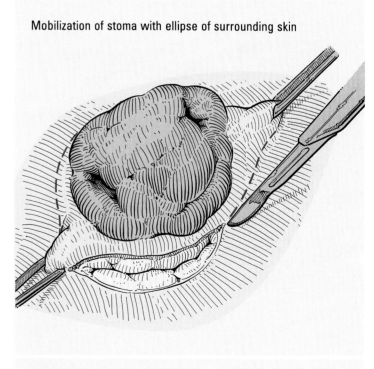

Mobilization of stoma with ellipse of surrounding skin

Fig. 5.140

5.76

Mobilization of bowel from abdominal wall

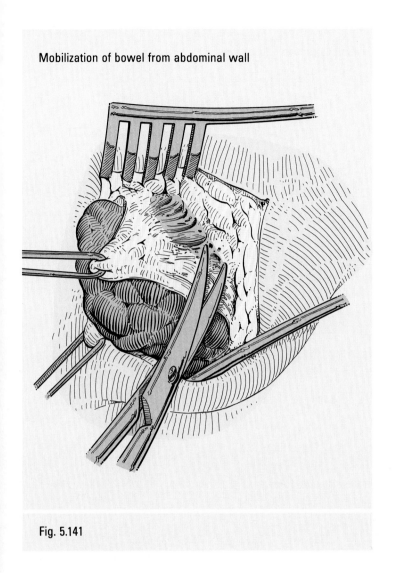

Fig. 5.141

Incision
Make an elliptical incision through the skin around the colostomy, with the long axis lying transversely.

Operative technique
1. Place Allis tissue forceps on the skin, one at each end of the ellipse (Fig. 5.140), and insert a self-retaining retractor into the incision.

2. Using dissecting scissors separate the subcutaneous fat from the serosa of the colon (Fig. 5.141); it is important to stay in this plane.

3. Dissection proceeds until the bowel is completely freed to the level of the peritoneum (Fig. 5.142). A finger in the lumen may facilitate this dissection and help define the anatomical plane.

4. If the stoma is oedematous, excise the edges to reveal the two lumina of the proximal and distal colon. If the edges are not oedematous, the skin ellipse is excised at the mucocutaneous junction.

5. Anastomose the two ends of the colon using a single layer of interrupted absorbable sutures (i.e. 3/0 Polydioxamone). This involves placing stay sutures at each end (Fig. 5.143). If

Applying gentle traction on stoma until freed to level of peritoneum

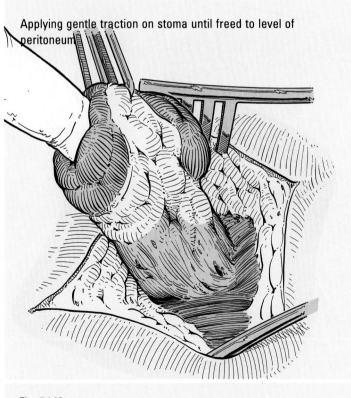

Fig. 5.142

Closure of stoma with bridge retained

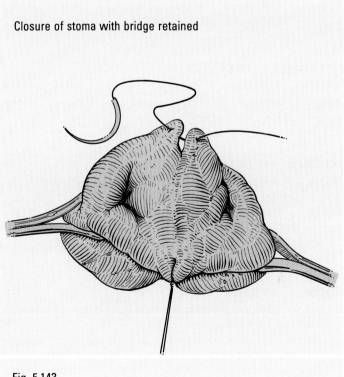

Fig. 5.143

the posterior wall has not been excised, place the first of these sutures at the margins of this posterior bridge. If, however, it was necessary to completely excise the stoma (see step 4), the back wall is anastomosed at this point with interrupted, all-layer sutures (Fig. 5.144).

6. Oppose the ends that will form the anterior wall with a layer of interrupted Lembert sutures which are supported and checked by passing a finger beneath the suture line. This prevents inadvertent apposition of the anterior and posterior walls.

7. Verify the patency of the anastomosis by gently invaginating the index finger and thumb through it. When complete, the stay sutures are divided and the bowel is allowed to fall back into the peritoneal cavity.

Wound closure and dressing

1. Place a corrugated drain down to the anastomosis (Fig. 5.145).
2. Oppose the incised muscle with a continuous nylon suture and use an interrupted nylon suture to close the skin around the corrugated drain.
3. Apply an absorbant dressing.

CLOSURE OF A LOOP ILEOSTOMY

A loop ileostomy may be closed in a similar manner, if the following points are borne in mind:

1. It is more straightforward to excise the stoma and perform a standard end-to-end anastomosis, especially where the ileostomy is formed with a spout.

2. Fashion the anastomosis in either one or two layers (see the Introduction).

3. The arterial supply is better and there is less risk of jeopardizing the supply to the distal bowel.

POSTOPERATIVE CARE

Fluids are gradually reintroduced, followed by solids, as bowel sounds return and any ileus resolves. The drain is removed when the bowels have opened.

SPECIAL OPERATIVE HAZARDS

1. Failure to excise non-viable or oedematous bowel ends will predispose to anastomotic break down.
2. Damage to the marginal artery in loop colostomies sited to the left of the middle colic artery may prejudice the blood supply of the distal colon as far as the upper rectum.

COMPLICATIONS

1. Wound infection is a risk, but significantly less so following closure of a loop ileostomy.
2. Abscess or fistula formation follows anastomatic leakage. A fistula will resolve spontaneously if there is no distal obstruction.
3. Stricture formation at the site of the anastomosis.

Reconstruction of back wall

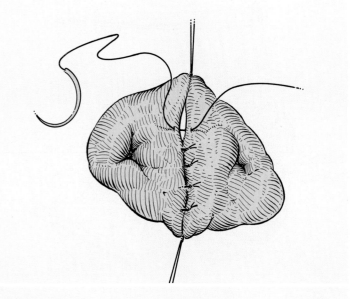

Fig. 5.144

Insertion of drain

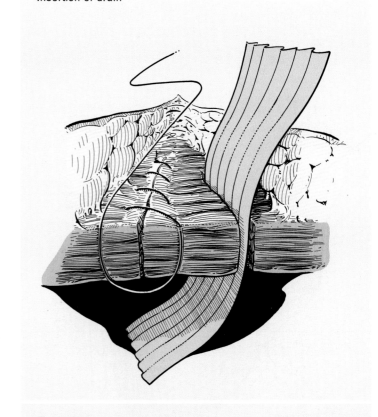

Fig. 5.145

6

Pelvic Surgery

Pilonidal Sinus

PREOPERATIVE ASSESSMENT

1. Patients present for surgery because of infection with intermittent discharge and pain, and sometimes abscess formation. An abscess needs to be drained and the granulation tissue curetted. This is performed using the 'blind' excision of an ellipse of tissue from the midline in the natal cleft; the sinus openings are rarely visible with an underlying abscess.

2. If the condition persists despite surgical drainage, elective excision of the sinus is required once the infection is quiescent.

RELEVANT ANATOMY

A pilonidal sinus develops following the implantation of hair into the skin of the natal cleft, and extends into the subcutaneous tissue overlying the coccyx or lower sacrum. There may be single or multiple openings in the midline (Fig. 6.1) and side branches are not uncommon. The sinus is lined by either stratified squamous epithelium, granulation tissue or a mixture of both.

OPERATION
Preparation

Under general anaesthesia the patient is placed prone on the operating table in the 'jackknife' position, although the left lateral position may be employed. The buttocks are then strapped apart and the surrounding skin is shaved, cleansed and draped.

A very careful inspection is made to identify all the openings of the sinus. This is helped by injecting methylene blue into an opening to delineate the ramifications of the sinus. A sinus probe is then gently inserted to identify the main tract.

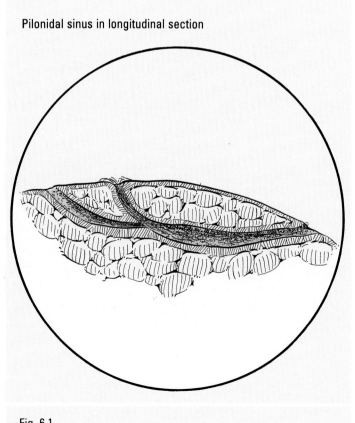

Pilonidal sinus in longitudinal section

Fig. 6.1

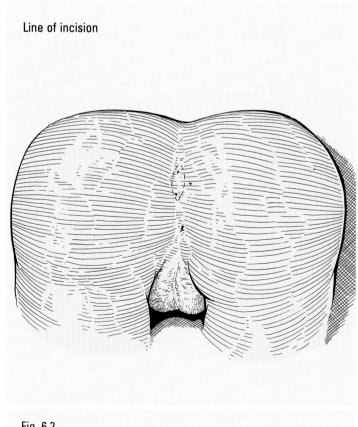

Line of incision

Fig. 6.2

The sinus is grasped and traction applied

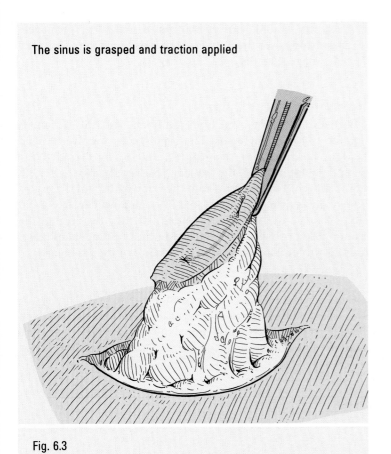

Fig. 6.3

The sinus is excised *en bloc* with sharp dissection

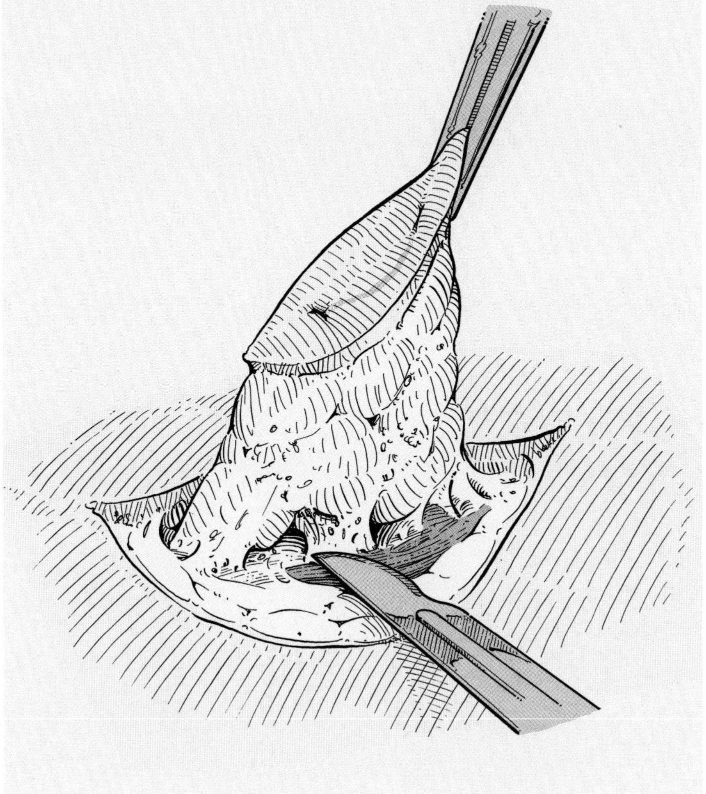

Fig. 6.4

Incision
Make an elliptical incision which includes all the midline cutaneous openings (Fig. 6.2).

Operative technique
1. By sharp dissection, the sinus with surrounding healthy tissue is separated from the underlying sacrococcygeal fascia and excised (Figs 6.3 and 6.4) with its nearby side channels.

2. Remaining side channels can be seen as they are stained blue and are dealt with by excision of a small disc of skin incorporating the opening. Excise or curette the track of the side channel using a narrow curette or a tiny brush to remove granulation tissue and loose hairs (Fig.6.5).

3. Curette the granulation tissue and diathermize the bleeding points of the main tract. Ensure all the hairs have been removed.

Wound closure and dressing
1. The wound is left open if either there has been recent infection or the resulting defect following excision is large. Even if there has not been a recent infection and the wound is small, it is not good policy to close by primary suture because of the danger of recurrent abscess formation under the flaps.

The openings of the lateral extensions are excised and the track 'cored out'

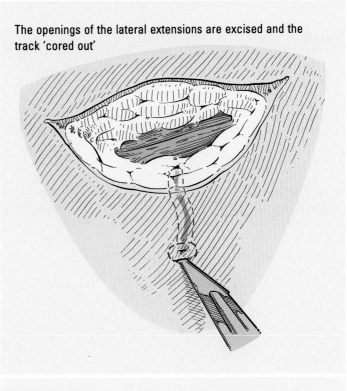

Fig. 6.5

The wound is packed

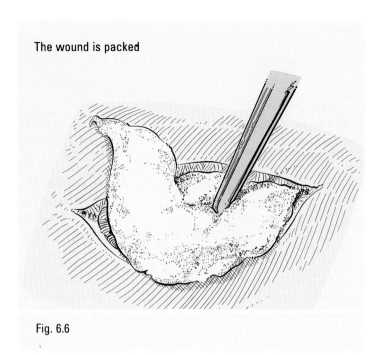

Fig. 6.6

2. Pack the wound with ribbon gauze soaked in proflavine cream and cover the dressing with a pad held in place with a T-bandage (Fig. 6.6).

POSTOPERATIVE CARE
The dressing is removed after 24 hours and the patient is allowed to have daily baths. The wound is covered with a pad held in position with firm-fitting underwear. Provided the wound looks healthy, the patient is allowed home after 48 hours and told to continue with the daily baths and dressings. The cavity is virtually painless, but the patient will need to avoid sitting on the wound. It is essential that the area around the wound is kept shaven and depilated whilst healing takes place, as ingrowth of hair will lead to recurrence of the problem.

COMPLICATIONS
Recurrent pilonidal sinus may occur if either small side channels have been overlooked at the initial operations or hair ingrowth is allowed during healing.

The rigid sigmoidoscope is 25 cm in length, and has a detachable eyepiece, a light source and a bellows to insufflate the rectum with air (Fig. 6.7). This instrument is used to examine the rectum and lower sigmoid colon.

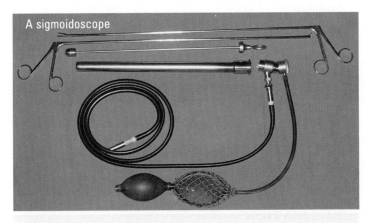

Fig. 6.7

PREOPERATIVE ASSESSMENT
1. Ensure that the patient is not arthritic, since hip flexion under anaesthetic may cause damage. Elect to perform the examination in the left lateral position in such patients.
2. If possible, a suppository is given on the morning of the procedure to evacuate the rectum.

RELEVANT ANATOMY

The rectosigmoid junction, where the rectum commences and the sigmoid colon loses its mesocolon, lies opposite the third piece of the sacrum. The sigmoid colon forms a sharp angle at the rectosigmoid junction as it swings out on its mesentery.

The rectum is approximately 12 cm long and its longitudinal muscle is shortened at three levels to give rise to three lateral curvatures (Fig. 6.8); the upper and lower being convex to the right and the middle convex to the left. As a result of these curvatures, horizontal folds (valves of Houston) consisting of mucous membrane and circular muscle project into the lumen of the rectum; the upper and lower on the left side and the middle fold on the right (Fig. 6.9).

The anal canal is approximately 4 cm in length and passes downwards and backwards to the anal orifice, making an acute

The rectum, viewed from the front

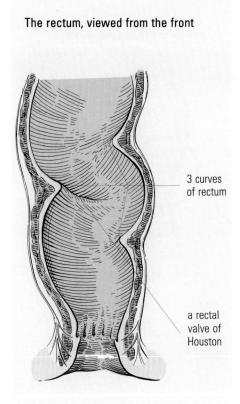

3 curves of rectum

a rectal valve of Houston

Fig. 6.8

Direction of introduction of sigmoidoscope

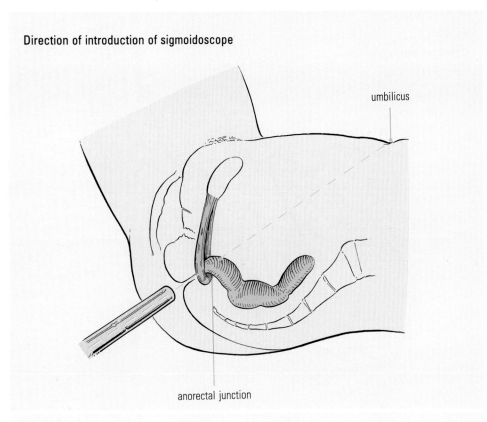

umbilicus

anorectal junction

Fig. 6.9

angle with the rectum at the anorectal junction (Fig. 6.9).

A more extensive description of the anatomy of this region is given on page 6.22 in Abdominoperineal Excision of the Rectum.

OPERATION
Preparation
For the procedure the patient is anaesthetized and placed in the Lloyd-Davis or left lateral position.

Operative technique
1. Perform a digital examination of the rectum.

2. Insert the well-lubricated sigmoidoscope into the anus, pointing it towards the patient's umbilicus (Fig. 6.9). Once in the rectum, the obturator is removed and the eyepiece and light source are connected. The remainder of the examination is performed with the rectum seen under direct vision (Fig. 6.10).

3. Pass the sigmoidoscope posteriorly, so that it is in line with the rectum, and the whole circumference of the rectal wall is visualized as the instrument is advanced. Circumvent the horizontal folds as the sigmoidoscope is passed through the rectum, and direct its tip in an anterior direction as it follows the curve of the rectum formed by the hollow of the sacrum.

4. At the rectosigmoid junction, avoid damaging the bowel by negotiating the sharp curve with great care, especially in the anaesthetized patient. This can be aided by careful manipu-lation and by gentle insufflation opening the bowel lumen as the sigmoidoscope is advanced into the sigmoid colon.

5. If a tumour is seen and it is possible, inspect the bowel to determine its proximal limit and exclude a second lesion higher up.

6. Biopsy any abnormal rectal mucosa and tumours using special biopsy forceps passed through the sigmoidoscope, with the eyepiece detached.

7. The best view is often obtained whilst withdrawing the sigmoidoscope when the bowel wall is again inspected. The commonest site for lesions to be missed is just above a horizontal fold (Fig. 6.11). Before removing the sigmoidoscope completely, the insufflated air is released by removing the eyepiece.

SPECIAL OPERATIVE HAZARDS
1. Perforation of the bowel may occur when taking a biopsy and the full thickness of the bowel is breached. More rarely the bowel is perforated by 'blind' insertion of the sigmoidoscope.
2. Persistent bleeding after a biopsy has been taken may require a diathermy probe to be passed through the sigmoidoscope to coagulate the bleeding site. Use minimal power so as to avoid bowel perforation.

COMPLICATION
Delayed haemorrhage from a biopsy site.

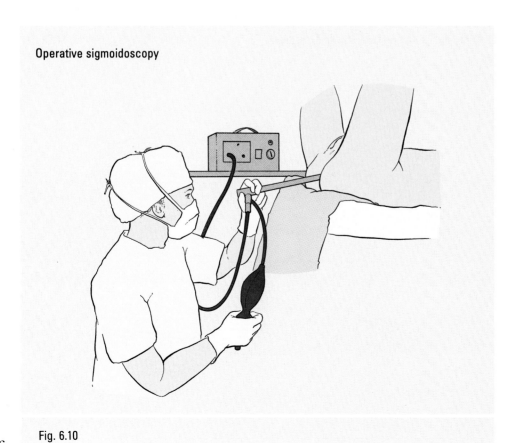

Operative sigmoidoscopy

Fig. 6.10

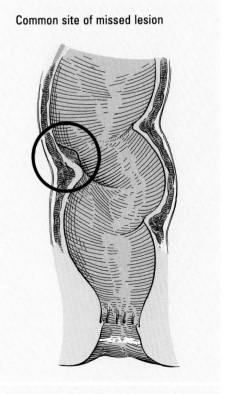

Common site of missed lesion

Fig. 6.11

Submucous Resection of Rectal Villous Adenoma

Peranal submucous resection is indicated for the excision of a sessile villous adenoma from the rectum.

PREOPERATIVE ASSESSMENT
1. Perform a rectal examination; this will reveal approximately half of the cases of villous adenoma. The lesion is usually soft, and often feels like velvet, with any areas of firmness, ulceration or tethering of the lesion to the underlying muscularis externa suggesting the possibility of malignant change. Biopsies cannot reliably exclude the presence of malignancy in some part of the lesion, although the accuracy can be improved by taking tissue from areas which feel suspicious.
2. Carry out careful sigmoidoscopy, as the majority of lesions are within the range of the rigid sigmoidoscope, and rectal lesions are more reliably demonstrated with this instrument than by either barium enema or colonoscopy.

3. A barium enema should be performed in all cases, as the development of a villous adenoma indicates the possibility of a field change in the colonic epithelium, in which synchronous lesions may be present and metachronous lesions may develop.

RELEVANT ANATOMY
Villous adenomas arise in the epithelium of the rectum and do not penetrate the basement membrane to invade the underlying lamina externa unless foci of malignancy are present. The epithelium and lamina externa constitute the mucosa, which is separated from the underlying submucosa by the muscularis mucosa. The submucosal plane lies between the muscularis mucosa and the muscularis externa, and it is in this plane that the lesions are excised (Fig. 6.12). Lesions containing foci of invasive malignancy may be excised using this technique provided that the muscularis externa is not penetrated by the tumour.

OPERATION
Preparation
An enema should be given on the morning of surgery to empty the rectum. Antibiotics are not routinely prescribed. The operation is performed under general anaesthesia and the patient is placed in the lithotomy position. Use a Park's retractor to give good exposure of the rectum and infiltrate the submucosa beneath the lesion with a solution of saline containing adrenaline (1:400,000); this lifts the lesion away from the muscularis externa, and thus facilitates dissection in the correct plane as well as reducing bleeding.

Incision
1. Gently grasp the normal mucosa below the lesion with tissue-holding forceps and tent it up.
2. Make an incision at this position with a diathermy point and enter the distended submucosal plane (Fig. 6.12).

Operative technique
1. Develop the plane cranially, using either sharp dissection or cutting diathermy, and lift the lesion away from the underlying muscle (Fig. 6.13). Bleeding points should be coagulated or under-run.

2. Traction on tumour and mucosa must be gentle as both are friable, but it is usually possible to draw the upper rectum downwards as the dissection proceeds with the result that lesions extending up to 20 cm from the anal verge can be removed using this technique; this can be helped by traction on a stay suture placed below the lesion.

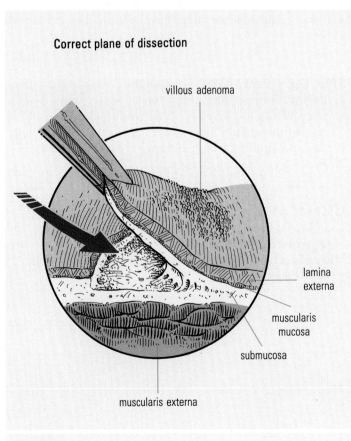

Correct plane of dissection

villous adenoma

lamina externa

muscularis mucosa

submucosa

muscularis externa

Fig. 6.12

3. Remove a cuff of surrounding normal mucosa with the lesion. It is preferable to remove the lesion in one piece, but this may not be possible with large lesions, particularly when they are circumferential.

4. The presence of invasive malignancy may have been demonstrated by biopsy; in other cases it may only become apparent as the submucosal layer is distended with saline and adrenaline, when the lesion does not lift away from the underlying muscularis externa because of tethering. Small (<2 cm diameter) areas of invasive malignancy arising in a villous adenoma can be removed by a modification of the technique of submucous resection where a disc of muscularis externa beneath the malignant area is removed in continuity, exposing extrarectal fat. This adaption is unsuitable for cases where tumour has penetrated the muscularis externa to invade perirectal fat.

Wound closure and dressing

1. In most cases the mucosal defect created by the removal of a benign villous adenoma may be left to heal by second

Diathermy is used to dissect in submucosal plane

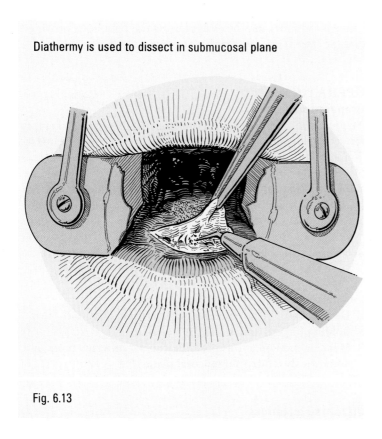

Fig. 6.13

intention. However, the incidence of postoperative bleeding is reduced if the defect is closed.

2. Where a circumferential benign lesion has been resected, mucosal continuity must be restored. This is achieved by placing longitudinal sutures in the muscularis externa, to fold this layer like a concertina and approximate the mucosal surfaces, which are also sutured. Absorbable sutures (e.g. Vicryl) mounted on a J-shaped needle are suitable for this purpose.

3. In cases of invasive malignancy where a disc of muscularis externa has been removed, the muscular defect must be closed with interrupted absorbable sutures.

4. Send the resected specimen for histological examination to confirm that the margins of excision are tumour-free.

POSTOPERATIVE CARE
Aperients, usually consisting of a bulking agent and a lubricant (e.g. liquid paraffin), are prescribed in the immediate postoperative period to ensure an early return of normal bowel habit. Prophylactic antibiotics are prescribed in cases where the muscularis externa has been breached.

Regular long-term follow-up is required as further benign or malignant lesions arise in the colon or rectum in one-fifth of cases. The majority develop at, or near, the level of the original lesion. Some recurrences are due to incomplete resection but others arise *de novo* as a manifestation of epithelial instability. In addition to regular sigmoidoscopic assessment of the rectum, examination of the remainder of the colon by either barium enema or colonoscopy is necessary at intervals which are dictated by each unit's policy, the particular circumstances of the case and the development of further symptoms or signs. During the first 5 years after resection, full examination of rectum and colon may be appropriate after 12 months and then at intervals of 2 years.

SPECIAL OPERATIVE HAZARDS
1. Perforation of the rectum must be recognized and repaired at the operation. If apparent postoperatively it can be successfully managed conservatively by keeping the patient nil-by-mouth and prescribing antibiotics.
2. Reactionary haemorrhage.

COMPLICATIONS
1. Secondary haemorrhage usually reflects an infection and may require re-exploration in theatre.
2. Stenosis occurs particularly with circumferential lesions.
3. Recurrence (see above).

Haemorrhoidectomy

PREOPERATIVE ASSESSMENT

1. Use a sigmoidoscope to exclude other rectal conditions such as a large bowel carcinoma which can precipitate the prolapse of piles and is an important cause of rectal bleeding.
2. Perform a barium enema or colonscopy in elderly patients with rectal bleeding.
3. The operation should not be performed in patients with inflammatory bowel disease. It should also be avoided during pregnancy since improvement usually follows delivery.
4. The patient is admitted on the day before surgery and a glycerine suppository is inserted that evening. A disposable enema is given on the morning of the operation.
5. Aperients are commenced on the day before surgery to allow easier evacuation and a regular bowel habit post-operatively.

RELEVANT ANATOMY

The anal canal is 4cm in length, running from the rectum to the anal margin, and is lined with epithelium. The membrane contains longitudinal folds (anal columns) which are joined by crescentic folds (anal valves) at the pectinate line (Fig. 6.14).

The blood supply to the rectum and anal canal is mainly from branches of the superior rectal arteries, reinforced by the middle and inferior rectal arteries which arise from the internal iliac arteries. The superior rectal artery, the continuation of the inferior mesenteric artery, divides into the right and left branches; the right branch further divides into anterior and posterior branches. These three terminal ramifications run downwards within the anal columns.

Venous blood drains via a submucosal plexus of veins. In a transverse section of the anal column the venous plexus is more pronounced, forming three venous cushions which are situated in a right anterior, right posterior and left posterior position; this corresponds to the position of the terminal branches of the superior rectal arteries (Fig. 6.15). These venous cushions assist in continence of flatus and are supported by smooth muscle fibres arising from the internal sphincter and elastic tissue which is widely distributed between the venous plexuses.

Haemorrhoids arise when the supporting structures become stretched allowing the anal cushion to prolapse unsupported. The venous plexus of each 'pile' (haemorrhoid) then becomes engorged with blood.

OPERATION

Preparation

General anaesthesia is used, supplemented by caudal anaesthesia to ensure postoperative pain relief for up to 12 hours. Epidural or low spinal anaesthesia can be used in the place of general anaesthesia for the elderly or patients unfit for this type of anaesthetic.

After placing the patient in the lithotomy position with the

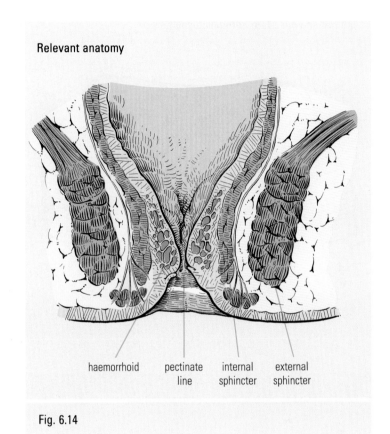

Relevant anatomy

haemorrhoid　pectinate　internal　external
line　sphincter　sphincter

Fig. 6.14

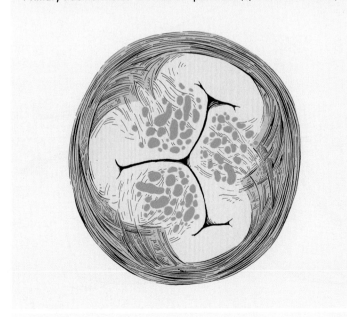

Primary haemorrhoids in classical positions (3, 7 and 11 o'clock)

Fig. 6.15

buttocks pulled to the edge of the table, the perianal skin is cleansed with a mild antiseptic (e.g. Hibitane) and the anal canal is cleansed using a sponge soaked in antiseptic solution.

The patient is then draped with leggings, and a towel that has a hole is placed across so as to allow exposure of the perineum.

One per cent lignocaine with adrenaline (1:300,000) is infiltrated into each haemorrhoid to define the tissue planes, reduce bleeding, and provide some postoperative analgesia (Fig. 6.16).

Operative technique

1. An anal stretch is performed gently if the anal canal is tight; this makes exposure of the haemorrhoid easier and reduces postoperative pain (see page 6.13 in Anal Dilatation).

2. Dunhill forceps are placed on the perianal skin just outside the mucocutaneous junction of each haemorrhoid cushion; these lie at 3, 7 and 11 o'clock. If skin tags are present they should be included. Traction is then exerted on the forceps to pull each haemorrhoidal mass into view.

3. A Burkett forceps is applied to the upper border of each haemorrhoid and traction on these forceps will show the junction between the haemorrhoidal mucosa and normal anal mucosa (Fig.6.17).

Infiltration with dilute adrenaline solution

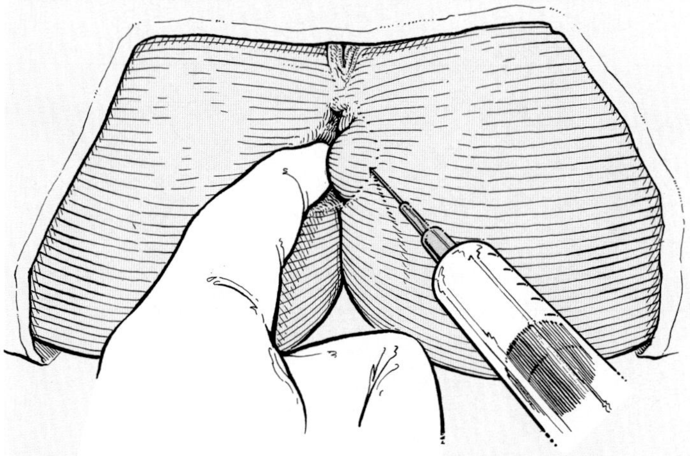

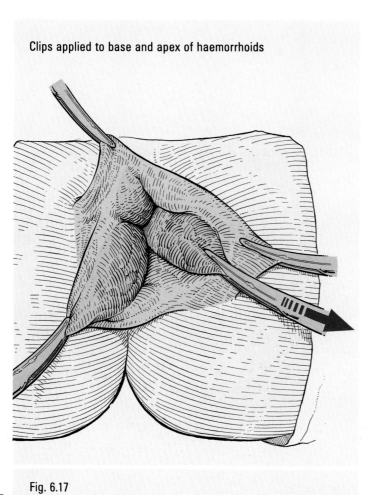

Fig. 6.16

Clips applied to base and apex of haemorrhoids

Line of skin incision

Fig. 6.17

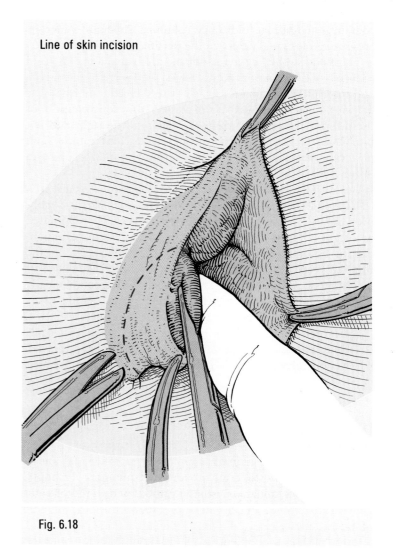

Fig. 6.18

4. The haemorrhoids are excised in turn. To avoid blood obscuring the operative field, start with the 7 o'clock haemorrhoid, then the 3 o'clock, and finally the 11 o'clock. The other haemorrhoids are held out of the way by attaching the forceps to the drapes with towel clips. Haemorrhoid excision proceeds by grasping the forceps in the palm of the left hand and inserting the index finger into the anal canal and pressing outwards to stretch the haemorrhoid over the pulp of the finger. Using curved Mayo scissors, a semicircle of skin is incised around the base of the haemorrhoid and then extended on either side of it onto the mucosal surface (Fig.6.18).

6. Sharp and blunt dissection removes the haemorrhoid from the underlying anal sphincter which is characteristically white in colour and must be seen before this dissection proceeds (Fig.6.19).

7. The dissection is tapered towards the apex of the pile, and once the pedicle is defined it is transfixed with a 00 catgut or similar absorbable suture(Fig.6.20). The knot is then tied on the luminal surface (Fig.6.21). It is important to avoid incorporating the anal sphincter in this stitch as this will lead to severe postoperative pain.

8. After the haemorrhoid is excised leaving a fairly long cuff of tissue distal to the ligature, traction is exerted on the ligature to draw down the pedicle so the haemorrhoidal bed can be seen and any bleeding points diathermized.

9. The two remaining haemorrhoids are dealt with in a similar fashion; in both cases adequate 'bridges' of normal skin and mucosa must be left between the dissected beds.

10. If secondary haemorrhoids are present they can be excised by dissection beneath the mucosal 'bridges', unless the bridges are narrow in which case dissection should be limited to the 'primary piles'. The wound may be trimmed to remove any skin tags.

11. The final result should resemble a three-leafed clover with triangular-shaped skin bridges (Fig.6.22).

Wound closure and dressing
1. The wounds are covered with paraffin gauze that is folded into triangles and tucked into the anus so it lies over the wound. An absorbable pad is applied and held in place with a T-bandage.

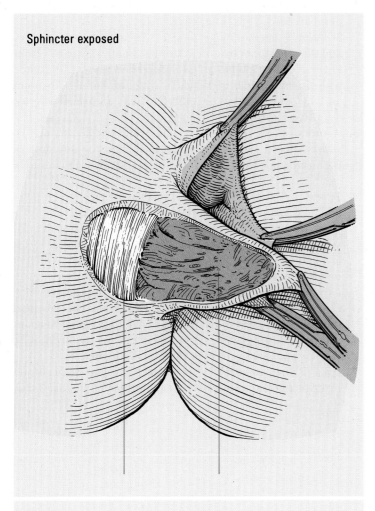

Sphincter exposed

Fig. 6.19

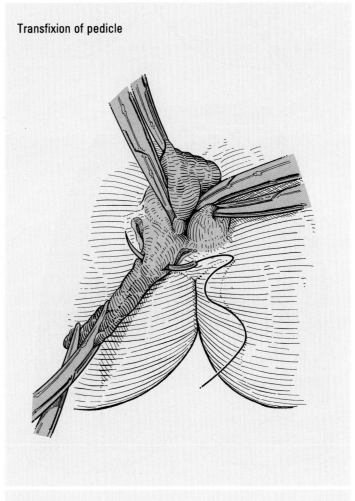

Transfixion of pedicle

Fig. 6.20

2. The insertion of sponge rolls and rubber tubes into the anus to stop postoperative bleeding is painful and can be avoided if the surgeon ensures that the wound is absolutely dry at the end of the operation.

Transfixion completed

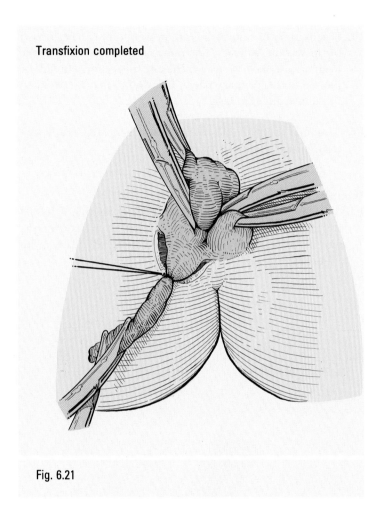

Fig. 6.21

Dress with paraffin gauze

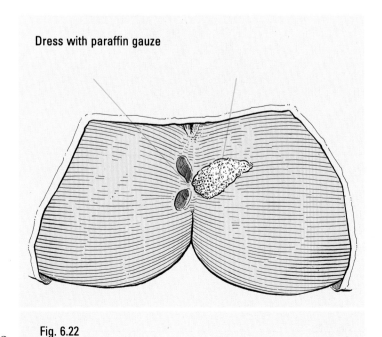

Fig. 6.22

POSTOPERATIVE CARE

The dressings are soaked off in the bath on the day following the operation. Subsequently, the patient should have a bath daily and wash carefully after each bowel action.

A rectal examination to check for stenosis is performed on the fifth postoperative day or after 2–3 weeks, depending on the surgeon's choice. If stenosis or sphincter spasm are present the patient is instructed on the use of an anal dilator.
patient is instructed on the use of an anal dilator.

The patient remains in hospital until the bowels can be opened comfortably, and is encouraged to follow a high fibre diet on discharge. Complete healing of the wound usually occurs within 6 weeks. The patient is warned to expect some discharge until healing is complete.

SPECIAL OPERATIVE HAZARDS

1. Damage to the anal sphincters.
2. Incorporating the sphincters in the transfixion ligature causing severe postoperative pain.

COMPLICATIONS

1. Reactionary haemorrhage due to bleeding from small vessels in the mucosal edge or the raw surface of the wound. It may be stopped by applying a gauze swab soaked in adrenaline solution (1:200,000), although diathermy may be required. Very rarely the ligature on the pedicle may slip and the bleeding can be profuse, in which case the patient is re-anaesthetized, returned to the theatre and the bleeding point secured.
2. Secondary haemorrhage tends to occur between the first and third postoperative weeks and is usually due to infection. If the bleeding point can be located it is under-run, otherwise the anal canal is packed with gauze for 24–48 hours and the patient placed on antibiotics (e.g. metronidazole and a cephalosporin).
3. Acute urinary retention results from poor pain control which should be corrected first. Catheterization may be required, and in a male patient prostatic disease needs to be excluded.
4. Faecal impaction may occur if the patient is not given adequate pain relief and aperients.
5. Anal stenosis during wound healing may indicate inadequate skin 'bridges', in which case the patient is taught to use a dilator. If the problem persists then the anus is dilated under anaesthesia.
6. Cross-healing results in adhesions between opposite wounds; this is prevented by passing regular firm stools. Once formed, the adhesions need to be broken down under general anaesthesia and prevented from re-occurring by prescribing regular aperients with or without anal dilators.
7. Anal fissures are due to poor healing and may be prevented by ensuring the wounds are clean and using an anal dilator if necessary.

Anal Dilatation

The rationale for anal dilatation is that spasm and contracture of the internal sphincter aggravate the venous congestion in prolapsing haemorrhoids and prevents an anal fissure from healing. Forced dilatation of the anal sphincter under general anaesthesia, followed by use of a lubricated plastic anal dilator twice daily for 3 weeks, will often relieve the patient's symptoms from haemorrhoids and permit a fissure to heal.

PREOPERATIVE ASSESSMENT
1. Dilatation is only performed after a trial period on a high-fibre diet and after aperients have failed to relieve symptoms.
2. Pain may preclude preoperative sigmoidoscopy if there is an anal fissure. In such cases, sigmoidoscopy is performed when the patient is anaesthetized prior to anal dilatation.
3. Two glycerin suppositories are given preoperatively.

RELEVANT ANATOMY
The anal canal is the continuation of the rectum where it passes through the pelvic floor. It ends at the anal verge (Fig. 6.23).

The circular muscle coat of the rectum becomes thickened and forms the internal sphincter, the lower border of which can be felt. The anal canal loses the longitudinal muscle coat which fans out intermingling with the lowest part of the external sphincter to insert into the perianal skin. The latter constitutes the corrugator cutis ani muscle.

The external sphincter is composed of a deep, a superficial and a subcutaneous portion. These are striated mucles which encircle the anal canal; some muscle fibres are a continuation of the fibres of the deep sphincter and merge with the fibres of the pelvic floor musculature. The external sphincter is also supported by the longitudinal muscle fibres which transverse the lowermost part of the external sphincter.

OPERATION
Preparation
General anaesthesia is employed, with or without a caudal block, and the patient is positioned in a lithotomy–Trendelenburg or left lateral position. A digital examination and sigmoidoscopy are performed to exclude other anal or rectal diseases.

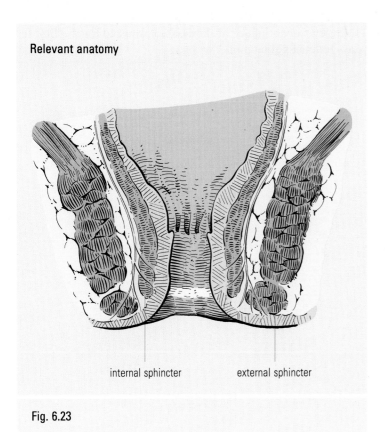

Relevant anatomy

internal sphincter   external sphincter

Fig. 6.23

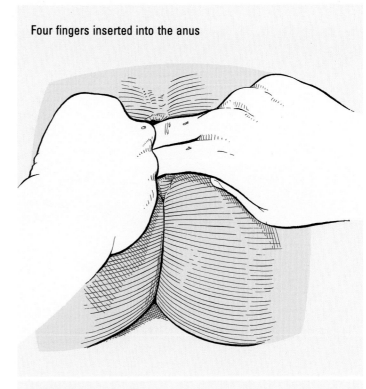

Four fingers inserted into the anus

Fig. 6.24

Operative technique

1. Insert a lubricated, gloved index finger into the anus. The constricting bands of the lower fibres of the internal sphincter can be easily felt.

Foam pack to reduce haematoma

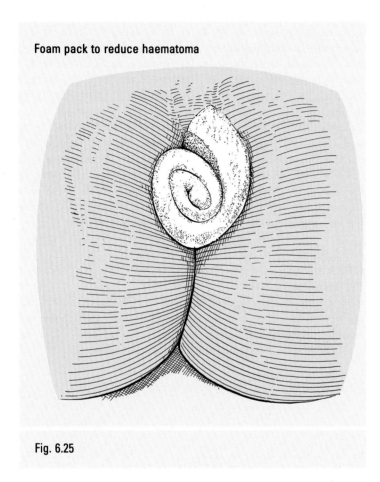

Fig. 6.25

2. Insert the index finger of the other hand into the anus and gently pull the fingers apart.

3. Insert two further fingers so that the constrictions are gently overcome. The stretch should be maintained for a minimum of 1 minute and pressure exerted at 3 and 9 o'clock to stretch break the constrictions at these points rather than at 6 or 12 o'clock which can impair continence (Fig. 6.24).

4. A 'four-finger' stretch is adequate to overcome the constriction, although some surgeons advocate inserting six or even eight fingers to provide adequate dilatation.

5. At the end of the procedure, insert a lubricated sponge roll into the anal canal to reduce haematoma formation (Fig. 6.25); a tape is attached to the roll to allow easy removal after 1 hour.

POSTOPERATIVE CARE

Commence bulk-forming aperients and instruct the patient in the use of an anal dilator. Discharge the patient on the day following surgery.

SPECIAL OPERATIVE HAZARDS
1. Damage to the external sphincter.
2. Perianal haematoma; this is rarely severe and is self-limiting.
3. Prolapse of the mucosa or haemorrhoids can occur after dilatation of the narrowed outlet.

COMPLICATIONS

Incontinence occurs when excessive dilatation has been performed and this is why a 'four finger' stretch is recommended. Transient incontinence of flatus is not unusual for the first few days following dilatation.

Lateral Subcutaneous Sphincterotomy

Lateral subcutaneous sphincterotomy is performed to allow a chronic fissure-in-ano to heal.

PREOPERATIVE ASSESSMENT
1. Exclude any fissures due to ulcerative colitis, Crohn's disease, tuberculosis or syphilis.
2. Aperients should be tried first to correct constipation. This often leads to healing of recent fissures.

RELEVANT ANATOMY
This is covered on page 6.13 in Anal Dilatation. An anal fissure may arise from the passage of hard stools which tear the anal mucosa below the pectinate line. This results in spasm of the anal sphincters encouraging fresh tears and preventing healing. Ninety per cent of anal fissures are situated in the midline posteriorly; the remaining 10% are situated anteriorly. An oedematous tag of mucosa, called a sentinel pile, may be found at the lower limit of the fissure at the anal margin.

OPERATION
Preparation
The patient is placed in the Lloyd-Davis or lithotomy–Trendelenburg position and the operation performed under general anaesthesia. A caudal block should not be used as this relaxes the internal sphincter making it difficult to define. The table is tilted head-down and elevated so that the anus is at eye-level when the surgeon is seated. The area is cleansed and draped. An examination under anaesthetic and sigmoidoscopy should be performed to exclude any other pathology and to confirm the diagnosis.

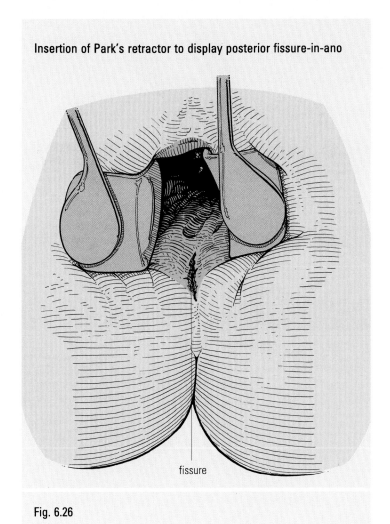

Insertion of Park's retractor to display posterior fissure-in-ano

fissure

Fig. 6.26

Rotate retractor prior to palpation of lower border of sphincter

lower border of sphincter

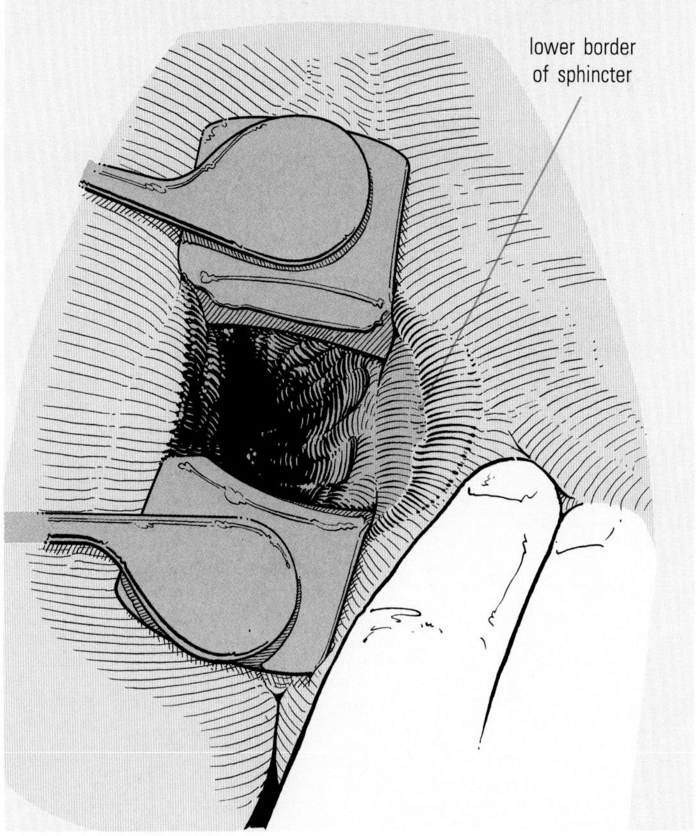

Fig. 6.27

Operative technique

1. Insert a Parks' anal retractor, open the blades and then inspect the fissure (Fig.6.26).

2. Rotate the retractor through 90° to demonstrate the internal sphincter, which is stretched and can be easily palpated as a firm band (Fig.6.27).

3. Via a small stab incision, insert a scalpel with a number 11 blade subcutaneously at the 3 o'clock position at the anal margin, parallel to the skin and with the blade facing down (Fig.6.28).

4. Rotate the blade through 90° so that the cutting edge faces the internal sphincter. Pressure on the scalpel will then cause the muscle fibres of the sphincter to divide, and this can be felt as the tension on the sphincter relaxes. The muscle is divided up to the pectinate line (Fig. 6.29).

5. Once the scalpel has been withdrawn the completeness of the sphincterotomy is checked by pressing a finger against the sphincterotomy site. This will rupture any residual fibres.

Wound closure and dressing

Bleeding is arrested by applying the corner of a strip of paraffin gauze against the wound and a sponge pad is inserted into the anus for 1 hour.

POSTOPERATIVE CARE

Aperients are prescribed together with a high-fibre diet.

SPECIAL OPERATIVE HAZARDS

Damage to the external sphincter muscle resulting in incontinence.

COMPLICATIONS

1. Haematoma formation is minimized if a foam pack is placed for 1 hour.
2. Abscess formation is uncommon and generally follows haematoma.
3. Recurrence of fissure; this is uncommon if the operation is performed correctly.

Insertion of scalpel subcutaneously

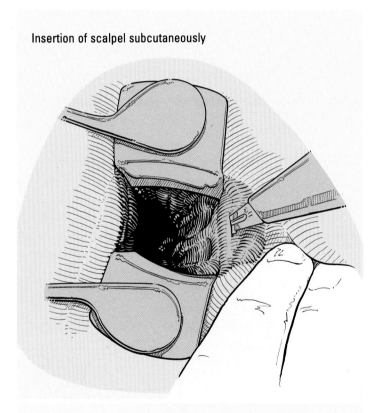

Fig. 6.28

Extent of sphincterotomy

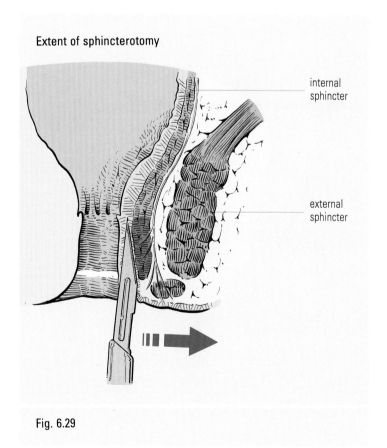

internal
sphincter

external
sphincter

Fig. 6.29

Submucous and intersphincteric abscesses originate from a blocked anal gland which then becomes infected. The intersphincteric frequently presents when it has extended caudally forming a perianal abscess or laterally to produce an ischiorectal abscess. The infection of the anal gland may have been borne by the blood or extended from the skin.

PREOPERATIVE ASSESSMENT
1. Discover if there is a history of inflammatory bowel disease or diabetes mellitus, as such patients are prone to this type of infection.
2. Determine whether the patient has had a previous abscess; this might suggest the presence of a fistula-in-ano.
3. If an abscess is suspected, surgery should not be deferred because there is a risk of fistula formation.

RELEVANT ANATOMY
The anal canal is approximately 4 cm long, commencing at the level of the levator ani. Midway along its length the anal columns of mucosa unite to form the anal valves along the pectinate (dentate) line (Fig. 6.30). Lying above each valve is a recess, called an anal sinus, and it is in the region of the sinuses that the anal glands open into anal crypts. These glands are branching structures, extending up and down between the mucosa and internal sphincter, and also penetrating the sphincter to extend radially into the intersphincteric plane.

Anorectal abscess formation occurs in one of the potential spaces around the anal canal; these are usually filled with areolar tissue or fat (Fig. 6.30). The submucous space lies between the mucous membrane and internal sphincter down to Hilton's white line, where the lower border of the internal sphincter can be palpated.

The perianal space is a continuation of the submucous space below the white line, and is separated from it by a dense submucous layer of connective tissue. The perianal space extends laterally as far as the most lateral of a series of radiating elastic septa which pass through the subcutaneous sphincter to create the corrugator cutis ani.

Lateral to the internal and external sphincters, and below the levator ani, lies the ischiorectal fossa containing adipose tissue. The two ischiorectal fossa communicate behind the anal canal, which should be taken into consideration when treating an abscess at this site as a 'horseshoe' abscess can form.

Relevant anatomy

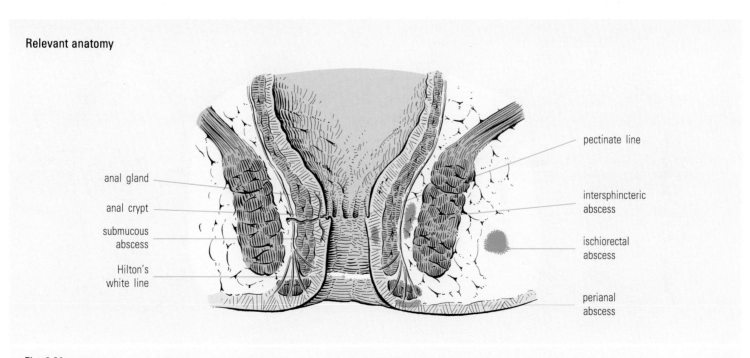

Fig. 6.30

Incision into abscess

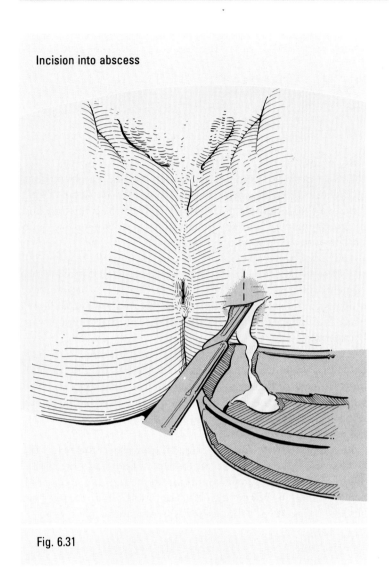

Fig. 6.31

OPERATION
Preparation

For all abscesses, the patient is anaesthetized and placed in the lithotomy position. A rectal examination with sigmoidoscopy is then performed to check for evidence of inflammatory bowel disease and fistulous openings. If abnormal mucosa is encountered it is biopsied. The anal canal, however, must not be probed to define a fistula, since it is very easy to create a false track through the friable inflamed tissues.

PERIANAL AND ISCHIORECTAL ABSCESSES
Incision

A cruciate incision is made over the point of maximum tenderness and fluctuance (Fig. 6.31).

Operative technique

1. The four skin flaps are excised to avoid premature closure and sent for histological examination (Fig. 6.32). In the case of an ischiorectal abscess the skin flaps should be generously eexcised, this allows the cavity to heal by secondary intention.

2. A sample of pus or a pus swab is sent for culture and microscopy.

3. All the loculi are broken down with a finger to ensure complete drainage. For an ischiorectal abscess, the horseshoe extension around the back of the anal canal is also sought and, if present, the ischiorectal fossa on the other side is also opened.

Saucerization of cruciate incision

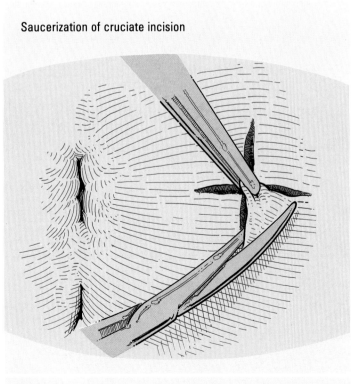

Fig. 6.32

Wick inserted into cavity

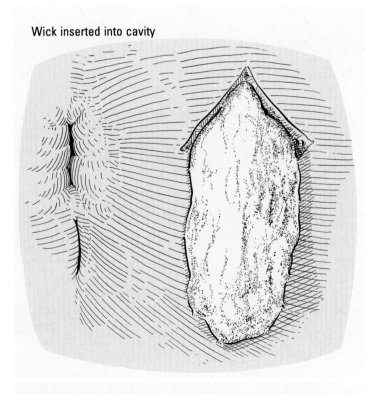

Fig. 6.33

Wound dressing

The wound is loosely packed with ribbon gauze soaked in proflavine cream (Fig. 6.33).

SUBMUCOUS ABSCESS

This has usually discharged already, presenting with the passage pus *per rectum*. If this has not occurred, it is opened into the anal canal using a diathermy needle and a Park's anal retractor.

INTERSPHINCTERIC ABSCESS

If it extends high up the anal canal, there may be difficulties in distinguishing it from a pelvirectal abscess above the levator ani. The diagnosis is made by rectal examination which reveals a tender lump at the dentate line. The intersphincteric abscess is then drained into the rectum.

POSTOPERATIVE CARE

Dressings are soaked off in a warm bath on the following day, and the wound is repacked. The dressings are changed daily and the patient is discharged when the dressing can be comfortably changed at home.

If a fistula is suspected, further examination is performed under general anaesthetic after 5 to 7 days. It is more easily dealt with once the acute inflammation has resolved.

SPECIAL OPERATIVE HAZARDS
1. Creating a fistula.
2. Damage to the sphincters or levator ani when exploring the abscess cavity.

COMPLICATIONS
1. Fistula-in-ano.
2. Constipation, in which case the patient should be started on a combination of faecal softener and bulk laxative while defaecation is painful and the abscess is healing.
3. Recurrent infection; this is more common with the deeply seated ischiorectal abscesses.

Fistula-in-ano

A fistula-in-ano is an abnormal communication between the perianal skin and the rectum or anal canal. It is usually secondary to anorectal sepsis and can be high or low according to its relationship to the sphincter mechanism (Fig. 6.34). The majority are of the low type and are treated by laying open since the remaining external sphincter will maintain continence. This operation is described below. High fistula should be managed in a specialist unit because to simply lay open the track would leave the patient incontinent. The definitive treatment of high fistulae requires dissection of tracks with division and reconstitution of the sphincters, usually with a defunctioning colostomy to divert the faecal stream. The insertion of a non-absorbable ligature or seton along the track, tying the ends together to retain it, allows reassessment of the fistula and its relationship to the sphincters in the awake patient and may also promote healing.

PREOPERATIVE ASSESSMENT

1. Perform a careful digital examination. The fistula can often be felt as a cord-like structure.

2. Use sigmoidoscopy with biopsy to exclude Crohn's disease, tuberculosis and malignancy.
3. A fistulogram may help to define the anatomy preoperatively.
4. Shave the perineum and evacuate the rectum on the day of the operation with a phosphate enema.
5. Perform a chest X-ray if tuberculosis is suspected.

RELEVANT ANATOMY

This is covered on page 6.17 in Anorectal Abscess.

Goodsall's rule states that fistulae with an external opening which lies in front of a horizontal line passing through the centre of the anus usually run radially, whereas external openings posterior to this plane tend to open into the bowel in the midline (Fig.6.35).

OPERATION

Preparation

Under a general or spinal anaesthetic the patient is placed in the lithotomy position and the perineum cleansed and draped after a preliminary examination using proctoscopy and sigmoidoscopy.

Operative technique

1. Identify the external opening of the fistula, which appears as a red, indurated, discharging swelling. Insert a Park's retractor into the anus and look for the internal opening following Goodsall's rule. By injecting methylene blue into the external opening the internal opening may become apparent as the dye comes out.

2. Pass a blunt probe into the external opening and pass it along the track until the tip can be seen to emerge into the anal canal; take great care and do not apply force as a false passage will ensue. If the probe will not pass through to the internal opening insert a second probe internally to meet the first (Fig. 6.36). Palpate the tissue overlying the probe to confirm that it is not a high fistula.

3. Follow the probe with a grooved dissector, then cut down onto it with a knife and excise a fillet of tissue so as to widely lay open the fistula along its length (Fig. 6.37).

4. Gently curette granulation tissue and any epithelium from the track. Some low fistula have a blind-ending intersphincteric extension which is drained by opening it with a pair of blunt sinus forceps.

Relevant anatomy

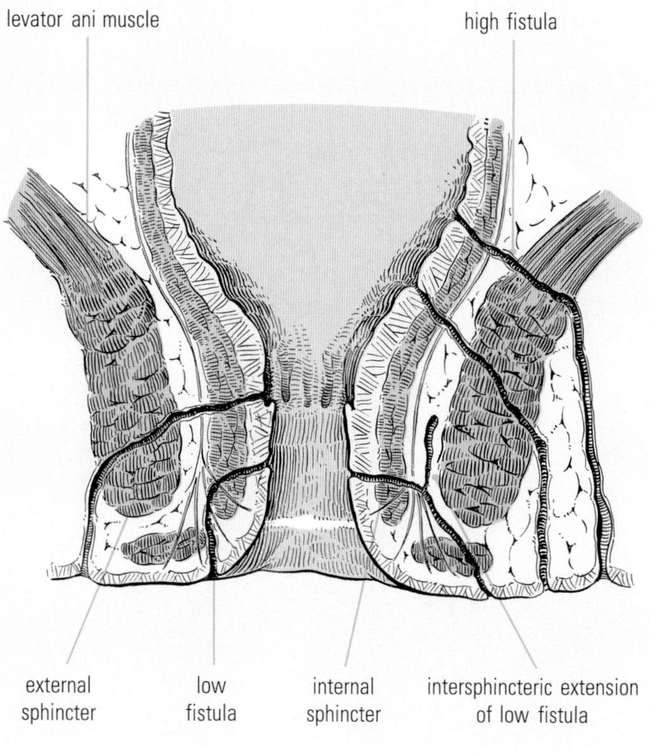

levator ani muscle — high fistula

external sphincter — low fistula — internal sphincter — intersphincteric extension of low fistula

Fig. 6.34

Wound dressing

Ensure haemostasis with careful use of diathermy but make no attempt to close the wound. Apply a non-adherent dressing such as paraffin gauze and cover this with an absorbent pad which is held in place with a T-bandage.

POSTOPERATIVE CARE
Administer faecal softeners and soak off the dressing in the bath on the following day. Cover the anus with an absorbent pad and advise the patient to wash their bottom with soap and water whenever their bowels have opened. Review the patient weekly in the clinic and perform a gentle digital examination to ensure that cross healing of the skin edges is not occurring. Extensive fistula may need to be redressed with a gauze wick if a large cavity persists; this may require a general anaesthetic.

SPECIAL OPERATIVE HAZARDS
1. Converting a low to a high fistula by forceful probing, particularly if there is a blind-ending intersphincteric extension.
2. Inability to define the internal opening. In such cases open the lower part of the fistula and look into the resulting cavity for traces of methylene blue or an area of friable granulation tissue.
3. Damage to external sphincter.

COMPLICATIONS
1. Recurrent fistula or abscess following inadequate drainage, failure to recognize the true nature of the track, an overlooked foreign body or inadequate postoperative supervision whilst healing is in progress.
2. Faecal incontinence due to damage to external sphincter.

Probes inserted into each opening

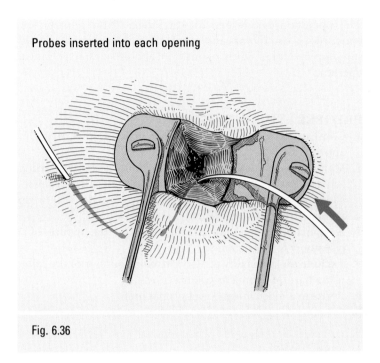

Fig. 6.36

Goodsall's rule

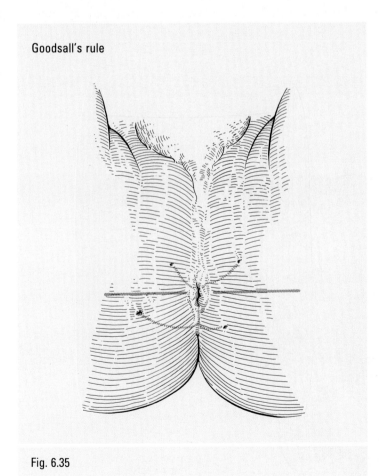

Fig. 6.35

Laying fistula open

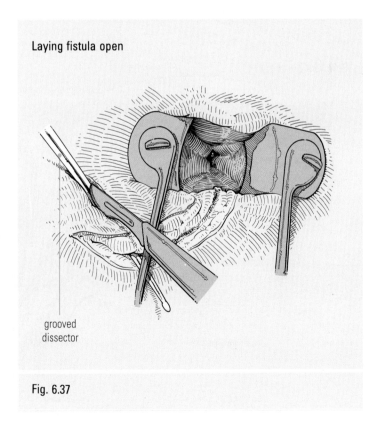

grooved dissector

Fig. 6.37

Abdominoperineal Excision of the Rectum

This operation is indicated for carcinoma of the anus or low lying rectal carcinoma and is generally performed by two surgeons operating synchronously; an abdominal and a perineal operator.

PREOPERATIVE ASSESSMENT

1. Confirm that a restorative operation is impossible or inappropriate.
2. Mark the site of the stoma, taking into account sporting activities, skin folds when seated and the position of a belt. Generally this will lie in the left iliac fossa midway between the iliac crest and umbilicus.
3. A stoma nurse should carefully explain the nature of a colostomy to the patient.
4. Exclude the possibility of a synchronous tumour of the colon using barium enema or colonoscopy.
5. Perform a mechanical bowel preparation.
6. Administer perioperative antibiotics.

RELEVANT ANATOMY

The distal continuation of the sigmoid colon, the rectum, commences within the concavity of the sacrum and lies upon the lower sacrum, coccyx and the midline raphé between the levatores ani; the rectosigmoid junction lies about 15cm from the anal verge. The three taeniae coli of the sigmoid colon spread out to form an outer longitudinal muscle coat and, unlike the sigmoid colon which is attached by the sigmoid mesocolon, the rectum has no mesentery. Its upper third is invested on three sides by peritoneum, its middle third is covered in front by peritoneum, and its lower third lies below the pelvic peritoneum (Fig. 6.38). Below, from the level of the pelvic floor, the rectum continues as the anal canal and the outer longitudinal muscle coat is replaced by circular external sphincters. The anal canal is surrounded by the fat of the ischiorectal fossae on each side. The anorectal junction is angulated forward by the puborectalis sling which is attached to the pubis. In front of the anal canal is the fibromuscular perineal body. In the male this lies behind the urethra and external urethral sphincter

Relevant anatomy

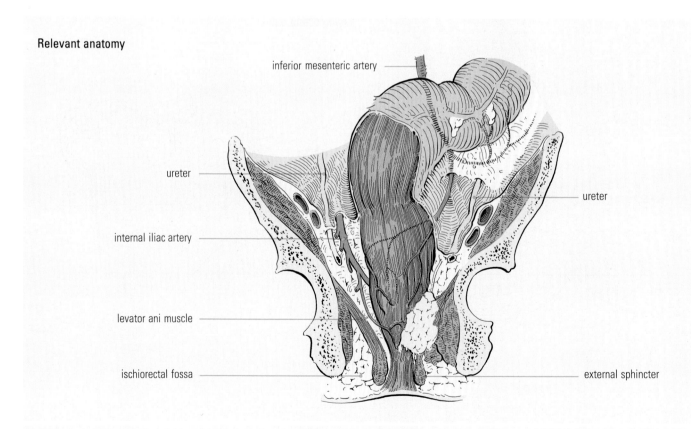

inferior mesenteric artery

ureter

ureter

internal iliac artery

levator ani muscle

ischiorectal fossa

external sphincter

Fig. 6.38

and below the recto-urethralis muscle which runs from the lower rectum to the junction of prostatic and membranous urethra. In the female the posterior wall of the vagina lies in front of the perineal body (Fig. 6.39). Above the pelvic floor, the rectum is separated from the bladder by the rectovesical pouch in the male and from the uterus by the pouch of Douglas in the female.

The rectum receives blood chiefly from the inferior mesenteric artery which, having given off branches in the root of the sigmoid mesocolon to supply the sigmoid colon, crosses the pelvic brim just medial to the left ureter, crossing the bifurcation of the left common iliac artery to become the superior rectal artery. It divides into a left and right anterior and posterior branches to supply the rectum, reinforced by the middle rectal arteries (from the internal iliac arteries) which reach the rectum through the lateral ligaments (condensations of the fascia surrounding the rectum) on either side. Posteriorly there are small arterial branches entering the rectum which arise from the median sacral artery which is the distal continuation of the aorta. These run in the fascia of Waldeyer, also called the mesorectum, which is a condensation of fibrous tissue lining the hollow of the sacrum; this helps to support the rectum. There is little anastomosis between these arteries.

The venous drainage is to the inferior mesenteric vein and hence to the splenic and portal veins, and also to the internal iliac veins via the middle rectal veins. The veins communicate freely within the rectal wall.

The lymphatic drainage follows the arterial supply. Lymph follicles in the mucosa drain to the pre-aortic nodes along the inferior mesenteric artery, and to nodes on the side walls of the pelvis and in the hollow of the sacrum along the middle rectal and median sacral vessels. All these lymph node groups should be removed when undertaking curative resection of rectal carcinoma.

OPERATION
Preparation
Place the patient in a modified lithotomy position as described by Lloyd-Davies. With a steep head-down tilt the legs are abducted, flexed to 30° at the hips and 45° at the knees (see page 6.49, Fig. 6.99). Remove the end of the table, bring the buttocks over the end supported on a sandbag, and insert a urinary catheter.

Insert a 00 silk purse-string suture to seal the anus, and clean and drape the abdomen and perineum leaving the proposed colostomy site exposed. In the male the scrotum is strapped up out of the way with adhesive surgical tape.

ABDOMINAL APPROACH
Incision
Enter the abdomen with a lower midline or left paramedian incision (see the Introduction). If the latter is used it must be clear of the proposed colostomy site.

Relevant anatomy (female)

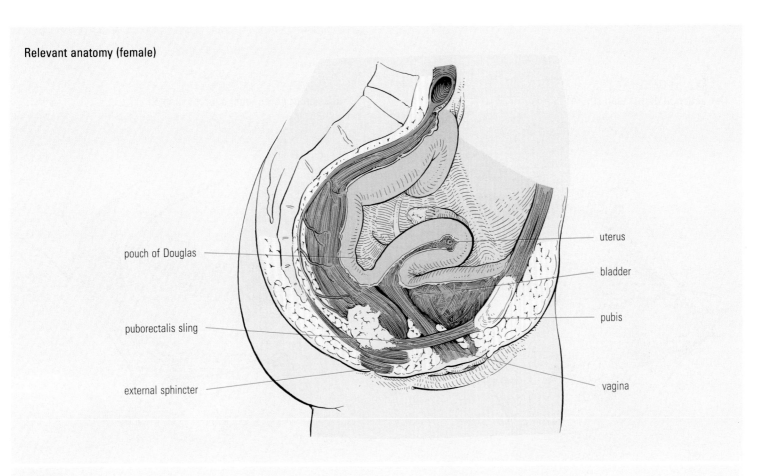

pouch of Douglas

puborectalis sling

external sphincter

uterus

bladder

pubis

vagina

Fig. 6.39

Operative technique

1. Perform a thorough laparotomy, paying particular attention to the growth, the draining lymph nodes and the liver. Pack the small intestine out of the way with a large wet swab.

2. Sew the uterus (or fundus of the bladder in the male) to the lower end of the wound for retraction (Fig. 6.40).

3. Divide the peritoneum along the lateral side of the descending and sigmoid colon whilst the bowel is drawn medially (Fig. 6.41). Similarly divide the peritoneum on the right side of the rectum (Fig. 6.42), and join the two peritoneal incisions across the front of the rectum at the level of the peritoneal reflection. Positively identify and preserve both ureters at the pelvic brim.

4. Identify the inferior mesenteric artery and vein as they cross the pelvic brim in the root of the mesocolon and separately ligate and divide them either here, or in a young person with curable disease, dissect proximally and ligate the inferior mesenteric artery at its origin from the aorta, immediately below the fourth part of the duodenum in order to excise as much lymphatic tissue as possible. Ligate and divide the vein at the same level.

5. Lift up the sigmoid colon so that the blood vessels in the mesocolon can be seen and select the point of bowel section such that the divided end will comfortably reach the proposed site of the stoma without tension. The mesocolon is divided, with ligation of the contained arteries, up to the point of bowel section (Fig. 6.43).

6. With forward traction on the sigmoid colon, mobilize the rectum from the hollow of the sacrum with scissors (Fig. 6.44), keeping close to the bone, and divide its lateral attachments until the lateral ligaments are reached. Anteriorly dissect the rectum from the uterus in the female, or in the male from the bladder until the seminal vesicles and prostate are reached. This dissection is generally easier in the female because of the wider pelvis.

7. Using a Lloyd-Davies clamp or a Roberts' forceps, clamp the lateral ligaments of the rectum (containing the middle rectal vessels), divide them close to the side wall of the pelvis (Fig. 6.45) and ligate them with an absorbable (e.g. 00 Vicryl) suture whilst the rectum is retracted to the opposite side.

8. The perineal operator will have reached the levator ani muscle from below (see later in this chapter) and the remainder of the mobilization including division of the remaining fascia of Waldeyer can be performed from above and below until the rectum is completely free.

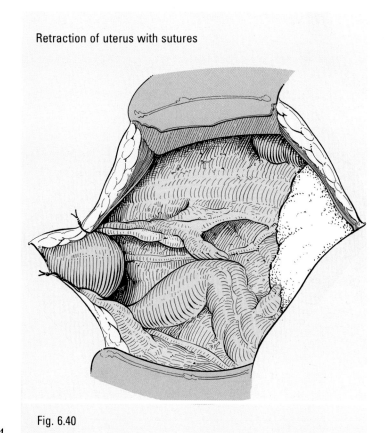

Retraction of uterus with sutures

Fig. 6.40

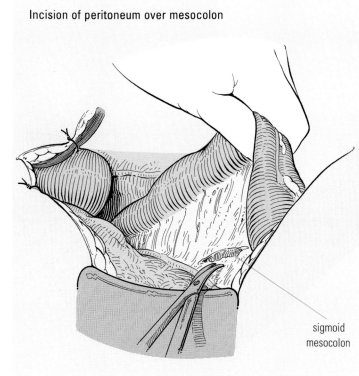

Incision of peritoneum over mesocolon

sigmoid mesocolon

Fig. 6.41

9. Apply de Martel crushing clamps to the bowel, divide it and remove the specimen. Tie a clean swab over the proximal divided end of the bowel.

10. Grasp the skin at the centre of the colostomy site with a Lane's tissue-holding forceps and excise a 3-cm disc with a knife (Fig. 6.46). Similarly excise the underlying disc of fat

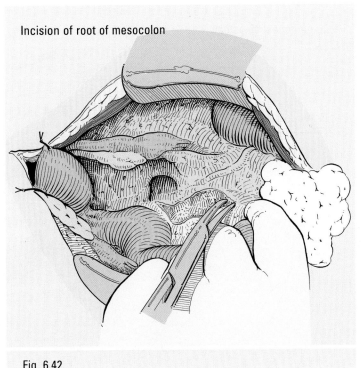

Incision of root of mesocolon

Fig. 6.42

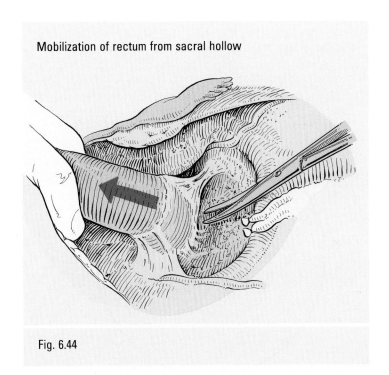

Mobilization of rectum from sacral hollow

Fig. 6.44

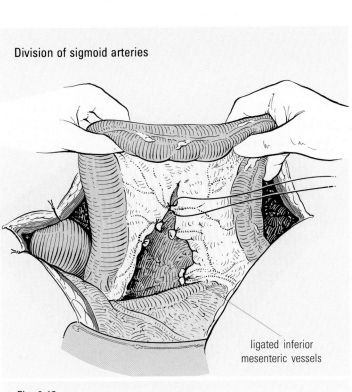

Division of sigmoid arteries

ligated inferior
mesenteric vessels

Fig. 6.43

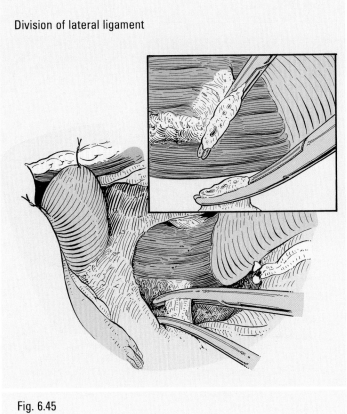

Division of lateral ligament

Fig. 6.45

6.25

and incise the aponeurosis in cruciate fashion with a knife (Fig. 6.47). Push two fingers through the exposed muscle until the peritoneum is reached. The index and middle fingers of the other hand are then pushed under the divided left lateral peritoneum and burrowed under the peritoneum of the left lateral abdominal wall until the other fingers are reached, so creating an extraperitoneal tunnel to the skin. Pass the clamped terminal colon through this tunnel, taking care not to twist it (Fig. 6.48). It must lie without tension, and if this cannot be achieved, mobilize

Excision of disc of skin at colostomy site

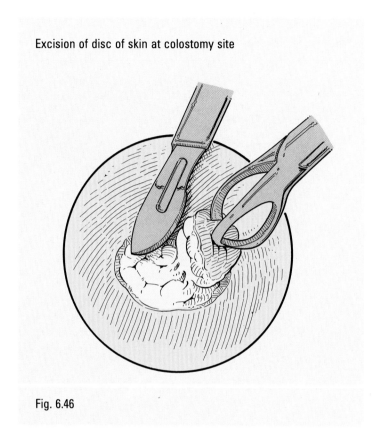

Fig. 6.46

Extraperitoneal colostomy

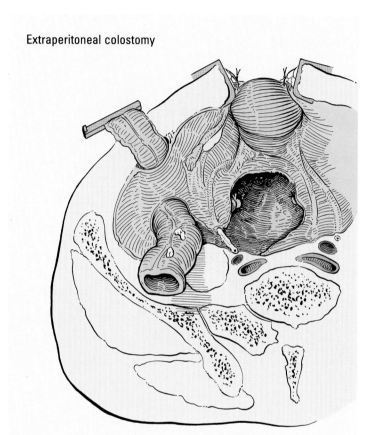

Fig. 6.48

Incision of aponeurosis

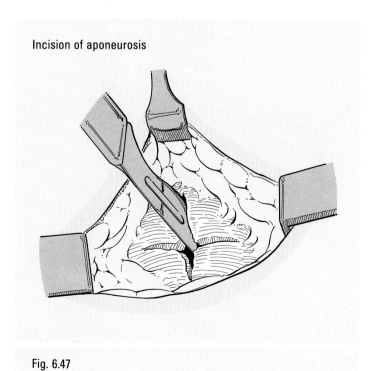

Fig. 6.47

Securing mucocutaneous sutures

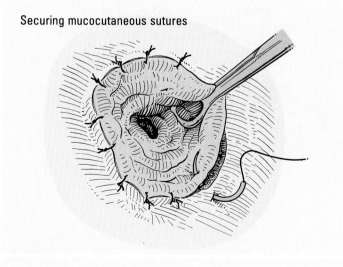

Fig. 6.49

6.26

the splenic flexure and draw the colon down to provide extra length.

11. Remove the sutures holding the uterus or bladder to the lower end of the wound and, if possible, close the peritoneum of the pelvic floor with continuous 2/0 chromic catgut. The peritoneal defect is often too large following adequate clearance of the tumour, and the omentum is then placed in the pelvis.

Abdominal wound closure and dressing

Insert a silicone drain and close the wound with continuous monofilament nylon, and the skin with interrupted nylon sutures. Apply a waterproof dressing.

Completion of colostomy stoma

1. Remove the swab from the colostomy which is still clamped, grasp the colostomy with two pairs of Babcock's forceps, and then remove the clamp with the crushed cuff of tissue by dividing it with a scalpel flush with the underside of the clamp.

2. Secure the colostomy by tacking the serosa of the bowel to the edge of the incised aponeurosis to prevent a paracolostomy hernia, and suturing the bowel edge to the surrounding skin with interrupted 2/0 chromic catgut sutures on a cutting needle (Fig. 6.49). Mucocutaneous apposition is important. When complete insert a finger into the stoma to check that the colon is not kinked and apply a transparent colostomy bag.

PERINEAL OPERATION

Incision

With the apex at the coccyx, make a narrow V-shaped incision around the anus, keeping a 2–3 cm margin on either side. In the male, extend the incision anteriorly to meet a short transverse incision at the level of the perineal body (Fig. 6.50). In the female, excise the posterior wall of the vagina (Fig. 6.51). Lane's tissue forceps are applied to the tissue to be removed.

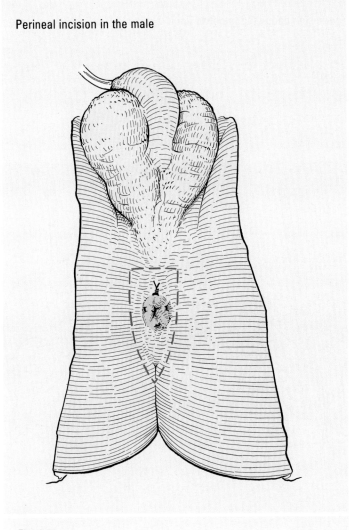

Perineal incision in the male

Perineal incision in the female

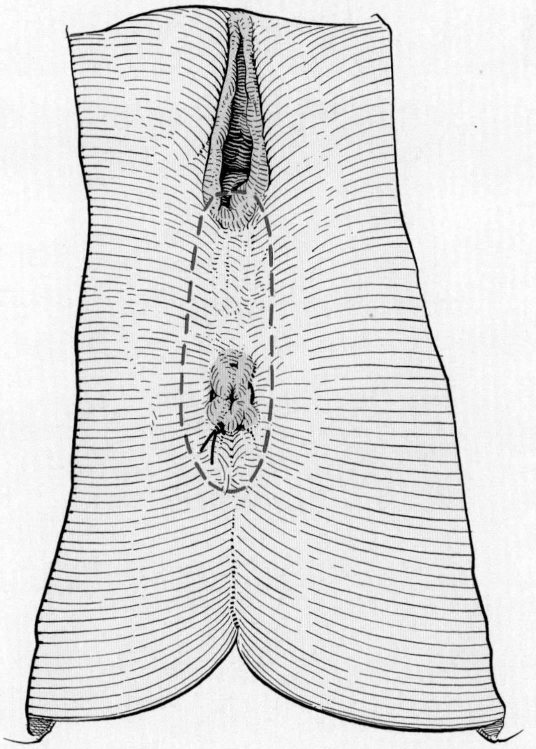

Fig. 6.50

Fig. 6.51

6.27

Operative technique

1. Laterally, deepen the incision through the ischiorectal fat outside the external sphincter (Fig. 6.52) until the pelvic floor musculature is visible, and insert a self-retaining retractor (Fig. 6.53). This region has a rich blood supply and bleeding should be stopped with ligatures or diathermy.

2. Anteriorly, in the female, extend the incisions in the posterior wall of the vagina on either side so they meet at the posterior fornix (Fig. 6.54). In a younger woman the vagina can be preserved by dissecting with care between it and the rectum. In the male, deepen the incision through the perineal body and behind the transversus perinei muscle (Fig. 6.55). Careful palpation for the catheter will locate the urethra. The plane of dissection in the male is between urethra and rectum, through the recto-urethralis muscle and anterior fibres of the coccygeus muscles.

   The posterior limit of the dissection is the coccyx, the lowest segment of which can be excised or left, according to preference.

3. Incise the attachments of the pelvic floor muscles to the coccyx and divide these muscles leaving a cuff attached to the rectum (Fig. 6.56). A finger hooked over the divided posterior edge of the levator may help at this stage.

4. Proceed with the dissection through the fascial attachments of the lower rectum in close collaboration with the abdominal operator, working from posterior to anterior until the rectum is free. It is withdrawn from above.

Perineal wound closure and dressing

Repair the muscles of the pelvic floor with an absorbable (e.g. Vicryl) suture (Fig. 6.57). Close the ischiorectal fat over a suction drain with chromic catgut (Fig. 6.58) and close the skin. A subcuticular stitch using an absorbable suture, such as 2/0 Vicryl, gives a more comfortable wound than interrupted sutures.

POSTOPERATIVE CARE

The patient is managed with intravenous fluids and a nasogastric tube until bowel sounds return and the colostomy has produced flatus. The patient is taught how to manage the stoma. Sutures are removed after 12 days.

Incision into ischiorectal fat

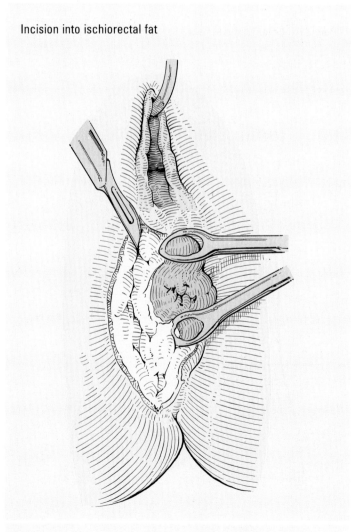

Fig. 6.52

Incision deepened to pelvic floor

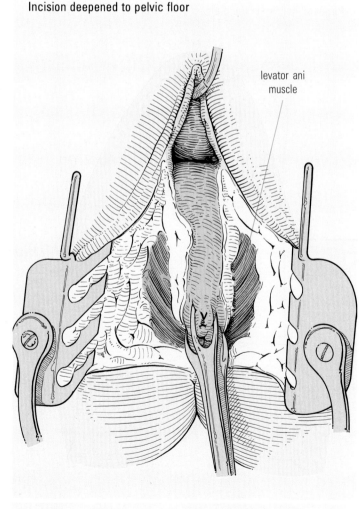

levator ani muscle

Fig. 6.53

6.28

Completed division of posterior vaginal wall

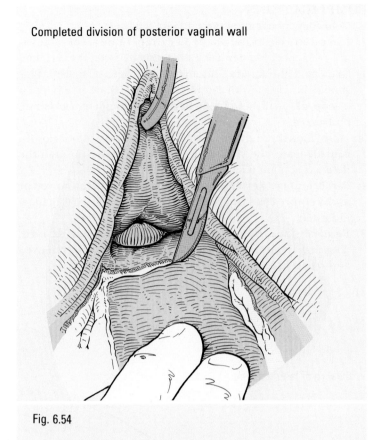

Fig. 6.54

Completed mobilization from the pelvic floor musculature

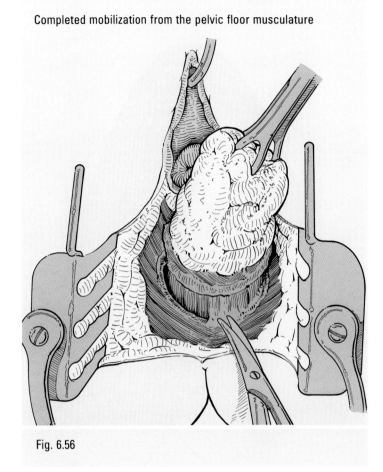

Fig. 6.56

Dissection in the male

levator ani muscle

transversus perinei muscle

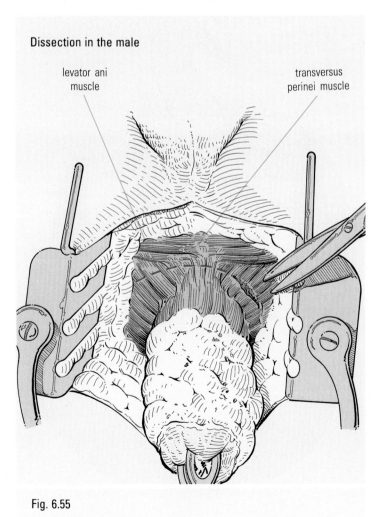

Fig. 6.55

Closure of pelvic floor

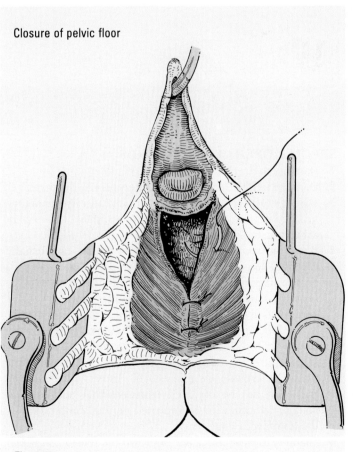

Fig. 6.57

6.29

Subcutaneous sutures

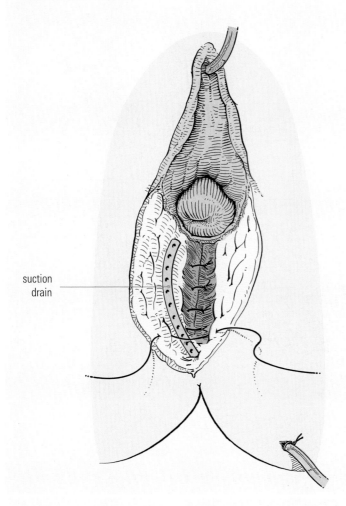

suction
drain

Fig. 6.58

COMPLICATIONS

1. Colostomy ischaemia, retraction or stenosis.
2. Lateral space entrapment; if an extraperitoneal colostomy is not fashioned, a potential space exists between the terminal colon and the lateral abdominal wall (lateral space). This should be closed with catgut (Fig. 6.59), since if left open a loop of small bowel can herniate through it, becoming obstructed.
3. Herniation through the pelvic floor; if the pelvic floor closure is inadequate, the small intestine can herniate through the defect (see point 6 in Special Operative Hazards).
4. Paracolostomy hernia; this is notoriously difficult to repair and requires resiting of the colostomy if treatment is indicated.
5. Perineal sinus; these generally heal if adequately drained. This may require excision of the coccyx if it was not removed at the first operation.

Closure of lateral space

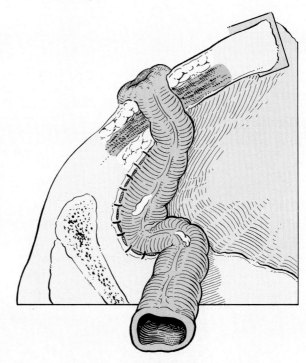

Fig. 6.59

SPECIAL OPERATIVE HAZARDS

1. Damage to ureters.
2. Damage to bladder or urethra, especially in the male.
3. Damage to inferior hypogastric nerves causing ejaculatory failure in the male. This may be unavoidable however in achieving an adequate surgical clearance.
4. Bleeding, usually from side walls of pelvis. This usually responds to packing.
5. Fixed tumours. These can usually be removed with *en bloc* removal, if need be, of part of the bladder, seminal vesicles and prostate in the male; and the uterus, tubes and ovaries in the female. If the tumour is truly unresectable, or the patient elderly or unfit, consider a loop colostomy or Hartmann's procedure (see page 6.36). Local symptoms from the growth are likely to be distressing, but some palliation can be obtained from external beam mega-voltage radiotherapy or repeated peranal fulguration of the lesion with diathermy.
6. Inability to close the pelvic floor without tension, in which case pack the wound and allow it to heal by second intention.

Anterior Resection of the Rectum

This procedure is indicated for the elective treatment of rectal cancers where an adequate clearance can be achieved below the growth to allow anastomosis.

PREOPERATIVE ASSESSMENT
1. Correct anaemia if present.
2. Warn patients with a low rectal tumour that a temporary colostomy may be necessary, and possibly a permanent colostomy if the final decision between anterior resection and abdominoperineal excision of the rectum is to be made at the time of the operation.
3. Administer antibiotics and, in elective cases, prepare the bowel.
4. Exclude a synchronous colonic carcinoma.
5. In the emergency situation (e.g. perforation or obstruction), consider performing an on-table wash-out of the colon with primary anastomosis, Hartmann's procedure, or simple defunctioning proximal colostomy for an obstruction.

RELEVANT ANATOMY
This is fully described on page 6.22 in Abdominoperineal Excision of the Rectum.

OPERATION
Preparation
Catheterize and place the patient in the Lloyd-Davies position (see page 6.49) with head-down tilt. Prepare and drape the entire abdomen and perineum.

Incision
Enter the abdomen through a midline or left paramedian incision, depending on the surgeon's personal preference and taking into account any previous incisions.

Operative technique

1. Perform a laparotomy, paying particular attention to the growth, the draining lymph nodes, and the liver.

2. The rectum is mobilized in an identical way to that described on page 6.24 in Abdominoperineal Excision as far as the division and ligation of the lateral ligaments (stage 7), and is as summarized below.

3. Mobilize the sigmoid colon by incision along either side of the peritoneum covering the sigmoid mesocolon; extend the two incisions to meet in front of the rectum at the level of the peritoneal reflection. Identify both ureters and spermatic or ovarian vessels.

4. Mobilize the root of the mesocolon from the posterior abdominal wall and, lifting it forward, ligate and divide the inferior mesenteric artery flush with the aorta, just below the fourth part of the duodenum. Tie the inferior mesenteric vein at the same level. In a palliative procedure, or in the elderly patient, the vessels can be divided at the pelvic brim.

5. Choose the point of proximal bowel section and divide the mesocolon up to that point. A more proximal site should be chosen in the descending colon if the inferior mesenteric vessels have been divided flush with the aorta. To allow the bowel to lie comfortably in the pelvis, mobilize the splenic flexure by division of the attachments of the colon to the spleen.

6. Draw the rectum forwards and mobilize it from the sacral hollow by dividing the presacral fascia with scissors. Ligate and divide the lateral ligaments.

Division of rectum with diathermy below a right-angle clamp

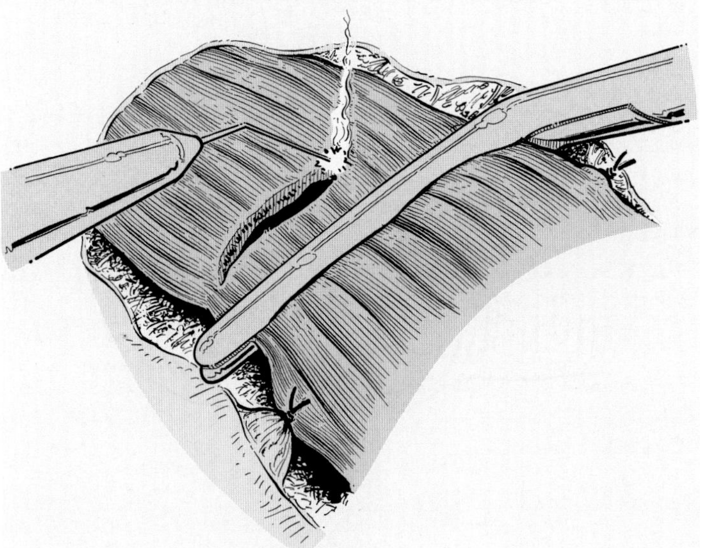

Fig. 6.60

6.31

Rectum held with tissue forceps

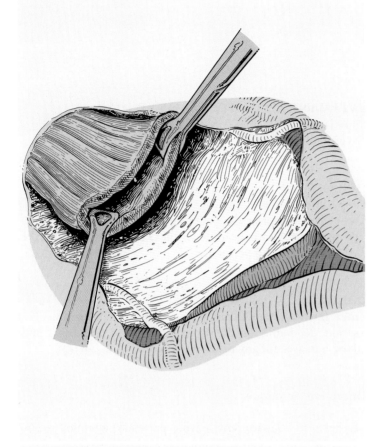

Fig. 6.61

Sutures for posterior layer of anastomosis in position

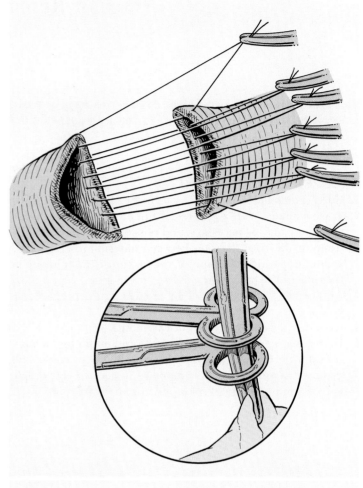

Fig. 6.63

Stay sutures inserted on either side

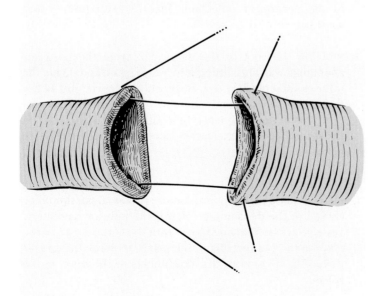

Fig. 6.62

Posterior layer of anastomosis complete

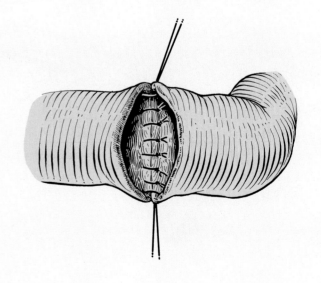

Fig. 6.64

7. With gentle upward traction on the bowel, the lower limit of the tumour will be palpable in the rectum. Further mobilize the rectum by sharp dissection until it is possible to place a clamp below the tumour, allowing at least 2 cm clearance. Apply a right-angled clamp.

Completion of anterior layer

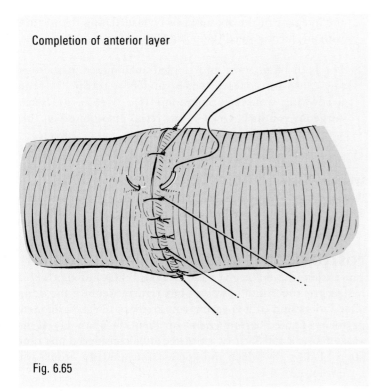

Fig. 6.65

Insertion of circumferential purse-string suture

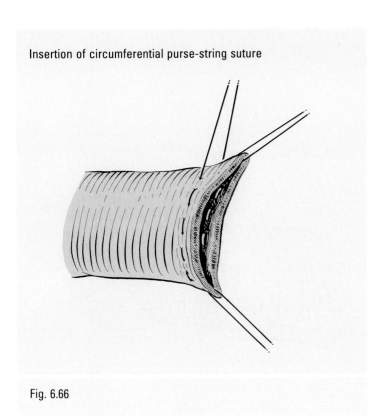

Fig. 6.66

8. Using a wide-bore catheter, wash out the rectum through the anus with a tumouricidal solution such as water or mercuric chloride.

9. Divide the anterior wall of the rectum below the clamp with cutting diathermy (Fig. 6.60). Place Babcock's forceps into each corner of the rectum and divide the posterior wall (Fig. 6.61).

10. Apply a non-crushing clamp to the bowel proximal to the proposed point of section, and a crushing clamp immediately distal to this point on the bowel; divide it with a knife flush with the crushing clamp and then remove the specimen with its two clamps. Fashion the anastomosis which can be either hand sewn or stapled; both these techniques are described below.

Either, for a hand sewn anastomosis
11. Place a suture (e.g. 3/0 PDS), from out to in, at each corner of the rectal stump and bring it out through the divided end of the proximal bowel, which is placed at the pelvic brim. Place a clip on the end of each suture and remove the Babcock's forceps (Fig. 6.62).

12. Insert further sutures at the midpoint of the back wall, and halfway between this and the corner stitch. The sutures should pass through all layers of the bowel wall, and with the exception of the first two will be tied within the lumen of the anastomosis.

13. Place and clip sutures in the intervening spaces; none of the sutures are tied at this stage. To prevent tangling, thread the clips along a Roberts forceps in the correct order (Fig. 6.63).

14. When all the sutures of the posterior wall are in place, slide the proximal colon down the sutures into the pelvis, until it is opposed to the rectal stump. The sutures must be kept taut.

15. Starting at one end, tie the sutures, leaving the sutures at each end long and clipped as stay sutures (Fig. 6.64).

16. Apply gentle traction on the sutures at each end and complete the anterior wall by inserting interrupted all-layer sutures (Fig. 6.65). The 'rule of halves' is used to prevent a dog ear being left.

17. With the anastomosis complete, fill the pelvis with saline, insert a sigmoidoscope into the anus and insufflate the rectum with air to test for leaks. If this is satisfactory, the soft clamp can be removed; if not insert additional sutures.

Or, for a stapled anastomosis
11. Insert non-absorbable stay sutures (3/0 polypropylene) into each side of the rectal stump (Fig. 6.66 and remove the Babcock's forceps.

12. Insert a non-absorbable 3/0 polypropylene purse-string suture into the rectal stump as illustrated (Fig. 6.66). Do not use an over-and-over stitch. Similarly insert a purse-string into the proximal colon.

13. Insert a sizer into the end of the bowel to gauge the width before inserting the appropriate sized stapling device, set fully closed, through the anus. Advance, and open it, until the head emerges completely from the rectal stump.

14. Tighten the purse-string and tie it around the central rod which separates the two components of the stapling cartridge (Fig. 6.67).

Purse string tightened around stapling device

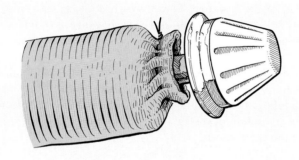

Fig. 6.67

Proximal bowel similarly secured around stapling device

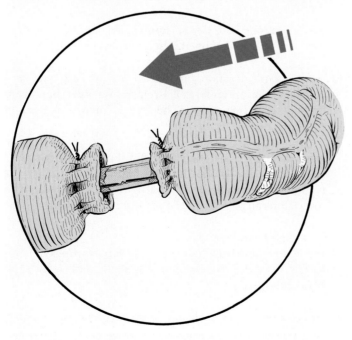

Fig. 6.68

15. Draw the proximal colon over the stapling head and tie the purse-string.

16. Close the device by tightening the knob on the handle, bringing the two ends of the bowel together (Fig. 6.68).

17. Release the safety catch on the stapling gun, and fire it by firmly squeezing the trigger. This introduces two concentric rings of staples into the bowel (Fig. 6.69), creating the anastomosis and excising two 'doughnuts' of tissue which contain the purse-string sutures from each end of the bowel. Check the 'doughnuts' to ensure they are complete. Test the integrity of the anastomosis by insufflating the rectum with air, having filled the pelvis with saline.

18. For both hand sewn and stapled anatomoses, if there is any cause for concern which cannot be rectified, create a covering transverse colostomy (see page 5.74). Some surgeons routinely cover a low rectal anastomosis in this way.

Wound closure

Place a silicone drain into the pelvis and close the wound with loop nylon. Nylon is used to suture the skin.

POSTOPERATIVE CARE

The patient should be given intravenous fluids and kept with a nasogastric tube until bowel sounds return. Remove the drain after 7 days and, if a covering colostomy has been fashioned, perform a limited barium enema on about the tenth day. If the anastomosis is satisfactory, closure can be considered any time after 14 days (by which time oedema around the stoma will have resolved).

Completed stapled anastomosis

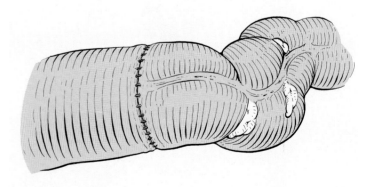

Fig. 6.69

SPECIAL OPERATIVE HAZARDS

1. Damage to ureters.
2. Impotence in the male resulting from damage to the hypogastric nerves.
3. Failure to draw the bowel fully over the stapling head can lead to incomplete 'doughnuts' which alert the surgeon to the possibility of a defect in the staple line. Unfortunately, this most commonly occurs posteriorly, and is therefore out of sight.
4. Splitting of the bowel can occur if too large a stapling head is used.
5. Failure of the stapling device.

COMPLICATIONS

1. Anastomotic stricture is usually due to ischaemia of the anastomosis secondary to tension.
2. Leakage or dehiscence of the anastomosis may lead to abscess or fistula formulation, and are commonly due to tension on the anastomosis. Peroperative contamination also predisposes to abscess formation.
3. Recurrence of tumour at the suture line may result from an inadequate margin of clearance or local implantation of tumour cells. Histological examination of the 'doughnuts' for tumour is an unreliable predictor of subsequent local recurrence.
4. Incontinence and urgency of defaecation is rarely due to sphincter damage and is usually due to the inability of the colon (as opposed to the rectum) to create the sensation of distention.

Hartmann's procedure is indicated for lesions of the upper rectum or sigmoid, where resection is required, but anastomosis is unsafe due to either inadequate preparation of the bowel or difficulty of access. This commonly occurs in emergency cases, for example a perforated diverticulum or obstructed carcinoma.

PREOPERATIVE ASSESSMENT
1. Ensure adequate resuscitation.
2. Prescribe intravenous antibiotics.
3. Decide whether this is the best operation under the circumstances. Alternative operations include resection with on-table wash-out and primary anastomosis, or a simple defunctioning colostomy in cases of obstruction. It is generally best to resect the diseased segment of bowel at the first operation. Remember that reversal of Hartmann's procedure can be very difficult.
4. Forewarn the patient that they will need a colostomy and mark the site.

RELEVANT ANATOMY
This is covered on page 6.22 in Abdominoperineal Excision of the Rectum. The principle of the operation is illustrated in Fig. 6.70.

HARTMANN'S PROCEDURE
Preparation
The patient is catheterized and placed in the Lloyd-Davies position. The skin is prepared and drapes applied to leave the lower abdomen, including the proposed colostomy site, exposed. The positioning of the drapes also allows a sigmoidoscope to be introduced.

Incision
Enter the abdomen through a midline or left paramedian incision (see the Introduction), depending on preference and previous incisions.

Operative technique
1. Identify the lesion and oversew any perforation to prevent ongoing contamination.

2. Perform a thorough laparotomy.

3. Mobilize the sigmoid colon by division of the peritoneum along its lateral side and draw the colon medially. Identify the left ureter and preserve it (Fig. 6.71); a soft rubber sling may be placed around it to aid this.

4. Continue the mobilization by incising the peritoneum on the

medial side of the sigmoid mesocolon, and divide the mesocolon with ligation and division of the sigmoid arteries until the diseased bowel can be resected with an adequate margin (Fig. 6.72). Usually the resection of the entire sigmoid colon is required. Distally the colon needs to be freed sufficiently to allow it to be closed off; this usually requires the upper rectum to be mobilized and may require division of the lateral ligaments of the rectum (see page 6.24 in Abdominoperineal Excision of the Rectum). Ideally, if there is adequate length of bowel beyond the lower resection margin, the distal bowel can be brought to the lower end of the abdominal wound and secured with mucocutaneous sutures as a mucous fistula. This is preferable as it is easier to reverse and there is no risk of the rectal stump leaking.

5. Divide the sigmoid mesocolon up to the edge of the bowel at the proposed point of bowel section. Ensure that the proximal end will reach the skin without tension.

Principle for Hartmann's operation

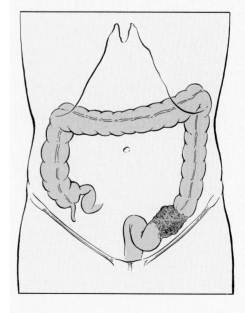

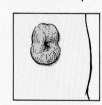

End colostomy

Closed off rectal stump

Fig. 6.70

6. Divide the proximal bowel between de Martel's clamps (Figs 6.73 and 6.74). The bowel beyond the distal resection margin is to be closed off.

7. Apply a right-angle clamp (e.g. Hayes clamp) distally and wash out the rectal stump via a sigmoidoscope using iodine solution. The rectal stump can either be closed off with hand sutures or by using a linear stapler. For the former, insert stay stitches on either side of the bowel distal to the right-angle clamp and divide the bowel flush with the lower edge

Mobilization of sigmoid colon

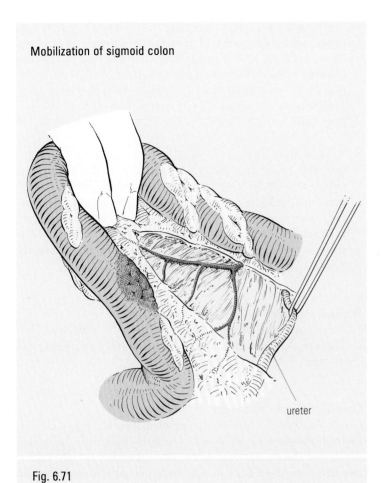

ureter

Fig. 6.71

Application of de Martel clamp

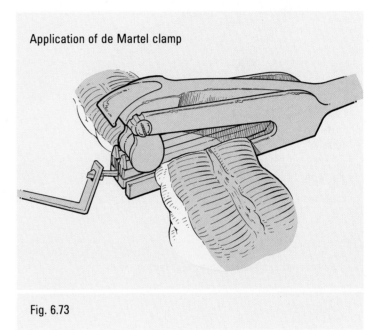

Fig. 6.73

Division of mesocolon

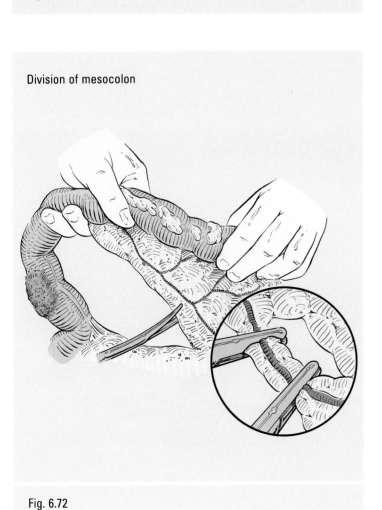

Fig. 6.72

Division of proximal bowel

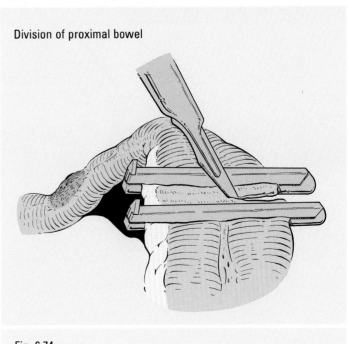

Fig. 6.74

6.37

Division of rectum

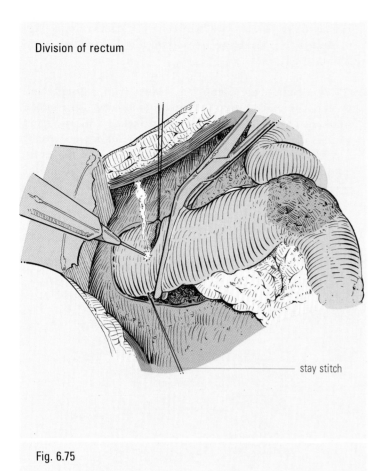

stay stitch

Fig. 6.75

of the clamp with diathermy (Fig. 6.75). The cut end is then closed with two layers of absorbable sutures, the second layer inverting and thus burying the first (Fig. 6.76). If a stapling device is to be used, this is applied beyond the clamp (Fig. 6.77) and fired, and the bowel divided with a knife immediately proximal to the device, before it is released (Fig. 6.78).

8. Apply Lane's forceps to the skin at the site of the colostomy (left iliac fossa) and excise a disc of skin with a knife. This exposes the underlying aponeurosis through which a cruciate incision should be made. Divide the underlying muscle and peritoneum and bring the proximal bowel, still clamped, out through the hole. An extraperitoneal route is not used as this makes subsequent reversal more difficult. Close the lateral space with 2/0 catgut (see page 6.30).

Wound closure
Perform thorough peritoneal lavage, insert a drain and close and dress the abdominal wound prior to completing the colostomy.

Completion of colostomy
Grasp the bowel with two pairs of Babcock's tissue-holding forceps and then divide it with a scalpel flush with the undersurface of the clamp (Fig. 6.79). The colostomy is fashioned as described on page 6.27 in Abdominoperineal Excision of the Rectum. Perform a gentle digital dilatation of the anus.

Two-layered hand-sewn closure of rectum

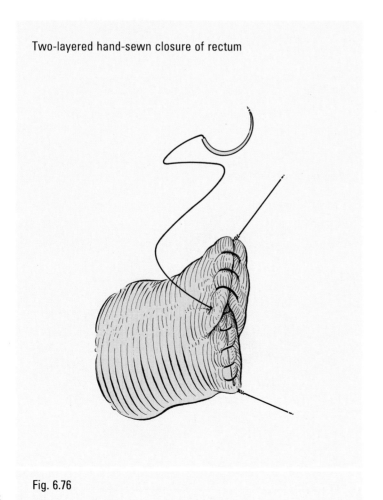

Application of linear stapler

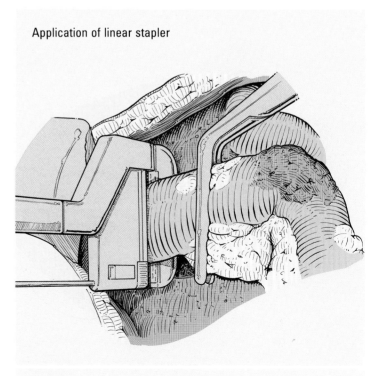

Fig. 6.76

Fig. 6.77

POSTOPERATIVE CARE

The patient is managed with intravenous fluids and a naso-gastric tube until the colostomy starts to work. Intravenous antibiotics should continue. After full recovery of at least 6 weeks elective reversal can be performed.

COMPLICATIONS

1. Colostomy stenosis, retraction and ischaemia. These problems occur when the colostomy has been placed under tension.
2. Paracolostomy hernia.
3. Leakage from the rectal stump. If it is not possible to close the rectum securely, it can be closed around a large silicone drain or Foley catheter which is brought out through the anterior abdominal wall.
4. An intra-abdominal abscess, either paracolic, subhepatic, subphrenic or between the small bowel loops. It follows contamination, which may have occurred preoperatively, and is indicated by a prolonged ileus, swinging fever, tachycardia and a high white cell count and requires drainage.

REVERSAL OF HARTMANN'S PROCEDURE

This can be difficult to perform because of pelvic adhesions; it is best to wait at least 6 weeks before considering reversal.

Preparation

Place the patient in the Lloyd-Davies position with the colostomy exposed, and apply the drapes to allow access to the anus.

Incision

Mobilize the colostomy (see page 5.76) and reopen the laparotomy incision.

Operative technique

1. Mobilize adherent small bowel loops that are present, and identify the rectal stump. Mobilize the proximal colon until the rectal stump and proximal colon can be brought together in the pelvis, without tension. If the location of the stump is difficult, a sigmoidoscope can be introduced to aid identification.

2. Dissection of the rectal stump must be kept to a minimum to avoid damage to its blood supply. Although a hand-sewn

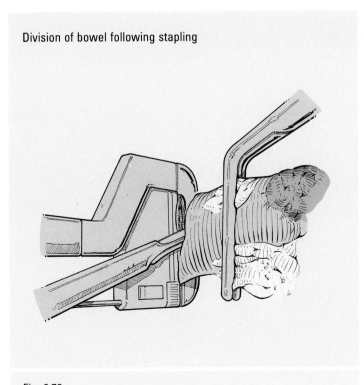

Division of bowel following stapling

Fig. 6.78

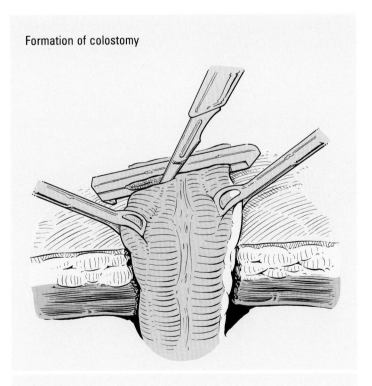

Formation of colostomy

Fig. 6.79

anastomosis can be performed, it is often easier and safer to use a stapling device. For this, introduce the gun through the anus with the distal anvil removed and use a knife to cut down onto the tip of the device, either through the anterior wall of the rectum or through the previous suture or staple line. Insert a purse-string suture into the proximal bowel. Screw the distal anvil onto the device and thread the proximal colon over the anvil. Tighten the purse-string suture

(Fig. 6.80). The gun can now be tightened up and fired to make the anastomosis. Check the integrity of the 'doughnuts' of tissue excised by the stapling device.

3. Test the integrity of the anastomosis by filling the pelvis with sterile saline and inflating the rectum with air via a sigmoidoscope with a soft clamp placed across the colon proximal to the anastomosis. A stream of tell-tale air bubbles indicates a leak which should be repaired with interrupted sutures.

4. Insert a silicone drain into the pelvis.

5. A covering colostomy in the right transverse colon may be indicated if there is any suspicion that the anastomosis might leak.

Wound closure and dressing
Close both the colostomy and the laparotomy wound with continuous nylon to the aponeurosis and interrupted nylon for the skin. Apply a dry dressing.

POSTOPERATIVE CARE
Intravenous infusion and the nasogastric tube are used until gastric emptying and bowel function recovers. The drain should remain for 7 days and sutures for 8–10 days.

SPECIAL OPERATIVE HAZARDS
1. Damage to adherent loops of small bowel whilst mobilizing rectum.
2. Damage to the ureter.

COMPLICATIONS
1. Leakage from the anastomosis with abscess or fistula formation.
2. Stenosis of the anastomosis.

Reversal of Hartmann's operation

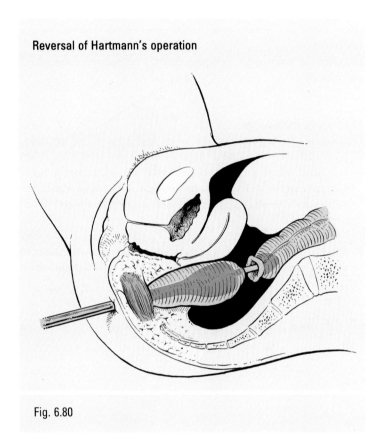

Fig. 6.80

Operations for Rectal Prolapse

An abdominal rectopexy in which the normal position of the rectum is restored and maintained is indicated for the treatment of full thickness rectal prolapse (Fig. 6.81). In elderly unfit patients a Delorme's operation, involving excision of the redundant rectal mucosa and plication of the underlying musculature, may be more suitable since it avoids the need for a laparotomy and can be performed under a spinal anaesthesia. Both operations are described below. Children with rectal prolapse should be treated conservatively since the curvature of the sacrum and rectum develop with growth and the prolapse spontaneously regresses.

PREOPERATIVE ASSESSMENT
1. Assess the patient, who is often elderly, for fitness for general anaesthesia.
2. Examine the rectum to demonstrate the weakness of the anal sphincter. In the majority of cases physiological studies are unnecessary.
3. Use sigmoidoscopy and a double-contrast barium enema to exclude any other large bowel disease.
4. Prescribe senna (e.g. Sennakot) to empty the bowel.
5. Warn men of the small risk of impotence or retrograde ejaculation. It should be explained to all patients that although the success rate for curing the prolapse is high, if incontinence is present it may persist. Postanal repair (see page 6.46) may be used subsequently to correct incontinence.
6. Prescribe one dose of a prophylactic antibiotic.

RELEVANT ANATOMY
The rectum is 12cm in length. Its upper third is covered with peritoneum in front and on each side, the middle third is

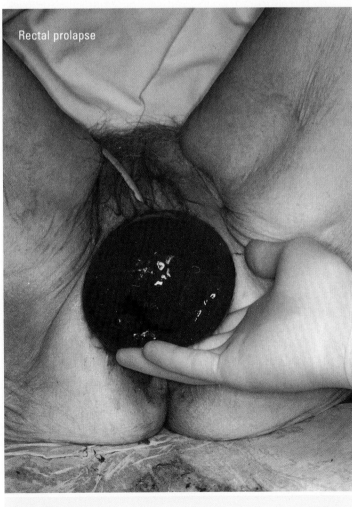

Rectal prolapse

Fig. 6.81

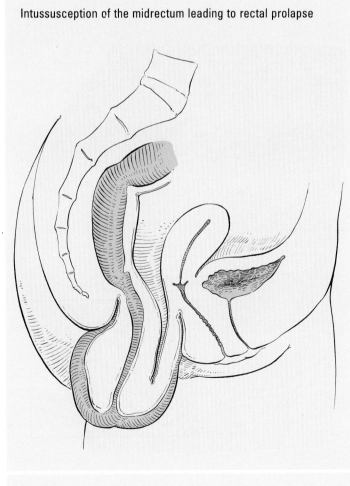

Intussusception of the midrectum leading to rectal prolapse

Fig. 6.82

Division of peritoneum over rectum

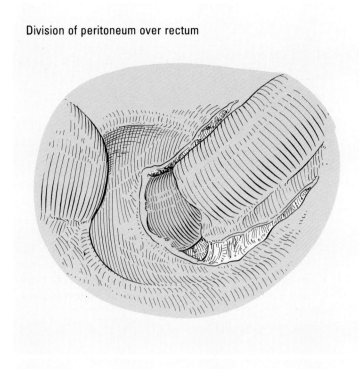

Fig. 6.83

Mobilization of rectum

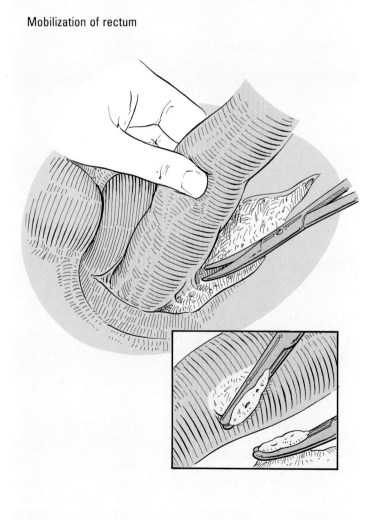

Fig. 6.84

covered only anteriorly and the lower third lies below the peritoneum of the pelvic floor. The rectum is attached to the presacral fascia by loose areolar tissue and is further supported by the lateral ligaments, which are condensations of fascia around the middle rectal arteries.

Complete rectal prolapse arises from intussusception of the midrectum through the anal orifice. In a large rectal prolapse the anterior part of the prolapse contains a peritoneal sac, a prolongation of the pouch of Douglas, constituting a sliding hernia of the anterior rectal wall through the anal canal (Fig. 6.82). In the majority of patients rectal prolapse is associated with weakness of the pelvic floor musculature which can be shown from electrophysiological studies to be due to an internal pudendal neuropathy, and is commonly thought to be the result of stretching the nerves during labour or from excessive straining when opening the bowels.

ABDOMINAL RECTOPEXY
Preparation
Under general anaesthesia a urinary catheter is inserted and the patient is placed in the Lloyd-Davies position; this enables a second assistant to stand between the legs. The table is tilted head-down and the abdomen is cleansed and draped.

Incision
Make a Pfannenstiel (see page 6.53) or lower midline incision (see the Introduction), insert a self-retaining retractor and pack the small bowel up out of the way with large gauze swabs. Retract the bladder and uterus with a St Mark's retractor held by the second assistant and carry out a laparotomy for coexistent disease.

Fixation of sling to lumbosacral disc

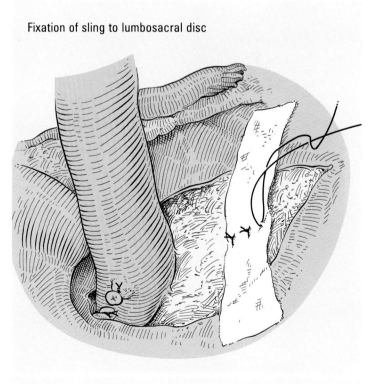

Fig. 6.85

Operative technique

1. Divide any adhesions from the sigmoid colon and mesocolon to the parietal peritoneum so the sigmoid colon can be pulled up clear of the pelvis. Incise the peritoneum on either side of the rectum with scissors from the level of the lumbosacral disc. Extend these incisions downwards into the pelvis, keeping medial to the ureters, and bring them across to meet at the front of the rectum (Fig. 6.83).

2. With gentle traction upward and forward on the rectum, divide the loose areolar tissue between the rectum and presacral fascia with scissors (Fig. 6.84). Keep close to the wall of the rectum to avoid damage to the hypogastric nerves and presacral veins.

3. Divide and ligate the lateral ligaments on each side close to the rectum (see inset to Fig. 6.84) and, with the rectum drawn up, anchor it to the sacrum. There are several methods available for maintaining the position of the rectum; the Ivalon sponge and Mersilene sling techniques are described in this chapter. They give similar long-term results. The former excites a local fibrous reaction binding the rectum to the sacrum, whereas the Mersilene sling, a modification of the operation described by Ripstein, constructs a suspensory sling for the mobilized rectum. The Ivalon sponge is easier to perform but carries a greater risk of complications.

Either, for the Mersilene sling
4. Cut a piece of Mersilene mesh into a 12 × 1 cm strip and, with the rectum held forward out of the way, anchor this strip at its midpoint to the lumbosacral disc with two or three non-absorbable sutures (Fig. 6.85).

5. Bring the two limbs of the sling loosely around the rectum and suture them to each other in front of the rectum (Fig. 6.86). The position of the rectum in the sling is maintained by suturing the lateral ligaments to the sling on each side (see Fig. 6.86). The mesh must not be tight around the rectum anteriorly and should allow the passage of a finger posteriorly between the sacrum and the rectum at the level of the sling.

Or, for the Ivalon sponge
4. Suture a sheet of polyvinyl alcohol (Ivalon) sponge to the presacral fascia between the sacral promontory and the third or fourth piece of the sacrum with four non-absorbable sutures. It is easiest to insert all the sutures first, then parachute the sponge down and tie it in place.

5. Wrap the sponge around the rectum and trim it so as to leave the anterior quarter of the rectum exposed. Secure the sponge to the rectal wall on each side with four non-absorbable seromuscular sutures (Fig. 6.87). It is essential not to completely encircle the rectum as the fibrosis induced by the sponge would create a rectal stricture.

6. Close the pelvic peritoneum with continuous chromic catgut, covering the rectopexy.

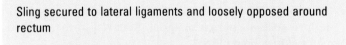

Sling secured to lateral ligaments and loosely opposed around rectum

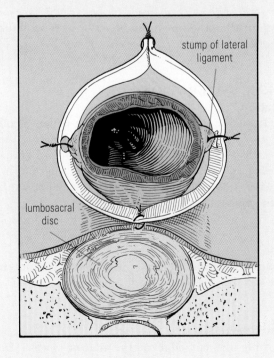

Fig. 6.86

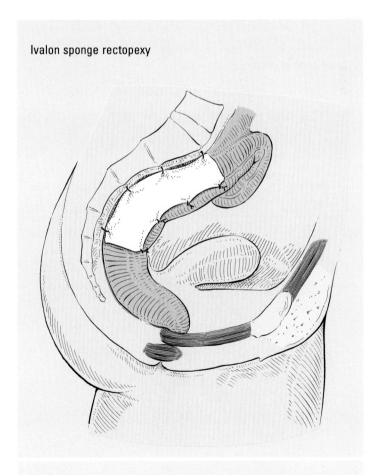

Ivalon sponge rectopexy

Fig. 6.87

6.43

Dissection in the submucosal plane

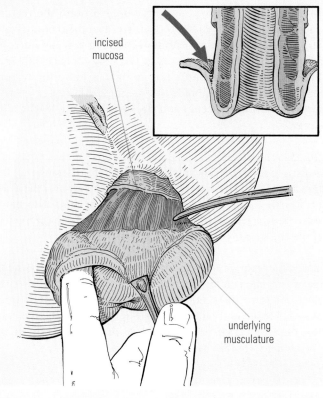

incised
mucosa

underlying
musculature

Fig. 6.88

Completion of dissection of mucosa

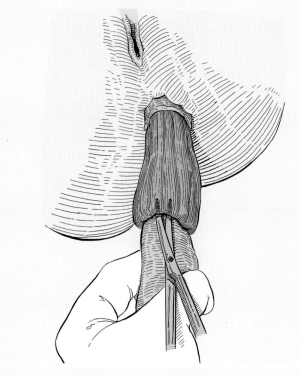

Fig. 6.89

Wound closure and dressing

A fine suction drain can be inserted behind the rectum and the wound closed with monofilament nylon, and the skin with interrupted nylon. A waterproof dressing is applied.

POSTOPERATIVE CARE

Oral feeding is recommenced when bowel function returns and, if used, the suction drain is removed after 24–48 hours. Aperients are given to ensure a soft, formed bowel motion. Sutures are removed on the eighth day.

SPECIAL OPERATIVE HAZARDS

1. Damage to the pelvic splanchnic (parasympathetic) nerves during mobilization of the rectum causing problems with incontinence.
2. Damage to the hypogastric nerves during mobilization of the rectum causing impotence in the male, but of little significance in the female.
3. Damage to the left iliac vein whilst inserting the needle into the lumbosacral disc.
4. Damage to the ureters.
5. Applying the Mersilene mesh sling too tightly around the rectum or completely encircling the rectum with an Ivalon sponge. This may lead to stenosis.

COMPLICATIONS

1. Persistent incontinence occurs in approximately 50% of patients following rectopexy, to a greater or lesser degree, and may require a postanal repair (see page 6.46).
2. Stricture formation.
3. Infection is rare but serious as it is unlikely to resolve in the presence of foreign material. Removal of the synthetic material may be required.
4. Persistant mucosal prolapse may be treated by banding or injection sclerotherapy if minor, or by ligation and excision if more pronounced.

DELORME'S OPERATION

Preparation

Under a general or spinal anaesthetic the patient is placed in the lithotomy position. The perianal area including the bowel lumen is cleansed and draped and the prolapse grasped and fully delivered with Duval's forceps. After checking with the anaesthetist, 1:300,000 adrenaline in normal saline is infiltrated under the mucosa of the prolapse.

Incision

The mucosa covering the prolapse is incised circumferentially with scissors, leaving a cuff about 5 mm wide.

Operative technique

1. Grasping the cut edge of the mucosa with a Duval or Babcock forceps, dissect the mucosa off the underlying muscularis in the submucosal plane, which is rendered relatively bloodless following the infiltration with dilute adrenaline (Fig. 6.88). When the apex of the prolapse is

reached the dissection is continued as far into the lumen of the prolapsed rectal segment as possible (Fig. 6.89), and the sleeve of mucosa excised.

Plication of muscle layer

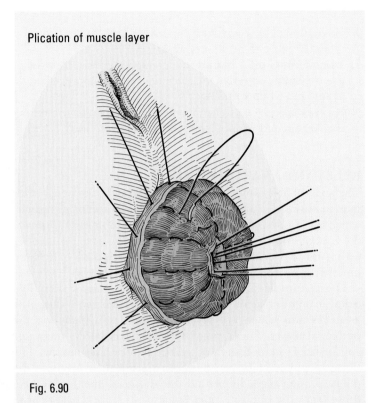

Fig. 6.90

2. Stop any bleeding with diathermy and insert a series of plicating absorbable sutures (e.g. 2/0 Vicryl), picking up the cut edges of mucosa and bites of the intervening denuded muscle tube (Fig. 6.90). Use twelve sutures inserted at the points of the clock face.

3. Reduce the tissue through the anus and then tie all the sutures. If tied first, reduction can be made unnecessarily difficult. No dressing is required.

POSTOPERATIVE CARE
Observe the patient for haemorrhage. Food and drink are normally allowed the following day, and glycerin suppositories are given on alternate days if the bowels have not worked.

SPECIAL OPERATIVE HAZARDS
1. Ulceration from prolonged exposure of the prolapse and previous sclerotherapy can make it difficult to find or stay in the submucosal plane.
2. Peroperative bleeding can be a problem. It is important to stop any visible bleeding before the tissue is reduced through the anus.

COMPLICATIONS
1. A reactionary haemorrhage may occur when the adrenaline wears off; secondary haemorrhage is usually due to local infection.
2. Incontinence may not be cured by the operation. The procedure can be usefully combined with a postanal repair in selected cases.

Postanal repair is indicated for the treatment of neurogenic faecal incontinence, which is associated with a gradual denervation of the external sphincter and puborectalis muscles. This operation plicates the muscles of the pelvic floor and external sphincter behind the anal canal, thus improving their action and reversing the changes that result in incontinence. Restoration of continence is achieved in 80% of cases.

PREOPERATIVE ASSESSMENT
1. Perform a digital examination of the anal canal and rectum to assess the resting sphincter tone, the increase in tone on maximal contraction, the length of the anal canal and the degree of preservation of the anorectal angle. Perineal descent may be visible when the patient is asked to strain.
2. Where complete rectal prolapse is present some form of rectopexy is indicated as a first procedure; if incontinence persists a postanal repair may be performed later.

3. Pelvic floor electromyography can be used to confirm and quantify pelvic floor denervation.
4. Lateral views on a barium enema and defaecating proctogram permits objective measurement of the anorectal angle at rest and when straining.
5. An enema is given on the morning of the operation to empty the rectum and prophylactic antibiotics prescribed.

RELEVANT ANATOMY
The anal canal is some 4cm long and lies below the pelvic floor musculature. It is surrounded by the internal sphincter muscle, which is a condensation of the circular smooth muscle fibres at the caudal end of the gastrointestinal tract. This in turn lies within the external sphincter, which is composed of striated muscle innervated via the pudendal nerves.

The rectum lies in the hollow of the sacrum and is cradled below in a gutter formed by the muscles of the pelvic floor (the levatores ani) which are also innervated principally via the pudendal nerves. The fibres of the medial free border of levator ani form a U-shaped sling called the puborectalis muscle. The fibres of puborectalis run posteriorly from their origin at the pubis, passing medially behind the anorectal junction to meet those from the opposite side. Some of its fibres coalesce with those of the upper part of the external sphincter posteriorly (Fig. 6.91). Muscle tone in the puborectalis sling causes angulation at the anorectal junction and maintains the anorectal angle at approximately 90° at rest and on straining. Waldeyer's fascia passes forwards from the anterior aspect of the lower part of the sacrum to the posterior aspect of the anorectal junction and provides support for the rectum.

Several factors contribute to the maintenance of continence: basal and voluntary anal canal sphincter pressure; length of the high pressure zone (sphincter length); anorectal angle; and raised intra-abdominal pressure forcing the anterior wall of the rectum against the top of the anal canal, closing it in a similar manner to a flap valve.

OPERATION
Preparation
Under general anaesthesia the patient is placed in the lithotomy position. The skin is prepared and towels are positioned so as to leave the perineum exposed.

The tissues behind the anal canal are infiltrated with a solution of saline containing adrenaline (1:400,000) to reduce bleeding and assist identification of, and dissection in, the intersphincteric plane.

Incision
Make a V-shaped incision 5–6cm behind the anus, with the apex pointing towards the sacrum (Fig. 6.92).

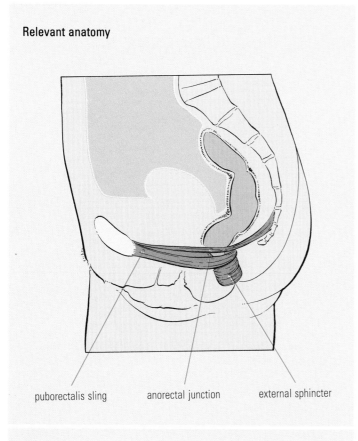

Relevant anatomy

puborectalis sling   anorectal junction   external sphincter

Fig. 6.91

Operative technique

1. Raise the skin flap and dissect to expose the subcutaneous aspect of the anal sphincters. The plane between internal and external sphincters is identified and developed behind the anal canal by sharp dissection (Fig. 6.93).

2. Proceed cranially with the intersphincteric dissection until the puborectalis and levator ani muscles are reached. Mobilize their medial borders.

3. Extend the plane anteriorly on either side of the anal canal so that when the dissection is complete the anal canal and rectum can be advanced anteriorly. At this stage divide Waldeyer's fascia as it limits the extent of anterior mobility of the rectum.

4. Retract the anal canal and internal sphincter anteriorly with a Langenbeck retractor so the medial borders of the levators, puborectalis and the external sphincter are displayed.

5. Plicate in turn each layer of muscle behind the anal canal. The method, which varies according to the preference of the surgeon, involves suturing deepest layer first, followed serially by each of the more superficial layers. Thus a layer of sutures is first placed between the levator ani muscles, taking a large bite of the muscle on each side (Fig. 6.94), and the suture is tied loosely to avoid strangulation of the tissues.

Developing the intersphincteric plane

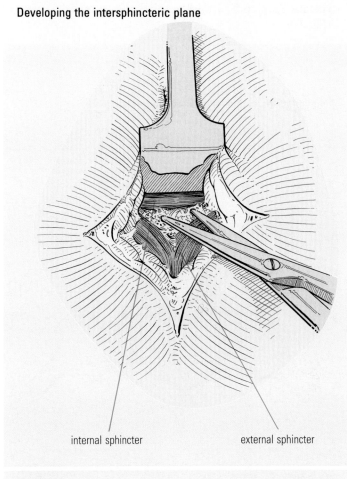

internal sphincter   external sphincter

Fig. 6.93

Position of incision

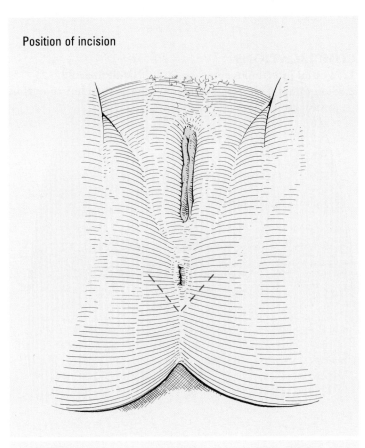

Fig. 6.92

The levatores ani are loosely sutured

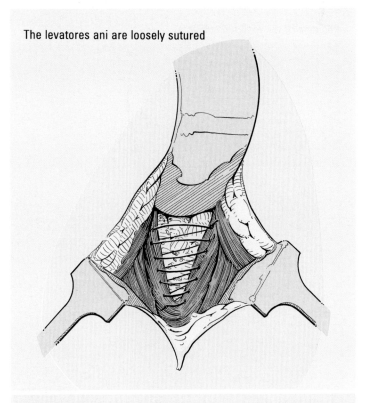

Fig. 6.94

Then a second layer of sutures similarly plicates the pubo-rectalis (Fig. 6.95), and a third the external sphincter (Fig. 6.96).

The suture material may be of nylon, or an absorbable material such as Vicryl, and each layer of sutures can be either interrupted or continuous.

Wound closure and dressing
1. Insert a suction drain to prevent any collection forming at the repair.
2. As the anus is advanced anteriorly by this procedure it may not be possible to close the incision without undue tension. In some of these cases the wound may be closed in the form of a 'Y' (Fig. 6.97), but, alternatively, the apex can be left open to heal by secondary intention.
3. Insert a urethral catheter.

POSTOPERATIVE CARE
The catheter is removed after 2–3 days, and the suction drain is removed when drainage ceases, usually after 2–3 days. Glycerine suppositories are given on alternate days to prevent straining. Alternatively, oral aperients can be given.

SPECIAL OPERATIVE HAZARDS
1. Siting the incision too close to the anus. With the advancement of the anus the wound may come to lie in the anal canal.
2. Damage to the rectum when mobilizing it from the upper surface of the levator ani muscle.
3. Difficulty in identifying the intersphincteric plane. Infiltration with dilute adrenaline or saline may help. The external sphincter is generally darker than the internal, but it becomes paler when degenerate.

COMPLICATIONS
1. Wound infection is common and difficult to avoid.
2. Sloughing of the apex of the 'V'; this is then left to heal by granulation.

Plication of the middle layer (the puborectalis)

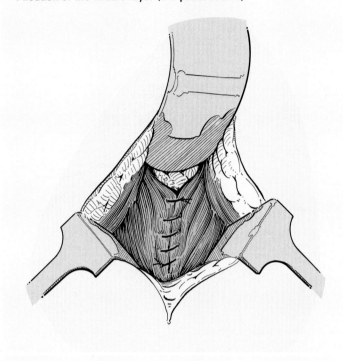

Fig. 6.95

Plication of the external sphincter

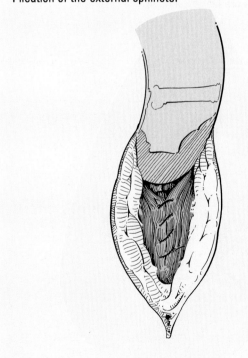

Fig. 6.96

V–Y plasty wound closure

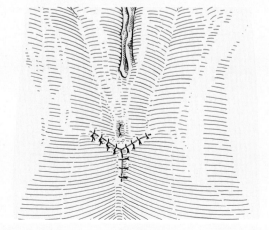

Fig. 6.97

In diseases affecting the entire colon, but restricted to the mucosa (e.g. familial adenomatous polyposis and ulcerative colitis), it is possible to remove all the diseased tissue and to create a reservoir to replace the rectum from loops of small bowel. Continence is maintained by preservation of the existing anorectal sphincter mechanism.

PREOPERATIVE ASSESSMENT

1. Confirm that the anorectal sphincters are adequate to maintain continence of loose effluent after the operation. If in doubt consider anorectal manometry.
2. Perform barium enema or colonoscopy to ensure that a carcinoma has not developed. This is not, however, an absolute contra-indication to a Park's pouch.

3. In cases of ulcerative colitis, check whether the dose of oral steroids can be reduced prior to surgery while ensuring adequate peroperative steroid cover.
4. Forewarn the patient that they may require a temporary ileostomy and mark the site on the skin with an indelible marker.
5. Prepare the bowel, if the patient has not undergone previous total colectomy, and prescribe antibiotic prophylaxis.

RELEVANT ANATOMY

The small bowel derives its blood supply from the superior mesenteric artery, which runs in the root of the small bowel mesentery; this mesentery is generally long enough to allow the small bowel to be brought deep into the pelvis. Crossing the pelvic brim, the inferior hypogastric nerves (necessary for potency in men) lie close to the peritoneal reflection of the mesorectum, and medial to the iliac vessels and ureter.

The dentate line marks the junction between the large bowel columnar epithelium and the squamous epithelium which is continuous with the skin (Fig. 6.98).

OPERATION

Preparation

Place the patient in a modified lithotomy position as described by Lloyd-Davies. With a steep head-down tilt the legs are abducted, flexed to 30° at the hips and 45° at the knees (Fig. 6.99). Place a sandbag under the buttocks and insert a urethral catheter.

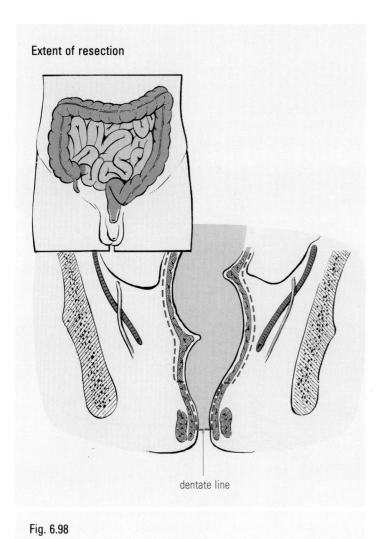

Extent of resection

dentate line

Fig. 6.98

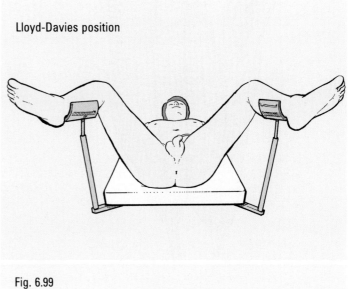

Lloyd-Davies position

Fig. 6.99

Incision

The abdomen is entered through a midline or a left paramedian incision according to personal preference.

Operative technique

1. Perform a total colectomy and mobilize the rectum with division of the lateral ligaments (for details see the chapters on total colectomy and anterior resection of the rectum).

2. Cross-clamp the rectum, wash out its lumen from below with saline, and then transect the rectum with cutting diathermy approximately 7–8cm from the anal verge.

3. Operating from below and using a Park's anal retractor and a headlight, infiltrate the submucosa with dilute adrenaline solution (1:300,000) to facilitate a mucosal proctectomy; this removes all the large bowel mucosa which is proximal to the dentate line, but preserves the muscular tube of the anorectal sphincters.

4. Fold back the distal small bowel on itself to form a 'W', and open it along its antimesenteric border (Fig. 6.100).

Completion of posterior wall

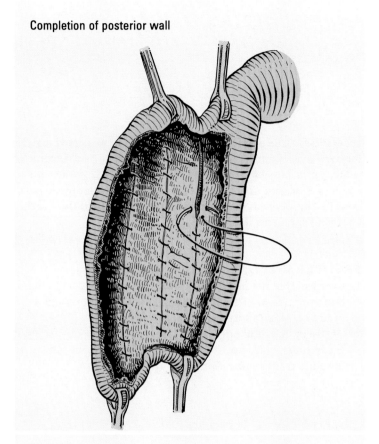

Fig. 6.101

Incision of antimesenteric border of ileum

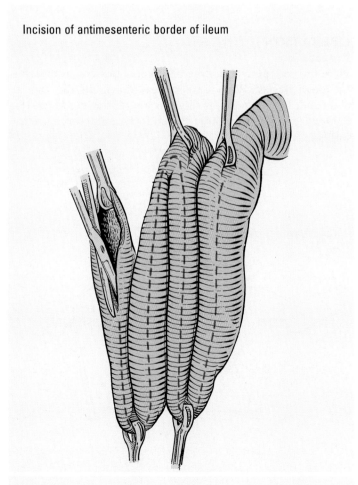

Fig. 6.100

Completed pouch

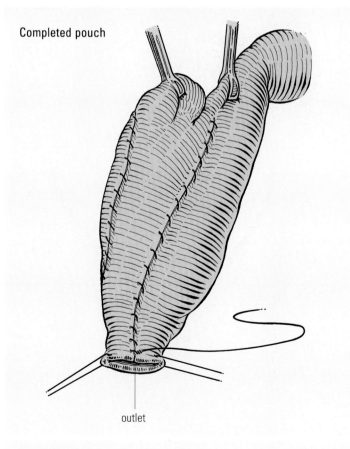

outlet

Fig. 6.102

5. Complete the posterior wall of the pouch by suturing the cut edges of adjacent loops together with running 3/0 absorbable stitches (Fig. 6.101). Complete the pouch by sewing the remaining two edges together. At the most dependent part of the pouch an opening is preserved that will admit two fingers (Fig. 6.102).

6. Use stay stitches to draw the completed pouch into the pelvis, and fashion a peranal, ileo-anal anastomosis between the opening in the pouch and the dentate line using interrupted 2/0 Vicryl sutures on a J-shaped needle (Fig. 6.103).

Wound closure

Redivac drains are inserted, one on each side of the pelvis, and if the ileo-anal anastomosis is to be defunctioned, a loop ileostomy is placed in the right iliac fossa.

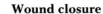

Peranal ileo-anal anastomosis

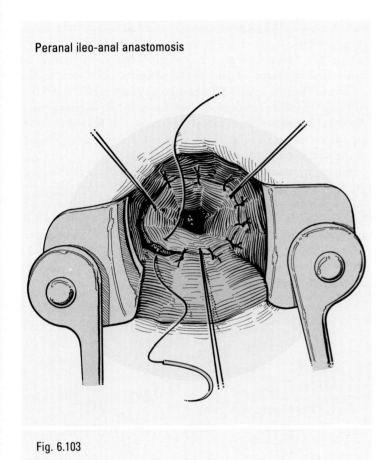

Fig. 6.103

SPECIAL OPERATIVE HAZARDS
1. Unrecognized carcinoma of the colon.
2. Damage to the ureters.
3. Damage to hypogastric nerves
4. Difficulty in bringing the pouch into the pelvis without tension on the mesentery.

COMPLICATIONS
1. Problems with incontinence, due to the more fluid consistency of stools, can generally be overcome with codeine phosphate or loperamide and retraining.
2. Complications from sepsis can be reduced by avoiding contamination, by maintaining good haemostasis and by washing out the rectum prior to the transection.
3. 'Pouchitis' is a condition that occurs in patients who have undergone this procedure for ulcerative colitis. The pouch undergoes inflammatory changes which can be diagnosed using sigmoidoscopy and biopsy; it usually responds to antibiotics.
4. In men, retrograde ejaculation can occur following damage to the inferior hypogastric nerves.

Ovarian Cystectomy and Oöphorectomy

A general surgeon dealing with emergencies must be able to deal with gynaecological causes of the acute abdomen. It is important to preserve ovarian tissue during the reproductive years.

PREOPERATIVE ASSESSMENT
1. In a female patient with acute abdominal pain always consider gynaecological disease.
2. Perform a careful pelvic examination and, if indicated, a pregnancy test.
3. Consider pelvic ultrasound or referral to a gynaecologist who may advise a diagnostic laparoscopy.

RELEVANT ANATOMY
The pelvic peritoneum is draped over the fundus of the uterus and the fallopian tubes, and laterally it extends to the side walls of the pelvis forming the double-leaved broad ligament (Fig. 6.104).

The ovaries lie on the side wall of the pelvis within the posterior leaf of the broad ligament; this is elongated to form the mesovarium which is attached to the circumference of the ovary. Within the broad ligament a fibromuscular condensation of tissue, the ligament of the ovary, attaches the ovary to the cornua of the uterus and then continues as the round ligament, running under the anterior leaf of the broad ligament to reach the deep inguinal ring. The broad ligament is folded over the top of the fallopian tube which is attached to the lateral aspect of the ovary at its inturned lateral extremity.

The ovarian artery comes directly off the aorta and crosses the ureter and pelvic brim to enter the lateral extremity of the upper border of the broad ligament (the infundibulopelvic fold) to reach the ovary. It gives off a tubal branch which anastomoses with the uterine artery within the broad ligament. The ovarian vein is a plexus of vessels which lie alongside the artery and ascend and coalesce to reach the inferior vena cava on the right and the renal vein on the left.

Relevant anatomy

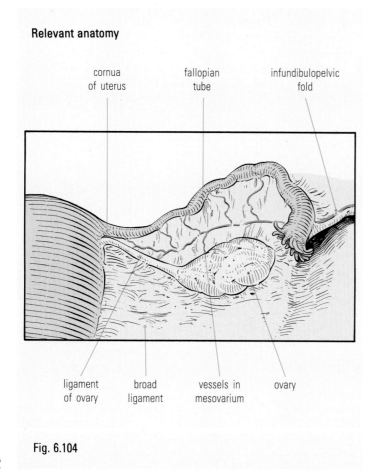

cornua of uterus · fallopian tube · infundibulopelvic fold

ligament of ovary · broad ligament · vessels in mesovarium · ovary

Fig. 6.104

Exposure of a cystic right ovary

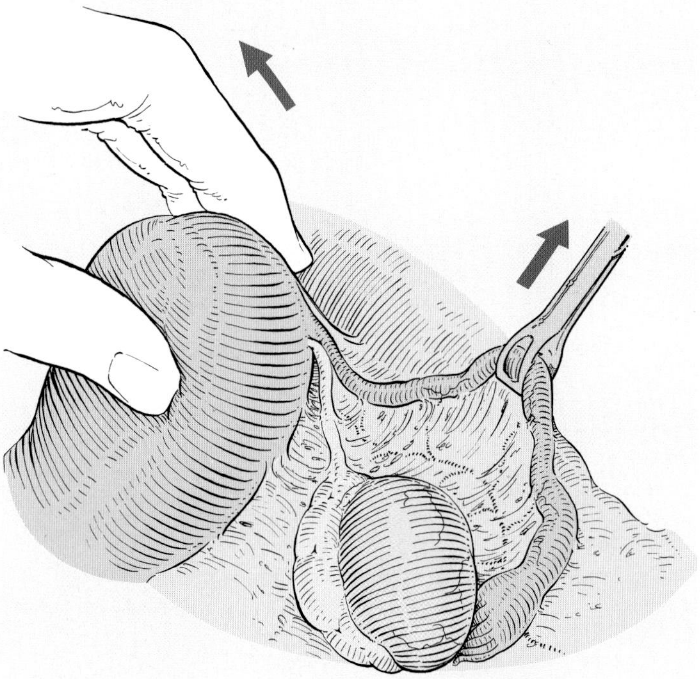

Fig. 6.105

OPERATION
Preparation
The anaesthetized patient is placed supine with head-down tilt and the lower abdomen is cleansed and draped. The bladder is emptied.

Incision
If a laparotomy incision such as a midline has already been made, extend this caudally to allow access to the pelvis. For an elective approach to the ovaries use a lower midline or Pfannenstiel incision, performed as follows. Make a slightly curved (convex downward) transverse lower abdominal incision and deepen it through the anterior rectus sheath. Lift and free the upper flap of rectus sheath in the midline using scissors, and then separate the recti in the midline and retract them laterally to expose the posterior peritoneum which is opened between clips. Insert a self-retaining retractor (e.g. a Doyen) and pack the bowel upward with a large moist swab.

Operative technique
1. To expose and inspect the ovary on one side, retract the uterus to the opposite side and lift the fallopian tube using a Babcock's forcep which is placed around it with its blades meeting at the mesosalpinx (Fig. 6.105). Inspect both ovaries. In the presence of an ovarian cyst carefully examine the peritoneum, omentum and liver for evidence of metastatic disease.

If there is none and the patient is of child-bearing years aim to preserve the ovary and excise only the cyst. Small follicular cysts in such patients are common and do not require excision or aspiration. In an older patient or if the cyst has replaced all the ovarian tissue, and in cases requiring oophorectomy for hormonal manipulation, excise the entire ovary. For cases of ovarian malignancy perform a hysterectomy with bilateral salpingo-oöphorectomy (see page 6.59) and excise the omentum.

2. To perform an ovarian cystectomy incise the capsule of the cyst with a knife at the point where it emerges from the ovary, taking great care not to puncture it (Fig. 6.106). Develop the plane using the scalpel handle or blunt rounded scissors between the cyst wall and the compressed surrounding ovary and gently work the cyst free (Fig. 6.106). Secure haemostasis and reconstruct the ovary by closing the hole left by the cyst with a series of concentric non-absorbable (e.g. 2/0 Prolene) purse-string sutures (Fig. 6.107). Repair the surface of the ovary with a running stitch.

3. If a large cyst has torted it will usually do so at the ovarian pedicle. In such cases the cyst and ovary are brick-red or black and usually the tube will have been dragged around it. Do not untwist the torsion but clamp it at its base and transfix the pedicle with a number 1 chromic catgut suture.

Circumcision of an ovarian cyst

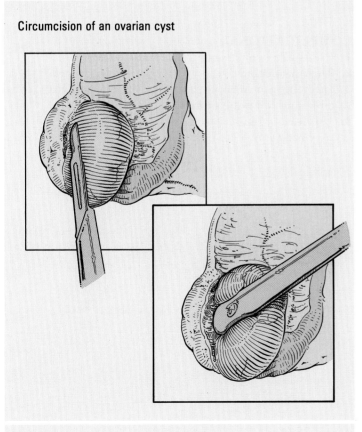

Fig. 6.106

Repair of defect in ovary

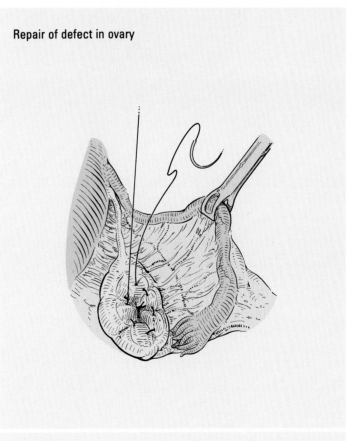

Fig. 6.107

4. To excise an ovary stretch the mesovarium by drawing the ovary away from the retracted tube and divide the mesovarium by clipping and tying. Keep close to the ovary, preserving the ovarian vessels which remain with the fallopian tube (Fig. 6.108). When the cornua of the uterus is reached the ovary will be attached by only the ovarian ligament which is divided and tied.

5. Open the specimen to get a better idea of its nature; papillary ingrowths and solid areas suggest malignancy. If doubt still exists regarding the nature of the cyst arrange for a frozen section examination.

6. If uncertainty exists regarding the state of the opposite ovary it should be bivalved by incising it on the side opposite the mesovarium (to preserve its blood supply) and inspecting its contents. Repair the ovary with a continuous non-absorbable suture (e.g. Prolene).

Wound closure and dressing
A drain is generally unnecessary. Close the peritoneum with catgut or nylon and the anterior sheath with loop nylon. Insert a Yeates drain if the patient is fat and close the skin with interrupted sutures. Apply a waterproof dressing.

POSTOPERATIVE CARE
Fluids are reintroduced the following day unless the small bowel has been extensively handled (e.g. if pelvic adhesions have been divided). Remove the Yeates drain after 48 hours. The sutures remain for 5 days for a transverse incision and 8 days for a midline incision.

SPECIAL OPERATIVE HAZARDS
1. Bleeding from the ovarian pedicle. The divided vessels tend to retract away between the leaves of the broad ligament, filling this space with haematoma. Blindly grasping for the vessels endangers the ureter, so either apply firm pressure for 5 minutes and incise the broad ligament to locate the bleeding point, or open the peritoneum over the ovarian vessels higher up and ligate them at this level.
2. Damage to the ureter.
3. Rupture of cyst. Seeding of cells from the cyst (even if histologically benign) can lead to pseudomyxoma peritonei with multiple mucin secreting lesions in the peritoneum.

COMPLICATIONS
1. Unsuspected malignancy in an excised cyst.
2. Pelvic haematoma.
3. Infertility or ectopic pregnancy from sepsis or tubal adhesions following surgery.
4. Unpleasant menopausal symptoms following bilateral oöphorectomy.

Excision of ovary

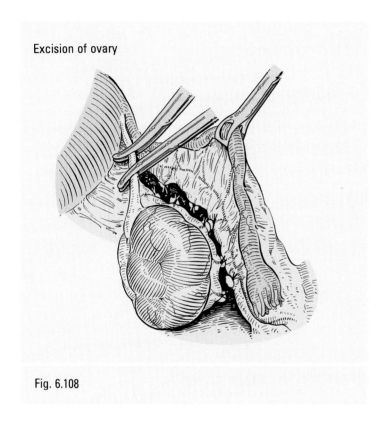

Fig. 6.108

Management of Ruptured Ectopic Pregnancy

PREOPERATIVE ASSESSMENT

1. Suspect an ectopic pregnancy if there is a history of a missed period or pregnancy and vaginal bleeding. The risk is increased in patients that have suffered pelvic inflammatory disease, have an IUCD, or have had a previous ectopic pregnancy. Consider laparoscopy and seek a gynaecological opinion.
2. Ascertain whether the patient has completed her family.
3. The diagnosis of haemoperitoneum may be confirmed by culdocentesis; under local anaesthetic, aspirating non-clotted blood through a 19G needle introduced into the pouch of Douglas via the posterior fornix of the vagina, which is viewed with a Sims speculum.
4. A ruptured ectopic pregnancy can cause catastrophic bleeding, although the presentation may be of more chronic lower abdominal pain. With acute rupture lie the patient flat, ensure adequate venous access and monitoring, com-

mence resuscitation and consider urgent exploration. The patient may remain hypotensive until the bleeding is dealt with.

RELEVANT ANATOMY

The fallopian tube lies between the leaves of the broad ligament at its upper margin. The fimbriated lateral end of the fallopian tube is apposed to the ovary. It continues as the dilated ampulla, and then tapers down to the narrowed isthmus before reaching the cornua of the uterus (Fig. 6.109). The tube is supplied with blood from the ovarian artery which runs below and parallel to the tube between the leaves of the broad ligament (the mesosalpinx) and meets the ascending uterine artery. It is within the fallopian tube that 99% of ectopic pregnancies occur, most commonly in the ampulla, fimbriated end and isthmus in that order. Ectopic pregnancy may undergo tubal abortion with

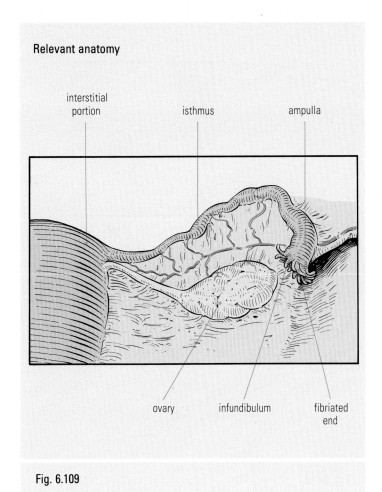

Relevant anatomy

interstitial portion | isthmus | ampulla

ovary | infundibulum | fibriated end

Fig. 6.109

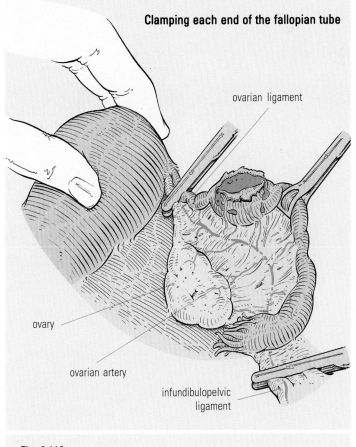

Clamping each end of the fallopian tube

ovarian ligament

ovary

ovarian artery

infundibulopelvic ligament

Fig. 6.110

Division of mesosalpinx

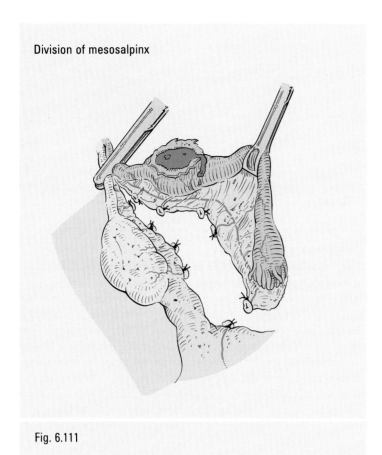

Fig. 6.111

extrusion of the conceptus through the tubal ostium, or may rupture through the side of the tube either into the peritoneal cavity or between the two leaves of the broad ligament.

Also see the Relevant Anatomy on pages 6.52 and 6.58.

OPERATION
Preparation
Place the patient supine with slight head-down tilt, and ensure that the bladder is empty by inserting a urethral catheter. Cleanse and drape the lower abdomen.

Incision
The abdomen may have already been opened for a diagnostic laparotomy. If so, extend the incision to allow access to the pelvis. Otherwise make a Pfannenstiel (see page 6.53) or lower midline incision (see the Introduction).

Operative technique
1. Evacuate blood and clots from the pelvis with a sump sucker, using a cupped hand as shown on page 8.17. Very rarely, autotransfusion of filtered citrated intraperitoneal blood is indicated.

Oversew cornua to uterus

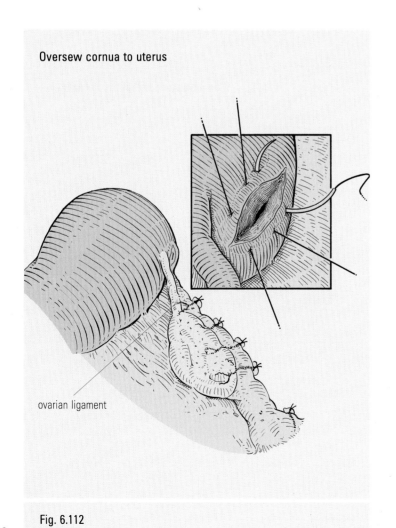

ovarian ligament

Fig. 6.112

Conservative surgery for ectopic pregnancy

Cuff salpingostomy

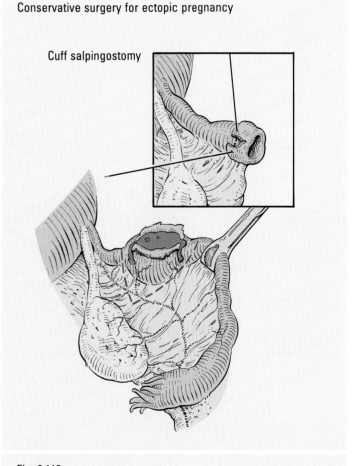

Fig. 6.113

2. Grasp the uterus, lift it into the wound and identify the side and site of the ectopic pregnancy. Inspect the other ovary and tube.

3. The safest option for the less experienced surgeon is to perform a salpingectomy on the affected side, preserving the ovary unless it is involved with the ectopic pregnancy. This is done by retracting the uterus to the opposite side and lifting the affected tube out of the pelvis to stretch up the infundibulopelvic ligament (and the contained ovarian vessels) which is clamped, as is the cornual end of the tube (Fig. 6.110). This will stop the bleeding. Divide and transfix the infundibulopelvic ligament with heavy chromic catgut between two clamps, and continue by dividing the mesosalpinx between the ovary and the tube until the cornua of the uterus is reached (Fig. 6.111). Excise the cornua of the uterus on the side of the ectopic pregnancy thus freeing the tube, and oversew the corner of uterus with interrupted 00 chromic catgut sutures (Fig. 6.112).

4. It may be preferable and possible to preserve the affected tube in selected cases of ectopic pregnancy, for example if the opposite side is abnormal. In such cases carefully milk the conceptus out of the fimbriated end, or open the tube along the border opposite the mesosalpinx with a knife, evacuate the conceptus and secure haemostasis with diathermy or fine catgut sutures. It is not necessary to close the tube. An alternative is to resect the damaged portion of tube with a wedge of the broad ligament (Fig. 6.113). In such cases repair the tube or evert the cut end of the tube with fine catgut sutures to create a cuff salpingostomy (see inset to Fig. 6.113).

Wound closure and dressing

Insert a drain into the pelvis, then close the wound with monofilament loop nylon and either interrupted skin sutures or a subcuticular stitch.

POSTOPERATIVE CARE

A nasogastric tube and intravenous fluids are required until gut function returns. The drain is removed after 24–48 hours, if dry, and the sutures are removed after 5 days for a Pfannenstiel and 8 days for a vertical incision. The patient must be counselled with regard to the likelihood of successful pregnancy and of a further ectopic pregnancy.

SPECIAL OPERATIVE HAZARDS
1. Rupture into the broad ligament. Open the ligament and evacuate the clot after dealing with the ectopic pregnancy.
2. Damage to the ureter when clamping the infundibulopelvic ligament.

COMPLICATIONS
1. Ten percent of patients will suffer a second ectopic pregnancy.
2. Only 60% of patients will go on to have a successful uterine pregnancy.

Whilst it is often appropriate to seek the advice of a gynaecologist when dealing with pathology in the female pelvis, a general surgeon should be capable of performing an abdominal hysterectomy for two reasons. Firstly removal of the uterus may be required as part of an *en bloc* excision of a malignancy of the large bowel or bladder, and secondly emergency hysterectomy may be required, for example, in a patient undergoing laparotomy for acute abdominal pain who is found to have ovarian carcinoma.

PREOPERATIVE ASSESSMENT

Clinical examination and CT scanning might suggest the involvement of the uterus with a pelvic malignancy.

RELEVANT ANATOMY

The pear-shaped muscular uterus is divided into a fundus above and the body below (Fig. 6.114). The upper part of the body meets the fundus at the two cornua from which the fallopian tubes extend outward on either side (the anatomy of the ovary and tube is considered on pages 6.52 and 6.55), and distally it tapers becoming the cervix which protrudes into the vagina. Anteriorly the lower part of the body and upper part of the cervix are adherent to the bladder base.

The anterior and posterior surfaces of the uterus are covered with peritoneum; this is reflected laterally as a double fold of peritoneum known as the broad ligament which encloses the fallopian (uterine) tube. The upper lateral extremity of the broad ligament, beyond the ovary and tube, forms the infundibulopelvic ligament which encloses the ovarian vessels. Posteriorly the peritoneum sweeps over the cervix and upper vagina and then back up over the rectum, forming the recess known as the pouch of Douglas. Anteriorly the peritoneum does not reach so deeply and is reflected over the bladder forming the uterovesical pouch above the level of the cervix.

Condensations of fibrous tissue extend posteriorly from the cervix on either side of the rectum to reach the sacrum as the uterosacral ligaments, and laterally from the cervix as the lateral ligaments which contain the uterine vessels. The round ligament runs forward from the cornua of the uterus to the deep inguinal ring, under the anterior leaf of the broad ligament which is tented up over it.

The uterus derives its blood supply from the uterine and ovarian arteries. The former arise from the internal iliac artery and crosses the pelvic floor in the base of the broad ligament,

Relevant anatomy

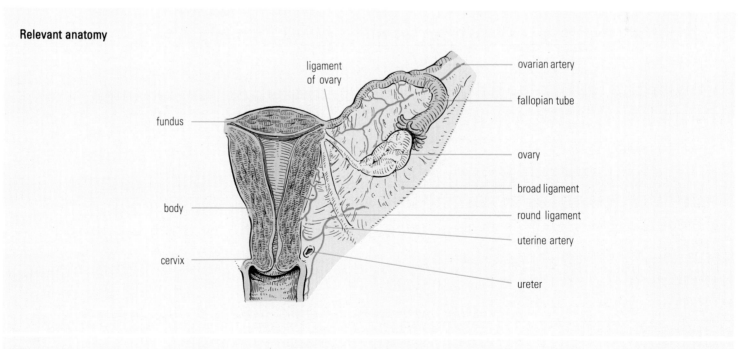

Fig. 6.114

crossing the ureter to reach the upper cervix where it sends a descending branch to supply the upper vagina and ascends between the leaves of the broad ligament, giving off branches to the uterus and anastomosing with the descending ovarian artery. The venous drainage of the uterus communicates freely with the venous plexuses of the bladder and rectum and flows into the internal iliac veins.

OPERATION
Preparation
The patient is placed supine with slight head-down tilt. The lower abdomen, perineum and vagina are cleansed, and a urethral catheter is inserted.

Incision
Elective abdominal hysterectomy is best performed through either a Pfannenstiel (see page 6.53) or lower midline incision (see the Introduction) if the diagnosis is in doubt. For the general surgeon, however, it may only become apparent that a hysterectomy is required after having entered the abdomen through some other laparotomy incision and this may need to be extended caudally to allow access to the pelvis. Insert a self-retaining retractor and use large packs to keep the bowel out of the pelvis.

Operative technique
1. Decide whether or not the ovaries are to be preserved. If the patient is suffering from ovarian malignancy both must be removed.

2. If the ovaries are to be removed, divide the round ligament and infundibulopelvic fold of peritoneum containing the ovarian vessels between clamps (Fig. 6.115). If the ovaries are to be preserved clamp and divide the fallopian tubes and round ligament on each side close to the cornua of the uterus (Fig. 6.116). Transfix the pedicles with number 1 chromic catgut, keeping the medial clamps on the uterus for retraction.

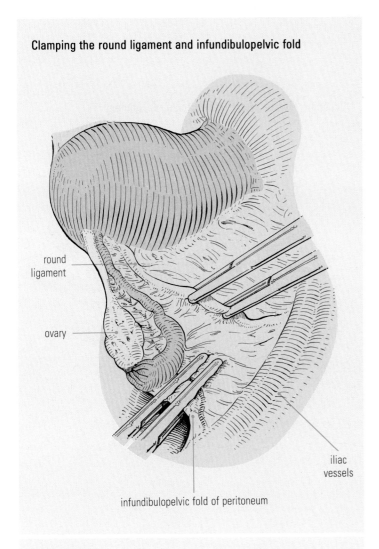

Clamping the round ligament and infundibulopelvic fold

round ligament

ovary

infundibulopelvic fold of peritoneum

iliac vessels

Fig. 6.115

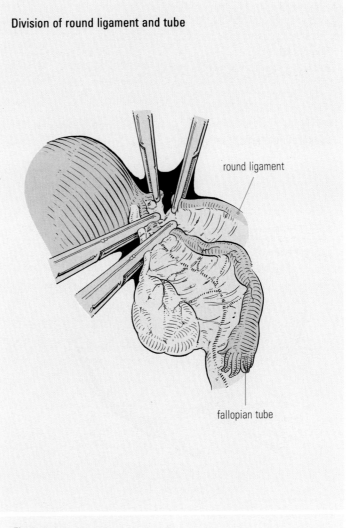

Division of round ligament and tube

round ligament

fallopian tube

Fig. 6.116

Division of broad ligament

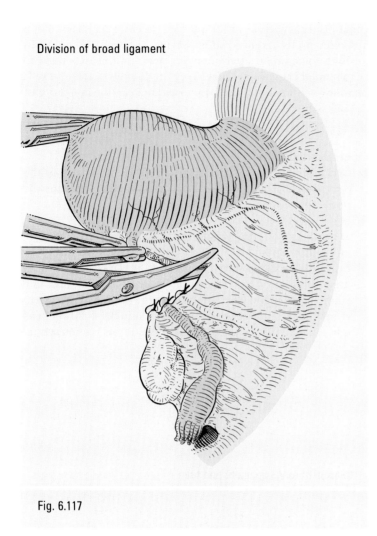

Fig. 6.117

Separating uterus from bladder

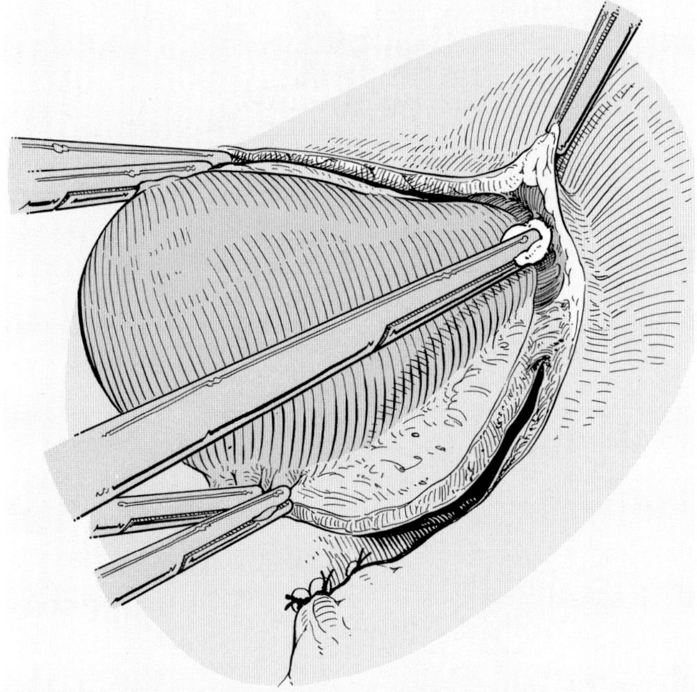

Fig. 6.118

3. Divide the anterior and posterior leaves of the broad ligament with scissors, keeping lateral to the uterine artery (Fig. 6.117).

4. Continue the peritoneal incision in the anterior leaf of the broad ligament across the front of the uterus just above the uterovesical pouch, and lift up the divided peritoneum over the bladder. Using a mixture of sharp and blunt dissection sweep the bladder and ureters down off the uterus (Fig. 6.118) to a level below the cervix, which can be located by palpation.

5. Apply a clamp to the uterine artery in the base of the broad ligament on each side, taking care to avoid picking up the ureter which passes under the artery. With the uterus retracted forwards place a second pair of clamps across the uterosacral ligaments and parametrium on each side behind and alongside the cervix (Fig. 6.119).

6. Grasp each corner of the vaginal vault with an Allis tissue-holding forceps and remove the uterus by circumferentially incising the vagina just below the level of the cervix (Fig. 6.120).

7. Transfix the divided lateral fornix of the vagina, leaving the stitch long so it can be used as a stay suture. Oversew the vault transversely with an over-and-over 00 catgut blanket stitch.

Clamping uterine artery and uterosacral ligament

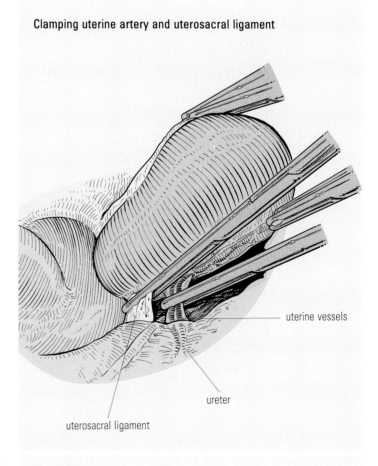

uterine vessels

ureter

uterosacral ligament

Fig. 6.119

6.60

Opening the vaginal vault

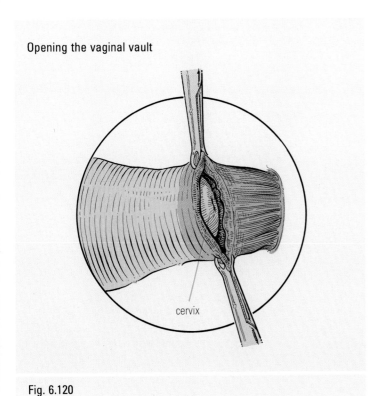

cervix

Fig. 6.120

Vaginal vault closed and remaining pedicles transfixed

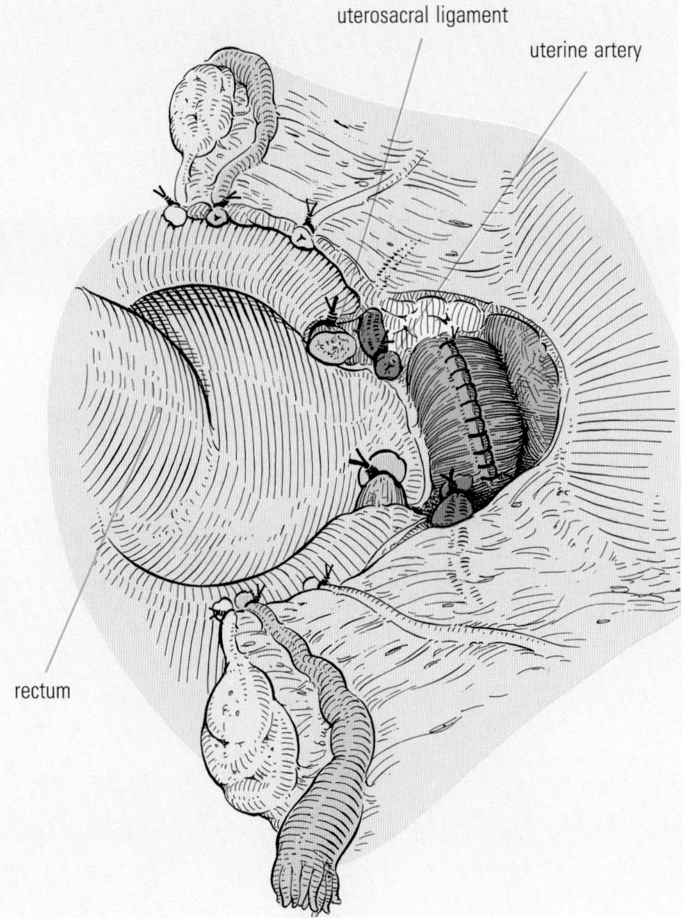

uterosacral ligament

uterine artery

rectum

Fig. 6.121

8. Transfix the pedicles contained within the remaining two clamps on each side with a catgut suture (Fig. 6.121).

9. If there is sufficient pelvic peritoneum, close it with a running 00 catgut stitch, although if the hysterectomy has been combined with excision of the bladder or rectum this will not be possible and the defect in the pelvic peritoneum remains.

Wound closure and dressing
Insert a fine suction drain into the pelvis and close the wound with monofilament nylon and the skin with interrupted sutures and clips. In obese patients a Yeates drain is left in the fat. Apply a waterproof dressing and swab the vagina clean of any blood clot.

POSTOPERATIVE CARE
Fluids are reintroduced when bowel sounds return, usually the following day. The drain is removed after 24–48 hours. The clips remain for 2 days while the sutures stay for 5 days for a Pfannenstiel incision and 8 days for a midline incision.

SPECIAL OPERATIVE HAZARDS
1. Damage to the ureters or bladder.
2. Dense pelvic adhesions, which increases the risk of damaging the ureters. Perform a subtotal hysterectomy in such cases, dividing and oversewing the uterus at the level of the isthmus after ligating and dividing the uterine arteries.
3. Oozing from the vagina. Occasionally this requires a vaginal pack for 24 hours.

COMPLICATIONS
1. Haemorrhage from a slipped tie or from the divided vaginal vault.
2. Infected pelvic haematoma.
3. Fistula formation, which can be ureterovaginal, vesicovaginal or rectovaginal.
4. Dyspareunia.

7

Surgery for Herniae

Infantile Umbilical Hernia Repair

PREOPERATIVE ASSESSMENT
1. As this hernia is common in black children the sickle cell status should be checked.
2. In the case of an emergency, look for evidence of an obstruction or strangulation with dehydration or sepsis.
3. If the child is in its first year of life the hernia should just be observed as some regress spontaneously.

RELEVANT ANATOMY
An infantile umbilical hernia results from a congenital defect that remains in the linea alba when the midgut returns to the abdominal cavity *in utero*. There is usually little or no subcutaneous fat between the overlying skin and peritoneal sac.

OPERATION
Preparation
The patient is placed supine and the skin is cleansed and draped.

Incision
A curved, transverse skin incision is made beneath the umbilicus (Fig. 7.1), and this incision is deepened to expose the anterior rectus sheath.

Operative technique
1. The sac is identified and its neck, which is emerging through the linea alba, is defined by sharp dissection around the lateral edges (Fig. 7.2).

2. The sac is often densely adherent to the overlying skin and attempts to separate them may result in devascularization or buttonhole damage to the skin. It is, therefore, preferable in some cases to open the sac leaving its apex attached to umbilical skin.

3. Clips are applied to the cut edge of the sac and its contents are reduced (Fig. 7.3). The sac is then closed with an absorbable 00 catgut suture. As the edges of the defect in the linea

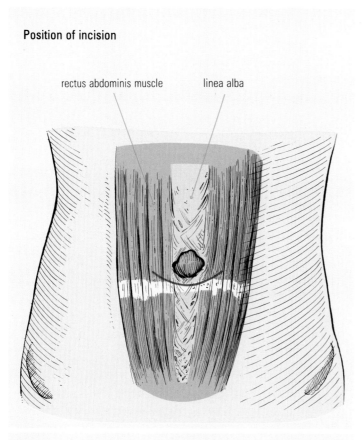

Position of incision

rectus abdominis muscle   linea alba

Fig. 7.1

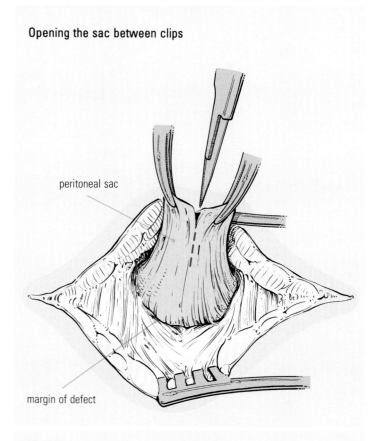

Opening the sac between clips

peritoneal sac

margin of defect

Fig. 7.2

alba are clearly defined and longitudinal, edge-to-edge repair can be completed using either monofilament or braided 00 nylon sutures (Fig. 7.4).

Wound closure and dressing
The deep surface of the umbilical skin is sutured to the rectus sheath with a single catgut stitch to avoid leaving a dead space (Fig. 7.5), and the skin closed with a subcuticular monofilament 00 nylon or polypropylene suture. Cover the suture with a simple sticky plaster.

POSTOPERATIVE CARE
The patient is usually well enough to be fully mobile and eating breakfast the next day and is generally allowed home. The skin suture is removed on the fifth or sixth postoperative day. It is pointless to instruct the mother to limit physical activity as this is impractical and the child will, in any case, return to normal activities as soon as the minor discomfort resolves.

SPECIAL OPERATIVE HAZARD
1. Devascularization of the umbilical skin.

COMPLICATIONS
1. Wound haematoma generally follows inadequate haemostasis. If there is concern that haematoma may form, apply a gauze pad and adhesive strapping to exert pressure.
2. Wound infection is uncommon and generally follows haematoma.
3. Recurrence.

Sac ready for closure with catgut

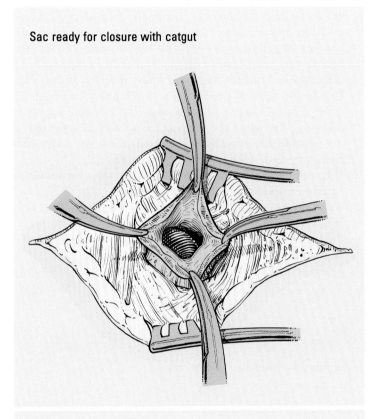

Fig. 7.3

Closure of defect with interrupted sutures

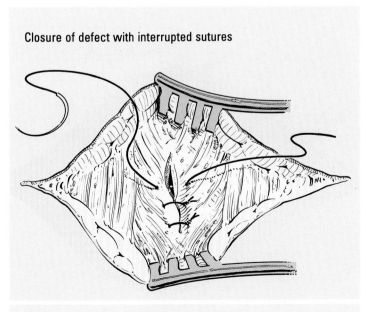

Fig. 7.4

Tacking umbilicus down to close dead space

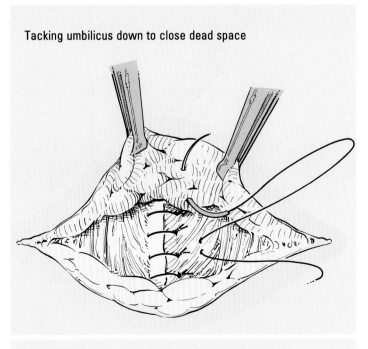

Fig. 7.5

7.3

Inguinal Herniotomy in Children

A hernia which appears in the first few months of life has a high risk of strangulation and should be operated upon as soon as possible.

RELEVANT ANATOMY

Inguinal herniae in infants and children are congenital in origin and due to a patent processus vaginalis (the peritoneal sac which descended with the testicle and has failed to close). Boys are affected ten times more frequently than girls and it is often associated with maldescent of the testis. Twenty per cent are bilateral. The sac may contain ectopic adrenal tissue, and the ovary in young girls.

The inguinal canal is much shorter in the child with the deep inguinal ring lying almost directly behind the superficial ring. The sac lies anterior to the vas and testicular vessels in boys (Fig. 7.6), within the cord coverings, and is related to the round ligament in girls.

PREOPERATIVE ASSESSMENT

1. If the child presents with a strangulated inguinal hernia, gentle reduction should be attempted first after adequate sedation and analgesia has been given with the child suspended in gallows traction, with the buttocks just off the bed. Gently compress the hernia from side to side with the fingers and thumb of one hand whilst applying gentle pressure to the apex of the hernia with the index finger of the other hand. If successful, the child is operated upon the following day when the oedema has settled. If reduction is not possible then the child is operated on as soon as any fluid and electrolyte disorders have been corrected.
2. Differentiate an inguinoscrotal hernia from a hydrocele by careful examination and transillumination.
3. Carefully examine both sides and mark the appropriate one. When reduced the sac can be felt if the cord is rolled under the finger where it crosses the pubis. Bilateral herniae should be repaired under the same anaesthetic.

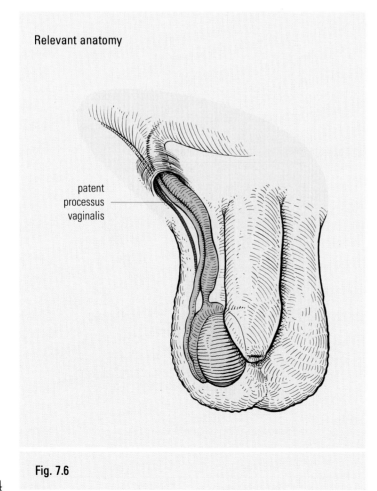

Relevant anatomy

patent processus vaginalis

Fig. 7.6

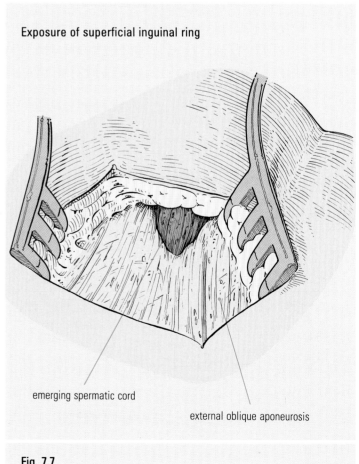

Exposure of superficial inguinal ring

emerging spermatic cord

external oblique aponeurosis

Fig. 7.7

OPERATION
Preparation
General anaesthesia is given and the child is placed supine on the operating table with the groin exposed, prepared and draped.

Incision
Make a skin crease incision, 2–3 cm in length, 1 cm above the medial part of the inguinal ligament.

Operative technique
1. Carefully divide the subcutaneous tissue and Scarpa's fascia by lifting the tissues with two pairs of forceps (one held by the assistant) and cutting between them with diathermy. Insert a small self-retaining retractor.

2. Locate the spermatic cord and define the superficial inguinal ring (Fig. 7.7). In an older child with a developed inguinal canal incise the external oblique aponeurosis laterally from the superficial inguinal ring.

3. Pick up the coverings of the spermatic cord with forceps and carefully open them longitudinally, by opening a haemostat,

to expose the contents of the cord including the hernial sac (Fig. 7.8). The sac appears white and opaque and its margin is usually well-defined compared to the surrounding tissue.

4. Apply an artery forcep to the margin of the sac, and gently sweep posteriorly the vas and testicular vessels in a boy (or the round ligament in a girl) with a non-toothed forcep (Fig. 7.9).

5. Open the sac to ensure that it is empty, transfix the neck with 4/0 catgut without twisting it and excise the sac beyond the ligature (Fig. 7.10). When released, the transfixed neck will slip away out of sight through the deep ring.

6. In a strangulated hernia, great care must be taken when locating and dissecting free the hernial sac as it is very easy to tear the sac or damage the cord structures or contained bowel. The sac is opened and the contents, if viable, are reduced. Should the contents be non-viable resection is necessary.

Wound closure and dressing
If divided, repair the external oblique aponeurosis with an absorbable (e.g. 2/0 Vicryl) suture. The subcutaneous tissue and

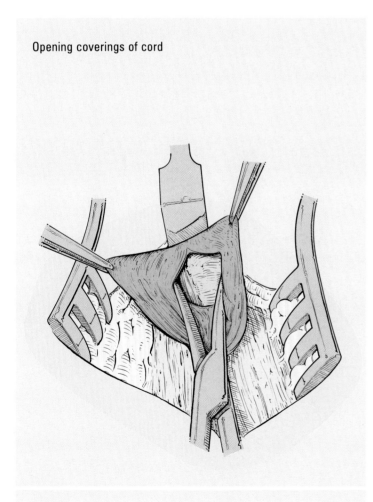

Opening coverings of cord

Fig. 7.8

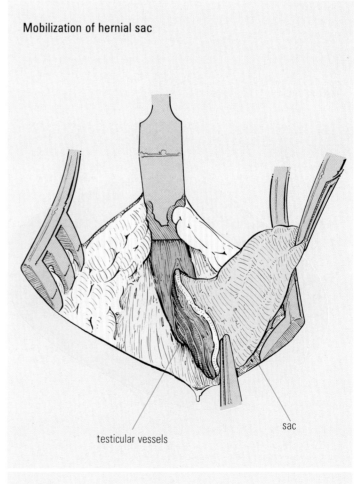

Mobilization of hernial sac

testicular vessels

sac

Fig. 7.9

7.5

Transfixion of sac

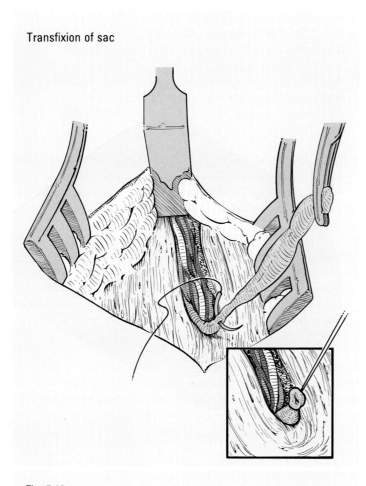

Fig. 7.10

Scarpa's fascia are closed in one layer with an absorbable (e.g. 2/0 Vicryl) suture and the skin is closed with a subcuticular absorbable stitch. Apply a waterproof dressing to the groin wound.

POSTOPERATIVE CARE
The child can usually be discharged home on the same day in elective cases. If the patient is operated upon as an emergency, discharge home is delayed until bowel activity returns to normal.

SPECIAL OPERATIVE HAZARDS
1. Damage to the vas or testicular vessels during the dissection.
2. Damage to the contents of the sac.
3. Tearing the sac; if the tear is close to the neck, mobilize more peritoneum from above whilst retracting the lateral border of the deep ring with a small Langenbeck retractor, so that the apex of the tear can be closed with the transfixion stitch (Fig. 7.11).

COMPLICATIONS
1. Wound haematoma or infection.
2. Testicular atrophy due to damage to the cord vessels.

Tear in sac

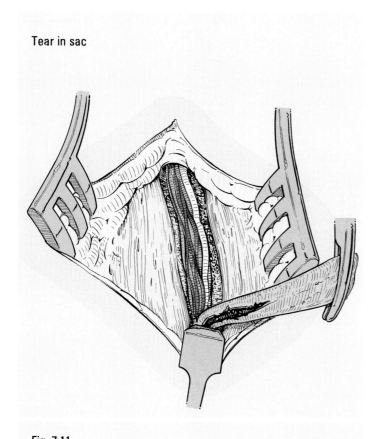

Fig. 7.11

PREOPERATIVE ASSESSMENT

1. Attempt to reduce any factors which increase the risk of recurrence (e.g. obesity, constipation, chronic cough or prostatic obstruction).
2. With a huge incisional hernia, preoperative reduction of the contents with a surgical truss will ensure that eventual repair of the hernia will not cause the patient ventilatory complications.
3. In cases of strangulation, ensure adequate resuscitation with attention to rehydration and correction of electrolyte disturbances. Pass a nasogastric tube.
4. Careful clinical examination is of the utmost importance in establishing the margins of the defect which are usually easy to define. Decide whether the hernia is single or multiple.

RELEVANT ANATOMY

An epigastric hernia arises through a weakness in the midline in the linea alba between the two rectus abdominus muscles somewhere along the line between the xiphisternum and the umbilicus. If small, the hernia will only contain extraperitoneal fat, covered with attenuated linea alba; with enlargement the peritoneum also herniates (Fig. 7.12). Even very small epigastric herniae can be painful.

An incisional hernia occurs through a previous surgical incision following failure of wound healing. The deeper layers generally disrupt in the early postoperative period, the skin remaining intact. It may be some time before the hernia becomes apparent. Factors that are likely to lead to a hernia include wound sepsis, debility, postoperative cough, abdominal distension, and poor technique of wound closure. Whilst any wound may be implicated, incisional herniae are less common through muscle-cutting incisions such as a grid-iron incision and occur most frequently through midline incisions.

OPERATION
Preparation

For an epigastric hernia repair the patient is placed supine on the operating table. This is generally also the case for an incisional hernia, although with a hernia through a loin incision the patient may need to be tilted on one side or even placed in the full lateral position to ensure good access. The skin is prepared and draped in the usual manner.

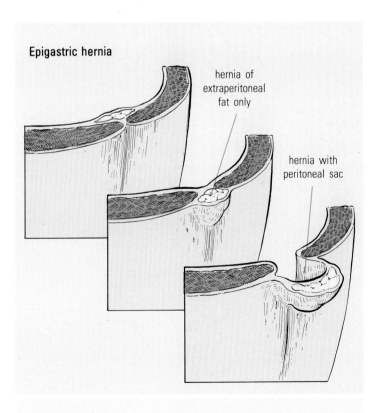

Epigastric hernia

hernia of extraperitoneal fat only

hernia with peritoneal sac

Fig. 7.12

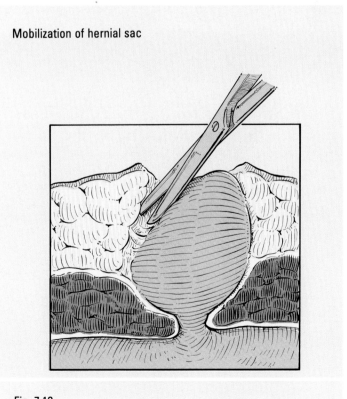

Mobilization of hernial sac

Fig. 7.13

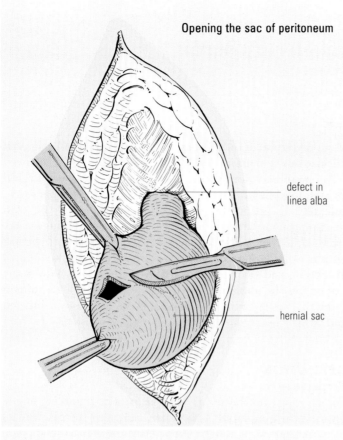

Opening the sac of peritoneum

defect in
linea alba

hernial sac

Fig. 7.14

Incision

Make a straight incision overlying the long axis of the defect, or excise a widened ugly scar. Care must be taken with an incisional hernia not to open directly into the peritoneal cavity, since the peritoneum may be adherent to the skin.

Operative technique

Small defects

1. Dissect the skin edges and superficial fat with scissors until the glistening hernial sac is identified. Keeping close to the wall of the sac and in the obvious plane between the sac and the surrounding tissues, clear the sac as far as its neck and carefully define the margins of the defect (Fig. 7.13).

2. Clean the sac of any extraperitoneal fat by blunt dissection and reduce its contents. If small, reduce the sac through the defect, but if it is larger, pick it up with two artery forceps, open it (Fig. 7.14), and then inspect and reduce its contents.

3. Transfix the neck with a 2/0 chromic catgut suture and excise the excess sac and extraperitoneal fat (Fig. 7.15).

4. Pick up the edges of the defect with forceps and reoppose them by suturing without tension using either an interrupted or a continuous stitch with a non-absorbable material such as nylon (Fig. 7.16).

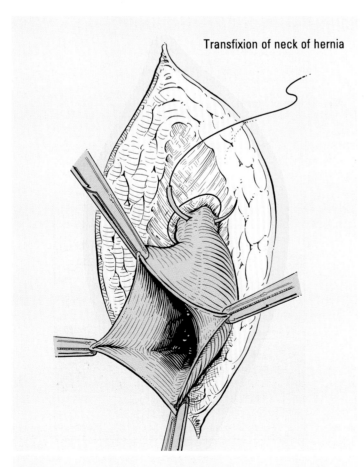

Transfixion of neck of hernia

Fig. 7.15

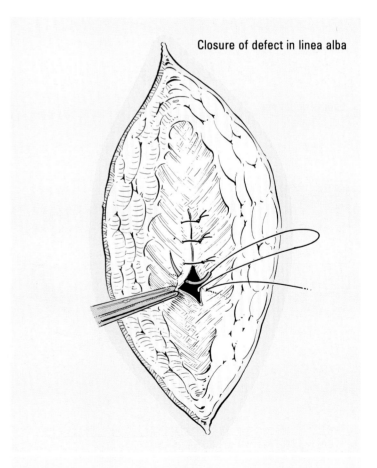

Closure of defect in linea alba

Fig. 7.16

Large defects

1. When making the incision, it may be obvious that there is an excess of stretched skin over the hernia. Resect it so as to allow comfortable wound closure without tension. At this stage be conservative since more skin can easily be removed later.

2. Mobilize the skin and subcutaneous tissues together from the underlying aponeurosis using scissors until healthy tissue is reached on all sides of the defect (Fig. 7.17).

3. Incise the attenuated tissues and peritoneum along one border of the hernia and dissect the intra-abdominal contents from the undersurface, so as to create a flap from the original hernial sac (Fig. 7.18). Similarly free the undersurface of the now exposed opposite margin of the defect.

4. If, following excision of all the scar tissue the margins of the defect can be brought together without tension, do this with continuous loop nylon. It may be necessary to make relieving incisions in the rectus sheath beyond. Should primary closure not be possible, a sheet of synthetic material (e.g. Prolene mesh) is used for the repair, as described below.

5. Using a continuous non-absorbable stitch, suture the edge of the defect to the edge of a sheet of synthetic material (Fig. 7.19).

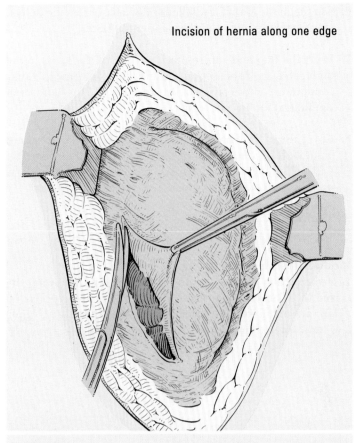

Incision of hernia along one edge

Fig. 7.18

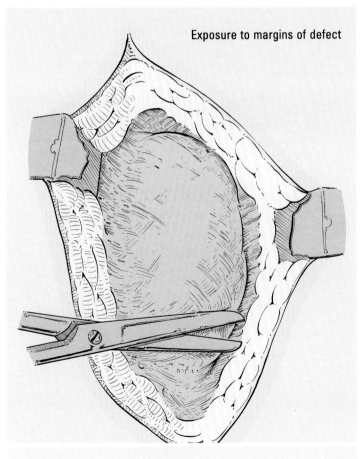

Exposure to margins of defect

Fig. 7.17

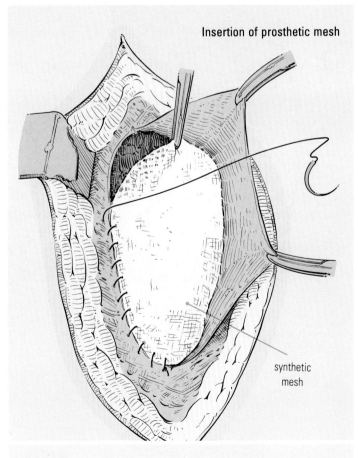

Insertion of prosthetic mesh

synthetic mesh

Fig. 7.19

6. Cut the mesh so that it will lie comfortably across the defect, reaching the opposite margin under the flap.

7. Evert the flap and suture the free edge of the mesh to the undersurface of the opposite edge of the defect with either continuous or interrupted sutures (Fig. 7.20). The mesh should be taut but not tight.

8. Cover the mesh with the flap, and suture the flap to sound tissue beyond the margin of the defect using 00 nylon (Fig. 7.21). This 'shutters' the mesh from the skin, as well as providing an additional, albeit weak, layer to the repair.

9. Ensure meticulous haemostasis.

Wound closure and dressing

Insert a suction drain to drain any haematoma following the repair of a large defect. Close the skin with interrupted 00 nylon; more skin can be excised at this stage if necessary. Apply a waterproof dressing.

POSTOPERATIVE CARE

If the bowel has been extensively dissected from the flap, or if the patient had been obstructed, ensure nasogastric suction is maintained until the aspirated volumes suggest that gastric emptying has recovered, thus reducing any postoperative distension. Remove the drain after 48 hours and the sutures after 10 days. Instruct the patient to avoid strenuous exercise for at least 3 months. Give prophylactic antibiotics if a mesh has been used.

SPECIAL OPERATIVE HAZARD

Damage to the contents of the hernial sac.

COMPLICATIONS

1. Wound sepsis; this can be difficult to eradicate if a synthetic mesh has been used and may require removal of the mesh.
2. Wound haematoma; this will predispose to infection.
3. Recurrence of hernia.

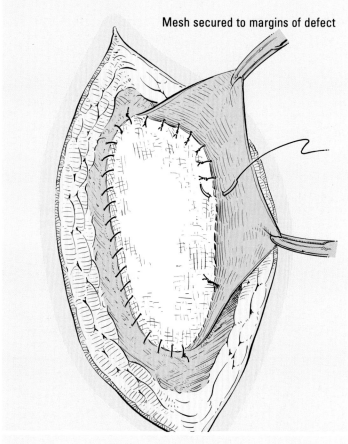

Mesh secured to margins of defect

Fig. 7.20

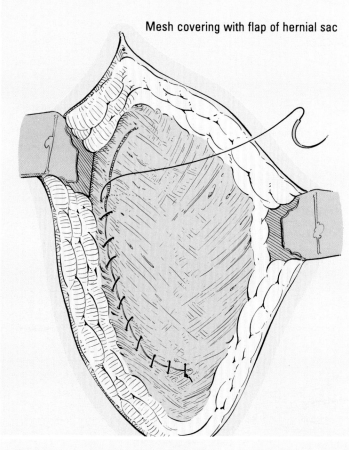

Mesh covering with flap of hernial sac

Fig. 7.21

Operative repair of an inguinal hernia is indicated for the control of symptoms and the prevention of strangulation.

PREOPERATIVE ASSESSMENT

1. Ensure that the clinical diagnosis is correct.
2. Exclude the possibility of either an additional hernia or intrascrotal pathology.
3. Check for chronic cough, chronic retention of urine and constipation, all of which predispose to an inguinal hernia and increase the risk of recurrence.
4. In cases of intestinal obstruction and strangulation, presenting with vomiting, pain and abdominal distention, ensure adequate resuscitation and rehydration. The principles of repair are the same in cases of strangulation, but the contents of the sac must be carefully inspected for viability prior to reduction.

RELEVANT ANATOMY

An understanding of the anatomy of the inguinal canal is essential (Fig. 7.22). It extends from the deep inguinal ring, a defect in the transversalis fascia lying 2 cm above the femoral pulse, and passes obliquely inferiorly, medially and anteriorly to end at the superficial inguinal ring, a defect in the external oblique aponeurosis which lies just above the pubic tubercle. The canal accommodates the ilio-inguinal nerve, the spermatic cord in the male, and the round ligament in the female. The principal constituents of the spermatic cord, which lies within the cremaster muscle and the internal spermatic fascia, are the vas deferens posteriorly, the testicular artery and the pampiniform plexus of testicular veins.

The floor of the inguinal canal is formed by the gutter-shaped inguinal ligament, which is derived from the upturned lower edge of the external oblique aponeurosis. The ligament passes from the anterior superior iliac spine to the pubic tubercle.

The inferior epigastric artery forms the immediate medial boundary of the deep inguinal ring. It arises from the external iliac artery and passes upwards into the rectus sheath. The posterior wall of the inguinal canal is formed laterally by the transversalis fascia. The fibres of the conjoint tendon, which lies in front of the cord laterally, arise from the internal oblique and transversus abdominis muscles and arch over the cord to form the medial part of the posterior wall of the inguinal canal, and insert onto the pubic crest.

Behind the cord a direct inguinal hernia will bulge through the transversalis fascia in the posterior wall of the canal. An oblique indirect inguinal hernia will pass through the internal ring, usually within the coverings of the cord, anterior to the vas deferens. The latter therefore arises lateral to the inferior epigastric vessels and passes obliquely along the inguinal canal into the scrotum.

OPERATION

Preparation

Place the patient supine and cleanse and drape the inguinal region. Inguinal hernia repair can be performed under general, spinal or local anaesthesia.

Incision

Make a skin crease incision 2 cm above the inguinal ligament, from above the pubic tubercle to above the femoral pulse. Open Scarpa's fascia to reveal the external oblique aponeurosis which is incised in the line of its fibres (Fig. 7.23). This opens the inguinal canal and reveals the ilio-inguinal nerve which is preserved. The presence or absence of an indirect sac is established and the strength of the posterior wall is assessed with a finger.

Operative technique

1. Mobilize the spermatic cord (Fig. 7.24) and identify the vas deferens, inguinal ligament, pubic tubercle and, if present, the indirect hernial sac.

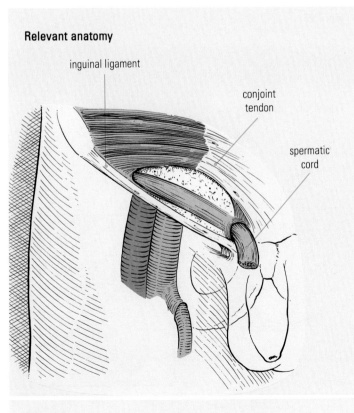

Relevant anatomy

inguinal ligament

conjoint tendon

spermatic cord

Fig. 7.22

2. If an indirect hernial sac is present, dissect the sac free from the cord (Fig. 7.25), pick it up with haemostats and open it; in a large hernia the fundus can be left undissected. Reduce the contents of the sac into the peritoneal cavity and clean the neck of the sac with a dental swab.

3. Twist the sac up to the neck and transfix the neck with 00 chromic catgut (Fig. 7.26). The remainder of the sac is then excised. Perform a Bassini repair to reinforce the posterior wall (see below).

For the repair of a small direct hernia (Fig. 7.27) use the

Incision of external oblique aponeurosis

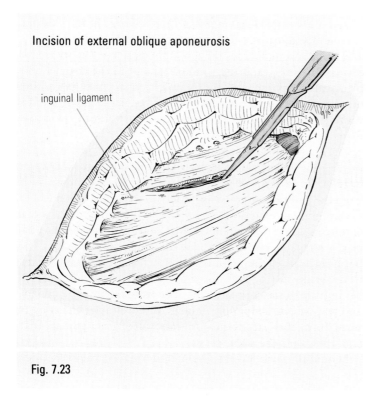

inguinal ligament

Fig. 7.23

Dissection of sac

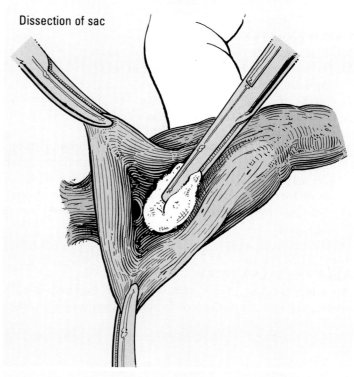

Fig. 7.25

Mobilization of cord

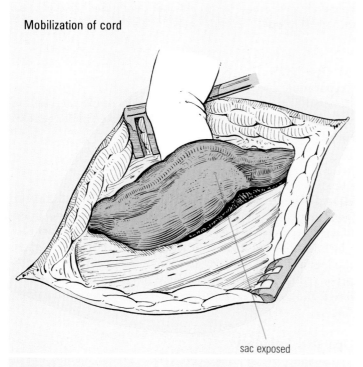

sac exposed

Fig. 7.24

Transfixion of sac

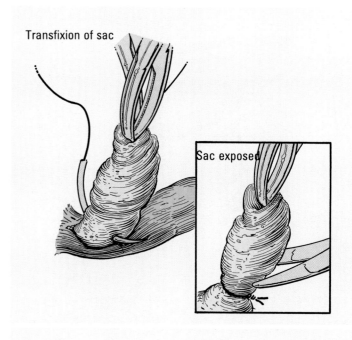

Sac exposed

Fig. 7.26

Bassini procedure with Tanner's slide. Larger defects may be difficult to repair adequately with this technique, due to attenuation of the tissues, and so a darn is inserted in the posterior wall of the inguinal canal to reinforce it. If the direct sac has a narrow neck, a herniotomy may be necessary with transfixion and excision of the sac. To reinforce the posterior wall of the inguinal canal, a non-absorbable suture such as 00 nylon suture is used either as a single ended or as a looped suture according to preference.

4. Place the first suture firmly into the periosteum overlying the pubic tubercle and through the medial end of the conjoint tendon, just at the insertion into the pubis.

5. Tie the suture, or lock it if the stitch is a loop, and run it laterally until the deep ring is reached, picking up the inner rolled edge of the inguinal ligament and opposing it to the conjoint tendon (Fig. 7.28). Use just enough tension to plicate the sac and avoid the inferior epigastric vessels which lie at the medial border of the deep ring. Sutures should not be placed deeply or they may puncture the bowel, bladder or femoral vessels. Do not strangulate the spermatic cord; it should be possible to insert the tip of a little finger into the deep ring alongside the cord after insertion of the suture.

7. Tie the nylon when the medial border of the ring is reached and perform a Tanner's slide by making a 4cm, vertical incision in the anterior rectus sheath so that the muscle can be seen bulging underneath. This is performed to relieve tension on the repair and discourage the stitches from

cutting out when the patient strains or coughs. To tighten the deep ring an additional suture can be placed lateral to the emerging spermatic cord.

8. If the posterior wall of the inguinal canal is very atrophic perform a darn between the lower border of the inguinal ligament and the firm tendinous portion of the conjoint tendon (Fig. 7.29). Ensure that the stitches are loose; they can be interlocked by taking each suture through the inguinal ligament and then under the last stitch before picking up the healthy conjoint tendon above. Avoid opposing these two structures as this would create tension causing the sutures to cut out. If the level of sutures in the tissue is varied with each stitch, producing a sawtooth pattern, the tissues should not split along the line of its fibres.

9. Tie off the suture once the pubic tubercle is reached and the darn is complete.

10. If the tissue is very poor or for large defects, use a sheet of synthetic material sewn to the margins of the defect to repair them.

Wound closure and dressing

Close the wound in layers with 00 chromic catgut using a continuous stitch for the external oblique aponeurosis as far as the emerging cord (i.e. to the lateral edge of the external inguinal ring) and the superficial fascia. Interrupted sutures are used for the skin and a dry dressing is applied.

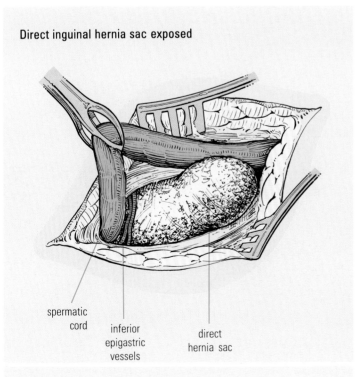

Direct inguinal hernia sac exposed

spermatic cord

inferior epigastric vessels

direct hernia sac

Fig. 7.27

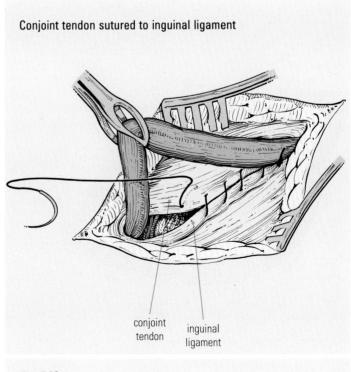

Conjoint tendon sutured to inguinal ligament

conjoint tendon

inguinal ligament

Fig. 7.28

POSTOPERATIVE CARE

The patient is allowed to get up the next day and discharged from hospital on the second day if all is well. The stitches are removed on the eighth day and the patient can return to normal activity, including work, after 2 weeks. Heavy lifting, however, is discouraged for 3 months, after which time the repair will be reinforced with mature collagen.

SPECIAL OPERATIVE HAZARDS

1. Damage to the vas deferens.
2. Damage to either the testicular artery or the pampiniform plexus of veins draining the testis.
3. Damage to hernial contents, such as bowel, bladder or omentum. This is a special risk if the hernia is found to be of a sliding and not a simple type. In sliding hernias, bowel or bladder form the posterior wall of the hernial sac and in such cases the sac must be excised and the viscera returned to the abdominal cavity.
4. Damage to the ilio-inguinal nerve will cause an area of sensory loss in the lower groin and scrotum.

COMPLICATIONS

1. Haematoma of the wound.
2. Infection of the wound.
3. Recurrence of the hernia; this can occur either before the wound has been closed or at any time after, even after many years. It may be due to either a haematoma or infection of the wound, or both, or may be due to a bad repair, poor tissues or excessive postoperative coughing or straining.

Completed repair

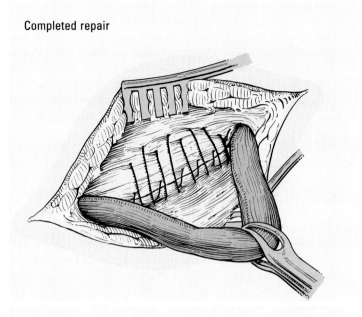

Fig. 7.29

4. Testicular atrophy from damage to the cord.
5. Development of a femoral hernia following the widening of the femoral canal by picking up the inguinal ligament during the repair.

Femoral Hernia Repair

A femoral hernia is a protrusion through the femoral canal, medial to the femoral vessels. The hernial sac may contain either omentum or bowel, and part of its medial wall may be formed by the bladder. When palpated the major component is usually extraperitoneal fat, but repair is advisable because the neck of the canal is narrow and its walls inelastic, resulting in a considerable risk of strangulation. The hernia is often irreducible. This type of hernia is less common than the inguinal variety and is four times more likely to occur in females than males. Most cases are found in the middle aged or the elderly. A Richter's hernia, where only one wall of the bowel protrudes into the sac, is particularly common in this site (inset to Fig. 7.30), and it is dangerous because peritonitis can occur without previous obstructive symptoms.

PREOPERATIVE ASSESSMENT
1. Ensure the clinical diagnosis is correct.

2. Ensure that the bladder is empty.
3. In cases of obstruction and strangulation pass a nasogastric tube and ensure adequate fluid resuscitation.

RELEVANT ANATOMY
The femoral canal lies behind the inguinal ligament, which forms its anterior boundary. Posteriorly is the pectineal line of the pubis, to which the pectineus muscle and its covering fascia (pectineal ligament of Astley Cooper) are attached. Medially the femoral canal is bounded by the crescentic edge of the lacunar (Gimbernat's) ligament, whilst laterally the femoral vein lies within the femoral sheath (Fig. 7.30). The femoral canal transmits the efferent lymphatic vessels from the leg and contains the lymph node of Cloquet which drains either the clitoris or the glans penis.

The femoral canal is the space into which the femoral vein can expand during exercise. The neck of a femoral hernia will

Relevant anatomy

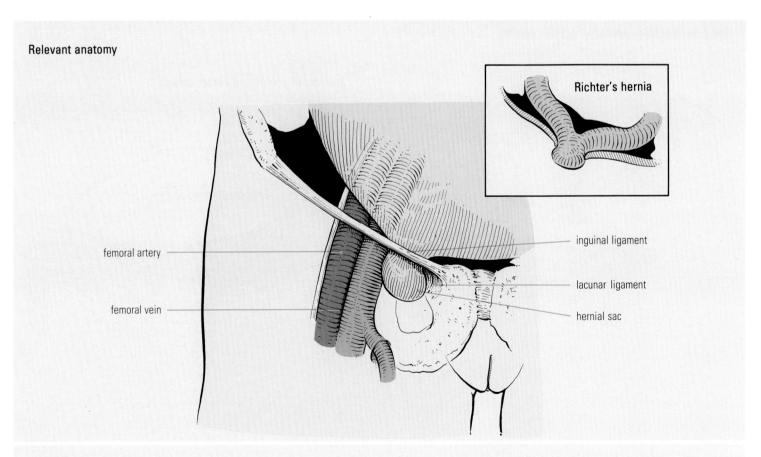

Richter's hernia

femoral artery

femoral vein

inguinal ligament

lacunar ligament

hernial sac

Fig. 7.30

7.15

Choices for skin incisions

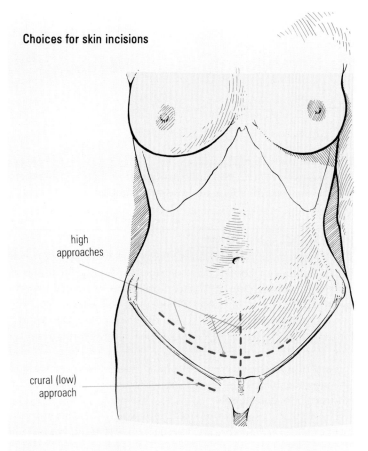

high
approaches

crural (low)
approach

Fig. 7.31

therefore lie below and lateral to the pubic tubercle. Once it has passed through the femoral canal, the hernia bulges into the femoral triangle. It may then turn up towards the inguinal ligament but it is prevented from overlying this by the attachment of fascia lata, unless it passes through the fascia via the cribiform opening for the saphenous vein. In 30% of patients, the obturator artery arises from the inferior epigastric instead of the internal iliac artery. The obturator artery will then pass to one side of the femoral canal, usually laterally. If it lies medially it is particularly vulnerable to surgical damage since it crosses the lacunar ligament, which may have to be divided in order to reduce the hernia.

OPERATION

There are three common approaches to the femoral canal (Fig. 7.31). The crural (low) approach described by Lockwood (see later in this chapter), which exposes the canal from below. It has the advantages of being relatively simple and can be performed under local anaesthesia, but has the major disadvantage that it is usually impossible to deal with strangulated contents. The inguinal operation, or high operation of Lotheissen, approaches the femoral canal from above. This dissection proceeds as for an inguinal hernia repair, except that the transversalis fascia is opened. The hernia is then reduced and its neck transfixed. The inguinal ligament is sutured to the pectineal ligament medially and the inguinal canal is then reconstituted. It has the disadvantage of disrupting a normal inguinal canal and does not provide access to strangulated contents as well as

Sac dislodged from defect, ready to be opened

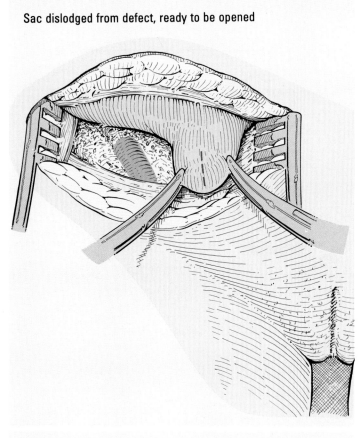

Fig. 7.32

Sac closed, margins of defect defined

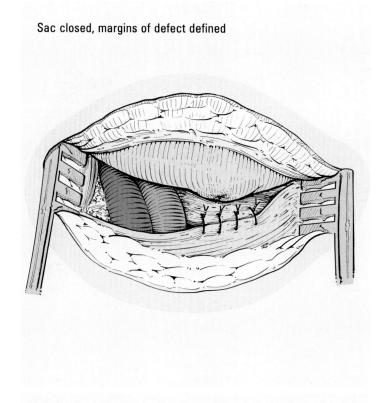

Fig. 7.33

the third option, the McEvedy (preperitoneal) approach, which will be discussed in detail next.

McEVEDY APPROACH

Preparation
The bladder should be emptied, and the anaesthetized patient placed supine before being cleansed and draped.

Incisions
1. A bilateral hernia can be approached through either a midline suprapubic or a Pfannesteil incision (Fig. 7.31). The rectus abdominis muscles are then separated in the midline to expose the peritoneum.
2. For a unilateral hernia make a transverse incision 6cm above and parallel to the inguinal ligament over the lateral border of the rectus sheath. Divide the subcutaneous tissues to expose the external oblique aponeurosis and rectus sheath.
3. Make a vertical incision in the lateral border of the rectus sheath and expose the peritoneum, which is not opened.

Operative technique
1. Using blunt dissection sweep the peritoneum and bladder away from the back of the anterior abdominal wall until the region of the femoral canal is exposed and the neck of the sac is identified. An excellent view can usually be obtained by this approach.

2. Apply gentle traction on the sac to reduce it, combined if necessary with pressure on the hernia from below. If reduction is difficult, the edge of the lacunar ligament can be divided.

3. Open the sac between haemostats (Fig. 7.32), taking care not to injure the bladder if it forms part of the medial wall. In cases with strangulation or obstruction inspect the contents and, if necessary, resect any non-viable bowel. If there is any doubt, wrap the bowel in a warm pack for 10 minutes and reinspect.

4. Transfix the neck of the sac with a catgut suture and excise any redundant peritoneum (Fig. 7.33).

5. Define the margins of the canal and close it medially by apposition of the inguinal and pectineal ligaments. It is essential that the most lateral suture is placed correctly. If it is placed too far laterally, the femoral vein may be obstructed, whereas if it is too medial, a recurrent hernia may develop. Gently retract the femoral vein laterally whilst the sutures are inserted. It is advisable to place all the sutures before tying them to confirm that positioning is satisfactory (Fig. 7.34). A non-absorbable suture (e.g. 00 Ethibond) is used and a J-shaped needle facilitates accurate placement. When completed, the femoral vein should not be constricted and the femoral canal should just admit the tip of the little finger (Fig. 7.35).

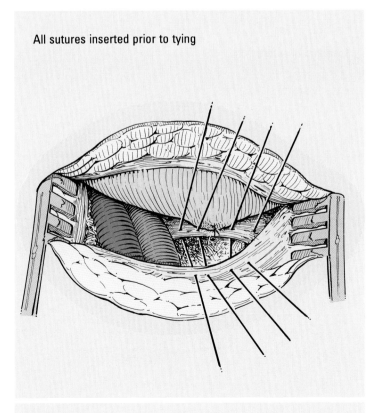

All sutures inserted prior to tying

Fig. 7.34

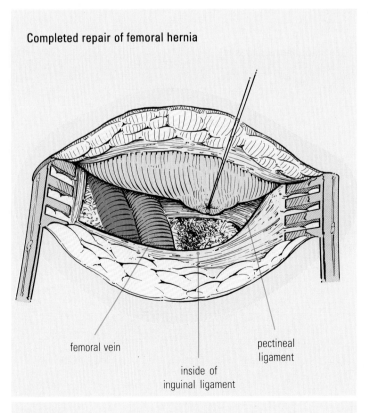

Completed repair of femoral hernia

femoral vein   pectineal ligament

inside of inguinal ligament

Fig. 7.35

7.17

Wound closure and dressing
Repair the rectus sheath with continuous loop nylon sutures. Close the subcutaneous tissues with catgut and the skin with interrupted or a subcuticular stitch. Apply a waterproof dressing. Drainage is unnecessary.

THE CRURAL APPROACH
Preparation
This is the same as above, but if necessary can be performed under local anaesthesia using infiltration with 1% lignocaine.

Incision
Make a skin crease incision just below the inguinal ligament overlying the hernia (Fig. 7.31). The smooth extraperitoneal fat is usually obvious. Insert a Travers' self-retaining retractor.

Operative technique
1. Dissect the hernial sac from the subcutaneous tissues.

2. Identify the boundaries of the femoral canal and the neck of the sac (Fig. 7.36).

3. Open the sac on its lateral side to avoid damage to the bladder. If the contents are gangrenous it may be impossible to perform a resection without opening the abdomen through a separate incision. If the contents are viable, reduce the contents and transfix the neck of the sac. Divide the lacunar ligament or split the neck of the sac if the reduction is difficult.

4. Retract the femoral vein laterally and suture the inguinal and pectineal ligaments as described for the McEvedy approach, but from below (Fig. 7.37).

Wound closure and dressing
Close the subcutaneous tissues and skin in separate layers. Again, drainage is unnecessary.

POSTOPERATIVE CARE
The patient is allowed up the following day, unless a bowel resection has been required, and is usually discharged within 2 or 3 days of surgery. The sutures should be removed on the seventh day and the patient is advised to avoid heavy lifting for 6 weeks if either the extraperitoneal or inguinal approach has been used.

SPECIAL OPERATIVE HAZARDS
1. Damage to the femoral vein, bladder or hernial sac contents.
2. Failure to identify a Richter's hernia.
3. Bleeding from an abnormal obturator artery.

COMPLICATIONS
1. Wound haematoma/infection.
2. Recurrence, which is very rare.

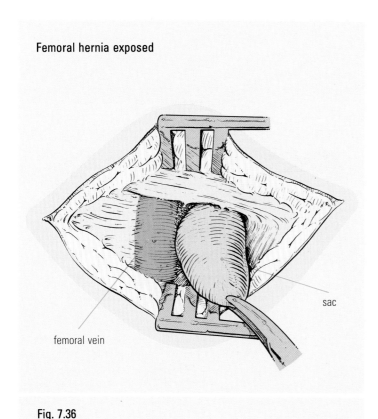

Femoral hernia exposed

sac

femoral vein

Fig. 7.36

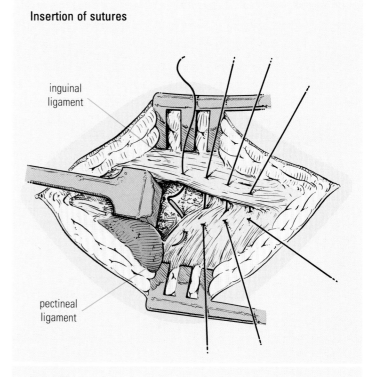

Insertion of sutures

inguinal ligament

pectineal ligament

Fig. 7.37

8

Surgery for Trauma

Burr Holes and Craniotomy for Trauma

PREOPERATIVE ASSESSMENT

1. Determine the site of the haematoma; the majority of haematomas occur on the same side as the dilated pupil or skull fracture, although hemiparesis can be a false localizing sign.
2. Most patients with an extradural haematoma have a lucid interval and then deteriorate. This type of haematoma can be seen as an elliptical clot on the CT scan.
3. The majority of patients with acute subdural haematomas are unconscious from the outset. Such haematomas can be seen as a crescent-shaped clot on the CT scan.
4. Acute subdural haematomas are often associated with intracerebral contusion or haematoma.
5. Question whether the patient is deteriorating too rapidly to be transferred to a neurosurgical unit. Performed efficiently and correctly, evacuation of an acute intracranial haematoma is life-saving procedure. However, the inexperienced surgeon may be ill-equipped to deal with bleeding from the contused brain, and may provoke further haemorrhage. This not only wastes valuable time by delaying the transfer to a specialist centre, but may compound the problem by poor siting of the flap, or by exacerbating brain swelling. In this respect the acute subdural haematoma can be much more difficult to treat than an extradural haematoma.

RELEVANT ANATOMY

The course and surface markings of the middle meningeal artery are shown in Fig. 8.1. It enters the skull via the foramen spinosum, located on the floor of the middle cranial fossa, approximately 2 cm medial to the junction between the middle and posterior thirds of the zygomatic arch. The site of bleeding is usually where the fracture line crosses the vascular marking seen on the skull X-ray. Occasionally, the fracture extends across the floor of the middle fossa and bleeding occurs near its origin. In either case, the expanding haematoma strips the dura from the inner table of the skull.

Bleeding into the subdural space occurs from either the disruption of cortical vessels, from the tearing of bridging veins entering the cortical venous sinuses, or from the sinus itself. The clot may spread to involve wide areas of the hemisphere because of the extent of the subdural space.

Relevant anatomy

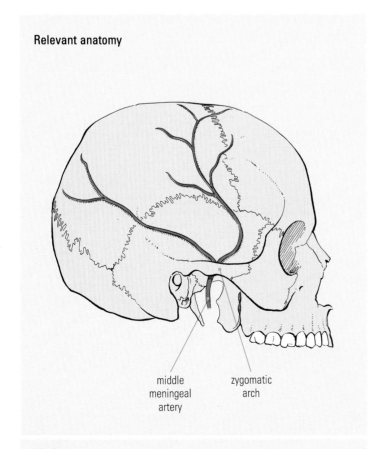

middle
meningeal
artery

zygomatic
arch

Fig. 8.1

Site of incisions for burr holes

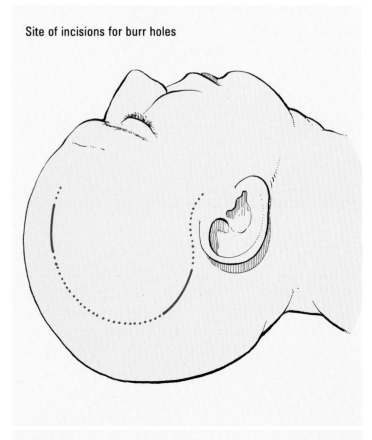

Fig. 8.2

OPERATIONS

Burr holes are used to locate the haematoma when the diagnosis is in doubt and also to verify its position. If increased exposure is required most neurosurgeons prefer to turn a flap, however inexperienced surgeons generally favour limited craniotomy.

BURR HOLES

Preparation

The scalp is shaved, cleansed and then draped over a wide area to allow increased exposure if this becomes necessary. An adhesive drape is convenient to hold the towels in place. The patient is placed supine with the head slightly elevated and turned to one side. A sandbag under the shoulders reduces rotation of the neck and therefore venous congestion. A skin marker can be used to mark the position of the incisions.

Infiltration of the subcutaneous and subgaleal layers with dilute lignocaine and adrenaline solution reduces bleeding, facilitates dissection, and may allow the operation to be performed under local anaesthetic.

Incision

1. Make a 3 cm incision cutting straight down to the bone in a position that can be incorporated into a craniotomy if necessary. Incisions near the base of the skull are made coronally, and those near the vertex sagittally. If an extradural haematoma is anticipated, site the incision in the temporal region. For subdural haematoma place the burr holes in the frontal and parietal regions (Fig. 8.2).
2. Strip the pericranium from the bone using a periosteal elevator.

Operative technique

1. Insert a small self-retaining retractor and open it widely; this will usually control scalp bleeding but diathermy can be used on any persistently bleeding vessels.

2. Using a 16-mm perforator on a Hudson brace, drill until the inner table of the skull is just perforated (Fig. 8.3). Do not lean on the brace in case the inner table gives way; gentle pressure is applied with the arm. Progress can be checked by removing the drill, but as the inner table is pierced the tip of the drill is no longer engaged in the bone and the feel of the drill changes. The skull is very thin in the temporal region.

3. Change to a reaming burr and enlarge the hole until the sides are parallel (Fig. 8.4).

4. Control bleeding from the bone edge with bone wax, and from the dura with light diathermy.

5. If an extradural haematoma is encountered either convert the exposure into a craniotomy (see later in this chapter), or enlarge the burr hole using bone nibblers until the bleeding point is identified and can be diathermized. When using the nibblers only take small bites as the thin bone below may fracture along the base of the middle cranial fossa.

6. If no clot is encountered pick up the outer layer of the dura with a sharp right-angled hook and lift it away from the

Burr hole deepened to inner table of skull

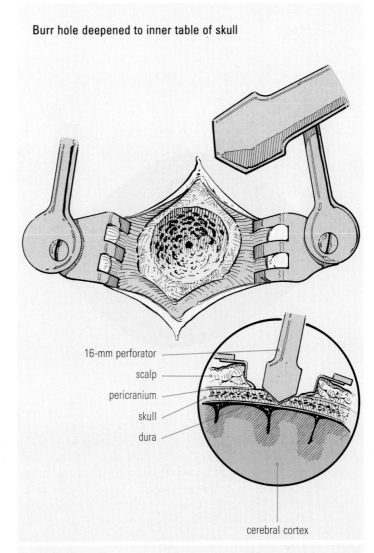

16-mm perforator
scalp
pericranium
skull
dura

cerebral cortex

Fig. 8.3

Enlarge hole with reaming burr

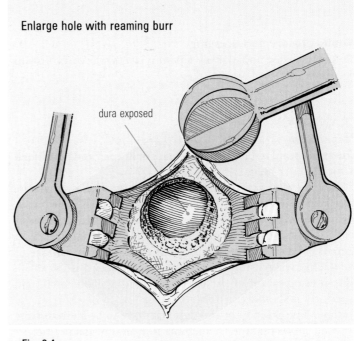

dura exposed

Fig. 8.4

Incision of dura

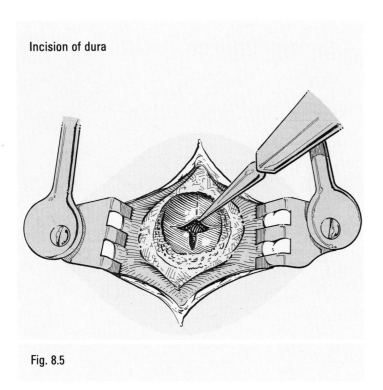

Fig. 8.5

cruciate fashion, and use diathermy on the dural edges (Fig. 8.5). Allow any clot to exude under its own pressure; the brain is soft enough to be removed with a sucker. If no clot is is soft enough to be removed with a sucker. If no clot is encountered, either place a second burr hole elsewhere, or explore the other side. Do not place a suction drain in the subdural space. If bleeding continues or the clot is not adequately evacuated, turn a flap.

7. Ensure haemostasis from the bone and dura. If a craniectomy has been performed hitch the dura up to the pericranium (see later in this chapter).

Wound closure and dressing

Closure of galea and skin in separate layers will control scalp bleeding.

CRANIOTOMY
Preparation

The entire scalp is shaved and the patient draped and positioned as for the burr holes.

Mark the flap with Bonney's blue. A large flap is advisable, particularly if an acute subdural haematoma is anticipated, because lobectomy may be required to achieve haemostasis from a burst lobe, or to provide an internal decompression if there is extensive brain swelling. The most common mistake of the inexperienced surgeon is to turn a flap which is too small. The inferior extent of the incision is the zygomatic arch, and anteriorly it should reach the hair line just to one side of the midline. The position of the flap may have to be altered if the CT scan shows that the haematoma is in an unusual position.

The subcutaneous and subgaleal layers are infiltrated with dilute adrenaline solution.

Incision
1. Incise the skin and galea in short lengths, with the surgeon's and the assistant's fingers exerting pressure either side of the wound to temporarily control bleeding until artery forceps are placed on the galea, or Raney clips are applied (Fig. 8.6). Do not cut straight down to the bone as the pericranium is required later to secure the bone flap.
2. Raise the scalp flap from the pericranium by gentle sharp dissection, and cover the flap with a moist swab.
3. Incise the pericranium and muscle using cutting diathermy, leaving a pedicle intact inferiorly to vascularize the bone flap. Insert two self-retaining retractors in the temporalis muscle and reflect the pericranium back to about 1 cm from the line where the bone will be cut.

Operative technique
1. Site the burr holes inferiorly on either side of the pedicle, and at intervals around the flap. Approximately five will be needed (Fig. 8.6).

2. Free the dura from the inner table of the skull using a blunt Adson dissector; this is essential in order to avoid tearing the dura and the underlying cortex when cutting the bone.

3. Using either a dural guide and Gigli saw, or an air-driven craniotome, cut between the burr holes. The saw should be

Sawing between burr holes with Gigli saw

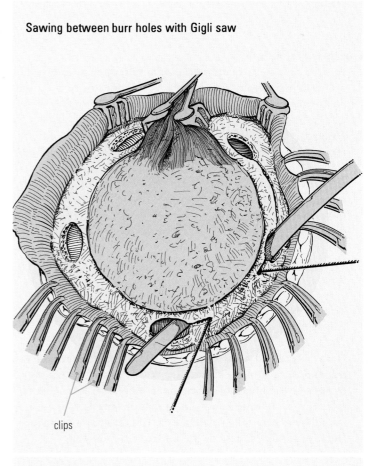

clips

Fig. 8.6

Flap reflected on pedicle of temporalis muscle

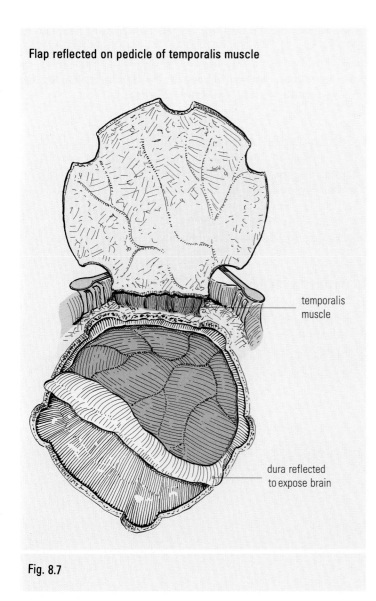

temporalis
muscle

dura reflected
to expose brain

Fig. 8.7

angled outwards to bevel the flap so that it will seat when it is replaced (Fig. 8.6). The bone at the base of the flap is not cut with the saw, but the edges are nibbled until the remaining bridge will fracture easily when the flap is elevated.

4. Elevate the flap, freeing the dura from the underside as it is raised, and nibble away the rough edges below where the bone was fractured with nibblers. Seal the flap with bone wax and cover with a damp swab.

5. Use diathermy to stop the bleeding from the middle meningeal artery and, if necessary, nibble away more bone.

6. If the clot has been removed and underlying dura is slack, indicating no underlying subdural haematoma, proceed with wound closure and dressing.

7. Otherwise, open the dura with a sharp hook and knife. The dural flap should be U-shaped, and based superiorly to avoid cutting across the veins draining into the superior saggital sinus (Fig. 8.7). Take care not to damage the underlying brain when opening the dura. Diathermize the dural edges.

8. Remove the clot by irrigation with warm Ringer's solution; do *not* use suction directly on the exposed brain. Coagulate bleeding points with bipolar diathermy or use silver clips, and when all bleeding is controlled, cover the cortex with a sheet of haemostatic gauze.

Wound closure and dressing
1. At the margins of the craniotomy hitch the dura up to the pericranium at intervals, thereby preventing the develop-

Sawing between burr holes with Gigli saw

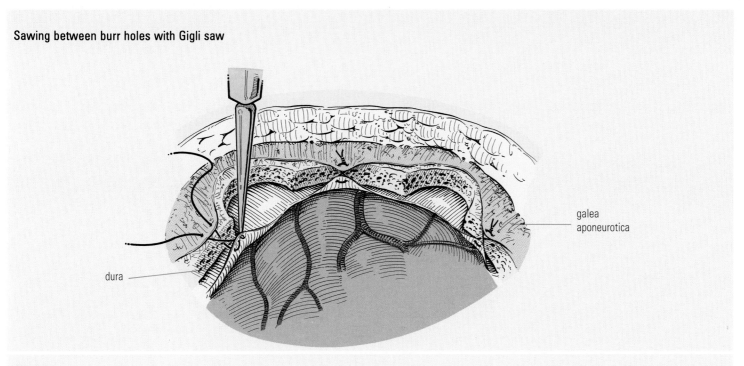

galea
aponeurotica

dura

Fig. 8.8

ment of a postoperative extradural haematoma (Fig. 8.8). Lift up the dura to avoid piercing the underlying brain and thereby provoke further bleeding, and then close with interrupted sutures. If the brain is very swollen replace the dura but do not close it. Make relieving incisions at the margins of the dural flap to reduce pressure on the brain where it may herniate through the defect.

2. Cover the dura with a sheet of haemostatic gauze and replace the bone flap. Use interrupted sutures to oppose the muscle and pericranium at intervals to hold the flap in place. If the dura is open and the brain is very swollen, the bone flap can be removed and the pericranium alone closed. The bone should be saved to act as a template for future cranioplasty. A suction drain is left in the subgaleal space, and the scalp closed in two layers.

3. Apply a firm head bandage.

POSTOPERATIVE CARE

A period of postoperative ventilation and fluid restriction will help to control cerebral oedema. Careful neurological observation is essential to check for evidence of further haematoma or brain swelling. Antibiotics may be given, but prophylactic anticonvulsants are not necessary following burr holes or evacuation of an extradural haematoma. The subgaleal drain is removed within 48 hours and the sutures at 7 days.

SPECIAL OPERATIVE HAZARDS

1. Incorrect positioning of the flap or burr holes.
2. Turning too small a flap.
3. Plunging with the Hudson brace.
4. Damage to the cerebral cortex when opening the dura, using suction, or inserting hitch stitches.
5. Failure to achieve meticulous haemostasis.

COMPLICATIONS

1. Further haematoma.
2. Cerebral oedema.
3. Infection.
4. Epilepsy.

Drainage of the Pleura and Pericardium

Intercostal drains can be inserted into the pleural space under local anaesthetic with ease and safety on the ward. Such drains are introduced to drain air or fluid. Routine postoperative drains do not need to be inserted by a closed technique and are considered in the sections on surgical access.

Pericardial drainage can be achieved easily under local anaesthesia by a small tube placed percutaneously into the pericardial cavity. Such a procedure will yield diagnostic information (blood after trauma or malignant cells in tumour involvement) or may give relief from cardiac tamponade.

PREOPERATIVE ASSESSMENT

1. Assess the indications for the use of intercostal or pericardial drains.
2. Determine the size of the drain required. When selecting intercostal drains there is a temptation to insert one that is too small. For draining pus or blood a large, 28 or 30 Fr drain is used, and even when draining an air space a large tube is best since air leaks can be considerable and drains excite a serous reaction which can itself lead to tube blockage.
3. Select the correct side and site for drain insertion. In an emergency drains may be inserted on clinical grounds alone, but usually a chest X-ray is taken before inserting intercostal drains.
4. Ensure an underwater seal is prepared and wall suction is available when using intercostal drains.
5. Evaluate the evidence for a clinically significant effusion (e.g. pulsus paradoxus) before inserting a pericardial drain. Echocardiography is used to confirm the degree of cardiac embarrassment, the position of the effusion and its consistency before using pericardial drains. Loculated effusions are better dealt with by formal pericardial fenestration.

RELEVANT ANATOMY

A knowledge of anatomy before using an intercostal drain will help minimize damage to intrathoracic structures. The intercostal drain should be inserted over the upper border of the rib below the space selected to avoid injury to the intercostal vessels and nerves which lie in the groove beneath each rib. Intra-abdominal structures will not be harmed if it is remembered that the domes of the diaphragm rise high up within the rib cage. The left hemidiaphragm with the spleen beneath it rises to the fifth rib at rest, and the right hemidiaphgram with the liver beneath it rises to the fourth space. A hemidiaphragm may be raised on the side of intrathoracic or abdominal disease and this may be hidden radiographically if an effusion is present.

The safest, easiest and most useful site of insertion for the intercostal drain is the fourth intercostal space in the midaxillary line. Drainage of localized collections may require the insertion of drains at specific sites and under such circumstances a tube may be guided using X-ray or ultrasound. Once an intercostal drain has been passed into the chest it may be directed as it is advanced into a basal position to drain fluid or into an apical position to drain air.

The pericardial sac lies in contact with the inner surface of the thoracic cage in its inferior part and is therefore easily tapped by a needle passed into it from just beneath the xiphisternum. Alternatively a small left anterior thoracotomy through the fourth intercostal space brings the surgeon down onto the pericardium directly, the lung being displaced laterally by its distension.

INTERCOSTAL DRAINAGE
Preparation

Ensure all your equipment including the underwater seal apparatus is to hand before starting and display a chest X-ray to identify the side requiring drainage.

Position the patient: for insertion into the midaxillary line the patient should lie supine with his arm elevated and his hand behind his head (Fig. 8.9). Give the patient a full explanation of the procedure and prepare a suitable area of skin with antiseptic.

Identify the chosen intercostal space (the second rib is easily located at the junction of manubrium and sternal body) and infiltrate it generously with 1% plain lignocaine. If the syringe is aspirated as it is advanced it will fill with fluid or air when it enters the pleural space.

Position of patient

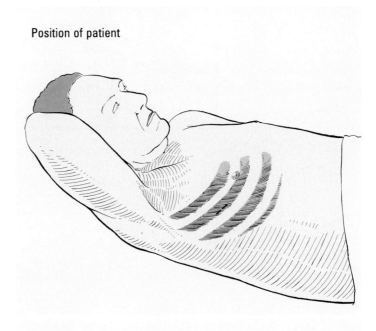

Fig. 8.9

Incision

Make a generous stab incision in the line of the intercostal space with a scalpel blade. This incision is deepened by a combination of blunt and sharp dissection using scissors or a haemostat until the pleura is reached and opened (Fig. 8.10). A finger may now be inserted into the thoracic cavity to confirm separation of the lung from the chest wall.

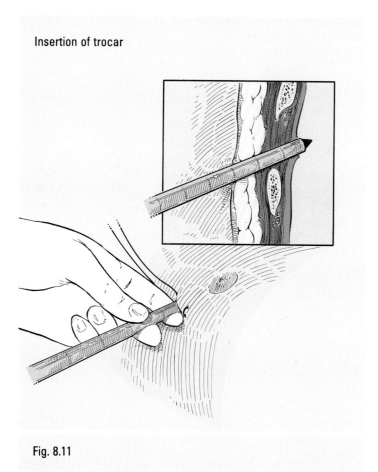

Deepening incision with a pair of scissors

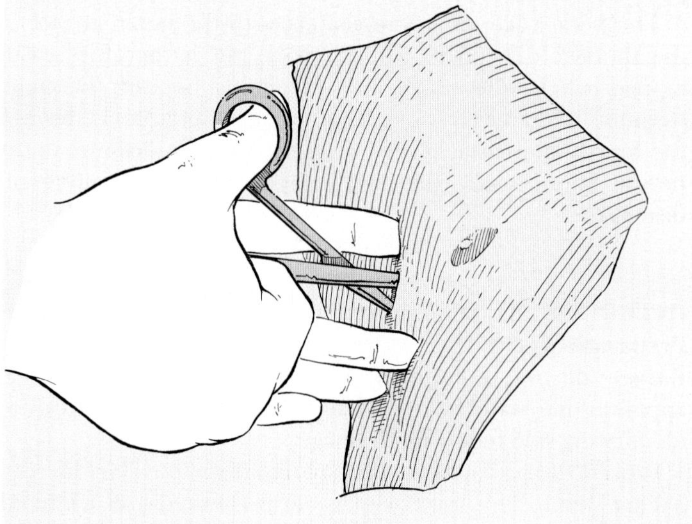

Fig. 8.10

Insertion of trocar

Fig. 8.11

Technique

1. Place a 00 braided nylon suture in the skin by the incision to tie the drain in position and a 3/0 nylon mattress suture with its ends left long and untied to close the incision when the drain is removed.

2. Take the selected drain: a flexible tube with end and side holes and a radio-opaque marker line. A trocar is present within the tube and this gives it rigidity for insertion and enables the tube to be 'directed' within the chest to apical or basal positions. The sharp point on the end of the trocar can inflict considerable damage and it is for this reason that a generous incision is made so that the tube may be inserted with minimal force (Fig. 8.11). As soon as the tube enters the chest withdraw the trocar slightly so that its point is guarded and direct the tube apically or basally as desired. Now advance the drain over the trocar.

3. Withdraw the trocar completely (Fig. 8.12) and connect the drain to rubber tubing leading to an underwater seal. There will now be a rush of air or fluid into the bottle and the fluid within the tubing will be seen to 'swing' with respiration.

4. Tie the tube in place and place a gauze dressing around the exit site of the drain.

5. A chest X-ray is taken to confirm satisfactory positioning of the drain and full expansion of the lung.

Management of chest drains

The drain should be connected at all times to an underwater

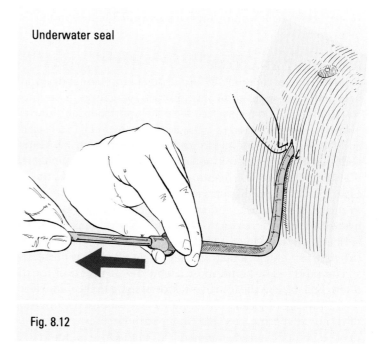

Underwater seal

Fig. 8.12

Drainage in progress

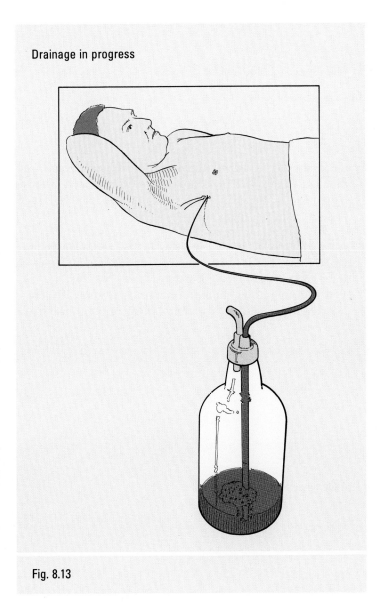

Fig. 8.13

being removed as soon as the new position has been achieved.

Drains are removed once postoperative blood loss has stopped, an effusion has drained, or the lung has expanded after a pneumothorax. When the tubes are draining air they should be left in place and on suction until the air leak stops. If there has been no leak for 36 to 48 hours and a chest X-ray shows the continued full expansion of the lung, the drains may be removed. There is no need to clamp the drains during this time.

When the time comes to remove the drain the patient is given an appropriate dose of an intramuscular opiate and inhales an oxygen/nitrous oxide mix. Cut the anchoring suture and withdraw the drain with a single swift pull during forced expiration. Use the nylon suture placed before the insertion of the drain to seal the hole and apply a gauze dressing. The sutures may be removed after 5 days.

SPECIAL OPERATIVE HAZARDS
1. Haemorrhage from intercostal vessels.
2. Damage to intrathoracic or intra-abdominal structures from injudicious use of the trocar.
3. Incomplete expansion of the lung due to misplacement of a drain or inadequate suction.

COMPLICATIONS
1. Tension pneumothorax due to clot within a drain or inappropriate use of clamps.
2. Introduction of infection into an effusion.

PERICARDIAL DRAINAGE FOR PERICARDIOCENTESIS
Preparation
A full explanation is given to the patient who is sat at 45° to the horizontal and the area of skin around the xiphisternum is prepared with antiseptic. The track is infiltrated with 1% plain lignocaine just to the left of the xiphisternum upwards and backwards at 45°. A definite 'give' in resistance will be felt as the pericardial cavity is entered.

Technique
1. Aspiration will now confirm the position of the effusion.

2. Introduce a wider bore needle or fine flexible catheter along this path.

3. Take samples or completely drain the effusion.

seal. This allows fluid and air to leave the chest but prevents air passing back in thus keeping the lung expanded (Fig. 8.13). A proprietary defoaming agent should be added to the fluid together with an antiseptic.

Drains should be routinely placed on suction with the free tube leading out of the underwater seal bottle connected to a high volume, low pressure suction device (wall suction is ideal) at 13 kPa.

Clamping drains increases the risk of a tension pneumothorax and this practice is therefore reserved for transferring the patient from the bed to a stretcher for transport, the clamps

Management of Abdominal Trauma

The successful management of trauma patients requires a methodical multidisciplinary approach to their assessment and treatment.

PREOPERATIVE ASSESSMENT

1. Assess and secure the airway, clearing any obstruction and ensuring adequate ventilation. A tension pneumothorax is drained and a sucking wound covered. Intubate and ventilate patients with flail wounds. Apply an oxygen mask if the patient has adequate self-ventilation.
2. Control external haemorrhage with pressure and cover compound fractures with iodine-soaked swabs.
3. Set up an intravenous infusion with a large-bore cannula in a peripheral vein and administer a balanced salt solution, or a colloid solution such as plasma if the patient is hypotensive. If peripheral venous access is difficult expose and cannulate the long saphenous vein at the ankle or insert a central line. Take blood for an urgent X-match.
4. Pass a nasogastric tube and insert a urinary catheter unless there are signs to suggest a urethral injury (see below).
5. Carefully examine the abdomen for signs of distention and peritoneal irritation.
6. Examine for neurological, vascular and orthopaedic injuries.
7. Perform the investigations indicated; these are listed below.

INVESTIGATIONS

1. An upright chest X-ray will yield information about the lungs, mediastinum, diaphragm, and show a pneumoperitoneum. A supine abdominal film may show retroperitoneal air, loss of psoas shadow and missile fragments.
2. CT scanning can be of great assistance in the diagnosis of abdominal trauma where physical examination is equivocal. Intravenous and oral contrast can be given and the examination allows evaluation of the solid abdominal organs, showing parenchymal disruption, contained haematoma and free fluid.
3. If there is an inability to void in cases with pelvic fractures, perform a urethrogram to exclude a urethral injury. This is suggested by blood at the urinary meatus and a high riding prostate on rectal examination. Do not insert a urethral catheter in such cases which may complete a partial rupture; instead use a suprapubic catheter.
4. An intravenous pyelogram should be performed in cases of haematuria. In the unstable patient a 'one shot' examination is used to check that there are two kidneys and that both are functioning without extravasation. Failure to visualize one kidney suggests a renal pedicle injury and an arteriogram is performed.
5. Patients with blunt abdominal trauma and equivocal abdominal findings or who are difficult to assess due to a head injury, or those with a persisting transfusion require-

ment should undergo diagnostic peritoneal lavage (see the next page). This procedure is contra-indicated in those patients with obvious trauma who cannot be stabilized; such patients require urgent laparotomy.

6. All high velocity missile injuries to the abdomen require laparotomy. Tissue disruption from the accompanying shock wave and cavitation may be extensive.
7. Penetrating injuries should undergo laparotomy if there is evisceration, pneumoperitoneum, shock or peritoneal irrita-

Abdominal paracentesis

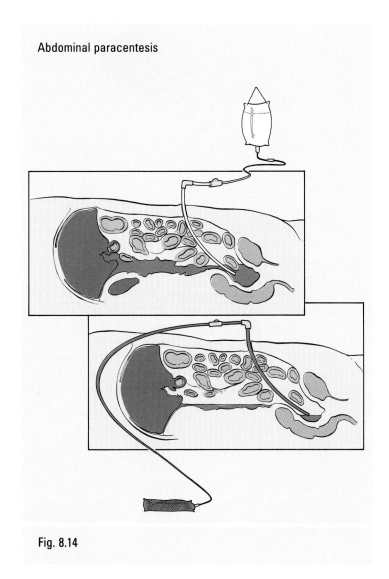

Fig. 8.14

tion. If none are present the wound is extended under local anaesthetic and locally explored under sterile conditions to allow its deeper limit to be established. If the peritoneum has been entered, diagnostic peritoneal lavage is performed.

RELEVANT ANATOMY

In trauma cases it is useful to regard the abdomen and chest as a single unit, sharing a common partition, the diaphragm. The abdominal cavity extends superiorly to the level of the nipples; missile and stab wounds which appear to have entered the chest may have damaged an intra-abdominal viscus, and chest wall trauma particularly associated with rib fractures may cause damage to the underlying abdominal organs, particularly the liver and spleen.

DIAGNOSTIC PERITONEAL LAVAGE

Preparation

With the patient supine cleanse the lower abdomen and apply drapes, leaving the midline from the umbilicus to the pubis exposed. Infiltrate the abdominal wall tissues with local anaesthetic (e.g. 1% lignocaine with 1:150,000 adrenaline). Open either a prepacked sterile temporary peritoneal dialysis catheter kit or a standard dialysis catheter.

Incision

With a scalpel make a 2–3 cm long midline incision one-third of the way between the umbilicus and the pubis and deepen it to the peritoneum if an open diagnostic peritoneal lavage is to be performed.

Operative technique

1. Under direct vision insert the lavage catheter into the abdomen and advance the catheter into the pelvis. Alternatively use one of the percutaneous paracentesis kits which are now available. These kits provide a needle which is inserted into the peritoneum and a guide wire which is fed down the needle. Withdraw the needle, thread a dilator over the wire, and then introduce the paracentesis catheter into the pelvis in Seldinger fashion over the guide wire. Another alternative is to nick the skin and insert a temporary peritoneal dialysis catheter which is supplied with a metal trocar.

2. Connect a syringe to the catheter and aspirate. If fresh blood is obtained close the skin and either perform a CT scan or arrange to perform an exploratory laparotomy.

3. If no blood is obtained connect an intravenous infusion apparatus to the catheter and instil approximately 10 ml Kg^{-1} of normal saline, up to a maximum of 1000 ml, into the peritoneal cavity (Fig. 8.14).

4. Gently rotate the patient from side to side to mix the lavage with any abdominal fluid and lay the infusion bag on the floor with the tap open to siphon back the lavage saline (inset to Fig. 8.14). Careful manipulation of the catheter should allow the return of nearly all of the fluid.

5. Remove the catheter.

Wound closure and dressing

If a formal incision has been made, close the peritoneum with an absorbable suture (e.g. Vicryl), and use layers of nylon for the fascia and skin. Apply a waterproof dressing.

POSTOPERATIVE CARE

The fluid is analysed by microscopy to look for blood cells (which may be obvious to the naked eye), organisms and food matter (indicative of a gastrointestinal injury), and assayed for amylase (raised in pancreatic injury) and bile (present in biliary injury).

A positive lavage is indicated by one or more of the following: >100,000 red cells per ml, >500 white blood cells per ml, vegetable matter, bacteria, bile, and amylase. The result may lead to an operation, though it is imperative to carefully observe patients following negative lavage as this will not necessarily exclude a retroperitoneal injury.

SPECIAL OPERATIVE HAZARDS

1. Damage to intra-abdominal structures. The risk of this is increased in pregnancy and with previous abdominal surgery which should be regarded as relative contra-indications. This is one drawback of percutaneous paracentesis with a trocar-mounted catheter.
2. Inadvertent infusion of fluid into the abdominal wall can occur if a percutaneous method is employed.
3. Missed injury. Diagnostic peritoneal lavage will not predict some retroperitoneal injuries (e.g. those to the duodenum, pancreas and kidney) and if there is a rupture of the diaphragm blood will enter the chest due to the negative pressure and can give a false negative result.

COMPLICATIONS

1. Abscess or fistula formation from damage to a viscus.
2. The introduction of fluid and possibly air into the peritoneum which can render the interpretation of subsequent CT or ultrasound scans more difficult.

LAPAROTOMY FOR TRAUMA

Preparation

The patient is placed supine, the skin cleansed from the jaw line to the knees and draped to expose the entire abdomen. Impaled foreign bodies are cleansed and included in the operative field.

Incision

Make a long midline abdominal incision from xiphisternum to pubis, although if the patient remains *in extremis* from torrential haemorrhage despite full resuscitation consider performing a preliminary anterior left thoracotomy to control the thoracic aorta prior to opening the abdomen since this will release any tamponade and may precipitate cardiac arrest.

Operative technique

1. If the left chest has been opened identify and mobilize the thoracic aorta behind the oesophagus by dividing the overlying parietal pleura. Place a sling around the aorta and

8.11

using a vascular clamp cross-clamp it as far distally as possible (Fig. 8.15).

2. With the abdomen opened, and with adequate retraction, examine any entry wounds on the inside of the peritoneum and rapidly evacuate intraperitoneal blood, scooping out clots by hand and aspirating with a sump sucker, using a cupped hand as shown on page 8.17. Insert large abdominal packs into the four quadrants whilst resuscitation continues.

3. Systematically examine the entire abdominal contents by removing each pack in turn, looking initially for bleeding sites, particularly from the liver and spleen, and spillage of the bowel contents from a ruptured viscus (the management of which is discussed in the next chapter). Examine both cupola of the diaphragm for rupture which is treated by primary repair with interrupted non-absorbable sutures such as Ethibond.

4. Injuries to the pancreas are easily overlooked unless actively sought by Kocherization of the duodenum, incision of the root of the transverse mesocolon to the left of the middle colic vessels and examination through the greater and lesser omenta.

5. Injury to the distal body or tail of the pancreas requires splenectomy and distal pancreatectomy. Mobilize the spleen in the usual fashion, but do not divide the pedicle. The spleen is then drawn medially and the damaged pancreas mobilized from the posterior abdominal wall and transected to the right of the injury. Oversew the divided pancreatic duct. If the pancreas is transected further to the right, drain the divided pancreatic duct from the distal segment into a Roux loop and oversew the other cut end (Fig. 8.16).

Extensive disruption of the duodenum, head of pancreas and bile duct may require pancreaticoduodenectomy. Isolated bile duct injuries are repaired over a T-tube with interrupted absorbable sutures.

6. Most renal injuries can be managed conservatively and exploration is only indicated for a renal pedicle injury or a rapidly enlarging retroperitoneal haematoma. In such cases a transabdominal approach is employed and it is essential to establish proximal control of the renal vessels prior to opening Gerota's fascia which will release any tamponade (Fig. 8.17). Incise the root of the mesentery with scissors and reflect it cranially to expose the abdominal aorta. Identify the left renal vein as it crosses the aorta and palpate the superior mesenteric artery. The renal arteries are close by

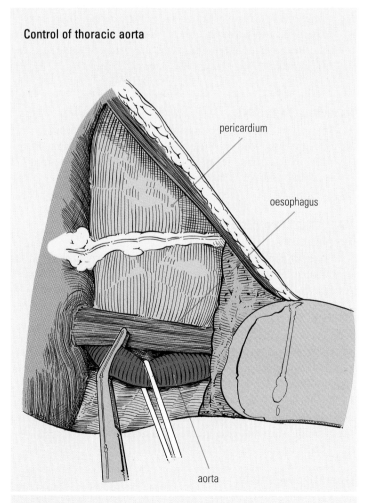

Control of thoracic aorta

pericardium

oesophagus

aorta

Fig. 8.15

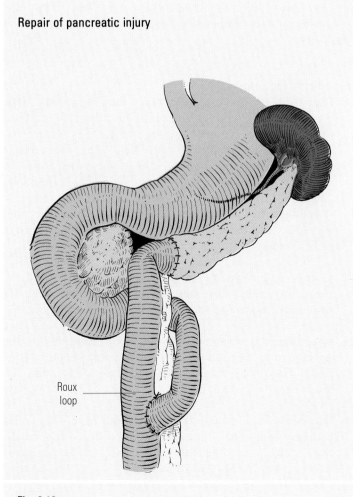

Repair of pancreatic injury

Roux loop

Fig. 8.16

on either side, the right crossing behind the inferior vena cava. The renal vessels may be multiple. The right renal vein is short, entering the right side of the inferior vena cava.

7. Use wet packs to soak up a retroperitoneal haematoma and allow visualization of the kidney which is repaired with or without partial nephrectomy, or removed. If there is a renal laceration repair any disruption of the collecting system with a running absorbable suture prior to closing the renal parenchyma and insert a nephrostomy tube to decompress the kidney.

8. Renal pedicle injury requires vascular reconstruction either by direct suture, repair with an interposition vein graft (using autologous saphenous vein) or autotransplantation onto the iliac vessels as for a renal transplant (see Chapter 128). If contemplating nephrectomy carefully examine the other kidney if a preoperative IVU has not been performed to demonstrate that the kidney is functioning on the other side.

Wound closure and dressing
Insert tube drains and close the wound with monofilament nylon, and the skin with interrupted nylon sutures unless there

is gross contamination in which case the superficial layers are left open and a saline-soaked gauze wick placed into the wound. If the wound is clean it can be closed a few days later by delayed primary suture. The superficial layers of stab wounds are generally left open as they are always potentially infected.

POSTOPERATIVE CARE
Patients suffering major trauma should be nursed in an intensive care unit with arterial and central venous monitoring. A nasogastric tube is retained until bowel function returns; a large retroperitoneal haematoma can cause a prolonged paralytic ileus. Intravenous antibiotics are administered and abnormalities of blood coagulation following massive blood transfusion vigorously corrected with clotting factors, platelet transfusion and intravenous calcium gluconate (to reverse citrate toxicity). The patient should be ventilated until haemodynamically stable; cases with chest trauma such as a flail segment may require more prolonged ventilation and may need a tracheostomy. Parenteral nutrition should be introduced in the early postoperative period since these patients are severely catabolic and rapidly enter negative nitrogen balance.

SPECIAL OPERATIVE HAZARDS
1. Missed injury, the greatest hazard, can only be avoided by meticulous laparotomy.
2. Massive haemorrhage, in which case consider packing and closing abdomen whilst the patient is resuscitated and clotting corrected.

COMPLICATIONS
1. Continuing haemorrhage requires the correction of clotting abnormalities and consideration of re-exploration.
2. Prolonged postoperative ileus may follow a retroperitoneal haematoma but is also a complication of intra-abdominal abscess formation.
3. Sepsis, from infected haematoma or anastomotic leakage. The latter may also lead to fistula formation. CT scanning is useful in localization of an abscess. A collection of pus should be drained either percutaneously under CT or ultrasound guidance, or by an open operation.
4. Large vessel damage can lead to arteriovenous fistula formation and high output cardiac failure.
5. Hypertension may follow renal trauma and necessitate nephrectomy.
6. Specific complications depend on the nature of the injury and are covered further in the appropriate chapters.

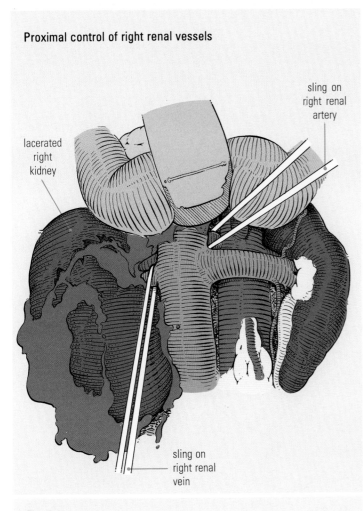

Proximal control of right renal vessels

sling on right renal artery

lacerated right kidney

sling on right renal vein

Fig. 8.17

Rupture of the bladder or gastrointestinal tract can follow a blunt or penetrating injury to the abdomen and may occur in isolation or in conjunction with damage to a solid viscus such as the liver or spleen. In civilian practice in the UK such injuries are usually blunt and follow road traffic accidents, whereas in military practice and in the USA, penetrating missile injuries are relatively more common.

PREOPERATIVE ASSESSMENT
The resuscitation and assessment of such cases is covered fully in the previous chapter.

RELEVANT ANATOMY
A penetrating injury can puncture any part of the gastro-intestinal tract, whereas in a blunt injury the damage is generally caused either by compression against the spine of, for instance the transverse colon, or by shearing in which case the regions particularly susceptible to damage are at the junction of fixed

(retroperitoneal) and mobile (intraperitoneal) segments of bowel (e.g. in the proximal duodenum, and just beyond the duodeno-jejunal flexure). The colon and rectum can be perforated at sigmoidoscopy and colonoscopy.

When a hollow viscus perforates the mucosa pouts out through the hole making it unlikely to seal spontaneously, with leakage and abscess formation.

Rupture of the bladder usually follows a blunt injury and may be intra- or extraperitoneal depending on whether the bladder was full or empty at the time of the injury. Extra-peritoneal rupture is uncommon without an underlying pelvic fracture. The same principles of management apply for cases of instrumental perforation (e.g. at cystoscopy).

OPERATION
Preparation
Place the anaesthetized patient supine and cleanse the abdomen, scrubbing clean any wounds and removing all particulate matter and debris. Apply drapes so as to expose the entire abdomen.

Debridement and closure of small bowel injury

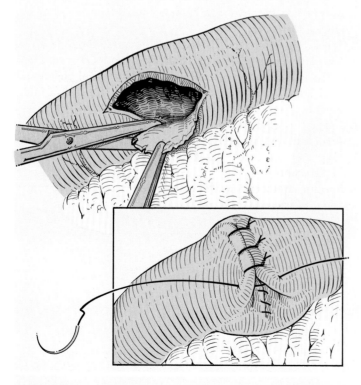

Fig. 8.18

Loop colostomy

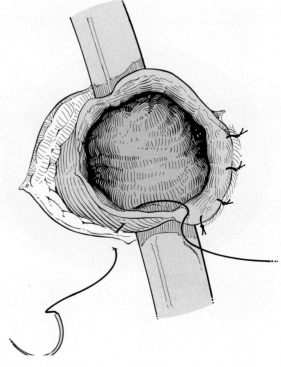

Fig. 8.19

Incision

Make a midline abdominal incision. In cases of penetrating injury avoid including the penetrating wound in the incision.

Operative technique

1. Perform a thorough laparotomy in all cases of trauma and examine the peritoneum carefully to locate the site of an entry wound. Attend to bleeding from a damaged liver or spleen first (see pages 4.28 and 8.17), and then systematically examine the entire gastrointestinal tract paying particular attention to the less obvious structures such as the retroperitoneal duodenum. Also inspect the mesentery, omentum, and retroperitoneal structures such as the pancreas and major vessels.

2. With lacerations to the stomach or small bowel, excise any excessive mucosa and trim back devitalized tissue until there is bleeding from the edges (Fig. 8.18) before closing the defect in two layers with an absorbable suture (e.g. Polydioxamone). Close tears transversely to prevent narrowing (see inset to Fig. 8.18). More extensive areas of damage to the small bowel and mesenteric tears leading to devascularized segments require resection with end-to-end anastomosis (see the Introduction). Duodenal injuries are debrided and small defects similarly repaired by direct suture, and defunctioned with a gastroenterostomy (see page 5.35) if the tissues are oedematous or the lumen narrowed; large defects should be drained into a Roux loop and in cases where the duodenum is widely devitalized a pancreaticoduodenectomy may be necessary.

3. Injuries to the colon and rectum are usually associated with peritoneal soiling, and primary repair is in general inadvisable. Following a thorough peritoneal toilet the damaged segment of colon can be mobilized and temporarily exteriorized, with or without repair of the defect, over a glass rod as for a loop colostomy (Fig. 8.19) (see page 5.74). This can be reversed after 2 weeks. More extensive colonic damage requires resection with exteriorization of both ends, which, if possible, are brought out together as a double-barrelled colostomy to simplify subsequent closure (Fig. 8.20). If a primary repair or resection is undertaken it should be performed in two layers and covered by a proximal colostomy or ileostomy for at least 14 days. Rectal injury is managed by mobilization of the rectum with division of its peritoneal attachments, and repair with a proximal covering loop colostomy.

4. If the bladder is ruptured, extend the incision to the pubis and dissect bluntly in the retropubic space to expose the defect which is debrided if necessary and repaired with two layers of continuous absorbable sutures. If there are pubic fractures there will be extensive haematoma mixed with extravasated urine in the extraperitoneal space. Visualization of the defect may be made easier by instilling sterile saline into the bladder via a urinary catheter and this technique can also be used to test the integrity of the repair. Following repair both extraperitoneal suprapubic and urethral catheters are inserted to allow irrigation of the bladder to remove blood clot, and a large silicone drain placed in the retropubic space (Fig. 8.21).

Double-barrelled colostomy

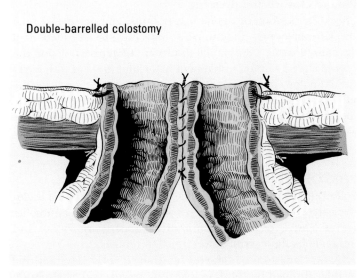

Fig. 8.20

Repair of ruptured bladder

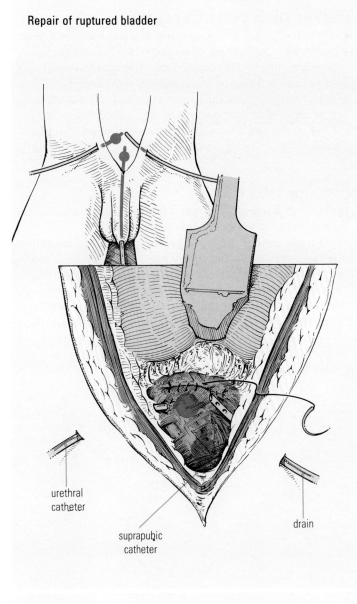

urethral catheter

suprapubic catheter

drain

Fig. 8.21

8.15

Wound closure and dressing

Check the position of the nasogastric tube and perform a final check for bleeding. Abdominal wounds must be debrided of all devitalized tissue. Abdominal drains are then inserted, and the wound closed with monofilament nylon and the skin with interrupted nylon. In the presence of gross contamination leave the superficial layers open and close them by delayed primary suture after 5–7 days if there is no sepsis. Secure a colostomy with interrupted mucocutaneous catgut sutures.

POSTOPERATIVE CARE

Following major trauma patients should be nursed in an intensive care unit until stable. Prescribe broad-spectrum antibiotics for at least 7 days and continue nasogastric aspiration and intravenous fluids until bowel function returns.

Colonic anastomoses should be drained for 7 days and the bladder drained for 14 days following repair, and a cystogram performed prior to removing the catheters.

A covering stoma can be reversed after 14 days if the repair or anastomosis which it is covering is radiologically intact.

SPECIAL OPERATIVE HAZARDS

1. Missed injuries. Traumatic injury requires a full and meticulous laparotomy in all cases. A positive search for damage must be made including entry into the lesser sac to palpate and see the pancreas and major vessels.
2. Failure to recognize the extent of an injury, in which case it is imperative to excise all the devitalized tissue. Never attempt to restore intestinal continuity with dubious tissue.

COMPLICATIONS

1. Delayed rupture of the bowel following a haematoma in the bowel wall or overlooked mesenteric injury.
2. Intra-abdominal sepsis. Despite continuing antibiotic therapy, there is a high incidence of postoperative sepsis, either from leakage from a suture line leading to abscess or fistula formation, from contamination alone, or from a missed injury (e.g. to the pancreas). The patient will be in negative nitrogen balance and requires parenteral nutrition.
3. Sloughing of the suprapubic tissues from urinary extravasation. Always thoroughly irrigate and drain the retropubic space in cases of bladder rupture.

Liver trauma is classified according to the extent of injury. A tear in Glisson's capsule may occur in isolation, or there can be an associated parenchymal laceration which may or may not be accompanied by major arterial or venous haemorrhage. In the most severe cases, extensive parenchymal damage is associated with injury to a major hepatic vein or the retrohepatic inferior vena cava. Such parenchymal lacerations are often stellate when caused by blunt trauma. Occasionally a parenchymal disruption occurs within an intact capsule and a subcapsular haematoma develops which may rupture subsequently into the peritoneal cavity, or into the biliary tree causing haemobilia.

As a result of the extensive portal blood flow to the liver, a parenchymal laceration may primarily result in venous haemorrhage. The rate of bleeding will diminish due to the effect of tamponade, provided that the abdominal wall and diaphragm are intact. This often allows for a period of resuscitation before surgery is undertaken. It may even allow patients to be treated conservatively as long as they remain stable after transfusion. Early surgery in an unstable patient will prolong the period of hypotension as the effect of tamponade is lost, and may significantly worsen the progress.

Evidence of continued bleeding or suspicion of an associated injury which cannot be treated conservatively such as a perforated hollow viscus are indications for surgery. In addition to correction of hypovolaemia, coagulopathy, electrolyte imbalance and the use of large volumes of cold-stored blood may complicate the case and require specific management.

When dealing with a major liver injury, skilled resuscitation, a well-stocked blood bank and an experienced surgical team are essential. The diagnosis of intra-abdominal bleeding is made by peritoneal lavage. CT scanning, when available, gives the best guide to the organs involved and the extent of damage.

When forced to operate in the acute situation, simple packing may achieve haemostasis and allow a period of 24–48 hours for correction of hypovolaemia, blood clotting and recovery of hypoxic injury to the myocardium. The packs can be removed semi-electively, if need be following transfer to a specialized unit.

PREOPERATIVE ASSESSMENT

1. Assess the patient for intra-abdominal haemorrhage, distended abdomen and abdominal wall bruising. Peritoneal lavage may be necessary.
2. Ensure adequate resuscitation, central venous access, and arterial, venous and urinary output monitoring.
3. Question whether surgery is necessary immediately or if the patient can be treated conservatively under close supervision initially.
4. Determine if the local facilities are adequate; if not the patient should be transferred to a specialized unit.
5. Examine the patient for evidence of other injuries.

RELEVANT ANATOMY

Details of the ligamentous attachments and vascular anatomy of the liver are covered on page 4.18 in Hepatic Lobectomy. The majority of liver trauma in the UK is caused by blunt injury, and involvement of other organs is common.

OPERATION

The purpose of surgery is to establish haemostasis, to remove devitalized tissue, and to repair damaged structures.

Preparation

With the patient supine and prior to anaesthetic induction the entire abdomen is exposed, cleansed and draped. Only when the surgeons are ready to start operating is a general anaesthetic administered as it may be accompanied by a drastic fall in blood pressure.

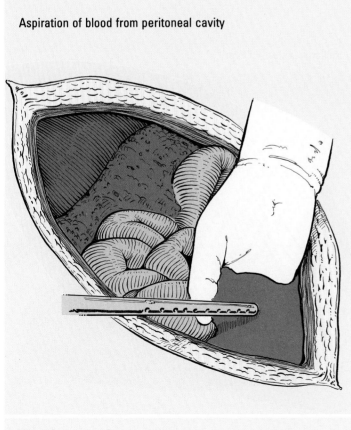

Aspiration of blood from peritoneal cavity

Fig. 8.22

Incision

A long midline incision is employed in cases of abdominal trauma because of the speed of exposure and the ease with which it can be extended to deal with other injuries.

Operative technique

1. Perform a rapid but thorough laparotomy to assess the extent of the injury and to determine the order of priority for treatment. A ruptured spleen is the most likely source of bleeding. Pack off any less serious injuries for attention later.

2. Evacuate large clots manually; pools of blood can be most efficiently removed by using the sump sucker within a cupped hand (Fig. 8.22).

3. Inspect the liver capsule for a tear. Palpate the diaphragmatic surface of both lobes to assess injury to the dorsal surface, and exclude an associated diaphragmatic rupture. Avoid extensive mobilization of the liver by division of the ligaments as this may open a deep fissured laceration and exacerbate bleeding.

4. A superficial tear which is not actively bleeding requires no further treatment. Evacuate all blood locally and reassess the area after a delay to check that haemostasis is secure.

5. Minor bleeding can usually be controlled by suturing of the capsule. When suturing take generous bites with catgut on a large atraumatic needle and do not stitch too tightly. Fibrin or collagen buttons reduce the risk of 'cutting out' (Fig. 8.23).

6. Stellate ruptures, particularly of the right lobe, may bleed profusely (Fig. 8.24). Pack the laceration with long gauze rolls and continue resuscitation (Fig. 8.25). Remove the packs when the patient has been stabilized and coagulation deflects are corrected (Fig. 8.26). If suturing is difficult or fails to control bleeding, repack the liver. Once haemostasis is achieved, place two large bore silicone drains nearby and close the abdomen with the packs *in situ*. Access to injuries to the posterior aspect and dome of the right lobe may require a thoraco-abdominal extension to the incision.

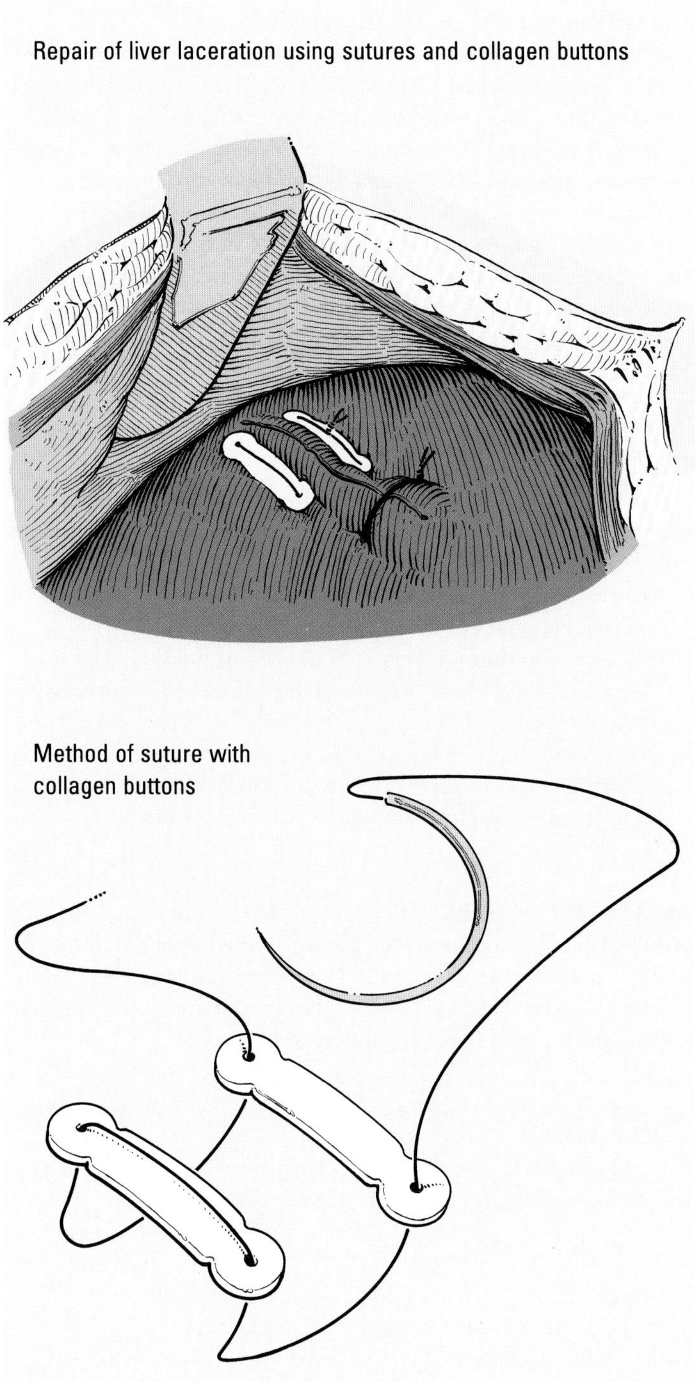

Repair of liver laceration using sutures and collagen buttons

Method of suture with collagen buttons

Stellate fracture of liver

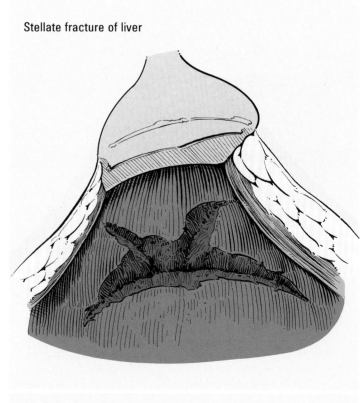

Fig. 8.23

Fig. 8.24

Insertion of gauze rolls

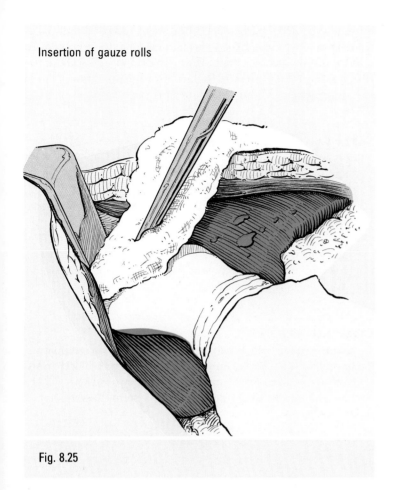

Fig. 8.25

7. Should packing fail to control the bleeding, apply a soft clamp to the porta hepatis (the Pringle manoeuvre) (Fig. 8.27). Ligate the appropriate branch of the hepatic artery if trial occlusion stops the bleeding. Frequently the hepatic arterial supply is anomalous; the left hepatic artery arises from the left gastric artery in 23% of cases, and the right hepatic artery from the superior mesenteric artery in 17% of cases. Remove the gall bladder if the cystic artery has been occluded. Following this it may be possible to remove the packs and complete haemostasis by suture of the capsule. If it fails, repack and close the abdomen as in stage 6.

8. Failure of the Pringle manoeuvre suggests there is bleeding from either a large hepatic vein or the inferior vena cava. If packing does not control this (if necessary from both sides of the liver), then a major resection is the only procedure likely to save the patient (see page 4.18 in Hepatic Lobectomy). Some surgeons employ vena cava shunts to isolate the retrohepatic inferior vena cava, whilst in a well-resuscitated patient temporary clamping of the inferior vena cava above and below the liver may be tolerated. After dividing the liver parenchyma by the finger-fracture technique and clipping the vessels on the cut surface, the venous tear is exposed and repaired using a continuous non-absorbable suture such as Prolene. The success of such a resection depends largely on the skill of the surgical and anaesthetic teams.

Removal of gauze rolls

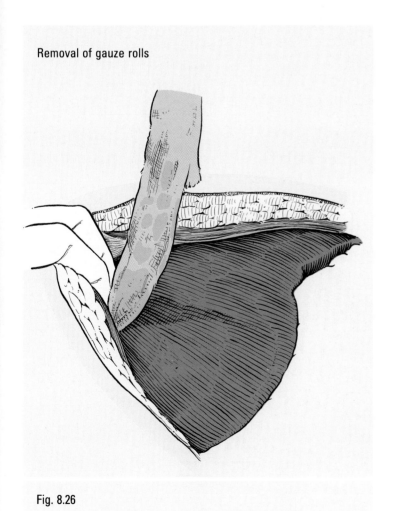

Fig. 8.26

Pringle's manoeuvre

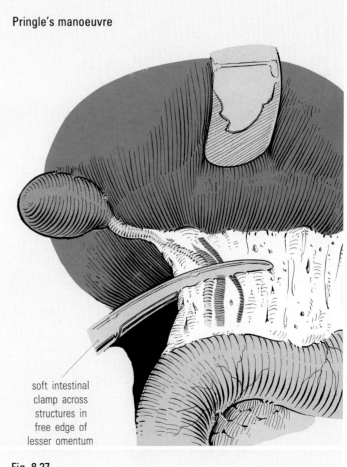

soft intestinal
clamp across
structures in
free edge of
lesser omentum

Fig. 8.27

8.19

9. If the abdomen has been packed and closed, the packs are usually removed around 48 hours if the patient is stable; facilities for major hepatic resection should be available. The packs are soaked with saline to loosen them and gently removed. Fresh packs are inserted for a further 10–15 minutes. Suture the capsule to complete haemostasis; if profuse bleeding is encountered, proceed with a major resection.

10. All liver injuries should be drained using large bore silicone tubes to allow for assessment of continued bleeding. Leakage of bile or other abdominal contents may also become evident. Elective drainage of the biliary tree is no longer undertaken.

Wound closure and dressing

Even if the packs are to remain *in situ*, close the wound with a loop nylon suture, and the skin with non-absorbable suture.

POSTOPERATIVE CARE

The patient is monitored in the intensive care unit, with particular attention to replacement of blood loss and correction of metabolic and coagulation abnormalities. A period of ventilation is usually required, particularly after major resection or if packs have been left *in situ*. Broad spectrum antibiotics are administered whilst the packs remain. Drains are removed on about the fifth day, and the sutures 7–10 days after the operation. Plan to re-explore after 48 hours to remove the packs.

SPECIAL OPERATIVE HAZARDS

1. Over zealous surgical treatment may exacerbate bleeding.
2. Failure to obtain adequate haemostasis before closing the abdomen.
3. Damage to the biliary or vascular tree resulting in devascularization of the liver, or a biliary fistula.
4. Failure to identify other injuries, particularly to retroperitoneal structures such as the duodenum or pancreas.
5. Air embolus in the hypotensive patient, since the venous pressure may be negative.

COMPLICATIONS

1. Haemorrhage, which may be exacerbated by coagulopathy.
2. Jaundice, this can be multifactoral (e.g. large blood transfusion, impaired liver function and biliary obstruction).
3. Bile leak, or bleeding into the biliary system (haemobilia).
4. Liver abscess.

9

Vascular Surgery

Techniques of Vascular Access

Whilst most methods of vascular access involve the percutaneous puncture of vessels, in selected instances a surgical approach is required. The following techniques are considered: the insertion of a tunnelled central venous line (e.g. Hickman line); the creation of an external arterio-venous fistula (Scribner shunt); and the creation of an internal arterio-venous fistula (Cimino–Brescia fistula). A tunnelled central line is usually inserted into the internal jugular vein, and exposure of the vessel prior to insertion is sometimes desirable (e.g. in children requiring long-term venous access such as for systemic chemotherapy).

Arterio-venous fistulae are created between an artery and vein, either at the elbow (e.g. brachial artery and cephalic vein), at the wrist (e.g. radial artery and cephalic vein) or at the ankle (e.g. posterior tibial artery and long saphenous vein). The former two are used for internal fistulae, the latter two for external fistula. A Cimino–Brescia fistula takes 4–6 weeks to mature (with arterialization of the vein) and should not be used prematurely for dialysis whereas a Scribner shunt can be used straight away for dialysis or haemofiltration.

In patients requiring long-term venous access in whom a Cimino–Brescia fistula is not possible, due to obliteration or inadequacy of the vessels, a synthetic graft (e.g. Teflon [PTFE], Dacron or Gore-Tex) can be interposed between a limb artery and vein, either straight (e.g. distal radial artery to median cubital vein) or looped (e.g. subcutaneously; based on the vessels in the cubital fossa or femoral triangle).

PREOPERATIVE ASSESSMENT

1. For the creation of a fistula, ensure that the vein to be used is patent. Use a tourniquet to locate it.
2. Ensure that the proposed artery is palpable.
3. Elect to perform a Cimino–Brescia fistula on the non-dominant arm, and before dialysis is actually needed; the fistula needs to be mature for dialysis and cannot be used immediately.
4. Under no circumstances perform a Scribner shunt in the arm if there is any possibility that long-term dialysis might be required because the forearm vessels must be preserved for the creation of a Cimino–Brescia fistula at a later date.
5. For insertion of a tunnelled central line (Hickman line), inform the X-ray department of the need for screening with an image intensifier, and ensure the operating table used is radiolucent to permit radiology.

RELEVANT ANATOMY

The internal jugular vein lies in the carotid sheath anterolateral to the carotid artery and vagus nerve, just behind the anterior border of sternomastoid, and receives the middle and inferior thyroid veins along its anterolateral surface. Sternomastoid is covered by skin and platysma (Fig. 9.1).

The cephalic vein runs along the radial border of the fore-

arm and lateral to the biceps muscle in the upper arm. It pierces the clavipectoral fascia to enter the axillary vein at the shoulder and is subcutaneous throughout its length. In the distal forearm the radial artery lies on the surface of flexor pollicis longus and the distal radius. In the mid-forearm it emerges from under bradioradialis to lie subcutaneously at the wrist (Fig. 9.2) before passing deeply into the hand between the two heads of the first dorsal interosseous muscle. It is accompanied by venae comitantes.

The posterior tibial artery runs between flexor digitorum longus and flexor hallucis longus in the lower leg and becomes subcutaneous at the ankle where it lies behind the medial malleolus, accompanied by its venae comitantes and the tibial nerve. It ends under the flexor retinaculum by dividing into the lateral and medial plantar arteries. The long saphenous vein is the continuation of the medial end of the dorsal venous arch of the foot and commences just in front of the medial malleolus, coursing toward the knee accompanied by the sensory saphenous nerve (Fig. 9.3).

Internal jugular vein

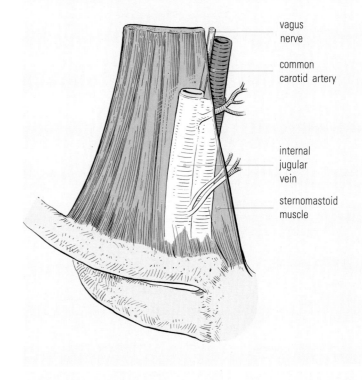

vagus nerve

common carotid artery

internal jugular vein

sternomastoid muscle

Fig. 9.1

TUNNELLED CENTRAL LINE
Preparation
The patient is placed supine, and the skin of the chest and neck on the side to be cannulated are exposed and cleansed. A head towel is applied.

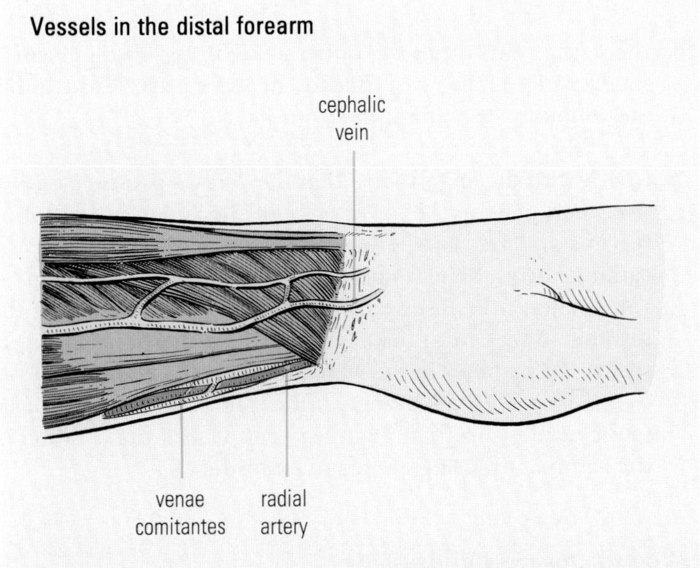

Incision
Make an incision in the lower skin crease of the neck, 2–3 cm long, centred over the carotid pulse, and a 5 mm stab wound at the proposed site of exit of the cannula over the upper chest, either medial to or lateral to the nipple.

Operative technique
1. Deepen the incision in the neck, dividing platysma until the sternomastoid muscle is reached.

2. With sternomastoid retracted laterally, the internal jugular vein is visible through the thin carotid sheath which is carefully lifted with dissecting forceps and opened with scissors. To improve access it is sometimes necessary to divide some of the medial fibres of sternomastoid.

3. Gently mobilize the internal jugular vein from the underlying carotid artery by passing a blunt right-angled forcep behind it. There are usually no tributaries entering the vein at this level. Place a soft rubber sling around the vein (Fig. 9.4).

4. Some cannulae are supplied with a tunnelling kit. If not, create a subcutaneous tunnel by pushing a Burkett forceps from the incision in the neck to the stab wound over the chest. Grasp the Hickman catheter with the forceps and

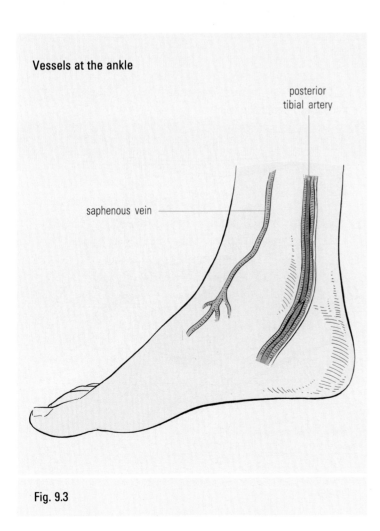

Vessels in the distal forearm

cephalic vein

venae comitantes   radial artery

Fig. 9.2

Vessels at the ankle

posterior tibial artery

saphenous vein

Fig. 9.3

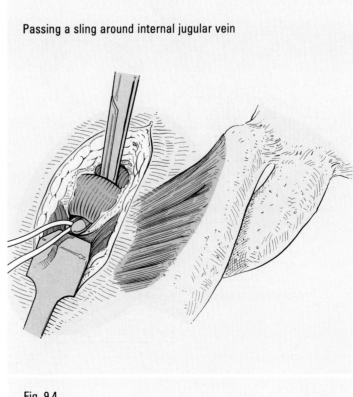

Passing a sling around internal jugular vein

Fig. 9.4

9.3

draw it through the tunnel (Fig. 9.5) until the cuff of the cannula lies under the skin not less than 1 cm from the entry point. Secure the emerging cannula to the skin with a silk suture. Flush each lumen of the catheter with heparinized

Draw catheter through tunnel

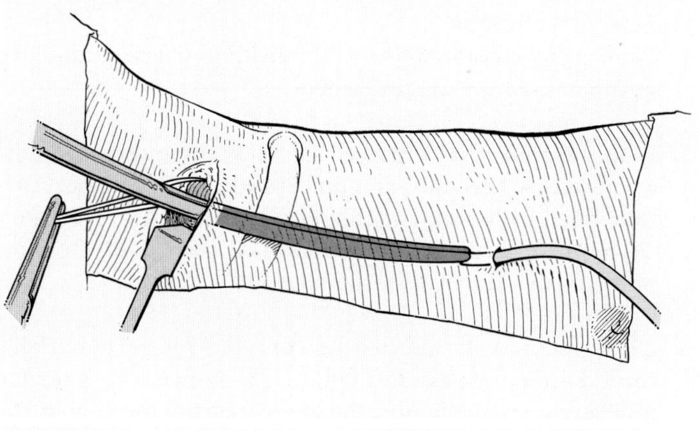

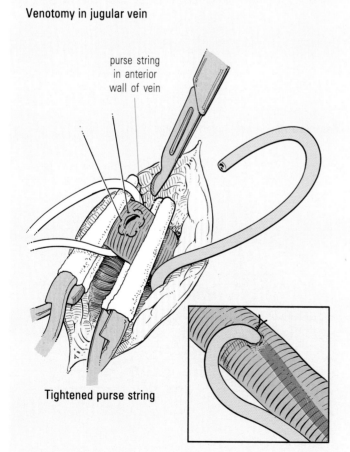

Fig. 9.5

Venotomy in jugular vein

purse string
in anterior
wall of vein

Tightened purse string

Fig. 9.6

saline. Using scissors cut the end off the Hickman line so it will lie in the superior vena cava or just inside the right atrium (the surface marking is the fourth intercostal space) when inserted.

5. Apply bulldog clamps to the proximal and distal jugular vein and insert a 6/0 or 7/0 vascular suture as a purse string into the anterior wall of the vein, starting at the 12 o'clock position (Fig. 9.6).

6. Incise the vein within the purse string using a scalpel with a small blade, taking care not to cut the suture. Ensure that the venotomy will admit the cannula.

7. Check with the anaesthetist that the venous pressure is positive, then pick up the lower edge of the venotomy with fine forceps and release the lower bulldog whilst threading the cannula through the venotomy and down the internal jugular vein. When fully inserted, with a gentle curve visible as the cannula arches in to the vein, gently tie the purse string to secure the catheter in the vein and ensure haemostasis (inset to Fig. 9.6). Flush all lumina of the cannula with heparinized saline and ensure that all are patent. Check the position of the cannula tip using an image intensifier.

Wound closure and dressing
Close the neck wound with subcutaneous catgut and use subcuticular or interrupted monofilament nylon sutures for the skin. Apply a dry dressing to the neck and antiseptic spray to the exit wound which is then covered with a dry dressing.

Venotomy in cephalic vein

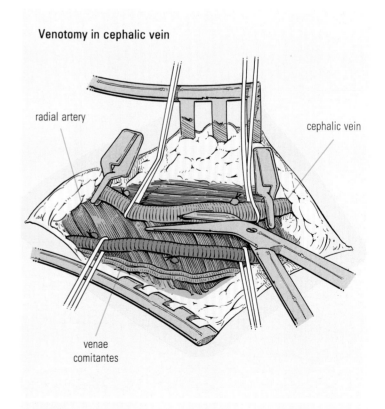

radial artery

cephalic vein

venae
comitantes

Fig. 9.7

POSTOPERATIVE CARE

It is prudent to take a postoperative chest X-ray as a permanent record of the position of the cannula. The sutures in the neck are removed after 3 days and the silk suture securing the cannula after 10 days by which time the ingrowth of fibrous tissue into the cuff of the cannula will prevent it from dislodging.

SPECIAL OPERATIVE HAZARDS
1. Bleeding as a result of damage to the jugular vein, which will usually stop if pressure is applied for 5 minutes.
2. Damage to the carotid artery or vagus nerve following forceful blind dissection behind the vein whilst it is being mobilized.
3. Air embolus which can be avoided by ensuring positive venous pressure prior to opening the vein.
4. Damage to the breast bud in the prepubertal female if the line is tunnelled behind the nipple.

COMPLICATIONS
1. Infection of the line, which usually results from subsequent bacteraemia rather than infection at the time of the insertion and may require removal of the line if it fails to respond to antibiotics. Infection around the entry site on the chest wall is minimized if the cuff on the cannula is at least 1 cm from the exit wound.
2. Cardiac arrhythmias if the tip lies in the right ventricle.
3. Blockage of the cannula.
4. Fracture of the cannula with embolization of the tip.
5. The cannula can tie itself into a knot, making removal difficult.

FORMATION OF CIMINO–BRESCIA FISTULA AT THE WRIST
Preparation
This procedure is generally performed under a regional anaesthetic (i.e. a brachial plexus block) with the patient awake. A general anaesthetic can be used in the very anxious patient, but this should still be combined with a brachial plexus block which produces advantageous venodilation. Additional local anaesthetic infiltration can be given if required. The patient is placed supine with the arm abducted at the shoulder and supported on an armboard. The forearm is cleansed and draped.

Incision
Make a 3–4 cm longitudinal skin incision in the distal third of the forearm midway between the radial artery and the cephalic vein.

Operative technique
1. Whilst an assistant lifts the skin edge with a pair of skin hooks, identify the cephalic vein and carefully mobilize it from the surrounding connective tissue.

2. Ligate and divide any small tributaries of the cephalic vein, until the exposed segment is free. Avoid picking up the delicate vein with forceps, using instead silk ties or slings to retract the vein.

3. Locate the radial artery by palpation and free it from its accompanying venae comitantes, again using silk ties or slings to apply traction to the artery rather than grasping it with forceps.

4. Mobilize the vessels until the artery and vein can be brought comfortably together without tension, ligating and dividing the branches as necessary.

5. Start a longitudinal venotomy with a scalpel and extend it to 1 cm using microvascular Pott's scissors (Fig. 9.7). Flush the proximal vein with heparinized saline through a plastic cannula to confirm its patency (Fig. 9.8). Occlude the vein proximally and distally with vascular clamps and make a parallel arteriotomy having similarly applied clamps to the artery. Flush the artery with heparinized saline.

6. Insert one end of a double-ended 6/0 polypropylene vascular suture (e.g. Prolene) from in-to-out into the distal end of the venotomy and the other end into the distal end of the arteriotomy, and tie them. Re-enter the lumen of the artery and complete the posterior layer of the anastomosis; initially use an over-and-over stitch picking up the opposed edges of the two vessels, but as the proximal end of the anastomosis is approached avoid picking up artery and vein together and pass the suture from inside the artery to out, and then from outside to in on the vein to ensure accurate placement of the stitches.

7. Having finished the corner of the anastomosis, complete half of the front layer and, leaving this suture on the outside, come back to meet it with the other end of the double-ended suture.

8. Remove the distal arterial clamp and once all the air has been flushed out, tie the suture and release the remaining clamps and the slings.

Flushing proximal vein

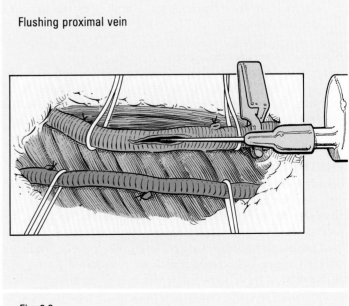

Fig. 9.8

9.5

Arteriovenous anastomosis

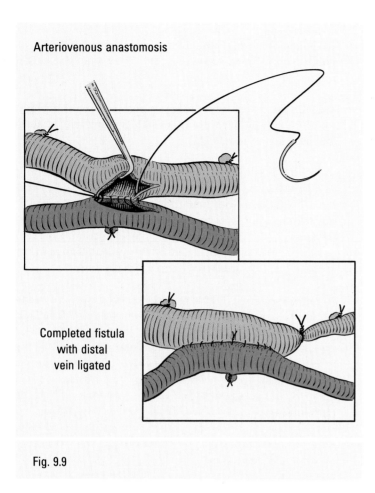

Completed fistula
with distal
vein ligated

Fig. 9.9

9. Ligate the vein distal to the fistula with silk (inset to Fig. 9.9). Divide it between ties if it will allow the fistula to lie more comfortably.

10. Apply gentle pressure for a couple of minutes by which time any bleeding should have stopped. It is rarely necessary to insert additional sutures for haemostasis, but if required it must be done with great care.

11. Confirm the patency of the fistula by feeling for the characteristic thrill or listening for a bruit over the proximal cephalic vein.

Wound closure and dressing
Insert a few interrupted subcutaneous sutures and close the skin with interrupted non-absorbable sutures, and apply a dry dressing. Use a waterproof skin marker to mark a point at which the thrill from the fistula is easily felt.

POSTOPERATIVE CARE
During the postoperative period the fistula must be carefully observed for patency by auscultation and palpation. Do not allow any form of tourniquet to be applied to that limb (e.g. for phlebotomy, or for blood pressure measurement) and avoid/ treat hypotension. Sutures are removed after a week. The fistula will mature in 4–6 weeks. If dialysis is required during this period it must be by some other means (e.g. peritoneal dialysis or haemodialysis via a central line or Scribner shunt). Show the patient how to check for patency and instruct them to reattend swiftly if the thrill disappears.

SPECIAL OPERATIVE HAZARDS
1. Damage to the intima leading to early failure from thrombosis.
2. Inability to comfortably oppose artery and vein, in which case consider dividing the distal vein to improve mobility, and performing an end-to-side anastomosis.
3. Vascular spasm. Topical application of papaverine is helpful in overcoming this.

COMPLICATIONS
1. Thrombosis, which is not an uncommon occurrence during or just after dialysis due to hypotension and damage to the intima of the vein. If diagnosed early, consider urgent re-exploration and pass a fine embolectomy catheter up the vein to remove clot. The long-term patency results are best for an end-to-side (vein to artery) rather than side-to-side or end-to-end anastomosis. The advantage of the described technique (side-to-side, but functionally end-to-side) is two-fold: keeping the distal vein intact stabilizes the vessels during the operation and, if re-exploration is required during the early postoperative period for thrombosis, the tie on the distal vein can be removed and an embolectomy catheter inserted without having to take the anastomosis apart.
2. Venous hypertension in the hand causes uncomfortable swelling and congestion of the hand with ischaemia of the fingertips. It is treated (and avoided) by ligation of the vein distal to the fistula.
3. Massive run-off through the fistula can lead to high output cardiac failure and necessitate ligation of the fistula.
4. Aneurysm and pseudo-aneurysm formation. This may occur at the suture line secondary to venous obstruction.

INSERTION OF A SCRIBNER SHUNT AT THE ANKLE
Preparation
This is performed under local or general anaesthesia. The lower limb is cleansed and draped, leaving the midcalf to fore-foot exposed. All the components of the shunt (e.g. two Teflon tips with introducers, two lengths of shaped tubing and a connector to go between them) must be close to hand.

Incision
Although a single incision can be made, it is easier to make two: one over the pulse of the posterior tibial artery and a second over the long saphenous vein just in front of and above the medial malleolus.

Operative technique
1. Identify the long saphenous vein and free it from the surrounding connective tissue and underlying saphenous nerve. Pass two silk ligatures around the vein and occlude it by gentle traction to these ligatures.

2. Make a transverse venotomy with a knife and insert the Teflon cannula of the shunt proximally into the vein mounted on its introducer (Fig. 9.10), which can double as a sizer. Secure the cannula by tying the proximal ligature. Ligate the vein distally with the second ligature, and then tie this around the cannula. Tie the two ligatures together (Fig. 9.11).

3. The Scribner tubing has a U-shaped bend in it and a 'step' at the point where it emerges from the skin. With the tubing lying on the skin see where the step will lie and make a stab incision through the skin at this site. Using an artery forceps develop a small subcutaneous pocket for the apex of the loop to lie in and thread the tubing through the stab wound. Flush the tubing with heparinized saline; and with pressure over the proximal vein to occlude it, remove the introducer from the cannula tip and insert the distal end of the cannula into the tubing.

4. Locate the artery by palpation, and free it from the surrounding venae comitantes. Similarly cannulate it (see point 2) before flushing with heparinized saline and applying a clamp to the emerging tube.

5. Insert the small connector between the two emerging tubes– having flushed out any air by allowing back bleeding and complete the circuit (Fig. 9.12).

Wound closure and dressing

Close the skin with interrupted non-absorbable sutures, and spray an antiseptic powder onto the exit sites. Clearly mark the venous and arterial limbs of the shunt and apply dry dressings to the wounds, leaving the shunt exposed.

POSTOPERATIVE CARE

The shunt can be used immediately for haemodialysis or haemofiltration by clamping both limbs of the tubing and removing the connector. When not in use, reconnect the tubes and remove all the clamps; the flow must be continuous through the shunt which is noticably warm to the touch when patent. Sutures can be removed after 8 days. Always ensure strict attention is paid to asepsis when manipulating the shunt.

SPECIAL OPERATIVE HAZARDS
1. Damage to the saphenous nerve or posterior tibial nerve.
2. Non-patency of the artery; to avoid this always ensure that the pulse is palpable prior to starting the operation.

COMPLICATIONS
1. Occlusion of the shunt, which may respond to milking the shunt, flushing with saline or embolectomy with a fine Fogarty catheter (see page 9.21). Intentionally clamping the shunt will cause the blood in the shunt and its feeding and draining vessels to clot; this is performed prior to removal of the shunt.
2. Infection; as with foreign material anywhere this can be difficult to eradicate and may require removal of the shunt. An infection localized to the exit wounds of the tubing may respond to local application of antiseptic/antibiotic preparations.

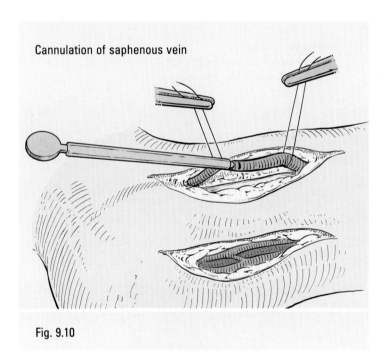

Cannulation of saphenous vein

Fig. 9.10

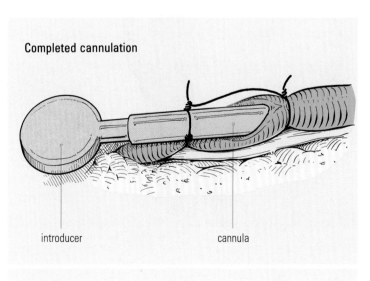

Completed cannulation

introducer   cannula

Fig. 9.11

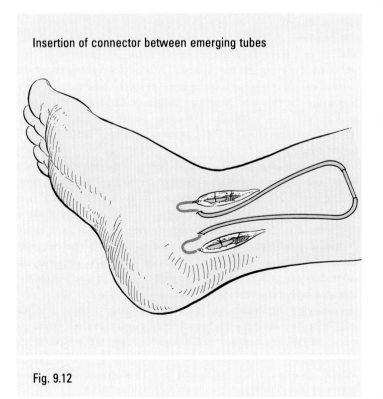

Insertion of connector between emerging tubes

Fig. 9.12

The procedure is indicated for patients with symptomatic carotid stenosis, presenting as transient ischaemic attacks or stroke. Complete occlusions should not be operated on.

PREOPERATIVE ASSESSMENT
1. Check for a bruit in the neck.
2. Carry out angiography, duplex ultrasound, or digital subtraction angiography to assess the extent of the occlusions.
3. Assess collaterals to determine the need for a shunt during surgery.

RELEVANT ANATOMY
The two most common sites for atheromatous plaques to cause stenosis are at the bifurcation of the common carotid artery and just beyond the origin of the internal carotid (Fig. 9.13).

The common carotid artery has no branches proximal to its bifurcation and lies within the carotid sheath, which also encloses the internal jugular vein, vagus nerve and internal carotid artery. The jugular vein lies lateral to the common carotid artery and proximal internal carotid artery, but spirals posteriorly to lie behind the artery at the skull base.

The surface marking for the common carotid is a line drawn from the sternoclavicular joint to its bifurcation at the upper border of the lamina of the thyroid cartilage (third cervical vertebra). It lies deep to the anterior border of the sternomastoid muscle. The posterior belly of digastric passes in front of the internal jugular vein and just above the bifurcation of the carotid artery.

The internal carotid at first lies lateral to the external carotid, and is relatively superficial. It then slopes posteriorly and medially, running up the side wall of the pharynx to enter the carotid canal; it has no branches in the neck. The carotid sinus is a bulge in the wall near the origin of the internal carotid, and it has a rich supply from the glossopharyngeal nerve. This nerve also supplies the carotid body which lies behind the bifurcation.

The hypoglossal nerve emerges between the internal jugular vein and internal carotid artery deep to the posterior belly of digastric. It then passes anterior to both the internal and external carotid at which point the ansa cervicalis arises from it and runs down the carotid sheath to supply the strap muscles. A useful landmark for the hypoglossal nerve is the common facial vein, which crosses it. Further cranially, the internal carotid is crossed by the pharyngeal branch of the vagus and the glossopharyngeal nerve.

Following occlusion of the internal artery, the collateral supply to the anterior and middle cerebral territory is via the circle of Willis. Further collaterals develop in longstanding carotid stenosis, principally via the ophthalmic artery. These vessels usually provide sufficient flow to maintain an adequate cerebral blood flow during carotid cross-clamping.

OPERATION
Preparation
Place the patient in a supine position with the neck slightly extended and the head turned away, but not so much that the sternomastoid muscle covers the carotid.

Incision
Incise the skin and platysma along the anterior border of sternomastoid from the angle of the mandible almost to the clavicle (Fig. 9.14).

Operative technique
1. Expose the great auricular nerve and external jugular vein and ligate and divide the vein.

Relevant anatomy

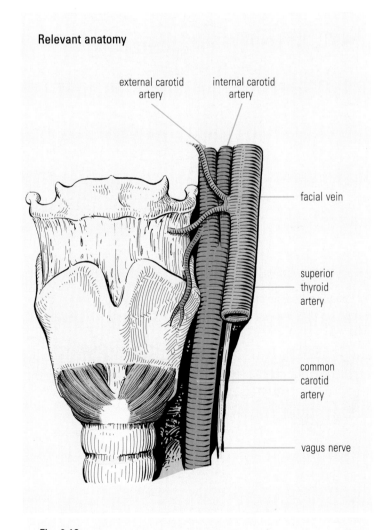

Fig. 9.13

2. Open the plane in front of the anterior border of sterno-mastoid and insert two self-retaining retractors. The internal jugular becomes visible, with the posterior belly of digastric crossing it above and the common facial vein entering it anteriorly.

3. Ligate and divide the common facial vein (Fig. 9.15) and enter the plane anterior to the internal jugular vein. Retract the vein, exposing the common carotid artery and its bifurcation.

4. Identify the hypoglossal nerve which lies deep to the posterior belly of digastric where it crosses the external and internal carotids. Identify and retract the descendens hypoglossi.

5. Dissect out the common carotid and its branches, keeping close to the wall of the vessels. Control the superior thyroid artery with a sling (Fig. 9.16). Manipulate the diseased segment as little as possible to reduce the risk of embolization, and avoid dissecting posteriorly in the region of the carotid sinus to spare its nerve supply.

6. Once the patient has been heparinized systemically apply soft clamps to the three arteries. Occlude the internal carotid first and then make an arteriotomy over the diseased segment with a scalpel; this is extended using Potts scissors.

Site of incision

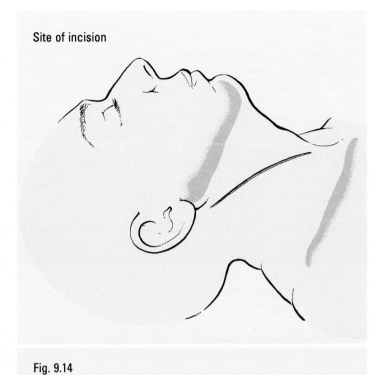

Fig. 9.14

Division of facial vein prior to exposure of carotid artery

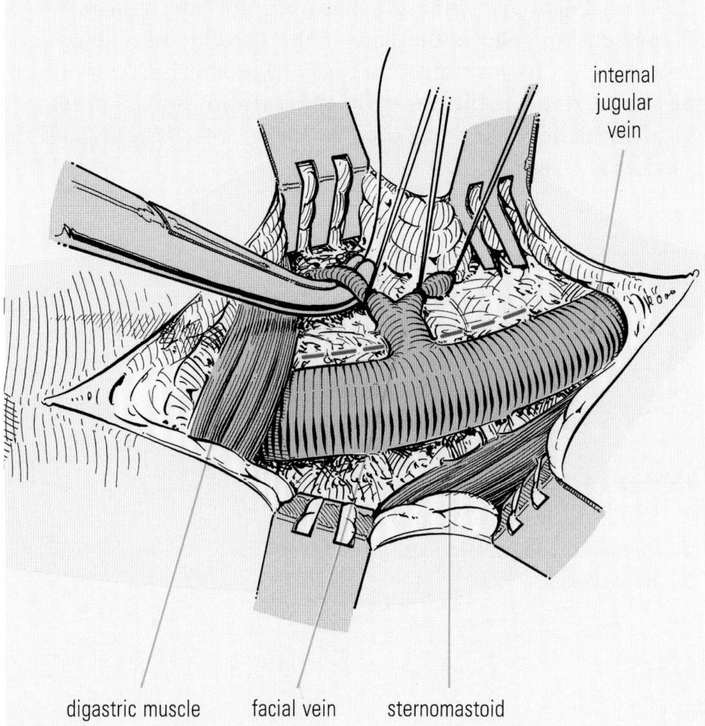

internal
jugular
vein

digastric muscle   facial vein   sternomastoid
muscle

Fig. 9.15

Exposure and control of carotid artery

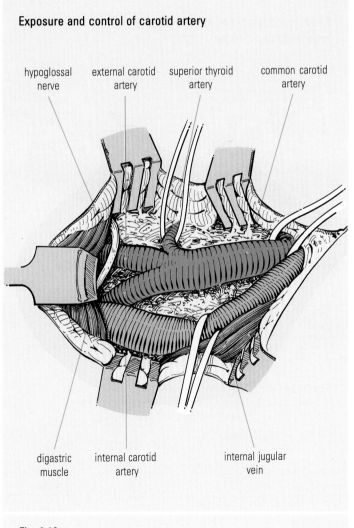

hypoglossal   external carotid   superior thyroid   common carotid
nerve   artery   artery   artery

digastric   internal carotid   internal jugular
muscle   artery   vein

Fig. 9.16

Good back bleeding from the internal carotid, when the clamp is removed, is indicative of an adequate collateral circulation, but a cerebral function monitor is more reliable.

If the distal collaterals are adequate

7. Use a Watson–Cheyne dissector to create a plane between the atheroma and the media (Fig. 9.17) and develop it both circumferentially and vertically until the plaque is cored out. It is essential that the intima is secure at the limits of the dissection or a flap may lift, especially distally, causing an occlusion.

8. Wash out any debris and close the arteriotomy with a continuous, non-absorbable, 5/0 suture (e.g. Prolene). On occasions a vein patch may be necessary to avoid producing a stenosis.

9. The order in which the clamps are released is important as this minimizes the risk of a cerebral embolus due to any remaining air or debris. Unclamp the internal carotid first, followed by the external carotid, and finally release the common carotid clamp whilst the origin of the internal carotid is occluded temporarily with a finger.

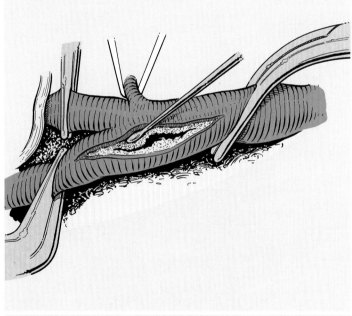

Dissection of plaque from distal common carotid and proximal internal carotid arteries

Fig. 9.17

If the distal collaterals are inadequate

7. In order to maintain cerebral perfusion a Javid shunt is required; this is a silastic tube which has bulbous ends to secure it inside the vessels. The essential factors are to exclude air, clot or debris from the system. After heparinization make the arteriotomy, as above, to a little beyond the full length of the stenosis.

8. Apply a clamp to the proximal end of the shunt. The distal end of the shunt is then inserted into the internal carotid and secured by a ring clamp.

9. Gently release the clamp on the shunt until all the air is expelled.

10. Place the proximal end in the mouth of the common carotid and release the clamp on the shunt again to fill its lumen with blood and remove any remaining air.

11. Advance the shunt into the common carotid and secure it.

12. Finally, slowly release the clamp on the shunt whilst checking for any air within it, complete the endartectomy, and remove the shunt prior to closing the vessel.

Wound closure and dressing

Drain the wound with either a small suction or corrugated drain and close the platysma and skin in separate layers with catgut and interrupted nylon, and apply a light dry dressing.

POSTOPERATIVE CARE

Fluctuations in blood pressure are common, particularly during the first 24 hours while the baroreceptor mechanism resets. Hypertension follows division of the carotid sinus nerve and responds to hypotensive therapy. Hypotension can usually be avoided by infiltration of the carotid sinus nerve with local anaesthetic. Remove the drain after 24–48 hours and the stitches at 5 days.

SPECIAL OPERATIVE HAZARDS
1. Cerebral ischaemia.
2. Embolization caused by a clot, debris or air.
3. Creating an intimal flap.
4. Damage to hypoglossal nerve.

COMPLICATIONS
1. Wound haematoma and infection.
2. Transient ischaemic attacks or stroke.
3. Restenosis.

Cervical Sympathectomy

A cervical sympathectomy involves the disruption of the sympathetic outflow to the upper limb by excising the sympathetic trunk below the fused inferior cervical and first cervical ganglion, and is performed for the relief of excessive upper limb sweating with good results. It can also be combined with repair of a subclavian aneurysm such as occurs with a cervical rib if multiple emboli have reached the hand. Its role in the treatment of Raynaud-type disorders is rather more controversial because the effect is often short lived. Intractible pain in the upper limb may be improved by cervical sympathectomy if it has responded to chemical sympathetic blockade; this should only be undertaken in collaboration with a pain control specialist.

PREOPERATIVE ASSESSMENT
1. In cases of upper limb ischaemia, perform plain X-rays of the neck and thoracic inlet to look for a cervical rib and arteriography to search for an associated obstruction or aneurysm formation in the subclavian artery.
2. Warn the patient of the possibility of developing a Horner's syndrome (i.e. ptosis and miosis of the ipselateral eye and reduced sweating of that side of the face).

RELEVANT ANATOMY
The scalenus anterior muscle runs forward and laterally from the anterior tubercles of the third to sixth cervical vertebrae to insert onto the scalene tubercle of the first rib; the phrenic nerve lies on its surface (Fig. 9.18). The subclavian vein runs in front of scalenus anterior and the subclavian artery runs behind it. The upper aspect of the subclavian artery gives rise to, from medial to lateral, the vertebral artery, the thyrocervical trunk and the costocervical trunk; the latter two can be divided if need be but the vertebral artery, lying just lateral to the cervical sympathetic chain, must be preserved. The internal thoracic (mammary) artery arises from the underside of the subclavian artery. On the left side the thoracic duct arches over the artery to enter the subclavian vein. The inferior cervical ganglion is usually fused with the first cervical ganglion to form the stellate ganglion which lies in front of the neck of the first rib. Lateral to it lies the supreme intercostal vein, the superior intercostal artery and, further lateral, the first thoracic nerve. The dome of the pleura keeps these structures applied to rib cage and the suprapleural membrane extends forward from C7 over the dome of the pleura.

OPERATION
Preparation
The patient is placed supine with head-up tilt and the head is rotated away from the side to be operated. The root of the neck is cleansed and draped. If a headlight is available it will improve visibility.

Incision
Make an incision approximately 6cm long a finger's breadth above the clavicle, starting over the lateral border of the sternomastoid muscle.

Operative technique
1. Deepen the incision through the platysma muscle and secure haemostasis. Retract or ligate and divide the external jugular vein.

Relevant anatomy

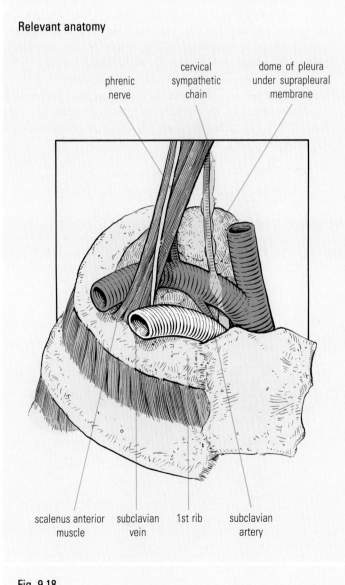

phrenic nerve · cervical sympathetic chain · dome of pleura under suprapleural membrane

scalenus anterior muscle · subclavian vein · 1st rib · subclavian artery

Fig. 9.18

2. Insert a self-retaining retractor, such as a Travers, and divide the lateral fibres of sternomastoid. The omohyoid muscle will be seen and is divided or retracted upward to improve access.

3. Visualize the phrenic nerve on the surface of scalenus anterior, gently pushing the subclavian vein downward if necessary. With care free the nerve from the muscle and place a soft rubber sling around it to gently retract it medially.

4. Working from lateral to medial, use scissors to divide the scalenus anterior muscle with a series of small snips (Fig. 9.19) to expose the subclavian artery which is controlled with a sling or tape (Fig. 9.20).

5. Retract the artery either upward or downward. To improve access the thyrocervical and costocervical trunks can be divided, but the vertebral artery must be preserved.

6. Gently free the suprapleural membrane posteriorly and sweep the dome of the pleura downwards with a dental swab, taking care not to open the pleura (if this happens there is a characteristic hiss as air enters the pleural space). Retract the lung apex and pleura downward with a malleable copper retractor and identify the stellate ganglion in front of the neck of the first rib. This must be preserved together with the rami arising from it (Fig. 9.21). It may be initially located by palpation with the tip of the index finger.

7. Remove the second and third thoracic ganglia together with the lower third of the stellate ganglion, dividing all their rami (Fig. 9.22), although some surgeons prefer to preserve the entire stellate ganglion.

Subclavian artery mobilized

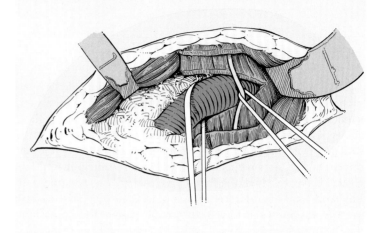

Fig. 9.20

Sympathetic chain displayed

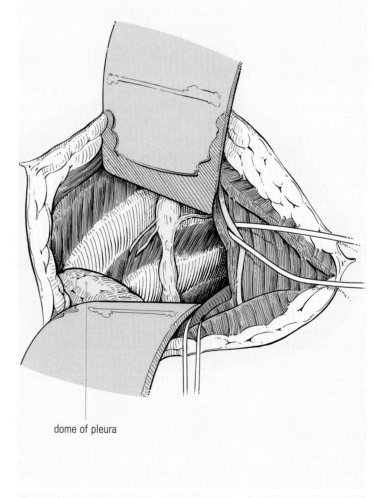

dome of pleura

Fig. 9.21

Division of scalenus anterior muscle

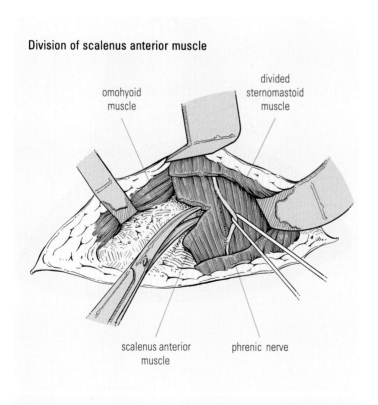

omohyoid muscle

divided sternomastoid muscle

scalenus anterior muscle

phrenic nerve

Fig. 9.19

Wound closure and dressing

If the pleura has been opened ensure that the lung is fully inflated, then close the pleura with a fine catgut suture and arrange a postoperative chest X-ray. The divided omohyoid, sternomastoid and scalenus anterior muscles need not be repaired. Insert a fine suction drain and close the skin and platysma as one layer with interrupted nylon sutures. Apply a waterproof dressing.

POSTOPERATIVE CARE

The drain is removed after 24 hours and the sutures after 5 days. An improvement in the hand should be noticeable immediately.

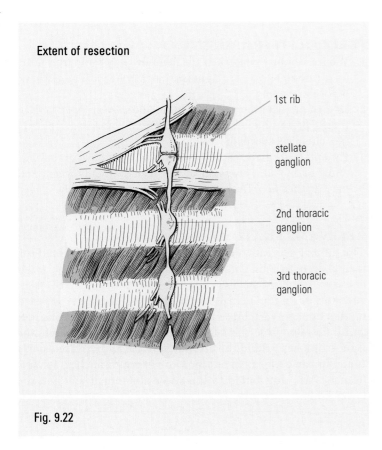

Extent of resection

1st rib

stellate ganglion

2nd thoracic ganglion

3rd thoracic ganglion

Fig. 9.22

SPECIAL OPERATIVE HAZARDS

1. Damage to the stellate ganglion causing Horner's syndrome.
2. Damage to the phrenic nerve, causing paralysis of the hemidiaphragm.
3. Damage to the thoracic duct. If this is recognized during the operation the duct should be ligated.
4. Damage to the apical pleura causing a pneumothorax.
5. Damage to the subclavian vessels or their branches.
6. Troublesome bleeding can follow damage to the intercostal vessels of the first space.
7. Unsuspected cervical rib, some of which are radiolucent fibrous bands. Excise any that are found.
8. Damage to the first thoracic nerve causing impaired function of the small muscles of the hand.

COMPLICATIONS

1. Recurrence of Raynaud symptoms.
2. Pneumothorax from opening the apical pleura. If noted postoperatively a chest drain is required if it is causing symptoms or increasing in size.
3. Lymphatic fistula from damage to the thoracic duct.

Lumbar Sympathectomy

Indications for lumbar sympathectomy include lower limb arterial insufficiency, traumatic arterial spasm, hyperhidrosis, acrocyanosis frigida, and causalgia. The extent of the sympathectomy depends on the degree of the denervation required. Excision of the second and third ganglia of either lumbar trunk leads to denervation of the ipselateral lower limb beyond the midthigh. If the buttock area needs to be included, the first ganglion must also be removed. However, it should be remembered that bilateral removal of the first lumbar ganglion is likely to interfere with ejaculation in the male.

PREOPERATIVE ASSESSMENT
1. Where doubt exists as to the benefit of a sympathectomy (e.g. causalgia) use a diagnostic block with local anaesthetic before operating.
2. Determine whether permanent ablation by an open operation is preferable to semi-permanent ablation using phenol (i.e. chemical sympathectomy).
3. Patients with diabetes mellitus are liable to have autonomic neuropathy, so if the skin of the feet is already warm and dry, further benefit from sympathectomy is unlikely.

RELEVANT ANATOMY
The lumbar sympathetic trunk enters the abdomen behind the medial arcuate ligament, and is entirely extraperitoneal. It lies anterior to the psoas fascia and the lumbar segmental vessels, and runs down the medial border of psoas, where it is attached to the lumbar vertebrae and transverse processes. The left trunk lies alongside the lateral border of the aorta, while the right trunk lies behind the inferior vena cava; there are usually four lumbar ganglia. In addition to visceral branches, somatic branches are distributed to the lower abdominal wall and the lower limb.

PROCEDURES
CHEMICAL SYMPATHECTOMY
A chemical sympathectomy is performed percutaneously under X-ray control and local anaesthesia. A needle is inserted midway between the spinous processes of L2 and L3, 3 cm from the midline. The cannula is advanced anteromedially until it strikes the lumbar vertebral body, and is then angled slightly laterally so that it skirts just anterior to the body. After aspirating to exclude venepuncture, local anaesthetic is instilled to test for satisfactory placement prior to phenolization. The skin temperature of the foot should rise.

OPERATIVE SYMPATHECTOMY
Preparation
The anaesthetized patient is placed supine with a sandbag under the ipselateral buttock. The abdomen and ipselateral loin are cleansed and draped.

Incision
Start the skin incision 3 cm lateral to the umbilicus, and extend it transversely for about 15 cm.

Operative technique
1. Divide external oblique in the line of the incision and open the lateral third of the anterior rectus sheath (Fig. 9.23).

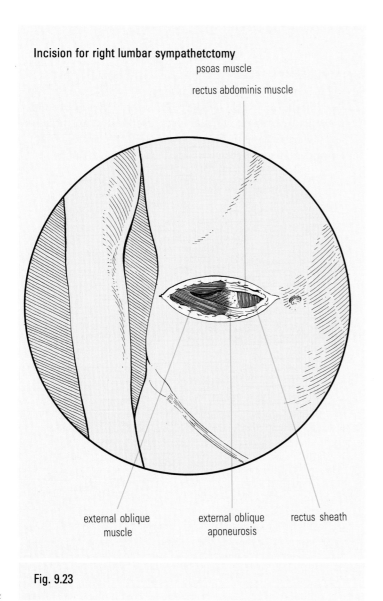

Incision for right lumbar sympathetctomy

psoas muscle

rectus abdominis muscle

external oblique muscle

external oblique aponeurosis

rectus sheath

Fig. 9.23

9.14

2. Displace the rectus muscle medially and open the lateral margin of the posterior rectus sheath to enter the extraperitoneal plane. Sweep the peritoneum from the deep surface of the transversus abdominus muscle by blunt dissection with an index finger. Using cutting diathermy divide the internal oblique and transversus abdominus muscles, taking care to preserve the neurovascular bundles and to stay out of the peritoneum.

3. Completely free the peritoneum laterally, and then sweep the peritoneum medially using a swab-on-a-stick, until the psoas muscle is identified; suture any tears in the peritoneum immediately, since if it is torn it will fill with air and billow into the operative field. The ureter will be displaced with the peritoneum and should be easy to identify. If in doubt, pinch it gently with non-toothed forceps and observe for peristalsis. The only other structure likely to be confused with sympathetic trunk is the genitofemoral nerve, but this lies more laterally over the body of psoas muscle, and contains no ganglia.

4. Using the index finger, identify the lumbar trunk as a thick band lateral to the aorta on the left, and behind the inferior vena cava on the right. Insert a Deaver retractor to complete the exposure, taking care to avoid damage to the inferior vena cava on the right (Fig. 9.24).

5. Carefully mobilize the second and third ganglia, hold them with Roberts' forceps, and excise them by dividing the trunk with scissors above the second and below the third ganglia (Fig. 9.25). Perform the Roberts' test: if the weight of a Roberts' forceps is sufficient to break the excised specimen, it cannot have been the entire trunk (Fig. 9.26).

Exposure of lumbar sympathetic chain

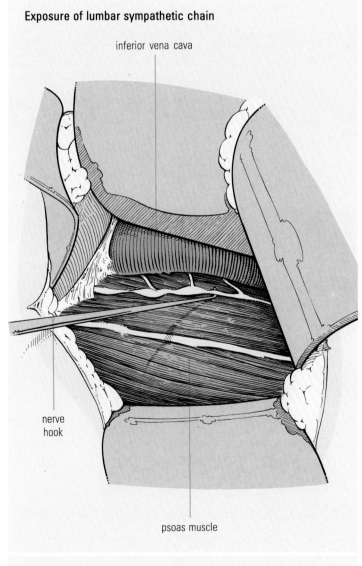

inferior vena cava

nerve hook

psoas muscle

Fig. 9.24

Cut chain with scissors

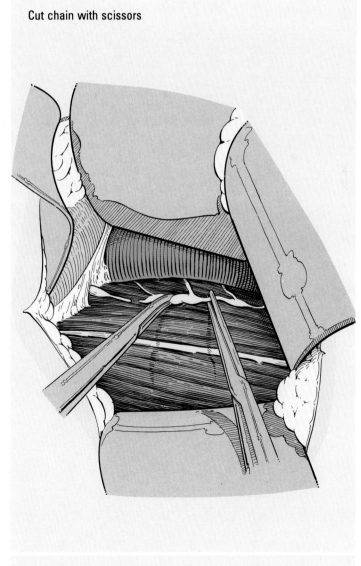

Fig. 9.25

Wound closure and dressing

Drainage is unnecessary. Close the abdominal muscles in two layers with 00 nylon, and the skin with subcuticular or interrupted sutures. Apply a waterproof dressing.

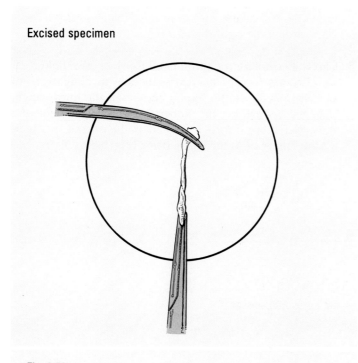

Excised specimen

Fig. 9.26

POSTOPERATIVE CARE

A temporary ileus may follow the retroperitoneal dissection, which is managed with a nasogastric tube and intravenous fluids. If an adequate operation has been performed, the foot should become warm and dry. Sutures are removed after 1 week.

SPECIAL OPERATIVE HAZARDS
1. Damage to the ureter, genitofemoral nerve or inferior vena cava.
2. Damage to the neurovascular bundles when dividing the internal oblique and transversus abdominus muscles.
3. Dissection in the wrong place.
4. Opening the peritoneum, in which case close the hole straight away with catgut.

COMPLICATIONS
1. A paralytic ileus may result, but usually settles quickly.
2. Post-sympathectomy pain may develop some weeks later, but is almost always self-limiting within a few months.
3. Bilateral removal of the first lumbar ganglion in the male will impair ejaculation.

Surgery for Varicose Veins

Surgery for varicose veins is commonly undertaken for cosmetic reasons. Medical indications include venous ulceration from chronic venous insufficiency. It is essential that the deep venous system of the leg is intact if one is considering interrupting the superficial venous system.

PREOPERATIVE ASSESSMENT

1. Suspect deep venous insufficiency if there is a history of previous deep vein thrombosis or trauma. Use Doppler studies or venography to investigate the deep veins.
2. Determine whether the valve of the saphenofemoral junction is competent and localize the level of any incompetent valve(s). Determine whether the varicosities involve the long or short saphenous systems or both. Incompetence at the sapheno-femoral junction can lead to the formation of a dilated saphena varix at this level.
3. Inquire about previous surgery or sclerotherapy to the veins.
4. Outline the veins with a permanent 'skin marker' while the patient stands on a stool in a well lit room, and mark the sites of the varicosities and incompetent perforating veins carefully. This is the most important step in the surgical treatment of varicose veins, yet is commonly delegated to an inexperienced junior house surgeon, which is unfair to both this doctor and the patient. The legs and groins are shaved.

RELEVANT ANATOMY

Varicose (i.e. tortuous and dilated veins) result from either a congenital incompetence of the valves in the superficial veins draining the lower limb (primary), or obstruction to the deep venous system of the lower limb, for example by venous thrombosis or a pelvic tumour (secondary). As the long saphenous system is most commonly affected, it is important for the surgeon to be familiar with the course of the long saphenous vein and the sites of its connections with the deep venous system.

The superficial venous drainage of the lower limb commences in the foot with a dorsal venous arch, which overlies the metatarsal heads and receives blood from the sole of the foot via branches which perforate the interosseous spaces. The dorsal arch continues medially as the long saphenous vein and laterally as the short saphenous vein, both of which run cranially in the subcutaneous tissues.

The long saphenous vein (Fig. 9.27) commences in front of the medial malleolus and runs up the medial side of the calf, passing just behind the bony prominence of the medial part of the knee joint. It then continues up the thigh to enter the medial side of the femoral vein just below the skin crease of the groin (Fig. 9.27). In the calf, the vein is accompanied by the saphenous nerve, a branch of the femoral nerve, which is sensory to the medial side of the calf and foot.

The long saphenous vein communicates with the deep venous system through two or three valved perforating veins in the

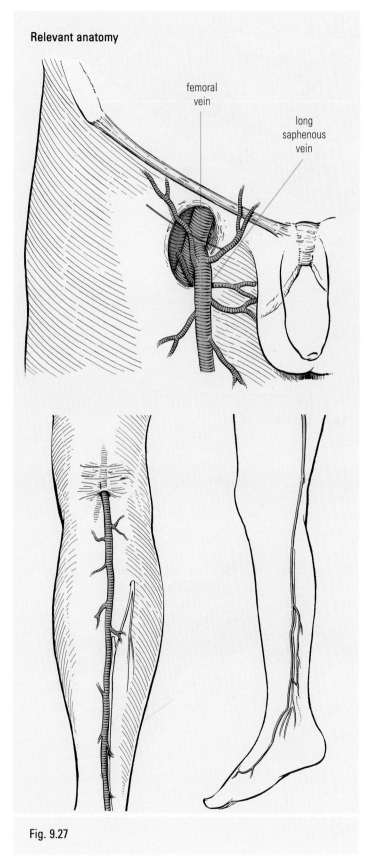

Relevant anatomy

femoral vein

long saphenous vein

Fig. 9.27

9.17

Exposure of long saphenous vein at the groin

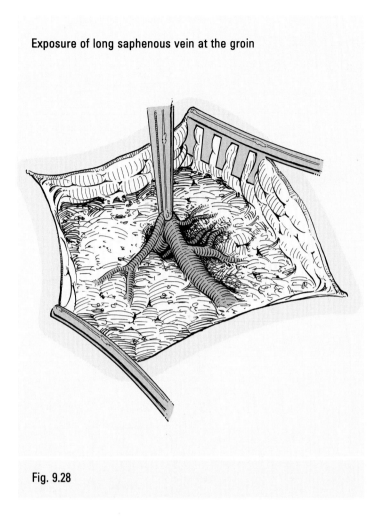

Fig. 9.28

Ligation of tributaries

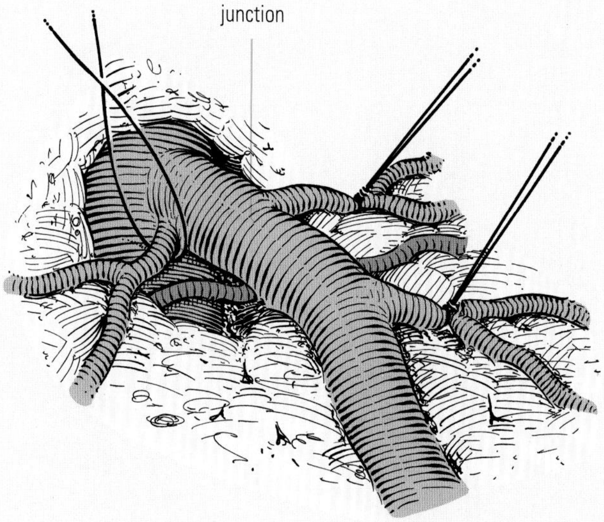

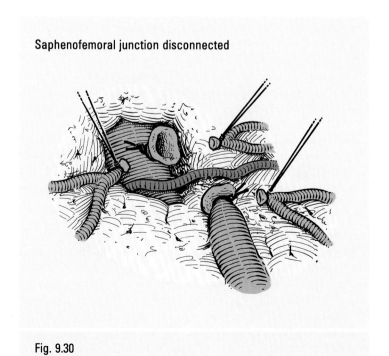

Fig. 9.29

calf, and one or two in the thigh. Close to the saphenofemoral junction, the long saphenous vein receives tributaries which drain the skin of the upper thigh and the skin of the inguinal and pubic regions.

The short saphenous vein (Fig. 9.27) is the continuation of the lateral end of the dorsal venous arch and passes behind the lateral malleolus and up the back of the calf, where it is associated with the sural nerve. It pierces the fascial roof the popliteal fossa to enter the popliteal vein. There are superficial connections between the long and short saphenous veins.

OPERATIONS
LONG SAPHENOUS VEIN
Preparation
The anaesthetized patient is placed supine. The legs are lifted by feet and the legs and groins cleansed and draped with a towel covering the genitalia and surgical gloves over the feet. The legs are abducted and head-down (Trendelenberg) tilt applied.

Incision
Make an incision obliquely over the saphenofemoral junction, over the saphenous vein in front of the medial malleolus, and short vertical stab incisions over the marked varicosities.

Operative technique
1. In the groin, carefully dissect the long saphenous vein and its tributaries and display the saphenofemoral junction (Fig. 9.28). Ligate and divide the tributaries with an absorbable suture (e.g. 00 Vicryl) (Fig. 9.29), and then ligate and divide

Saphenofemoral junction disconnected

Fig. 9.30

Exposure of saphenous vein at the ankle

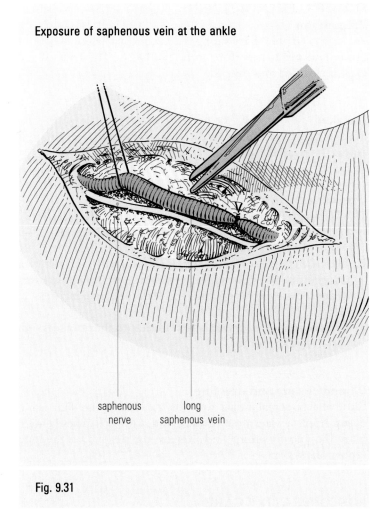

saphenous nerve   long saphenous vein

Fig. 9.31

Insertion of stripper

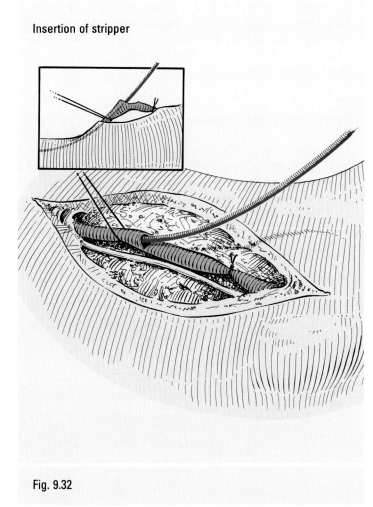

Fig. 9.32

the saphenous vein between 0 silk ties flush with the saph-enofemoral junction (Fig. 9.30). With a saphena varix it is sometimes safer to transfix the junction.

2. At the ankle, carefully free the origin of the long saphenous vein from the saphenous nerve, ligate it distally (Fig. 9.31), and partially divide it so that the stripper can be passed into the lumen (Fig. 9.32).

3. Negotiate the stripper up the vein, ensuring that it remains superficial throughout. At the knee it can be cut down onto and brought out through the skin if only the portion below the knee is to be stripped, otherwise it can be brought out at the groin where it will be seen through the wall of the ligated saphenous vein.

4. Use a 00-gauge silk ligature to secure the vein around the stripper at each end. Transect the vein at the ankle and open it at the thigh to allow access to the end of the stripper. The T-bar handle is attached and the stripper slowly withdrawn via the groin wound. As the stripper moves up the leg, pick up the varicosities through the stab incisions using a fine haemostat (Fig. 9.33) and avulse them by traction, with re-application of the haemostat close to the skin to allow the

Grasping tributary with haemostats

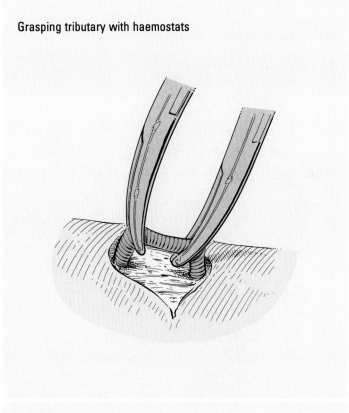

Fig. 9.33

9.19

maximum length of vein to be removed (Fig. 9.34). Perforating veins are formally dissected and ligated with silk. Firm pressure with a swab should be applied over the avulsion sites by an assistant. The stripper is pulled up until its distal end emerges from the groin (Fig. 9.35).

Wound closure and dressing
Close the fascia of the groin with an absorbable suture (e.g. Vicryl) and the skin with nylon sutures or staples throughout. Cover the groin wound with a sticking plaster and the leg wounds with Nobecutane spray and non-adherent gauze. The leg is bandaged firmly from the foot to the groin.

Avulsion of vein

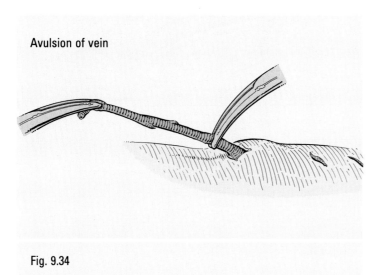

Fig. 9.34

Withdrawal of stripper

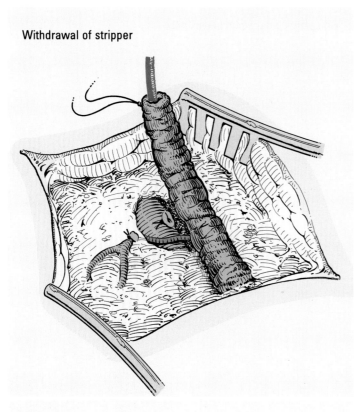

Fig. 9.35

SHORT SAPHENOUS VEIN
Preparation
To approach the short saphenous vein the patient is placed prone and needs therefore to be intubated. The back of the knee is cleansed and draped.

Incision
Make a 'lazy-S' incision over the short saphenous vein where it enters the popliteal vein.

Operative technique
1. Mobilize the short saphenous vein and control it with a sling. Ligate and divide any branches which enter the vein.

2. Extend the opening in the tough fascia of the popliteal fossa transmitting the short saphenous vein vertically with scissors to allow exposure of the junction with the popliteal vein.

3. Divide the short saphenous vein flush with the popliteal vein between silk ligatures.

Wound closure and dressing
Close the popliteal fascia with 00 Vicryl and the skin using nylon. Apply a waterproof dressing and, while still anaesthetized, place the patient supine and prepare for surgery on the long saphenous system.

POSTOPERATIVE CARE
The patient is mobilized the following day and given removable supporting bandages. Exercise (walking) is encouraged with the bandages on, and when resting the patient is advised to elevate the feet with the bandages off for the first 6 weeks.

> ### SPECIAL OPERATIVE HAZARDS
> 1. Damage to the femoral vein.
> 2. Damage to the saphenous nerve; this usually occurs at the ankle and will cause sensory loss over the medial side of the foot.

COMPLICATIONS
1. Slipping of the ligature on the saphenofemoral or saphenopopliteal junction; use of a suture ligature should eliminate this hazard which, should it occur, is an indication for urgent re-exploration.
2. Wound infection, particularly infection of the groin wound.
3. Haematoma; some bruising is inevitable, but can be minimized by peroperative pressure on the avulsion sites, and the correct application of bandages.
4. Recurrence of varicosities; if varicosities are visible immediately after the operation it is likely that one or more sites of valve incompetence have been overlooked, whereas later recurrences reflect the underlying valvular weakness in the superficial venous system.

Femoral Embolectomy

Femoral embolectomy is performed to remove an arterial embolus from the arterial tree of the lower limb, and can be adapted to remove a saddle embolus from the lower aorta.

PREOPERATIVE ASSESSMENT

1. Ensure that the clinical diagosis is correct as it is easy to mistake it for arterial thrombosis. If in doubt or if the history is several days long request an emergency arteriogram.
2. Give $1\,mg\,kg^{-1}$ body weight intravenous heparin.
3. Check the cardiovascular system for hypertension and ischaemic heart disease, particularly a recent myocardial infarction, and uncontrolled atrial fibrillation. Document all lower limb pulses.
4. Does the patient have diabetes?

5. Decide whether to operate under local or general anaesthetic.

RELEVANT ANATOMY (Fig. 9.36)

When the arterial lumen proximal to the common femoral artery is occluded the femoral pulse is lost. In a fat patient this can make identification of the femoral arteries quite difficult and a knowledge of the anatomy of the femoral triangle is essential if vital structures are to be preserved.

The common femoral artery emerges from under the inguinal ligament at the mid-inguinal point, halfway between the pubic tubercle and the anterior superior iliac spine (Fig. 9.36). The femoral vein lies immediately medial, and the femoral nerve immediately lateral, to the artery at this point. The long saphenous vein pierces the cribriform fascia and drains into the

Relevant anatomy

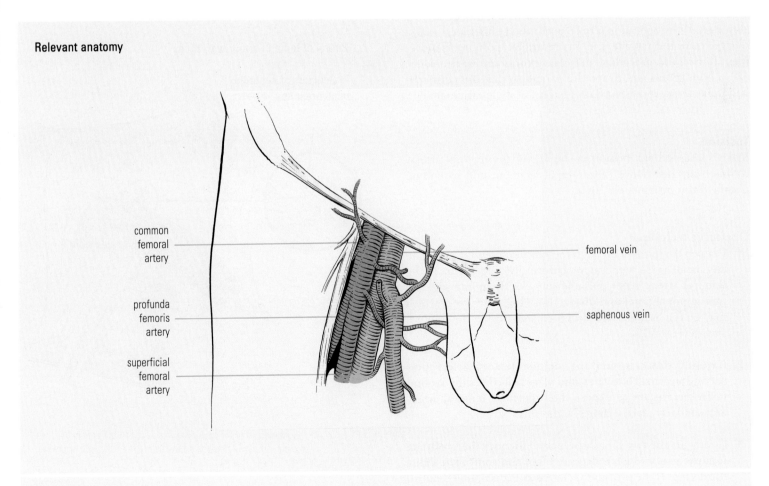

common
femoral
artery

profunda
femoris
artery

superficial
femoral
artery

femoral vein

saphenous vein

Fig. 9.36

anteromedial aspect of the femoral vein, approximately 3–4 cm below the inguinal ligament. At this point the long saphenous vein receives several named tributaries, including the superficial circumflex iliac and superficial epigastric veins, which may need to be ligated and divided before the common femoral artery can be fully exposed. Once the common femoral artery has been identified, dissection along the artery within the femoral sheath will avoid any risk of damaging the adjacent femoral vein and nerve.

The common femoral artery usually gives off four branches, the superficial circumflex iliac, the superficial epigastric, the superficial external pudendal and the deep external pudendal arteries, before dividing into the superficial femoral artery and profunda femoris arteries approximately 5 cm below the inguinal ligament. In an ischaemic limb these branches should be preserved as they may provide a collateral circulation. The profunda femoris artery usually arises from the lateral or deep aspect of the common femoral artery and occasionally two profunda arteries may be found.

OPERATION

Preparation

If the patient is in great pain or is very agitated or confused it is preferable to use general anaesthesia. However, if the patient is co-operative but in a poor general condition it is better to use local anaesthetic such as 1% lignocaine or 0.25% bupivicaine. In either case an anaesthetist will be required in the operating theatre to monitor the patient's condition and administer an appropriate anaesthetic or sedative whilst the surgeon operates.

Place the patient in a supine position with the legs slightly abducted. If the operation is to be performed under local anaesthetic ensure the patient is in a comfortable position as movement during the procedure may cause considerable problems. Clean both groins and drape the patient so that the perineum and pubis are covered but both femoral triangles are exposed.

Incision

Make a longitudinal incision in the line of the femoral artery, commencing just above the inguinal ligament and extending distally for approximately 10 cm.

Operative technique

1. Deepen the incision through the subcutaneous fat and ligate any small veins with catgut before dividing them. If the femoral artery is not pulsatile stay exactly in line with the mid-inguinal point and dissect down onto the artery which may be felt as a hard cord immediately within the femoral sheath (Fig. 9.37).

2. Carefully dissect around the common femoral artery, preserving any small branches, and place a silicone sling around it. Dissect distally to expose the superficial femoral artery and similarly place a sling around this.

3. Gently lift the two slings upwards to identify the profunda femoris artery which is dissected free and controlled with a third sling. If the profunda femoris artery is double, control both branches (Fig. 9.38).

Exposure of femoral artery

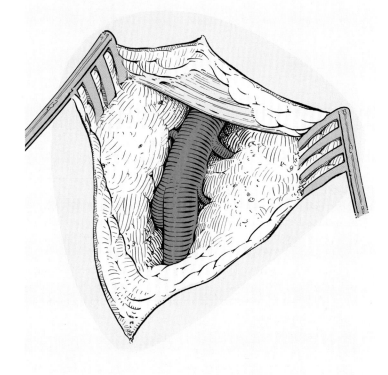

Fig. 9.37

Control of femoral artery with slings

Techniques of securing small branches

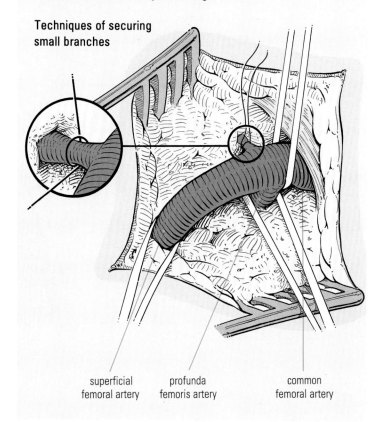

superficial femoral artery   profunda femoris artery   common femoral artery

Fig. 9.38

4. If the femoral arteries are pulsatile, apply an arterial clamp to the common femoral artery and paediatric or heavy bulldog clamps to the superficial and profunda femoris arteries (Fig. 9.39). If the arteries are not pulsatile, clamps need not be applied but they should be close to hand.

5. Palpate the common femoral artery and identify an area of its wall which is not too hard or rigid. If possible make an oblique arteriotomy in the common femoral artery (Fig. 9.40).

6. If the arteries were pulsatile carefully release the proximal, common femoral clamp to establish that the inflow is good. If pulseless, then pass an appropriately sized (e.g. 4 or 5 Fr) Fogarty embolectomy catheter proximally for 10–15 cm, inflate the balloon to the volume printed on the catheter and gently withdraw it (Fig. 9.41). As the thrombus and clot are extruded control the artery with the silicone sling to prevent an uncontrolled gush of blood. If the flow is not excellent repeat the procedure until there is no more clot and a powerful jet of blood. Place an arterial clamp on the common femoral artery. If an adequate inflow cannot be established summon help.

7. Pass a smaller embolectomy catheter down the superficial femoral artery as far as possible (ideally the catheter should pass to the ankle) and inflate the balloon just sufficiently to produce slight resistance and withdraw any clot (Fig. 9.42). Adjusting the volume in the balloon by pressure on the inflating syringe allows it to fit snugly into the vessel and gives slight resistance when it is withdrawn. Repeat this

until good back bleeding is obtained. If the catheter will not pass distally because the vessel is severely atherosclerotic then it is likely that the diagnosis is incorrect and the patient has suffered an acute thrombosis of a stenosed artery.

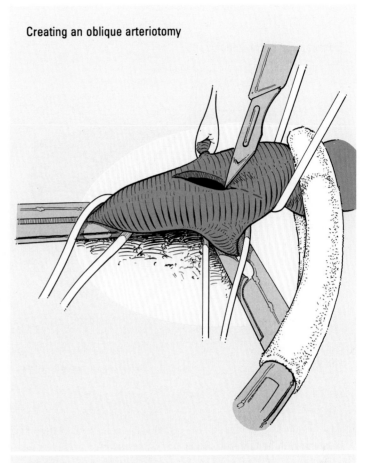

Creating an oblique arteriotomy

Fig. 9.40

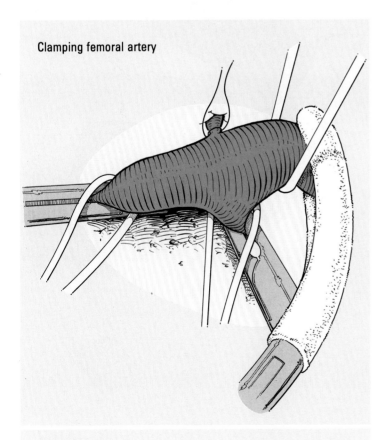

Clamping femoral artery

Fig. 9.39

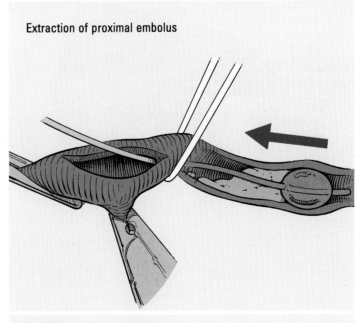

Extraction of proximal embolus

Fig. 9.41

9.23

8. Repeat the process for the profunda femoris artery. Flush 20ml of heparinized saline down the superficial femoral and profunda femoris (Fig. 9.43) and place clamps on each vessel.

9. Send samples of embolus for culture and histological examinations.

10. Check that the other femoral pulse is still easily palpable. If not, then a clot or thrombus from the aortic bifurcation has probably been dislodged down the contralateral iliac arteries and an embolectomy will have to be performed via that groin.

11. For a saddle embolus, expose the femoral arteries on both sides and pass an embolectomy catheter up one side into the aorta, with the femoral artery on the other side occluded with a clamp. Repeat from the other side with the first side clamped. It is important to clamp the other side to prevent the embolus dislodging into the lower limb arteries.

12. Repair the arteriotomy with a continuous, non-absorbable (e.g. 6/0 Prolene) suture, passing the needle from outside inwards on the upper edge so that the needle then passes from the inside outwards on the lower edge; this reduces the possibility of raising a distal intimal flap which may lead

Extraction of distal embolus

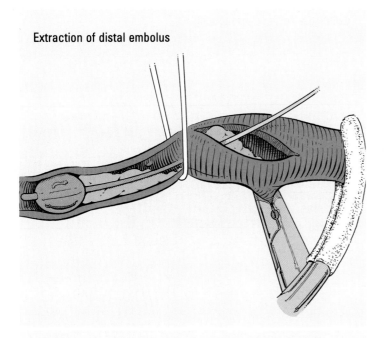

Fig. 9.42

Flushing with heparinized saline

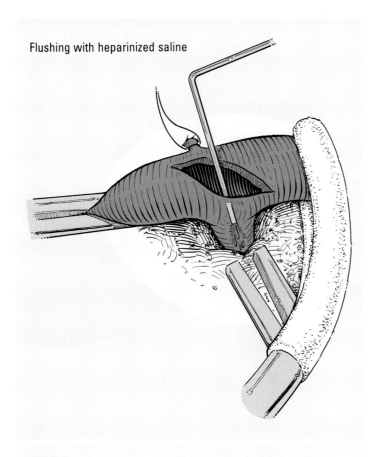

Fig. 9.43

Closure of arteriotomy

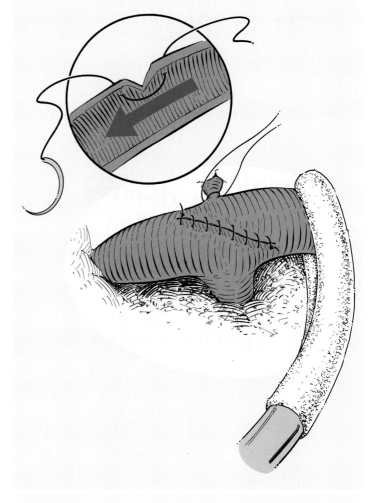

Fig. 9.44

Use of vein patch to repair arteriotomy

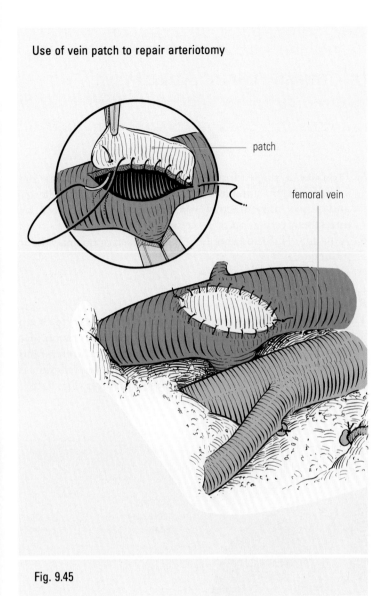

patch

femoral vein

Fig. 9.45

to a dissection (Fig. 9.44). If there is any risk of narrowing the vessel at the arteriotomy site, make a patch from a piece of adjacent vein and stitch this into the defect with a running suture (Fig. 9.45). When placing the sutures, again sew from the inside of the artery out to prevent raising an intimal flap. Under no circumstances use the long saphenous vein as a patch as it may be required for a reconstructive bypass.

13. Release the distal clamps to allow retrograde filling of the vessels with blood. Remove the proximal clamp, place a dry swab over the suture line and wait for the bleeding to stop. This may take some minutes and it is better to be patient than to place further sutures which may damage the vessel.

Wound closure and dressing

1. Insert a suction drain and close the wound with catgut for the fascia and nylon for the skin.

2. Check that the foot is adequately perfused at the end of the operation.

POSTOPERATIVE CARE

Unless there is a specific contra-indication the patient should remain systemically heparinized fro 3–4 days and then be converted to warfarin. A cause for the embolus should then be sought, likely origins being the left atrial appendage, endocardium, the mitral or aortic valve and the thoraco-abdominal aorta. The result of culture and histological examinations of the embolus should be checked. The duration of warfarin treatment will depend on the underlying cause of the embolus. The suction drain should be removed when drainage has become minimal and the patient is mobilized as soon as possible. Sutures can be removed on the eighth to tenth day depending on healing.

SPECIAL OPERATIVE HAZARDS

1. Damage to the femoral vein or nerve.

2. Dislodgement of embolus into the contralateral limb. This requires an embolectomy on the other side.

3. Production of an intimal flap and consequent dissection and occlusion of the vessel.

4. Failure to extract embolus or to establish good back bleeding is associated with a poor outcome. Consider an on-table arteriogram and, if appropriate, proceed to a bypass (see page 9.42 on femoropopliteal bypass).

COMPLICATIONS

1. Wound haematoma and infection.

2. Ischaemic gangrene of toes, foot or lower leg if the embolectomy was incomplete. 'Trash foot' results from small emboli occluding the vessels in the foot.

3. Lymphocele or lymphatic fistula in the groin.

Elective Repair of Infrarenal Abdominal Aortic Aneurysm

An otherwise fit patient with an aortic aneurysm of 6cm in diameter has a 75% chance of rupture within 18 months. Whilst mortality from elective repair is less than 5%, and mortality from rupture exceeds 50% with many dying before they reach hospital.

PREOPERATIVE ASSESSMENT
1. Check the cardiovascular system; a specialist opinion may be required on the state of the myocardium.
2. The respiratory system should be assessed.
3. Investigate renal function.
4. An arteriogram and/or CT scan are needed to confirm that the aneurysm is infrarenal and to determine whether the iliac arteries are aneurysmal.
5. Prescribe a single dose of prophylactic flucloxacillin and gentamicin (or suitable alternative if the patient is allergic and/or has unsatisfactory renal function) to be given on anaesthetic induction.
6. A mannitol infusion should be commenced upon anaesthetic induction.

RELEVANT ANATOMY
To repair an abdominal aortic aneurysm it is necessary to clamp the aorta above the aneurysm and to clamp the common iliac arteries distally. This places the duodenum, the ureters and major veins at risk, so a clear knowledge of the anatomy is essential to avoid damaging any of these structures (Fig. 9.46).

Relevant anatomy

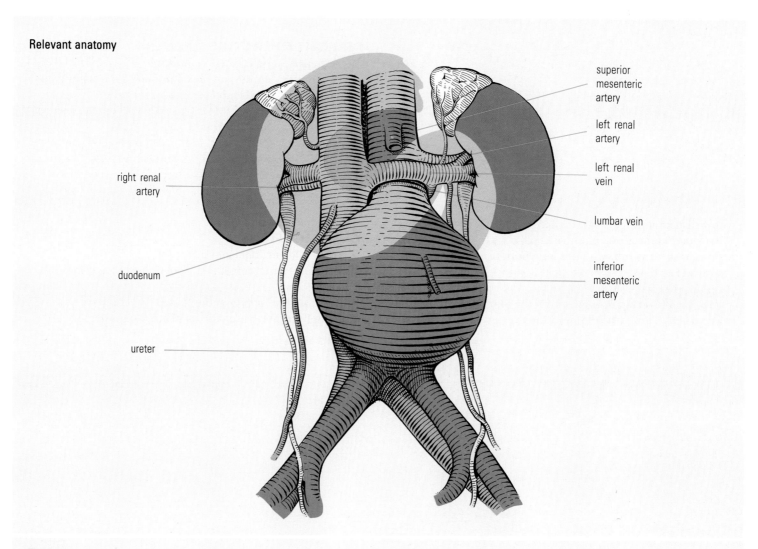

right renal artery

duodenum

ureter

superior mesenteric artery

left renal artery

left renal vein

lumbar vein

inferior mesenteric artery

Fig. 9.46

9.26

The third and fourth parts of the duodenum lie immediately anterior to the aortic wall, at the level of the renal arteries. The duodenum is often adherent to the aortic wall, especially if the aneurysm is inflammatory, and must be carefully dissected free before the neck of the aneurysm can be identified. As the duodenum is reflected to the right, the inferior mesenteric vein, which is stretched over the left side of the aneurysm, passes posterior to the duodenum and anterior to the neck of the aneurysm. If the vein prevents adequate access to the neck of the aneurysm it will require ligating and dividing.

The left renal vein is anterior to the aorta at the level of the renal arteries. If the neck of the aneurysm is very close to the renal arteries it will be necessary to mobilize the left renal vein in order to gain sufficient space to apply an aortic clamp; it is rarely necessary to ligate and divide the left renal vein. There is usually a lumbar vein draining into the back of the left renal vein, immediately to the left of the aneurysm neck, and this vein can be easily torn whilst applying the aortic clamp. Great care should be taken to avoid damaging this lumbar vein, and it is best to suture ligate and divide it if difficulties arise.

The common iliac veins lie immediately behind the common iliac arteries and the ureters pass anterior to the bifurcation of the common iliac arteries. Both these veins and the ureters are liable to be damaged when the iliac arteries are clamped. The common iliac arteries are commonly tortuous in patients with aneurysmal disease but they can be cross-clamped without dissecting them from the underlying veins; persistent attempts to circumferentially dissect these arteries when the vein is adherent may result in a hole in the vein and torrential haemorrhage. If the arteries are clamped before their bifurcation the ureters are not placed at risk.

The inferior mesenteric artery arises from the front of the aorta 4–5 cm above the aortic bifurcation and will therefore arise from the front of an abdominal aortic aneurysm. In patients with an aneurysm, the inferior mesenteric artery is often thrombosed and the left colon receives its blood supply via the marginal artery of Drummond. However, if the artery is patent, it will need to be oversewn to stop back bleeding when the aneurysm sac is opened. A few surgeons recommend re-implanting patent arteries into the aortic graft, which prolongs a major operation but reduces the risk of ischaemic necrosis of the colon; this is uncommon but potentially lethal.

OPERATION
Preparation
Place the patient supine with both arms abducted, and a urinary catheter inserted to monitor urine production. Full cardiorespiratory monitoring with an electrocardiograph, and central venous, arterial and pulmonary wedge pressure lines are essential.

Clean the skin of the entire abdomen from nipples to mid-thigh and drape the patient so that both groins are in the operative field. Use an adhesive drape to hold the towels in the desired position (Fig. 9.47).

Incision
Make a midline incision from the xiphisternum to the symphysis pubis. Use two self-retaining retractors to hold the wound open (Fig. 9.48).

Position of drapes and skin incision

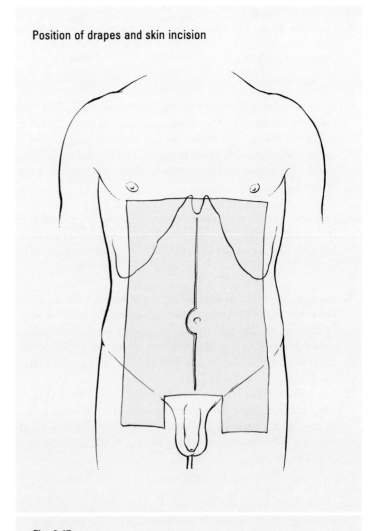

Fig. 9.47

Transverse colon reflected upward to expose aneurysm

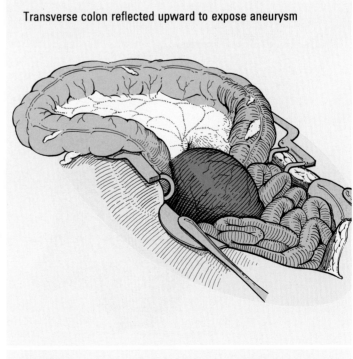

Fig. 9.48

9.27

Operative technique

1. Perform a careful laparotomy (see page 5.2) to confirm that the aneurysm is confined to the aorta and to exclude any other pathology.

2. Reflect the root of the small bowel mesentery by incising its peritoneal attachment to the posterior abdominal wall from the caecum to the duodenojejunal flexure. Identify and protect the right ureter. If the duodenum is adherent to the aneurysm wall carefully dissect it free before placing the small bowel in a sterile polythene bag to prevent damage or dessication.

3. Examine the neck of the aneurysm and its relationship to the renal arteries, the left renal vein and the vena cava. Identify and ligate the inferior mesenteric artery close to its origin (Fig. 9.49).

4. Expose the common iliac arteries and dissect sufficiently to allow vascular clamps to be placed across the full diameter of each vessel. Do not attempt to dissect around the entire circumference of the iliac arteries. Some surgeons do encircle the aorta above the neck of the aneurysm with a tape.

5. If a knitted graft is to be used, remove 50 ml of blood from the patient using a sterile syringe and ask the scrub nurse to save it. All patients are systemically anticoagulated with 1 mg kg^{-1} body weight of intravenous heparin, allowing 3 minutes for the heparin to circulate before clamping the aorta and iliac arteries (see Fig. 9.50). Take care not to damage the vena cava or lumbar and iliac veins.

6. Incise the aneurysm longitudinally (Fig. 9.50) and remove all the thrombus from the lumen, oversewing any bleeding lumbar arteries, the median sacral and the inferior mesenteric artery (if not ligated earlier) from within the aortic lumen, with silk sutures (Fig. 9.51).

7. Extend the incision in the aneurysm upwards to the anterior aspect of its neck and downwards as far as the distal ring which embraces the orifices of both common iliac arteries. At both the upper and lower limits of the incision cut the aorta laterally for a quarter of the circumference on each side, thereby leaving the posterior half of the circumference intact (see inset to Fig. 9.50). Do not completely transect it at either end.

8. Measure the diameter of the aortic lumen and select a suitably sized, straight Dacron graft. Stretch the graft to open the corrugations and cut the required length. If a knitted graft is used, preclot it at this stage by introducing the blood that had been previously removed.

9. Using a double ended 2/0 vascular suture, commence the upper anastomosis in the midline of the posterior wall by taking a double bite through the neck of the aneurysm,

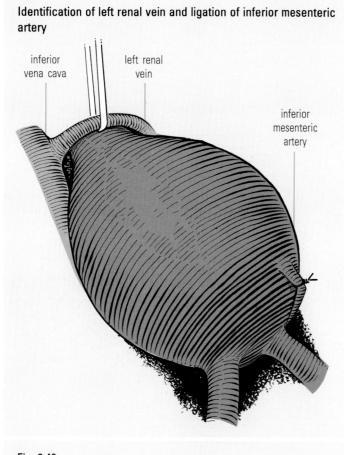

Identification of left renal vein and ligation of inferior mesenteric artery

inferior vena cava

left renal vein

inferior mesenteric artery

Fig. 9.49

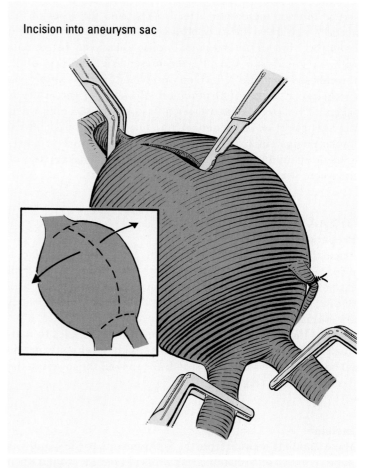

Incision into aneurysm sac

Fig. 9.50

from the top downwards (Fig. 9.52). Use each end of the suture to place two or three loose stitches through the aneurysm neck and the graft, and then parachute the graft into position whilst applying tension on the sutures.

10. Continue the posterior wall of the upper anastomosis using each end of the suture to complete a quarter of the suture line, taking double bites of the aortic wall throughout (Fig. 9.52). Ensure that your assistant keeps adequate tension on the suture.

11. Complete the anterior wall of the upper anastomosis by suturing the graft to the cut edge of the aorta so that each end of the suture reaches the midline. Again take double bites of the aortic wall and ensure that tension on the suture is maintained throughout. Securely knot the two ends together where they meet.

12. Place a Craford clamp across the graft and, having warned the anaesthetist, test the anastomosis by partially releasing the aortic clamp. The graft is then lifted up in order to inspect the posterior wall of the anastomosis. Make sure you are satisfied that the anastomosis is adequate, particularly posteriorly, because you will no longer have access to it after this point in the operation. Significant bleeding points along the suture line are secured with further interrupted sutures.

13. Use a second double ended 3/0 non-absorbable suture (e.g. Prolene) to fashion the distal anastomosis in a similar manner, taking double bites of the aortic wall from the bottom upwards (Fig. 9.53). It may be necessary to use a

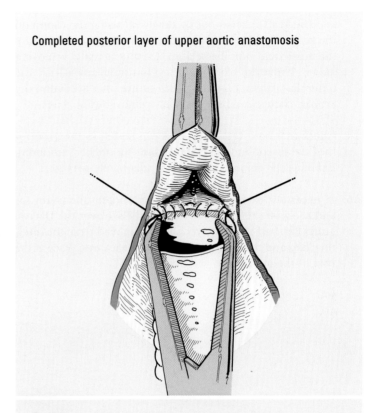

Completed posterior layer of upper aortic anastomosis

Fig. 9.52

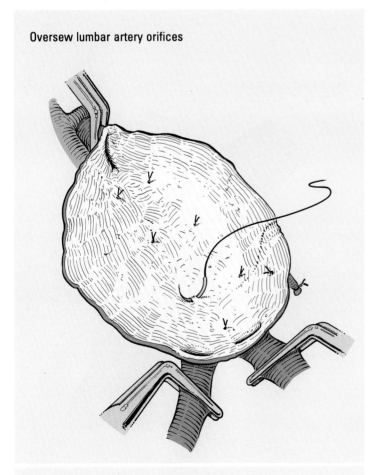

Oversew lumbar artery orifices

Fig. 9.51

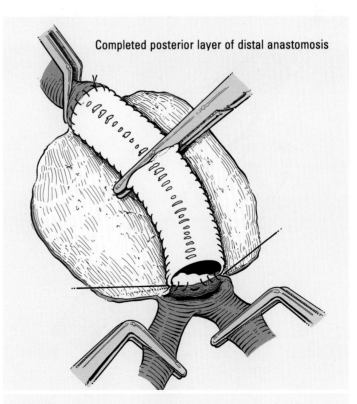

Completed posterior layer of distal anastomosis

Fig. 9.53

9.29

bifurcation ('trouser') graft to either the iliac vessels, or to the femoral vessels exposed in the groin with oversewing of the proximal ends of the iliacs, if the aneurysm extends beyond the aortic bifurcation (see page 9.35). Before closing the anterior wall of the distal anastomosis release the iliac clamps for a few seconds to allow back bleeding and then reapply the clamps. Once the anaesthetist has been warned and the graft flushed out by slowly releasing the clamp on the graft, close the distal anastomosis and completely release the aortic and one iliac clamp, without actually removing either. When the blood pressure has stabilized release the other iliac clamp. Providing both suture lines are sound the arterial clamps can be completely removed (Fig. 9.54).

14. Check that both femoral pulses can be felt in the groin; if they are absent femoral embolectomy should be considered. Examine the colon to ensure it is adequately perfused.

15. If necessary excise some of the redundant aneurysm sac and use a 00 catgut suture to close the sac over the Dacron graft (Fig. 9.55). The bowel is then removed from the intestinal bag and the peritoneum sutured back into place at the root of the mesentery.

Wound closure and dressing

Drains are not usually required and only serve as a potential route for infection. Close the wound with a continuous monofilament nylon to the linea alba, catgut for fascia and subcuticular or interrupted non-absorbable sutures (e.g. Prolene) for the skin before covering the wound with a waterproof dressing.

POSTOPERATIVE CARE

The patient should remain intubated and ventilated for the first 12 hours after operation and will therefore be nursed in an intensive care unit for 24–28 hours until extubated and adequately self-ventilating. Cardiac, respiratory and renal function will be carefully monitored during this period and the circulation to the legs should be regularly assessed, although pedal pulses often do not return for 6–12 hours.

The urinary catheter and cardiovascular monitoring lines should be removed as soon as they are no longer essential for the recovery of the patient, as they represent potential routes for infection which could lead to infection of the graft. Prophylactic antibiotics should be discontinued after 24 hours unless there is a specific indication to continue them.

Both anastomoses completed

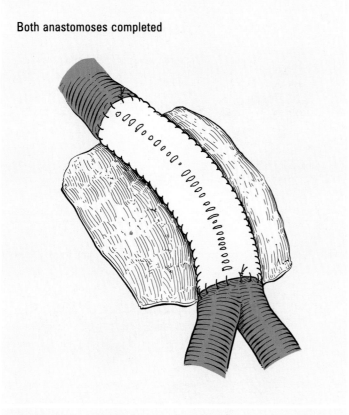

Fig. 9.54

Sac closed over graft

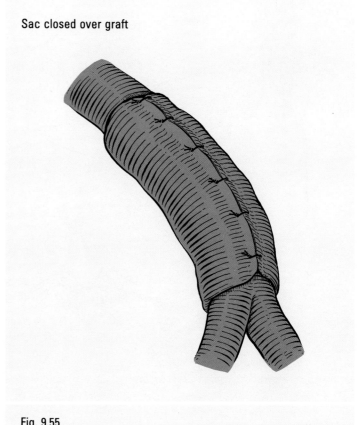

Fig. 9.55

SPECIAL OPERATIVE HAZARDS

1. Damage to the vena cava.
2. Damage to the left renal vein.
3. Bleeding from a torn lumbar vein.
4. Bleeding from a damaged iliac vein.
5. Injury to a ureter.
6. Distal emboli of thrombus.
7. Occlusion of one or both renal artery orifices.

COMPLICATIONS

1. Reactionary haemorrhage as blood pressure rises.
2. Myocardial infarction.
3. Trash foot from distal emboli.
4. Necrosis of the left colon if the marginal artery is not patent.
5. Renal failure.
6. False aneurysm formation from the upper anastomosis which can fistulate into the duodenum.
7. Graft infection following bacteraemia.

Repair of Ruptured Aortic Aneurysm

Rupture of an aortic aneurysm is rapidly lethal unless treated surgically.

PREOPERATIVE ASSESSMENT

1. Perform a chest X-ray and ECG. A ruptured aortic aneurysm may by mistaken for a severe myocardial infarct and the hypotension can render the aneurysm impalpable. Often the diagnosis is obvious and further investigation is not appropriate if it is likely to delay treatment. If the diagnosis is unclear consider a CT or ultrasound scan.
2. Commence an intravenous infusion and cross-match twelve units of blood, but transfuse sparingly at this stage since a sudden rise in blood pressure may cause further bleeding.
3. Transfer the patient to the operating theatre and continue resuscitation there, ensuring adequate venous access for rapid transfusion and adequate monitoring of arterial and venous pressure and urine output.
4. If available, prepare a cell saver/rapid transfuser for use.

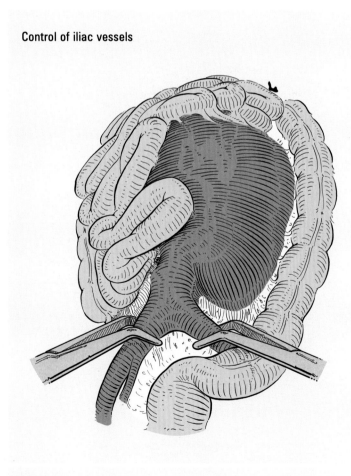

Control of iliac vessels

Fig. 9.56

RELEVANT ANATOMY

The aorta overlies the spinal column as it passes between the crura of the diaphragm to enter the abdomen lying under the floor of the lesser sac. Anteriorly it is related to the crura, the pancreas, the duodenum and the left renal vein. At the level of L2 it gives off the renal arteries and at L4 the inferior mesenteric artery. Paired lumbar arteries from the aorta pass posteriorly.

Abdominal aneurysms generally arise below the renal arteries. Rupture of the aneurysm anteriorly into the peritoneal cavity is usually rapidly fatal; posterior rupture is slightly more favourable since the surrounding tissue may contain the extravasated blood for a time. Occasionally an aneurysm can rupture into the duodenum.

Also see page 9.26 on the Elective Repair of Infrarenal Abdominal Aortic Aneurysm.

OPERATION

Preparation

The patient is anaesthetized on the operating table with the surgeon scrubbed and gowned and prepared to start immediately, and the abdomen cleansed from the nipples to the knees and draped to expose the entire abdomen and both femoral regions. With the situation thus partially under control this is a good time to stabilize the patient and ensure that all the required monitoring is instituted before proceeding. The induction of anaesthesia can be associated with a precipitous fall in blood pressure as the abdominal wall muscles relax and any tamponade is lost.

Incision

Make a midline incision from the xiphisternum to the pubis (see the Introduction). A retroperitoneal rupture appears like a large aubergine lifting forward the small bowel mesentery and sigmoid mesocolon. With an intraperitoneal rupture, blood will pour from the wound when the peritoneum is opened.

Operative technique

1. With an intraperitoneal rupture or in a seriously hypotensive patient the first priority is to establish proximal control of the aneurysm. If on the other hand the patient is stable at this stage the common iliac arteries can be located by palpation of their pulses prior to occluding the aorta and exposed by dissection of the overlying peritoneum and haematoma. It is unnecessary to encircle the arteries since this might damage the underlying iliac veins. Place the clamps in position with the jaws on either side of the vessels ready to occlude the lumina (Fig. 9.56).

2. To establish proximal control it is necessary to place an aortic clamp such as a DeBakey across the aorta below the

renal arteries, having mobilized the left renal vein upwards. Often, preliminary control of the aorta higher up is necessary before approaching the neck of the aneurysm. A useful method is to compress the upper abdominal aorta against the spine with a swab-on-a-stick (Fig. 9.57), or to clamp the aorta well above the renal arteries having opened the lesser omentum between the liver and stomach, divided the peritoneal floor of the lesser sac, and identified the aorta (by palpation) between the crura of the diaphragm although this approach can be difficult (Fig. 9.58). The neck of the aneurysm can then be dissected and clamped below the renal arteries. Do not attempt to encircle the aorta but place a clamp across it, from side-to-side, from the front. Another method of control, useful for an intraperitoneal rupture or following control of the proximal aorta, is to pass a large Foley catheter up the lumen of the aorta and inflate the balloon to occlude the lumen, having occluded the main channel of the catheter with a clamp (Fig. 9.59).

3. Establish distal control by clamping the common iliac vessels, and expose the aneurysm by dissection through, or reflection of, the root of the mesocolon or small bowel mesentery. Take care not to damage the contained blood vessels.

4. Open the aneurysm and oversew the orifices of the lumbar and inferior mesenteric arteries, then proceed as for an elective case using either a straight or bifurcation graft (see page 9.28). If a Foley catheter has been used to occlude the aorta the graft can be threaded over this and having completed the upper suture line, the balloon deflated, the catheter withdrawn, and a clamp applied to the graft prior to anastomosis of the lower end.

Exposure of supracoeliac aorta

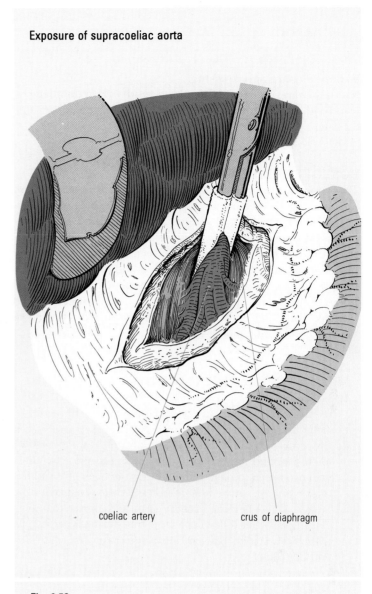

coeliac artery   crus of diaphragm

Fig. 9.58

Control of aorta with pressure

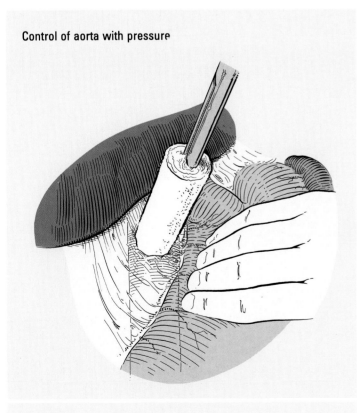

Fig. 9.57

Intraluminal control of aorta

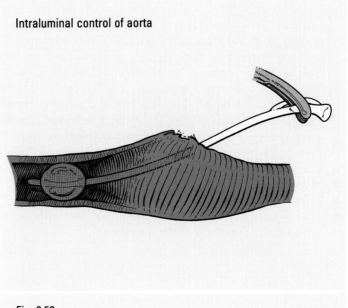

Fig. 9.59

5. Check the blood supply to the sigmoid colon before closing the abdomen.

Wound closure and dressing

No drains are inserted. Close the wound with monofilament nylon with nylon sutures or staples for the skin, and apply a dry dressing.

POSTOPERATIVE CARE

The patient is ventilated postoperatively in the intensive care unit and observed carefully for signs of bleeding such as a persistent tachycardia and abdominal distention etc. Elect to re-explore if signs of bleeding persist. Carefully observe the peripheral pulses and condition of the feet, looking for evidence of ischaemia. Monitor the urine output and biochemical parameters of renal function and give prophylactic antibiotics for 48 hours. Leave a nasogastric tube *in situ* until bowel function returns. Following extubation the patient can be returned to the ward and gently mobilized.

SPECIAL OPERATIVE HAZARDS

1. Ischaemia of the left side of the colon which may need, in rare cases, reimplantation of the inferior mesenteric artery into the graft.
2. Bleeding commonly occurs from around the top of the aneurysm and may result from damage to the left renal vein or from a lumbar vein entering the back of it rather than from the suture line. If necessary the renal vein can be tied off. Otherwise pack the area and ensure that any clotting disorder following a large transfusion is corrected with fresh frozen plasma, intravenous calcium chloride and platelets.
3. Damage to the ureters which may be difficult to identify because they are involved in the haematoma.

COMPLICATIONS

1. Reactionary haemorrhage.
2. Acute renal failure may follow prolonged hypotension, renal ischaemia from applying a clamp above the renal arteries, or damage to the renal artery orifices following completion of the upper suture line. An early renogram will confirm whether the perfusion of the kidneys is adequate or not.
3. 'Trash foot' following the passage of small emboli of blood clot and fragments of thrombus into the femoral vessels. Complete ischaemia of a leg is managed by femoral embolectomy. If no forward flow can be established, it might be necessary to re-explore the lower end of the graft and failure to revascularize a limb may require amputation.
4. Myocardial infarction.
5. Infection of the graft.
6. False aneurysm formation is usually from the upper suture line and may rupture into the duodenum.

Surgery for Occlusive Aorto-iliac Disease

Atheromatous disease of the lower abdominal aorta and iliac arteries can be fairly localized, or a manifestation of generalized atherosclerosis. In cases of vascular insufficiency of the lower limbs the more proximal lesion should generally be attended to first. Localized stenoses may be amenable to percutaneous balloon angioplasty, whilst more extensive disease requires a surgical approach.

An endarterectomy may be employed for localized disease of the aorto-iliac segment, but the long-term patency is better with a bypass graft, which is technically easier to perform and can be employed for more extensive disease. It is our department's policy to anastomose the distal end of the graft to the common femoral artery exposed at the groin. The external iliac artery, although accessible through the abdominal incision, is a narrower vessel which is often affected by progression of the occlusive disease. An aortofemoral bypass can be performed on one side only but in cases of bilateral disease (even if only one side is symptomatic) it is advisable to perform an aortobifemoral bypass since progression of the disease on the good side is highly likely.

The aorta can be approached by an extraperitoneal dissection via an oblique incision sweeping the peritoneum medially, similar to the method employed to expose the vessels for a renal transplant (see page 11.61). The transperitoneal approach is described below.

PREOPERATIVE ASSESSMENT

1. Calf claudication suggests disease of the femoral artery whereas buttock claudication with impotence (Leriche's syndrome) is suggestive of aorto-iliac disease. Perform Doppler studies and arteriography to define the lesions and the state of the distal vessels.
2. Careful preoperative anaesthetic assessment is essential as these patients frequently suffer from coronary artery disease and chronic bronchitis from smoking. A cardiological opinion may be merited in selected cases.
3. Instruct smokers to stop smoking.
4. Look for and control diabetes mellitus. In diabetics, commence a sliding-scale insulin infusion to cover the operation and postoperative period.
5. Prescribe prophylactic antibiotics.

RELEVANT ANATOMY

The abdominal aorta lies to the left of the inferior vena cava and bifurcates into the common iliac arteries at the level of the fourth lumbar vertebra, with a caudal extension (the median sacral artery) continuing in the midline. Posteriorly the aorta gives off paired lumbar arteries, laterally it gives rise to the renal arteries at the level of L2 and the gonadals at L3, and anteriorly the inferior mesenteric artery comes off just below the duodenum (Fig. 9.60). The aorta lies on the lumbar spine

and common iliac veins and is overlain by the duodenum, the left renal vein and lower down by the root of the mesentery and loops of small bowel. In occlusive disease collateral vessels develop to supply the leg, receiving blood from the lumbar arteries, and the mesenteric circulation via the middle rectal and internal iliac arteries.

The aorta bifurcates into common iliac arteries which divide into the internal and external iliac arteries. The latter pass under the inguinal ligament on each side to become the common femoral artery which divides into the superficial femoral and profunda femoris arteries.

OPERATION
Preparation
The operation is performed under a general anaesthetic. The patient is placed supine with the legs slightly apart and the heels protected from pressure by supporting the legs under the

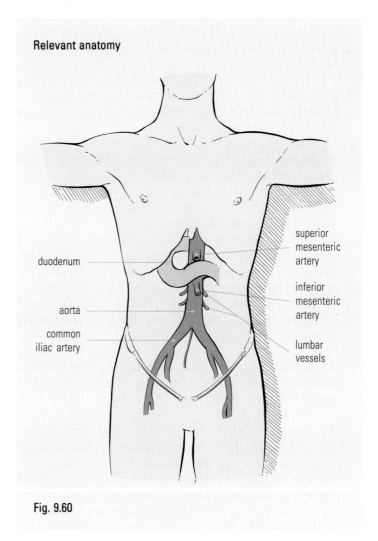

Relevant anatomy

duodenum

aorta

common iliac artery

superior mesenteric artery

inferior mesenteric artery

lumbar vessels

Fig. 9.60

achilles tendon. A urinary catheter is inserted and the skin cleansed from the nipples to the knees. Towels are applied to expose the entire abdomen and both groins and the genitalia are covered.

Incision

Enter the abdomen through a long midline incision from the epigastrium to the pubis (see the Introduction) and insert a self-retaining retractor. Expose the femoral vessels by making vertical incisions in each groin starting just above the mid-inguinal point and extending downwards for about 10cm.

Operative technique

1. Perform a preliminary laparotomy to exclude any other disease. Draw the transverse colon and omentum upward, divide the peritoneal reflection lateral to the caecum which is then lifted up, and incise the tented peritoneum where it covers the root of the mesentery with scissors (Fig. 9.61). Continue the dissection in this plane, mobilizing the mesentery from the front of the aorta but leaving the inferior mesenteric artery undisturbed to the left, and draw the duodenojejunal flexure to the right until the aorta is exposed to the level of the renal vein (Fig. 9.62). The right common iliac artery will have been exposed by this manoeuvre; the proximal part of the left is exposed by displacing the root of the sigmoid mesocolon laterally, while more distally this vessel is revealed by dividing the lateral peritoneal attachment of the sigmoid colon and drawing it medially. The common, superficial and profunda femoris arteries are exposed as described on page 9.21 and controlled with rubber slings.

2. Carefully palpate the vessels, assessing the degree of atheroma and the presence or absence of pulses to confirm the findings of arteriography.

3. Establish proximal control of the aorta by dissecting it free posteriorly below the level of the renal arteries and encircle it with a tape. Avoid damaging the inferior vena cava on the right side of the aorta. The lower aorta is similarly controlled just above the bifurcation.

4. Select a bifurcation or 'trouser' graft of the appropriate diameter for the vessels. If it needs to be preclotted (some types of knitted prosthesis require this) take the blood and preclot the graft according to the manufacturer's instructions. Ask the anaesthetist to give 1mgkg^{-1} body weight heparin intravenously.

5. Apply vascular clamps (e.g. DeBakey's) to the proximal aorta and distally unless the occlusion is complete in which case this is unnecessary.

6. Suture the proximal end of the bypass graft either end-to-side to the front of the aorta or end-to-end to the transected end of the aorta. The latter should only be performed for cases of complete occlusion. For the end-to-side option make a vertical arteriotomy in the front of the aorta; for the end-to-end suture divide the infrarenal aorta. Control troublesome back bleeding from lumbar arteries and the inferior mesenteric artery with bulldog clamps. If the atheromatous disease extends proximal to this level, establish control of the upper abdominal aorta with firm pressure (see page 9.33), release the upper clamp and remove the plaques by grasping them with forceps until a powerful flow of blood is achieved (Fig. 9.63). Reapply the upper aortic clamp.

7. If the aorta has been transected, oversew the cut distal end with a continuous 2/0 vascular suture.

8. Using scissors cut the proximal end of the graft. Avoid having the stem above the bifurcation of the graft too long in order to prevent splaying and sharp angulation with kinking of the lower limbs of the graft. Cut the proximal end obliquely for an end-to-side anastomosis, matching the size of the cut end and arteriotomy for size.

9. Perform the proximal anastomosis using a double-ended 2/0 vascular suture such as polypropylene (e.g. Prolene),

Mobilization of root of mesentery

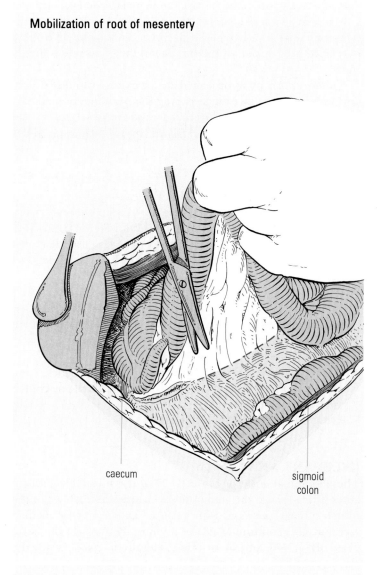

caecum   sigmoid
                                 colon

Fig. 9.61

starting posteriorly for an end-to-end anastomosis and inferiorly for an end-to-side (Fig. 9.64). Ensure that the knots are on the outside. Upon completion of the anastomosis, flush out the graft by partially opening the upper aortic clamp, then occlude each limb of the graft with a Crafoord clamp. Pack swabs around the anastomosis and then examine the suture line for persistent bleeding, which is controlled with carefully inserted additional sutures. Remove the aortic clamp(s) completely.

10. Using blunt dissection with a finger create a retroperitoneal tunnel on each side so that each limb of the graft can reach the femoral vessels. These tunnels lie anterolateral to the external iliac and common femoral arteries, and on the left side it runs under the root of the sigmoid mesocolon. Introduce a Roberts' forceps from below to grasp the limb of the graft and draw it through the tunnel (Fig. 9.65). Ensure that the graft is not being compressed by the inguinal ligament which should be divided if it is tight.

Removal of atheromatous plaque through arteriotomy

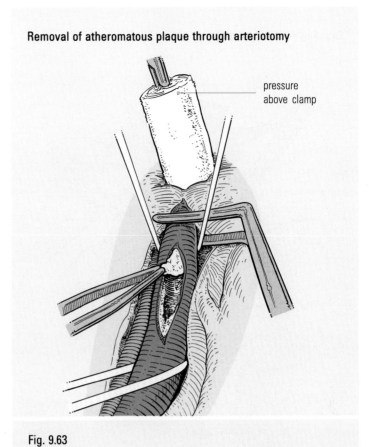

Fig. 9.63

Exposure of infrarenal aorta

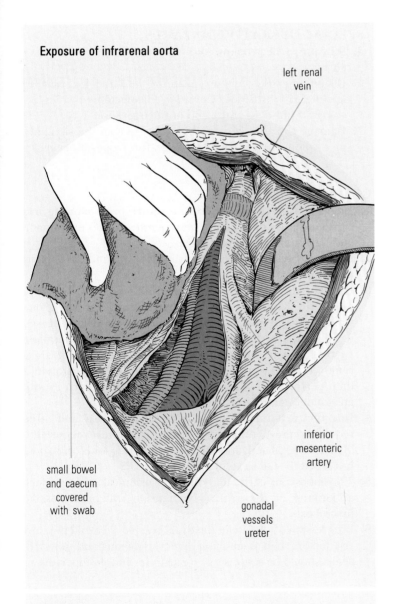

Fig. 9.62

Completed proximal anastomosis

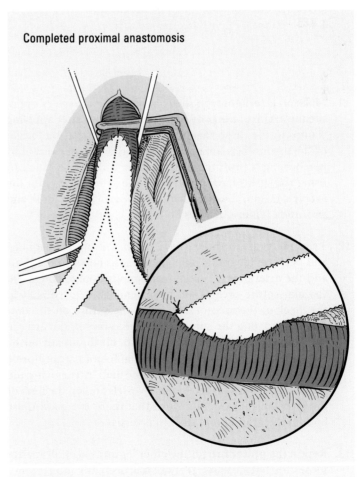

Fig. 9.64

Drawing right limb of graft into groin

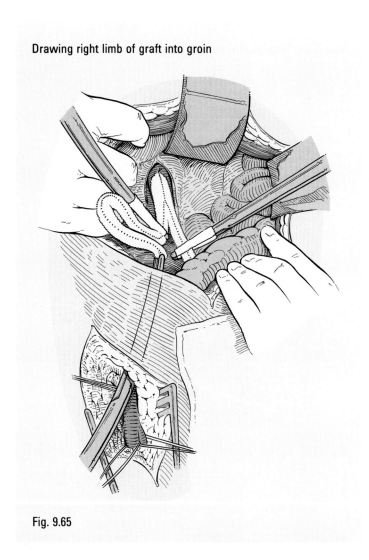

Fig. 9.65

11. Make an arteriotomy in the common femoral artery opposite the origin of the profunda femoris artery after applying clamps to the three femoral vessels. Check that the origin of the profunda is not diseased. If it is, widen the origin by performing a profundaplasty, either with a vein patch or using the graft, having extended the arteriotomy into the artery's origin. Ensure that the superficial femoral and profunda femoris arteries both back bleed freely.

12. Trim the graft to the correct length, cutting it obliquely, and perform an end-to-side anastomosis between the graft and the arteriotomy using a continuous double-ended 4/0 vascular suture such as polypropylene. Start proximally at the 'heel' of the anastomosis, tying the suture on the outside and passing the sutures from in-to-out on the arterial side to prevent lifting an intimal flap. Flush out any air by releasing the clamp on the superficial femoral artery prior to tying the suture. Revascularize the limb by removing the remaining clamps on the femoral vessels and on the limb of the graft on that side. Confirm that there is a good pulse both in the graft and in the distal vessels.

13. Repeat the procedure for the other leg and check all anastomoses for haemostasis. If there has been any interference with the inferior mesenteric artery check that there is no problem with the vascularity of the colon.

9.38

Wound closure and dressing
Ask the anaesthetist to pass a nasogastric tube, checking its position in the stomach if a transperitoneal approach has been used. Insert fine suction drains into each groin and close the groin wounds with 2/0 catgut to the deep fascia and staples or interrupted nylon sutures for the skin. Close the abdominal wound without drains using monofilament nylon and sutures or staples for skin. Cover the wounds with waterproof dressings. Examine the feet and record which pedal pulses, if any, are palpable.

POSTOPERATIVE CARE
During the postoperative period routine observations must include examination of the condition of the feet including the presence or absence of pedal pulses.

Intravenous fluids and nasogastric aspiration are continued until bowel function returns; the retroperitoneal dissection can lead to an ileus which takes several days to settle. The patient should receive intravenous antibiotics for 48 hours. The drains are removed after 24–48 hours and the patient is then mobilized. The staples or sutures are removed after 8–10 days.

SPECIAL OPERATIVE HAZARDS
1. Damage to the vena cava or iliac veins when encircling the aorta.
2. Dislodging atheromatous material into the leg vessels leading to 'trash foot'. Consider embolectomy if a leg is cold and pulseless at the end of the operation.
3. Damage to the ureters and blood vessels in the sigmoid mesocolon when tunnelling the graft retroperitoneally.

COMPLICATIONS
1. Haemorrhage can occur from a suture line following increases in the blood pressure postoperatively. It is uncommon but may require re-exploration.
2. Prolonged lymphatic leak or lymphocele from the femoral dissection.
3. False aneurysm can occur from the proximal or distal anastomosis; the latter presents as a pulsatile mass in the groin, while the former often goes unnoticed until it ruptures, usually into the duodenum. Treatment is by re-exploration. In the presence of an aortoduodenal fistula the graft is removed and the aorta closed off. Limb revascularization is then performed via an extra-anatomical route such as with an axillobifemoral graft.
4. Infection around the graft is difficult to treat and often requires removal of the graft if prolonged intravenous antibiotics or local irrigation around the graft with antibiotics has failed to lead to resolution.
5. Thrombosis, if early, may reflect a technical problem such as kinking of the graft. Hypotension will predispose to thrombosis.
6. Progression of disease in the distal vessels. To avoid this, any risk factors such as smoking, hyperlipidaemia and polycythaemia should be aggressively treated pre- and postoperatively.

Extra-Anatomical Bypass

Elderly and unfit patients with lower limb ischaemia in whom direct reconstruction of the aorto-iliac system is not feasible might be suitable for revascularization via an extra-anatomical route. The techniques of femorofemoral and axillobifemoral bypass are outlined below. The latter may also be employed if an aortic graft has had to be removed (e.g. for septic complications).

PREOPERATIVE ASSESSMENT
1. Careful assessment of cardiovascular and respiratory system.
2. Perform Doppler studies and arteriography of the arterial tree.
3. If a femorofemoral ('cross-over') graft is being contemplated the disease must be unilateral or a 'steal' syndrome might develop in the donor limb. When performing an axillo-femoral graft, always take the graft onto both femoral arteries to maintain the high flow in the graft which is necessary to maintain graft patency.
4. Prescribe prophylactic antibiotics.

RELEVANT ANATOMY
The anatomy of the femoral vessels is considered on page 9.21. The subclavian artery becomes the axillary artery where the vessel enters the apex of the axilla at the outer border of the first rib. The first part of the axillary artery, which is employed for axillofemoral bypass, lies medial to pectoralis minor, and deep to pectoralis major, the clavipectoral fascia and the mid portion of the clavicle (Fig. 9.66). It gives off branches which supply the pectoral muscles and is crossed by the cephalic vein which pierces the clavipectoral fascia to enter the upper surface of the axillary vein. The artery lies above and lateral to the axillary vein and is surrounded by the axillary sheath. The brachial plexus is intimately related to the second part of the axillary artery.

OPERATIONS
FEMOROFEMORAL CROSS-OVER GRAFT
Preparation

Under a general anaesthetic the patient is placed supine and catheterized. The lower abdomen, perineum and thighs are cleansed and drapes are applied so as to expose both groins but to cover the genitalia.

Incision

Make a vertical incision over each femoral artery, 7–10cm in length, to allow exposure of the common femoral artery up to the inguinal ligament.

Operative technique
1. Divide the deep fascia, open the sheath over the artery and insert a self-retaining retractor (e.g. a Travers). Identify and dissect the superficial femoral, common femoral and profunda femoris arteries on each side and control them with rubber slings. Any small side branches are encircled with a silk ligature to occlude them but they should not be ligated or divided (Fig. 9.38 on page 9.22).

2. Confirm the presence of a good pulse on the side from which the graft is to run. An 8mm Dacron graft is generally suitable and a reinforced variety is usually preferred. Some types of graft require preclotting which is performed in accordance with the manufacturer's instructions; others such as gelatin-treated grafts do not. Using the index fingers of each hand or Roberts' forceps, working from each incision, create a tunnel in the suprapubic tissues which may be deep to the recti and extraperitoneal (passing under the inguinal ligaments) or subcutaneous. Insert the forceps down the tunnel from the ischaemic leg to the other leg, grasp one end of the graft and draw it through the tunnel (Fig. 9.67). Ensure that the graft lies between the femoral vessels comfortably without any tension or kinks.

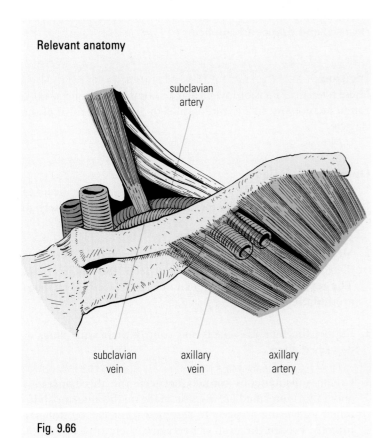

Relevant anatomy

subclavian artery

subclavian vein

axillary vein

axillary artery

Fig. 9.66

3. Ask the anaesthetist to anticoagulate the patient with $1\,\mathrm{mg\,kg}^{-1}$ of heparin and once sufficient time has elapsed for the heparin to circulate (at least 3 minutes) apply vascular clamps to the three vessels on the donor side. Paediatric or angled DeBakey clamps and bulldogs are particularly suitable.

4. Make an arteriotomy at a convenient site in the common femoral artery to match the obliquely cut end of the graft. Starting at the heel of the arteriotomy, and with the knot on the outside, perform a side-to-end anastomosis between the graft and the arteriotomy using a double ended 4/0 polypropylene suture (e.g. Prolene) and sewing from the

Insertion of femoro-femoral graft

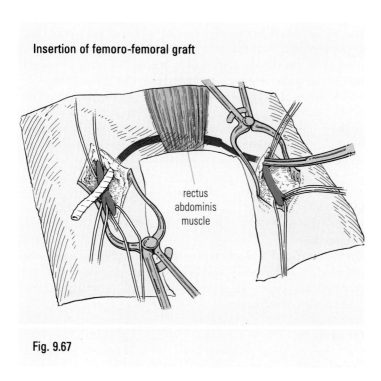

rectus
abdominis
muscle

Fig. 9.67

Anastomosis of graft to common femoral artery

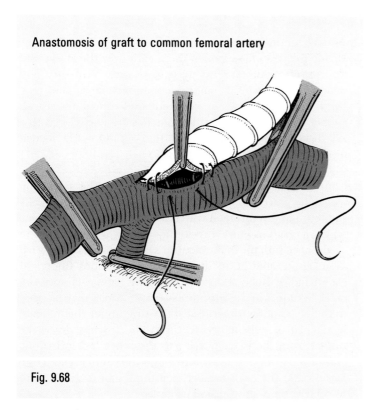

Fig. 9.68

proximal end along each side of the anastomosis to the distal end where the two ends are tied. Alternatively use two double-ended sutures, and work from each end of the arteriotomy towards the middle of each side (Fig. 9.68). To avoid raising an intimal flap always insert the needle from in-to-out on the artery, taking particular care at the ends of the anastomosis. Allow the graft to fill with blood by releasing one of the distal clamps, then place a clamp across the graft near to the anastomosis and, having placed swabs around the anastomosis, release the remaining clamps on the common femoral and profunda vessels. After 5 minutes remove all swabs and check for haemostasis. Persistent bleeding points can be secured with additional sutures.

5. Select the site for the anastomosis in the ischaemic limb, based on the arteriogram findings in conjunction with careful palpation of the vessels and make an arteriotomy. This is usually in the common femoral artery, and can be extended into the origin of the profunda femoris. Apply vascular clamps to the arteries on this side.

6. Cut the graft to the correct length obliquely and perform the second anastomosis in similar fashion to the first. Flush any air out of the graft and check that there are no clots forming prior to tying off the suture by transiently loosening the clamp on the graft. Once the suture is tied, remove all the clamps and apply gentle pressure with swabs for 5 minutes before inspecting the anastomosis for bleeding.

AXILLOBIFEMORAL GRAFT
Preparation
The patient is positioned as described for the femorofemoral graft. In addition the arm on the side to be operated is abducted to 90° on an arm board and the root of the neck and chest are cleansed and drapes are applied.

Incision
Make a vertical incision over each femoral artery, and a horizontal incision just below and parallel to the middle third of the clavicle.

Operative technique
1. Deepen the skin incision through the clavicular head of pectoralis major. Incise the axillary sheath with scissors to expose the axillary artery.

2. Mobilize the artery with ligation and division of its branches, if necessary, and careful dissection from the axillary vein. The cephalic vein is rarely encountered. Place rubber slings around the artery.

3. Expose the femoral vessels and control them with slings as described above.

4. Create subcutaneous tunnels between the three incisions and a short intermediate incision made on the anterior abdominal wall using a specially designed tunneller or Roberts' forceps. Preclot the graft if necessary, then draw each limb of the graft in turn into its tunnel by grasping its end with

Axillo-bifemoral graft

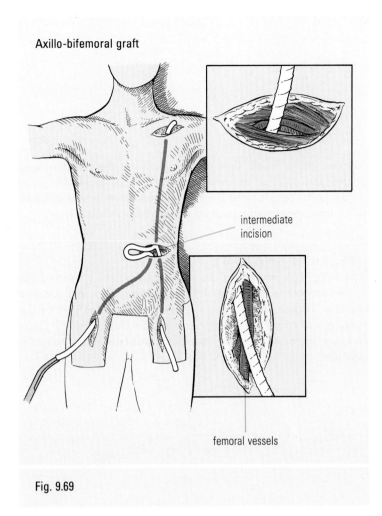

intermediate
incision

femoral vessels

Fig. 9.69

the Roberts' forceps and withdrawing the forceps from the track. The bifurcation of the graft will thus lie under this intermediate incision (Fig. 9.69).

5. With the graft in position, heparinize the patient and apply vascular clamps to the axillary artery. Make a longitudinal arteriotomy in this vessel.

6. Anastomose the proximal end of the graft to the arteriotomy with a double-ended 4/0 polypropylene suture (e.g. Prolene). Remove the distal, then the proximal clamps on the axillary artery and once good flow down the graft has been confirmed, clamp the proximal end of the graft and flush with heparinized saline.

7. Finally, clamp the femoral vessels on each side in turn and anastomose the distal ends of the graft to these vessels as for a femorofemoral graft (described previously in this chapter). Upon completion of all three anastomoses the clamps are removed.

Wound closure and dressing

Insert a fine suction drain into each wound. Close the deep fascia or muscle with an absorbable suture such as catgut and the skin with interrupted nylon sutures or staples. Connect vacuum bottles to the drains and cover the wounds with water-proof dressings. Check the vascularity of the hand or foot of the donor limb before unscrubbing.

POSTOPERATIVE CARE

Continue prophylactic antibiotics if there are infected ulcers. Remove the drains on the second postoperative day once drainage is <25 ml over 24 hours and gently start to mobilize the patient. If the patient was previously continent the catheter can then be removed, but if not it is kept until the groin wounds are healed.

Record on a chart the colour and condition of the feet together with the presence or absence of pedal pulses and Doppler pressures. Consider arteriography and re-exploration if sudden deterioration suggests an occlusion in the graft or in the femoral artery in the good leg. Sutures or staples remain for 8–10 days.

Patients undergoing axillofemoral bypass are instructed to avoid tight fitting clothing, particularly belts and bras since these can occlude the graft.

SPECIAL OPERATIVE HAZARDS

1. Difficulty in identifying the pulseless femoral artery in the ischaemic leg. Its position on the other side may serve as a clue; the artery emerges from under the inguinal ligament at the mid-inguinal point (halfway between the anterior superior iliac spine and symphysis pubis). The artery can usually be felt as a firm cord.
2. Damage to the femoral vein or femoral nerve following failure to identify the artery, and dissecting to one or other side of it.
3. Damage to the axillary vein if performing an axillo-femoral graft.
4. Bleeding from the tunnel, which should be controlled with pressure.
5. 'Trash foot' following embolization of debris into the foot. This is less common than with aneurysm surgery. Larger pieces of debris and any clot which has been allowed to form may be extracted using a Fogarty balloon catheter but a shower of smaller fragments may reach the small vessels in the foot. Always apply vascular clamps with great care and flush out vessels prior to revascularization.

COMPLICATIONS

1. Thrombosis of the graft. If this occurs early on it is likely to be due to technical factors such as kinking or an unrecognized intimal flap, or poor case selection with inadequate run-in or run-off. The situation may be salvageable by urgent re-exploration. Late occlusion may follow progression of the atheromatous disease. An axillofemoral graft can be occluded by tight fitting clothing particularly around the waist.
2. Infection around the graft, even with prolonged courses of antibiotics, is very difficult to eradicate without removal of the foreign material. It can lead to a secondary haemorrhage from an anastomosis.
3. Lymphatic collection or leak can be reduced by avoiding over-extensive mobilization of the artery and by excising any lymph nodes which are damaged in the dissection. These are generally self-limiting and aspiration should be avoided. Most resolve within 2–3 months.
4. 'Steal' syndrome from the diversion of blood; this is more common in the leg than the arm.
5. Haemorrhage and false aneurysm formation at one of the suture lines.

Femoropopliteal Bypass

Occlusion of the superficial femoral artery can be bypassed using the patient's own saphenous vein if there is reasonable 'run off' at the knee.

PREOPERATIVE ASSESSMENT
1. Check the cardiovascular system for hypertension and ischaemic heart disease.
2. The respiratory system should be assessed for chronic airways disease.
3. Use Doppler studies and arteriography to evaluate the arterial system of the lower limb.
4. Ensure that the saphenous vein is not varicose.
5. Prescribe a single dose of prophylactic flucloxacillin and gentamicin (or a suitable alternative if the patient is allergic or has poor renal function) to be given on anaesthetic induction.
6. Commence diabetic patients on an insulin sliding scale.

RELEVANT ANATOMY
The long saphenous vein runs subcutaneously in front of the medial malleolus and passes upward, behind the medial femoral condyle. It then swings forwards along the medial part of the thigh into the femoral triangle and pierces the cribriform fascia to enter the femoral vein just below, and lateral to, the pubic tubercle.

Relevant anatomy

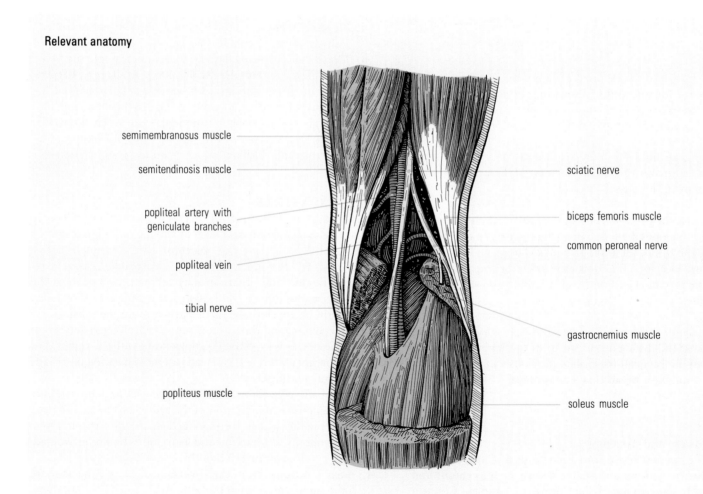

semimembranosus muscle

semitendinosis muscle

popliteal artery with geniculate branches

popliteal vein

tibial nerve

popliteus muscle

sciatic nerve

biceps femoris muscle

common peroneal nerve

gastrocnemius muscle

soleus muscle

Fig. 9.70

Site of groin incision

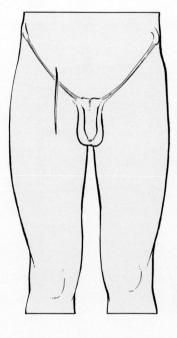

Fig. 9.71

Clean the skin of the entire limb, groin and lower abdomen with the appropriate antiseptic solution and drape the patient so that the leg can be freely moved if required. If there are infected ulcers on the foot, wrap the foot in sterile drapes. Display the arteriograms.

Operative technique

1. Make a longitudinal incision over the femoral vessels commencing just above the inguinal ligament and extending distally for approximately 15 cm (Fig. 9.71).

2. Dissect the saphenofemoral junction and inspect the long saphenous vein; if the vein appears to be adequate for use as an arterial bypass continue to dissect the vein distally to the limit of the wound (Fig. 9.72). Avoid extensive undermining of the skin flaps which may then necrose. If the vein is unsuitable a synthetic graft (e.g. P.T.F.E.) can be used.

Exposure of long saphenous vein at groin

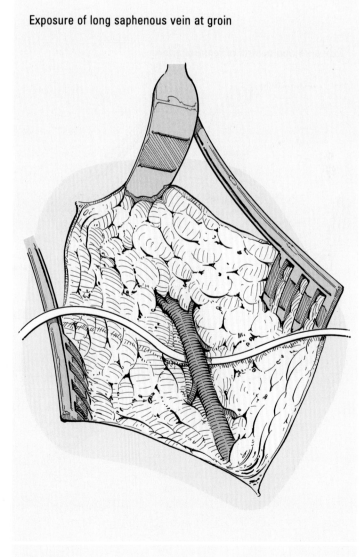

The common femoral artery lies between the femoral vein and the femoral nerve, being medial to the vein and lateral to the nerve. It commences where the external iliac artery passes under the midpoint of the inguinal ligament. The common femoral artery divides into the profunda femoris and superficial femoral arteries approximately 5 cm distal to the ligament; occasionally there are two profunda arteries. The common femoral artery usually has four small branches, the superficial circumflex iliac, the superficial epigastric, the superficial external pudendal and the deep external pudendal arteries.

The popliteal artery enters the popliteal fossa through the adductor hiatus. At this level the artery is medial to the sciatic nerve, but as the artery passes distally it curves laterally becoming anterior to the nerve, so that at its distal part the artery lies lateral to the tibial nerve. At all levels the femoral vein is between the artery and nerve (Fig. 9.70). Thus, if approached from the medial side the artery is most easily and safely identified in the proximal popliteal fossa, and dissection close to the arterial wall will then avoid damage to either the vein and/or the nerve.

OPERATION
Preparation
Place the catheterized patient supine with the affected limb externally rotated and slightly flexed at the hip and knee. Support the leg in this position by placing sandbags under the knee and against the sole of the foot.

Fig. 9.72

9.43

3. Ligate and divide the tributaries of the saphenous vein in the femoral triangle and then dissect the common, superficial and profunda arteries. Ensure that the entire common femoral artery is displayed to the level of the inguinal ligament so the proximal arterial clamp can be applied. Place a soft silicone sling around each vessel and preserve any small arterial branches, controlling them with heavy silk ties looped twice around each vessel but not tied (Fig. 9.73).

4. Expose the long saphenous vein by the knee through a longitudinal incision commencing behind the medial femoral condyle and extending distally for approximately 20 cm, in line with the posterior border of the tibia.

5. Identify the long saphenous vein and ensure that it is of adequate size at this level. Dissect the vein to the distal limit of the incision, and ligate and divide all the tributaries.

Exposure of saphenous vein

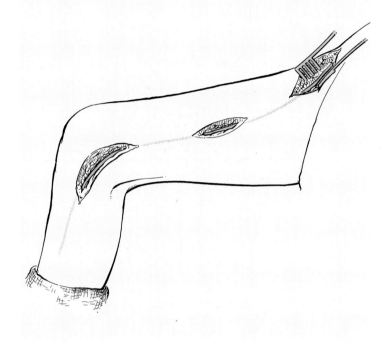

Fig. 9.74

Exposure and control of femoral artery

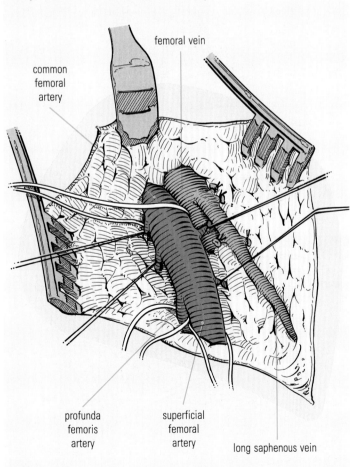

common femoral artery

femoral vein

profunda femoris artery

superficial femoral artery

long saphenous vein

Fig. 9.73

Control of the popliteal artery

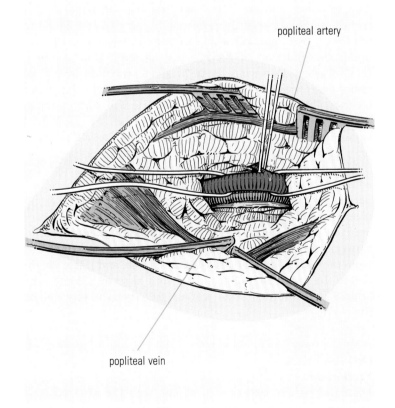

popliteal artery

popliteal vein

Fig. 9.75

6. Make a third incision, 10–15cm long, on the medial aspect of the thigh midway between the other two incisions. Identify the long saphenous vein and ligate and divide all the tributaries (Fig. 9.74); skilful use of Langenbeck's retractors will allow dissection of the vein beneath the skin bridges.

7. Ligate the long saphenous vein at the saphenofemoral junction and at the distal limit of the dissection. Once the vein has been marked for subsequent orientation and removed, gently flush it with heparinized saline. Use a ball-tipped needle to prevent intimal damage and check for leaks; these are repaired with 6/0 vascular sutures placed in the long axis of the vein to prevent narrowing of the lumen. It is then laid out straight and spots of Bonney's blue marked along its length to avoid twisting. The vein should be stored in a saline-soaked swab.

8. At the distal incision by the knee, deepen the dissection behind the sartorius and in front of the gracilis tendon, to enter the fat of the popliteal fossa. Using Browse retractors to improve access to the fossa, identify the neurovascular bundle and dissect the venae comitantes off the popliteal artery, taking care to preserve geniculate branches of the artery. Place soft silicone slings around the popliteal artery and control the geniculate branches (Fig. 9.75). Decide on a

suitable site for the distal anastomosis by palpating the vessel and reviewing the arteriograms.

9. Use a tunneller or sigmoidoscope to create a passage from the popliteal fossa upwards to the femoral triangle and draw the *reversed* vein through the tunneller, grasping the end with great care using long alligator forceps so as not to twist the vein (Fig. 9.76).

10. Having studied the arteriograms, establish the site for the proximal anastomosis by palpating the femoral vessels and choosing an area with the least atherosclerotic calcification.

11. Systemically anticoagulate the patient with $1\,\mathrm{mg\,kg^{-1}}$ body weight of intravenous sodium heparin. Allow a few minutes for the heparin to circulate and then use bulldog clamps (or tension on the slings) to occlude the popliteal artery at positions proximal and distal to the site chosen for the distal anastomosis. If clamps remain in place for much more than an hour it is wise to give a further dose of sodium heparin at $0.5\,\mathrm{mg\,kg^{-1}}$.

12. Make a 2–3cm longitudinal arteriotomy starting with a knife and extending it using Pott's scissors. Check the popliteal artery to ensure that the distal vessel is patent and

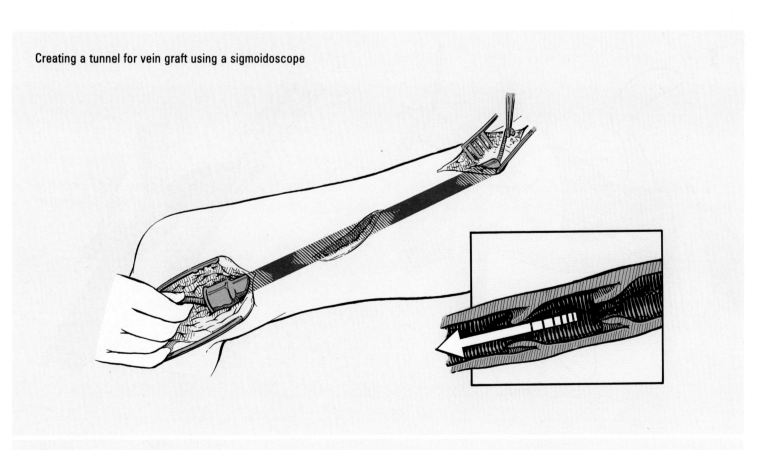

Creating a tunnel for vein graft using a sigmoidoscope

Fig. 9.76

Starting distal anastomosis

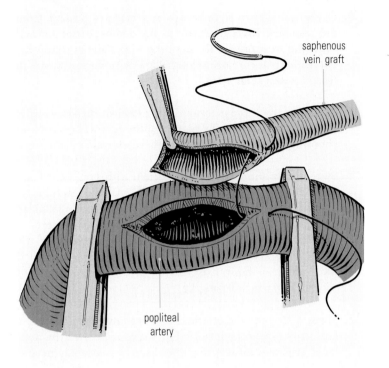

Fig. 9.77

some back bleeding is present. Spatulate the end of the vein and anastomose it end-to-side to the artery using a double ended 5/0 vascular suture, commencing at the proximal cleft of the arteriotomy (Fig. 9.77). Suture the back wall of the anastomosis first, complete the distal corner and use the second needle to complete the front wall (Fig. 9.78). If the popliteal artery has a narrow lumen it is easier to avoid producing a stenosis by using interrupted sutures at the distal cleft of the arteriotomy. Whichever technique is employed, the needle should always be passed through the arterial wall from within its lumen, to avoid raising an intimal flap.

13. Straighten the leg and determine the length of vein that will be required to reach the proximal anastomosis. Reposition the leg and clamp the common, profunda and, if patent, superficial femoral arteries with arterial clamps. Make a 2–3 cm longitudinal arteriotomy at the chosen site (Fig. 9.79) and spatulate the proximal end of the vein.

14. Anastomose the vein end-to-side to the femoral artery using a double-ended, continuous 4/0 vascular suture. Commence at the distal cleft of the arteriotomy and complete the medial side of the anastomosis first (Fig. 9.80), using the second needle to complete the lateral aspect of the anastomosis and taking care not to stenose the lumen of the vein.

Completing distal anastomosis

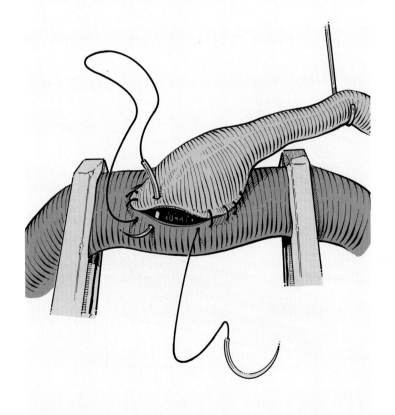

Fig. 9.78

Arteriotomy in common femoral artery

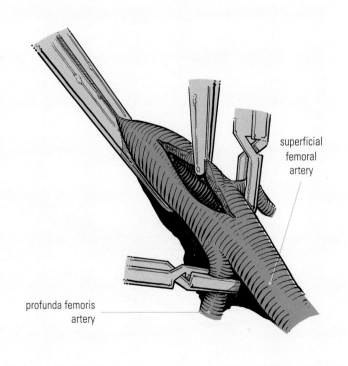

Fig. 9.79

Suturing the graft to femoral artery

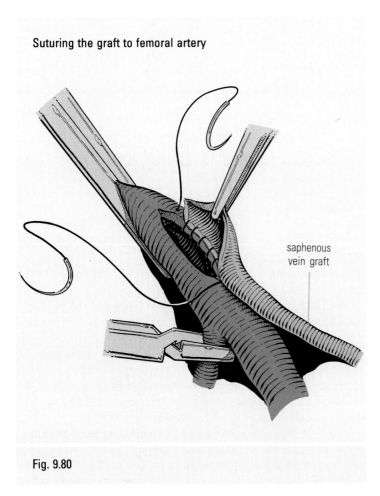

saphenous vein graft

Fig. 9.80

Completed proximal anastomosis

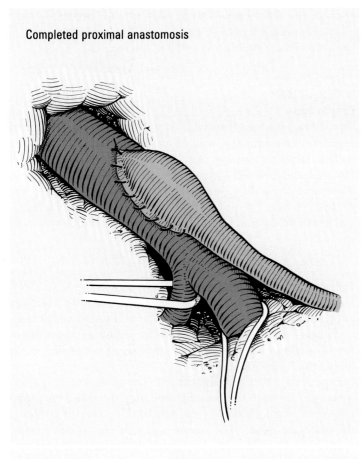

Fig. 9.81

Again, always pass the needle through the arterial wall from within its lumen. Before tying the suture remove the clamps from the popliteal artery and release the clamps on the femoral vessels to flush out air and allow the vein to fill with blood. Tie the suture and check the anastomoses for leaks (Fig. 9.81). If a second surgeon is present, it is possible to perform both anastomoses at the same time.

15. Close significant leaks with interrupted vascular stitches; tiny leaks will usually stop spontaneously if the area is gently packed with a gauze swab. On the rare occasion when it becomes necessary to reverse the heparin, give 1 mg protamine sulphate for every 1 mg heparin administered.

Wound closure and dressing
Place suction drains in the groin and popliteal fossa and close the wounds in two layers using a 00 catgut suture for the fascia and a subcuticular suture or staples for the skin.

POSTOPERATIVE CARE
The suction drains can be removed when drainage has become minimal, which is usually within 48 hours. After the removal of drains, the patient should be mobilized as soon as possible in order to minimize the risks of venous thrombosis, broncho-pneumonia and pressure sores. Sutures or staples can be removed after 8–14 days depending on wound healing. Some surgeons routinely prescribe anti-platelet agents such as aspirin or dipyridamole.

SPECIAL OPERATIVE HAZARDS
1. Damage to the femoral vein when dissecting the sapheno-femoral junction.
2. Damage to the femoral nerve when dissecting the femoral artery. To avoid this, do not dissect around the artery laterally.
3. Damage to the popliteal vein.
4. Poor quality or absent saphenous vein. Consider using the contralateral vein, or a synthetic graft.

COMPLICATIONS
1. Wound haematoma and infection.
2. Lymphocele or lymphatic fistula.
3. Sloughing of the skin from undermining when dissecting the saphenous vein.
4. Haemorrhage from an anastomosis; this may occur with a technically imperfect anastomosis immediately after the operation when the blood pressure rises. A secondary haemorrhage is likely to occur after several days if a wound becomes infected.
5. Thrombosis of the graft results from an inadequate inflow or run off, a hypercoagulable state or a technically inadequate anastomosis.

Femorodistal Bypass

In patients with ischaemic disease of the lower limb but with a diseased popliteal vessel which is unsuitable for femoropopliteal bypass, the more distal vessels may be patent and suitable for a femorodistal bypass graft, ideally using *in situ* saphenous vein.

PREOPERATIVE ASSESSMENT
1. Use Doppler studies and radiology of the lower limb arteries including the foot to define the state of the arterial tree. As a general rule proximal disease should be treated first.
2. Ensure that the long saphenous vein on that side is present, healthy and patent. Use Doppler studies or venography if

doubt exists. Mark the position of the saphenous vein on the skin with an indelible marker.
3. Prescribe prophylactic antibiotics and commence diabetic patients on a sliding scale of insulin.

RELEVANT ANATOMY
The course of the saphenous vein is considered on page 9.42 in Femoropopliteal Bypass.

The popliteal artery crosses the lower border of the popliteus muscle and divides into the anterior and posterior tibial arteries. The anterior tibial artery passes between the tibia and fibula and descends, with its venae comitantes and the deep peroneal nerve, on the interosseous membrane deep to tibialis anterior, extensor digitorum longus and extensor hallucis longus in the extensor compartment of the lower leg emerging onto the dorsum of the foot as the dorsalis pedis artery.

The posterior tibial artery is accompanied by its venae comitantes and the tibial nerve as it courses through the flexor compartment of the leg superficial to flexor digitorum longus and tibialis posterior. In its upper part it lies deep to the soleus and gastrocnemius muscles, but lower down it is covered only by skin and deep fascia. It passes behind the medial malleolus to enter the foot. Proximally it gives off the peroneal artery which descends lateral to it between the fibula/adjacent interosseous membrane and flexor hallucis longus.

OPERATION
Preparation
The arteriograms are displayed on an X-ray viewing box. Under a general anaesthetic a urinary catheter is inserted and the patient is placed supine. Any ischaemic ulcers are carefully cleansed and covered with a transparent waterproof dressing. The entire leg is then cleansed from the groin to the toes and draped to cover the perineum but expose the inguinal region and groin. A surgical glove is placed over the forefoot to cover the toes.

Incision
Make a vertical incision over the femoral artery as for a femoropopliteal bypass and continue the incision distally over the long saphenous vein to beyond the knee according to the proposed site of anastomosis, leaving short bridges of intact skin in the line of the incision if possible.

Expose the proposed distal vessel. The posterior tibial artery is exposed through the same incision used to expose the saphenous vein; this incision lies just behind the posterior border of the tibia (Fig. 9.82). The soleus muscle needs to be retracted away from the tibia in the upper calf; lower down the artery is only covered by skin and fascia. The peroneal artery can also be approached through this incision but further distally it is more

Exposure of posterior tibial artery

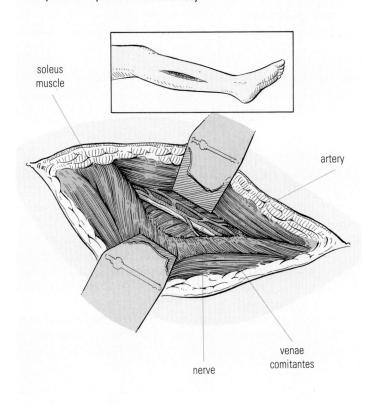

soleus muscle

artery

venae comitantes

nerve

Fig. 9.82

9.48

easily exposed via an anterolateral incision, excising a portion of the fibula (Fig. 9.83). An anterolateral incision is also used to expose the anterior tibial artery. This artery is located between the tibialis anterior and extensor digitorum longus in the upper leg and between tibialis anterior and extensor hallucis longus in the lower leg (Fig. 9.84).

Operative technique

1. Mobilize a segment of the distal vessel and carefully ligate any veins which cross it. Control the vessel with soft rubber slings and confirm that it is suitable for anastomosis.

2. Dissect the common femoral, superficial femoral and profunda femoris arteries at the groin and control each with a rubber sling (see page 9.44).

3. Follow the saphenous vein proximally and identify the saphenofemoral junction. Starting at the top, work along the saphenous vein individually ligating each tributary entering it with fine silk ligatures. It is unnecessary to mobilize the vein fully. In the lower thigh and calf look out for perforating veins connecting the saphenous vein to the deep venous system. Mobilize the distal end of the vein to allow it to comfortably reach the proposed site of distal bypass. To reach the anterior tibial artery the vein needs to be brought across the leg by tunnelling it through the flexor compartment, and through the interosseous membrane via a generous hole.

4. Ligate the saphenous vein at the saphenofemoral junction with silk and divide the vein beyond the ligature.

5. Ask the anaesthetist to administer $1\,mg\,kg^{-1}$ body weight of heparin intravenously and after 3 minutes apply vascular clamps to the common femoral, superficial femoral and profunda femoris arteries. Make an arteriotomy over the distal common femoral artery. Inspect the profunda origin for stenosis, widening the orifice with a vein patch (profundaplasty) if it is present.

6. Anastomose the obliquely divided proximal end of the saphenous vein to the arteriotomy (see page 9.46), release the clamps, and then apply gentle pressure with a swab until

Exposure of peroneal artery

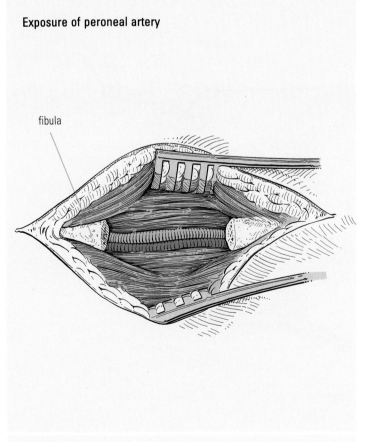

fibula

Fig. 9.83

Exposure of anterior tibial artery

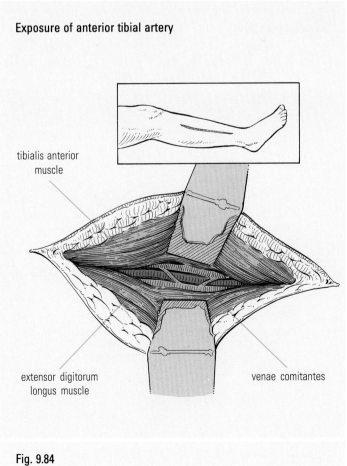

tibialis anterior muscle

extensor digitorum longus muscle

venae comitantes

Fig. 9.84

any bleeding from the suture line has ceased. Blood will flow down the graft to the level of the first valve and stop. Insert a valve disruptor (Fig. 9.85) into the distal end of the graft and advance it into the femoral artery before gently withdrawing the disruptor which will remove the valve cusps as they are encountered. As each valve is disrupted, the blood will flow as far as the next valve. When all the valves have been dealt with there should be a powerful jet of blood from the end of the graft. Apply a soft bulldog clamp to the graft.

7. Perform an arteriotomy in the distal artery with a knife, and extend its length to approximately twice the diameter of the vein using Pott's scissors, controlling forward and back bleeding by gentle traction to the slings rather than with clamps. Cut the end of the graft obliquely, spatulate it to match the arteriotomy and cut off the corners. Perform the distal end-to-side anastomosis between the end of the graft and the calf vessel with a 6/0 polypropylene double-ended suture (Fig. 9.86). With small vessels consider using interrupted sutures either throughout or at the apices of the arteriotomy; otherwise use a continuous running stitch with stay sutures at the proximal and distal ends of the arteriotomy. Always pass the needle from in to out on the arterial side to prevent lifting an intimal flap.

8. Upon completion of the distal anastomosis, release tension on the slings and allow back bleeding to expel any air prior to tying the suture. Release the clamp on the graft and place a swab over the anastomosis for a couple of minutes to allow any bleeding to stop; avoid inserting additional sutures unless bleeding from a point on the suture line is persistent. Check for a pulse in the artery beyond the anastomosis. Some surgeons recommend an on-table arteriogram at the end of the procedure.

Wound closure and dressing
Insert a suction drain over each anastomosis and close the subcutaneous tissues with chromic catgut and the skin with interrupted nylon or staples. Apply a light gauze dressing to the wound.

POSTOPERATIVE CARE
The suction drains are removed after 24–48 hours when drainage has ceased and the patient is then mobilized. Some swelling of the leg is almost inevitable and controlled with a lightweight support stocking. A Doppler ultrasound scan can be used to check for an audible pulse in the vessel at the level of the ankle or foot. Staples or sutures are removed after 10–14 days. Avoid prolonged knee flexion for at least 2 weeks. Some authorities recommend anticoagulation or oral antiplatelet drugs (e.g. aspirin and dipyridamole) postoperatively.

Disruption of valves

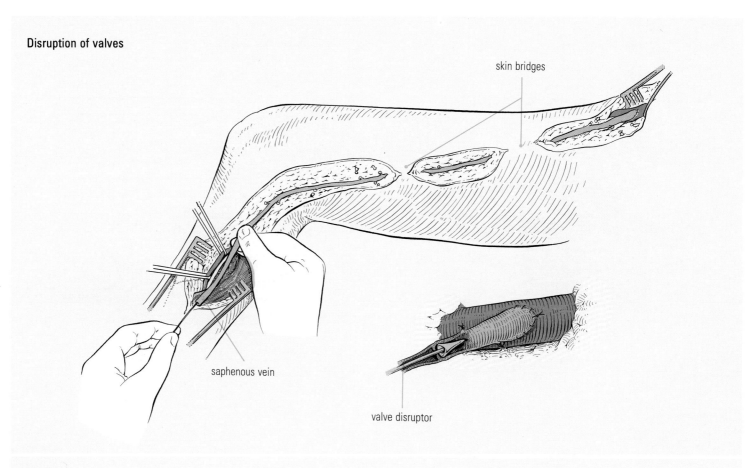

skin bridges

saphenous vein

valve disruptor

Fig. 9.85

Distal anastomosis

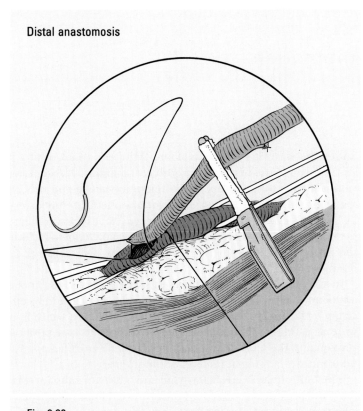

Fig. 9.86

COMPLICATIONS

1. Graft thrombosis occurring in the early postoperative period requires re-exploration. Embolectomy alone is rarely beneficial since the formation of clot usually indicates a technical problem with the graft such as an intimal dissection. Late thrombosis follows intimal hyperplasia in the graft and progression of the arteriosclerosis in the distal artery.
2. Lymphocele or lymphatic leakage from the groin can be troublesome but will usually resolve spontaneously.
3. Sloughing of the skin edge may follow undermining when exposing the vein. It is important to keep the incision over the vein and leave short bridges of intact skin along the incision line if possible.
4. Deep venous thrombosis.

Above Knee Amputation

The object of an above knee amputation is to ablate a limb that has been made useless by gangrene, ischaemia, infection, trauma or a tumour, and to construct a stump that will aid locomotion. This latter objective requires it to be pain-free, with healthy skin and muscle covering the divided femur.

PREOPERATIVE ASSESSMENT

1. These patients are usually elderly and suffering from generalized atherosclerosis, therefore their cardiovascular system should be carefully checked.
2. An assessment of the respiratory system is also important as they are often heavy smokers.
3. Prophylactic antibiotics should be given with the premedication to avoid infection by *Clostridium* species.
4. Commence sliding scale insulin in diabetics.

RELEVANT ANATOMY

The major vessels of the thigh will require ligation, although the femoral artery is often occluded due to atheroma. The femoral artery passes from the apex of the femoral triangle, under the sartorius muscle and into Hunter's canal, which it leaves through the hiatus of the adductor magnus. The femoral vein is medial to the artery in the femoral triangle and behind the artery in Hunter's canal. Anterior and medial to the artery in Hunter's canal is the saphenous nerve. As it is best to ligate the vessels in Hunter's canal, care should be taken not to include the saphenous nerve in the ligature as this will cause post-operative pain.

In the distal part of the thigh the sciatic nerve lies on the adductor magnus, under the semitendinosus muscle and biceps femoris. The nerve can be identified as a white cord which is as wide as a finger. It should be cleanly transected at a position proximal to the level of amputation in order to avoid a painful neuroma developing at the end of the stump.

The bulky quadriceps, hamstring and adductor muscles (Fig. 9.87) will provide a good cover for the divided femur if adequate is left after cutting. Remember, more can always be cut off but you cannot replace muscle or skin that has already been removed. Sufficient deep fascia should be preserved to cover the muscle, as exposed muscle will become adherent to overlying skin and predispose it to friction ulcers.

Cross-section through thigh

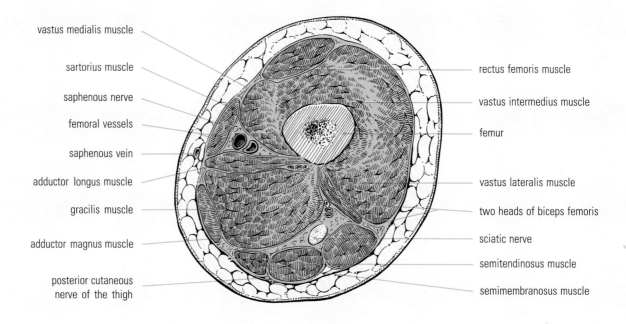

vastus medialis muscle

sartorius muscle

saphenous nerve

femoral vessels

saphenous vein

adductor longus muscle

gracilis muscle

adductor magnus muscle

posterior cutaneous nerve of the thigh

rectus femoris muscle

vastus intermedius muscle

femur

vastus lateralis muscle

two heads of biceps femoris

sciatic nerve

semitendinosus muscle

semimembranosus muscle

Fig. 9.87

OPERATION

Preparation

Place the patient supine with a sponge or skin pad under the good heel to relieve the pressure. Prepare the limb from the calf to the groin. Wrap the calf and foot in sterile towels and drape the patient so that the limb is freely mobile. Use a cutoff drape under the thigh to ensure that the perineum is excluded from the operative field.

Mark anterior and posterior skin flaps with a skin marker (Fig. 9.88), bearing in mind that the femur will be divided at a position 20–25 cm distal to the greater trochanter and sufficient skin must be left to cover the stump.

Incision

Use a scalpel to incise the skin down to the deep fascia.

Operative technique

1. Clip, divide and ligate the long saphenous vein (Fig. 9.89).

2. Identify the sartorius muscle and divide it as far distally as possible (Fig. 9.90).

Division and ligation of saphenous vein

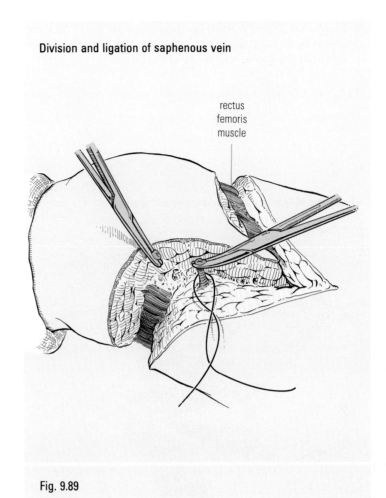

rectus femoris muscle

Fig. 9.89

Position of bone section and skin flaps

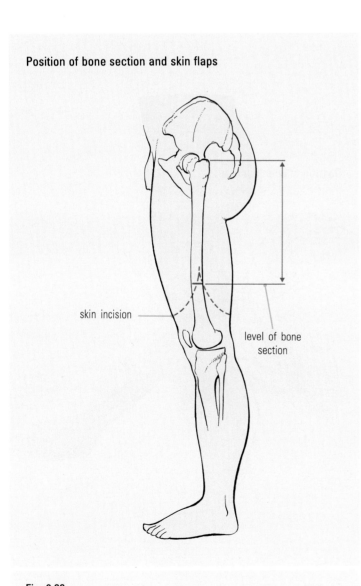

skin incision

level of bone section

Fig. 9.88

Division of sartorius muscle

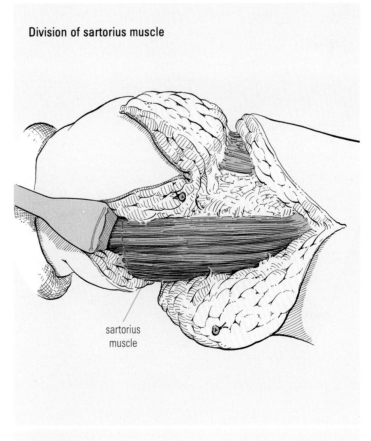

sartorius muscle

Fig. 9.90

3. Display the femoral artery in Hunter's canal (Fig. 9.91), then clamp, divide and ligate the femoral artery and vein making sure that the saphenous nerve is not included (Fig. 9.92).

4. Cut all the muscles of the thigh at the distal limit of the incision and stop excessive bleeding with catgut ligatures. Identify the sciatic nerve, pull it down, and cleanly transect it above the level of amputation (Fig. 9.93).

5. Incise the periosteum of the femur and use a periosteal elevator to strip periosteum proximally for approximately 4–5cm (Fig. 9.94).

6. Place a shield on the femur to protect the muscles before using a saw to divide it. Saw vertically through the femur (Fig. 9.95).

7. Use a rougine to smooth the edges of the transected femur (Fig. 9.96).

Wound closure and dressing
1. A 00 catgut is used to suture the periosteum over the end of the femur and suture the sartorius transversely across the end of the bone to the iliotibial tract. Insert a suction drain and position it over the sartorius.
2. Use a 0 catgut to suture the deep fascia so that the quadriceps and hamstring muscles oppose in an anterior–posterior direction (Fig. 9.97). The muscles should oppose easily without tension on the sutures.

Exposure of femoral vessels in subsartorial canal

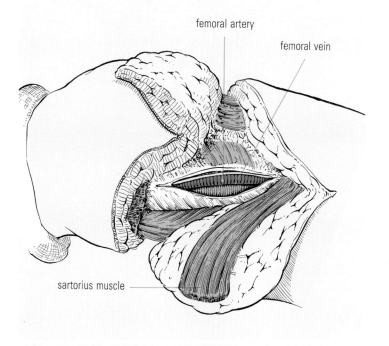

Fig. 9.91

Division of femoral artery

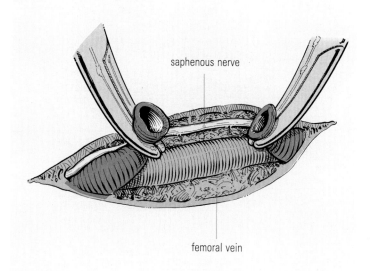

Fig. 9.92

Division of sciatic nerve

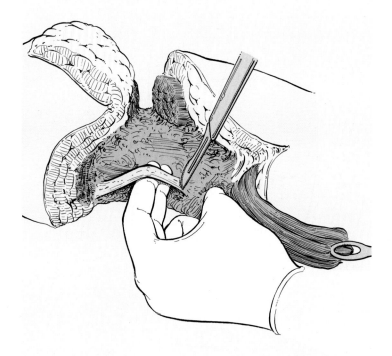

Fig. 9.93

Stripping periosteum off femur

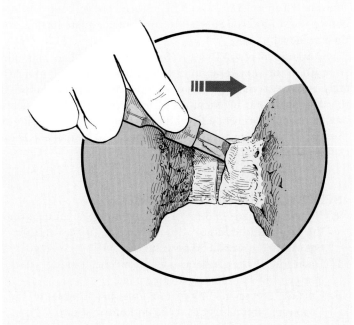

Fig. 9.94

Filing sharp edges of divided femur

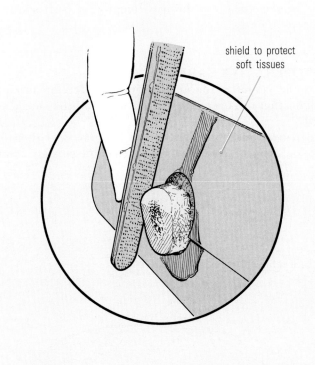

shield to protect
soft tissues

Fig. 9.96

Division of femur using Gigli saw

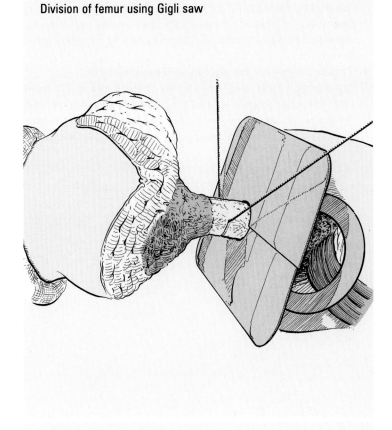

Fig. 9.95

Oppose anterior and posterior muscle groups over sartorius muscle

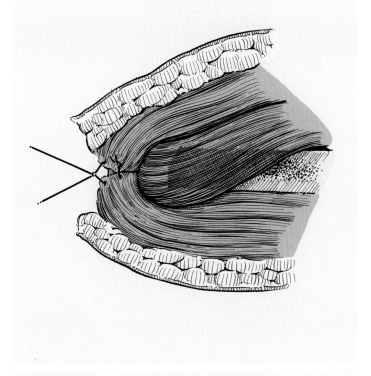

Fig. 9.97

3. Close the skin with a subcuticular polypropylene suture (Fig. 9.98). Again there must be no tension on the skin flaps.
4. Apply a gauze dressing and a crepe stump bandage, but do not bandage tightly as this may compromise perfusion and venous drainage.

POSTOPERATIVE CARE

It is quite common for male patients to develop urinary retention after this operation and a urinary catheter should be inserted.

The patient will be confined to bed for a few days after the operation and great care should be taken of the pressure areas;

Closure with subcuticular suture

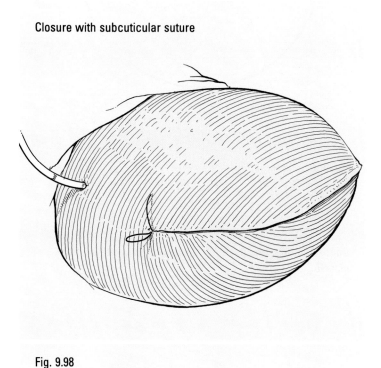

Fig. 9.98

sacral pressure sores can rapidly develop in these elderly and immobile patients, and a pressure sore on the heel of the remaining limb is a potential disaster.

The suction drain is removed as soon as it is dry, which is usually within 48 hours, while prophylactic antibiotics are continued for several days. The sutures are left for 14 days before the wound is inspected to confirm adequate healing for their removal.

Postoperative physiotherapy for the chest and to maintain strength in the remaining limb should be commenced immediately. As soon as the immediate postoperative pain has subsided the patient should be encouraged to lie prone at least twice a day, in order to prevent a fixed flexion deformity developing at the hip. Arrangements for limb fitting should be made as soon as the patient is well enough.

SPECIAL OPERATIVE HAZARDS

1. If an inadequate amount of skin or muscle is left to cover the stump of the femur without tension, further shortening of the femur will be necessary.
2. Inclusion of the saphenous nerve in the femoral artery ligature will cause postoperative pain.
3. Cutting the sciatic nerve too long predisposes to the formation of a neuroma at the end of the stump.

COMPLICATIONS

1. Urinary retention.
2. Wound infection; nowadays *Clostridium welchi* is fortunately uncommon but should nevertheless be considered in any amputee who rapidly becomes toxic, and the stump inspected for crepitus.
3. Wound breakdown is due to inadequate perfusion in severe peripheral vascular disease with iliac artery occlusion. It necessitates more proximal amputation and carries a grave prognosis.
4. Pressure sores on the sacrum or remaining heel.
5. Stump pain from the wound may require minor analgesia but settles fairly quickly, however phantom pain, which takes longer to settle, can occasionally persist. Patients whose pain persists after 2 weeks should be referred to a pain clinic.

Burgess-Type Below Knee Amputation

The object of the operation is to ablate useless tissue and to construct a useful organ of locomotion, that is a stump on which a prosthetic limb can be usefully employed. The latter will only be achieved if a viable posterior musculocutaneous flap can be placed over the transected end of the tibia. Such a stump is usually 15–20cm long and necessitates transection of the tibia in its upper third, approximately 14cm distal to the knee joint.

PREOPERATIVE ASSESSMENT

1. Assess the respiratory system for chronic airways disease and the cardiovascular system for hypertension and ischaemic heart disease.
2. If the patient is diabetic, control must be adequate and perioperative management of insulin should be discussed with the anaesthetist.
3. As it is most likely that the amputation is being performed for lower limb ischaemia, prescribe benzyl penicillin to commence with the premedication. If there is infection of necrotic tissue, add antibiotics as indicated by the culture reports.

4. Transcutaneous oxygen tension may help to predict if the amputation will heal.
5. Can the vascularity of the limb be improved (e.g. angioplasty, sympathectomy)?
6. Arrange a preoperative visit to a limb fitting specialist and a specialized physiotherapist.

RELEVANT ANATOMY

The upper part of the tibial shaft is triangular in cross-section (Fig. 9.99) and its subcutaneous surface is easily palpated. At this level the lateral, extensor surface is covered by the tibialis anterior muscle and the posterior, flexor surface is covered by a combination of the tibialis posterior, flexor digitorum longus and soleus muscles; the latter being the most superficial. The fibula is also triangular in cross-section in its upper third, but all three surfaces are covered by muscles. The lateral surface is covered by the peroneal muscles, the medial surface by the extensor and tibialis posterior muscles, and the posterior, flexor surface by the flexor hallucis longus and soleus muscles. The gap between the tibia and fibula at this level is bridged by the interosseous membrane.

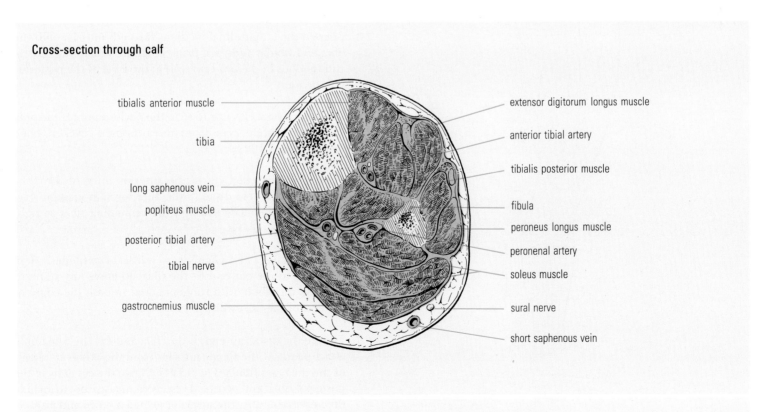

Cross-section through calf

tibialis anterior muscle

tibia

long saphenous vein

popliteus muscle

posterior tibial artery

tibial nerve

gastrocnemius muscle

extensor digitorum longus muscle

anterior tibial artery

tibialis posterior muscle

fibula

peroneus longus muscle

peronenal artery

soleus muscle

sural nerve

short saphenous vein

Fig. 9.99

There are three neurovascular bundles in the leg at this level: anterior to the interosseous membrane and covered by the extensor muscles are the anterior tibial vessels and nerve; the posterior tibial vessels and nerve lie between flexor digitorum longus and flexor hallucis longus; and the peroneal vessels lie on the tibialis posterior muscle, deep to flexor hallucis longus.

In the upper calf there are several structures to be identified in the subcutaneous tissues: the long saphenous vein, accompanied by the saphenous nerve, which lies parallel to and just behind the subcutaneous border of the tibia; the short saphenous vein which lies in the midline posteriorly; and the sural nerve lying just lateral to the short saphenous vein. Occasionally these latter two structures lie beneath the deep fascia at this level.

OPERATION

Preparation

The operation is usually carried out under general anaesthesia, although it may be performed under an epidural block or spinal anaesthetic, with sedation.

The patient is placed supine, the leg is cleaned from midthigh

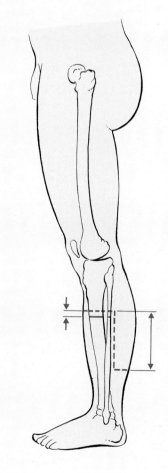

Position of bone section and skin flap

Fig. 9.100

to ankle and a cut-off towel is used to exclude the perineum from the operative site. The foot should be wrapped in a separate towel and further drapes placed so that the leg is free to be moved and remains exposed from midthigh to lower calf. A tourniquet is not employed as it is essential to confirm good bleeding from the flaps if the wound is going to heal.

Use a marker to plan the skin incisions (Fig. 9.100).

Incision

1. The anterior incision encompasses half of the circumference of the leg, 2 cm proximal to the proposed level of tibial transection. Parallel incisions then pass down both sides of the calf for a distance of approximately one and one half times the diameter of the calf. The posterior incision encompasses the remaining half of the circumference.
2. These incisions will produce a posterior flap, slightly longer than required, which can be precisely trimmed later in the operation.
3. If the skin does not bleed move to a more proximal level of amputation.

Operative technique

1. Identify, ligate and divide the long saphenous vein where it crosses the line of incision (Fig. 9.101). Do not include the saphenous nerve in the ligature as this will cause postoperative pain.

2. Extend the anterior incision squarely down through the muscles of the anterior compartment until the fibula is encountered. Ligate the anterior tibial vessels with either catgut or synthetic resorbable ligatures, and gently draw the associated nerve down and cleanly transect it with a knife. Avoid incorporating the nerve into the vascular ligature.

3. Deepen the longitudinal incisions through muscle, onto the tibia and fibula, and then transect all the remaining muscle and tendons in the posterior calf at the level of the posterior skin incision.

4. Use a periosteal elevator to strip the periosteum off the tibia to approximately 2 cm from the proposed level of bone section (Fig. 9.102).

5. Make a 45° bevelled cut in the anterior third of the tibia, approximately 2 cm distal to the anterior skin incision (Fig. 9.103), and then saw through the remaining tibia at right angles to its long axis.

6. Use bone shears or a Gigli saw to transect the fibula 2–3 cm proximal to the cut end of the tibia. Remove any spurs of bone on the fibula with rongeurs, and smooth the edges of the end of the tibia with a file.

7. Elevate the distal cut end of the tibia and cut the remaining attachments of the flexor muscles from the posterior aspect of the tibia and fibula (Fig. 9.104). Ligate the cut ends of the posterior tibial and peroneal vessels taking care not to include the nerves. Identify the sural nerve, pull it down and transect it cleanly so that the end retracts and does not lie over the end of the stump when the flap is sutured in place.

Division and ligation of saphenous vein

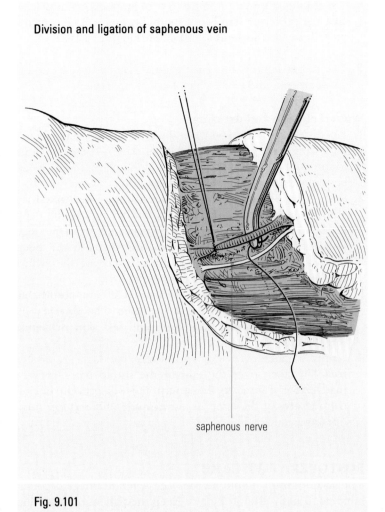

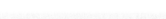
saphenous nerve

Fig. 9.101

Division of tibia with bevelling of anterior border

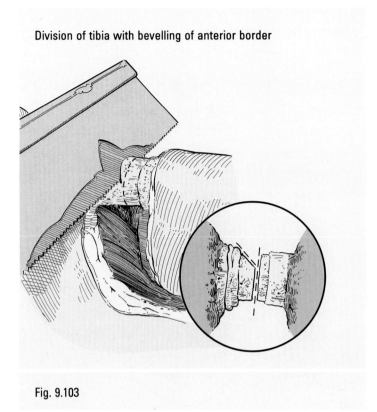

Fig. 9.103

Stripping periosteum off tibia

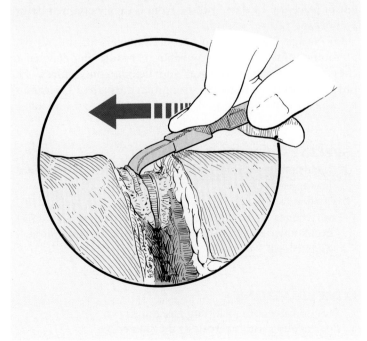

Fig. 9.102

Posterior compartment exposed by drawing distal tibia forwards

tibialis anterior muscle

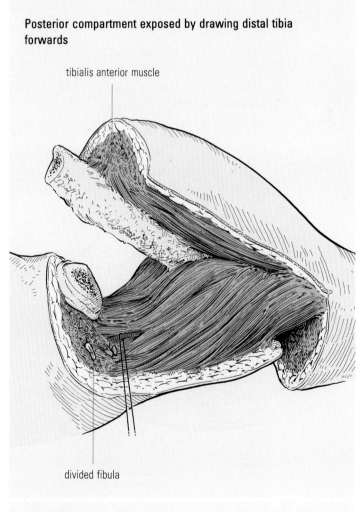

divided fibula

Fig. 9.104

Filleting posterior musclar flap

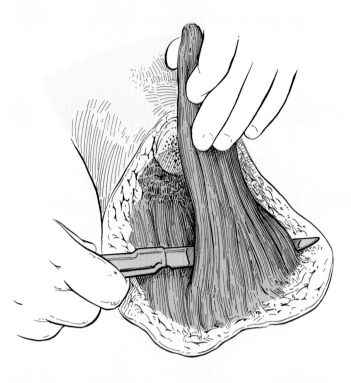

Fig. 9.105

Bone end covered with long posterior flap

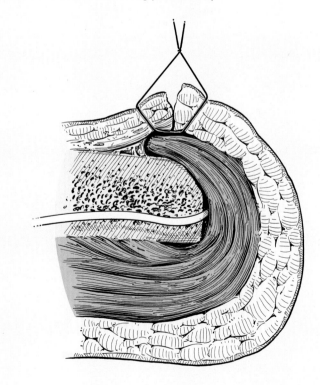

Fig. 9.106

8. Use a long amputation knife to trim away excess muscle so that the posterior flap is not too bulky and will lie over the end of the tibia without any skin tension (Fig. 9.105).

9. Use catgut ligatures to ensure good haemostasis from any small arteries and veins which have been divided.

Wound closure and dressing
1. Place a vacuum drain between the muscle and the tibial end, and bring it out through the lateral skin 5–10cm proximal to the wound; do not suture the drain in place, so that it can be removed without a change of dressing.
2. Suture the posterior flap in position using interrupted re-absorbable sutures, with buried knots, to appose the deep fascia over the muscle to the deep fascia anterior to the tibia. Ensure there is no muscle herniating through the deep fascia as this may cause adherence of overlying skin which may lead to problems with the prosthesis.
3. Use either a subcuticular or interrupted 3/0 non-absorbable sutures (e.g. Prolene) to close the skin. The former will produce more precise apposition and less skin ischaemia (Fig. 9.106).
4. Apply a gauze dressing and stump bandage. A plaster backslab taken over the end of the stump helps prevent inadvertent trauma to the stump and will prevent flexion contractures at the knee. It also considerably reduces post-operative pain.

POSTOPERATIVE CARE
The suction drain should be removed when drainage becomes minimal, usually after 1–2 days. Keep the patient on penicillin for 72 hours unless there is a particularly high risk of clostridial infection, when advice should be sought from a microbiologist. The backslab should be left undisturbed for a week unless the patient develops a fever, complains of pain or the wound begins to smell, at which point the entire dressing should be removed to allow inspection of the stump. The skin suture(s) should be left in place for 14 days and the wound then examined before authorizing suture removal.

Encourage the patient to become mobile with the aid of a physiotherapist as soon as possible to reduce the chances of chest infection, pressure sores and flexion contractures. The physiotherapist can also help strengthen the patient's remaining leg which will have to bear all the weight when first walking.

SPECIAL OPERATIVE HAZARDS
1. Inclusion of sensory nerves into a ligature causes severe postoperative pain.
2. Inadequate blood supply to the flaps, from vascular in-sufficiency or undue tension, will predispose to wound breakdown and may require a revised amputation at a higher level.

COMPLICATIONS
1. Wound infection, including gas gangrene.
2. Poor healing with necrosis of the skin edges.
3. Phantom pains.
4. Flexion contractures at the knee which makes rehabilitation difficult.

Conservative Amputations of the Lower Limb

Limited amputations of the foot and ankle are generally performed to dispose of non-viable or infected tissues resulting mainly from peripheral vascular disease particularly when associated with diabetes which may predominantly affect the small vessels. Less common indications are trauma and tumours.

The advantages over a below knee amputation are that the patient can still negotiate small distances without a prosthesis after a Syme's amputation and after a digit or ray amputation a prosthesis is not required.

PREOPERATIVE ASSESSMENT

1. Consider expectant treatment (auto-amputation) in cases of distal disease where it has been possible to improve the general condition of the patient or the local conditions in the limb (e.g. following lumbar sympathectomy).
2. Check peripheral vascular disease when considering a Syme's amputation, since amputation at a higher level may be more appropriate. A palpable posterior tibial pulse or an ankle/arm index of 0.35 or 0.45 in diabetics is considered adequate for a Syme's amputation.
3. Treat active infection with systemic and topical antibiotics and prescribe peroperative antibiotics ensuring cover against clostridia.
4. Use an X-ray to exclude osteomyelitis of the underlying bones.
5. Seek and treat concurrent cardiorespiratory disease and advise smokers to stop smoking. Ensure optimal diabetic control.

RELEVANT ANATOMY

The blood supply to the foot is from the anterior and posterior tibial arteries which feed either end of the plantar arch from which the digital arteries arise. These run with the digital nerves, the terminal sensory branches of the posterior tibial nerve, on the plantar aspect of the foot. Each nerve supplies one web space, dividing in the distal foot to supply the adjacent sides of the neighbouring toes. In general the plantar skin has a better blood supply, is thicker and is better adapted to weight bearing than the dorsal skin and this should be borne in mind when planning flaps.

It is advisable to leave a stump of metatarsal rather than to perform a disarticulation since this preserves the intermetatarsal ligament and improves the stability of the foot; similarly it is better to leave a stump of the proximal phalanx. If the big toe is disarticulated the long flexor tendons are sutured to the joint capsule to preserve the balance of the forefoot and the position of the sesamoid bones.

The tibia and fibula articulate with the talus which articulates with the underlying calcaneum at the subtalar joint. In performing a Syme's amputation the tough weight-bearing heel fat pad which covers the posterior part of the calcaneum is preserved.

This is enclosed between the superficial connective tissue and the deep fascia which may be breached when dissecting the pad off the calcaneum if the dissection is not kept in the subperiosteal plane. The blood supply to the heel runs laterally and revision of 'dog ears' may render the flap ischaemic by dividing these vessels.

OPERATIONS
AMPUTATION OF A TOE OR METATARSAL RAY
Preparation

These operations can be performed under general or regional anaesthesia. The patient is placed supine, the foot and ankle are cleansed and draped, and a 'shut-off' towel is wrapped around the back of the foot. A pneumatic tourniquet is omitted in the presence of peripheral vascular disease.

Incisions

Make a raquet-shaped incision starting on the dorsal surface of the forefoot 1 cm proximal to the metatarsophalangeal joint for a toe amputation (Fig. 9.107), and 1 cm proximal to the tarsometatarsal joint for a ray amputation. Extend it distally to the

Incisions employed for toe and metatarsal ray amputations

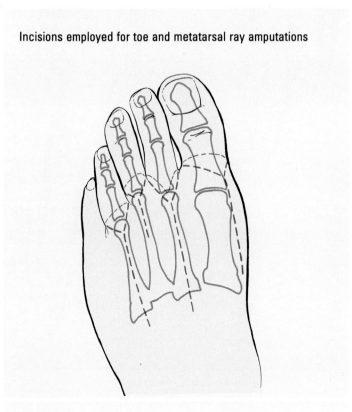

Fig. 9.107

flexor crease, encircling the toe. A wedge of the plantar skin can also be excised in a ray amputation. For the big toe start the incision superomedially and extend it laterally towards the plantar surface. A mirror image of this incision is used when amputating the little toe. All the toes can be removed simultaneously through an incision forming a plantar based flap, which upon completion is sutured to the dorsal incision just anterior to the metatarsophalangeal joint line.

Operative technique

1. Deepen the incision and cleanly divide the long flexor and extensor tendons under tension with a knife and, except for those related to the big toe, allow them to retract. The tendons that were attached to the big toe are held with clips.

2. Identify the neurovascular bundles lying deep to the plantar skin on either side of the toe and divide the nerve branches supplying the toe cleanly, preserving the innervation of the neighbouring toes when performing a ray amputation. Cauterize or ligate the vessels (Fig. 9.108).

3. Divide the remaining attachments to the bone with a knife and, using bone-cutting forceps, divide the bone at the base of the proximal phalanx for a toe amputation and the metatarsal shaft for a ray amputation (Fig. 9.108). The amount of bleeding from the transected bone is usually small.

4. After disarticulation of the big toe stitch the long tendons to the joint capsule of the metatarsophalangeal joint with an absorbable suture such as 00 Vicryl.

5. Secure haemostasis.

Wound closure and dressing
Close the wound with interrupted nylon sutures over a fine suction or corrugated rubber drain if there is oozing or infection and apply a non-absorbant gauze dressing followed by wool and a crepe bandage.

SYME'S AMPUTATION
Preparation
The patient is placed supine under general or regional anaesthesia with the foot overhanging the end of the operating table. The lower leg and foot are cleansed and draped. A sterile surgeon's glove can be placed over the forefoot if the toes are gangrenous and the proposed incision lines are marked on the skin surface with indelible ink.

Incision
Make an incision from the tip of the lateral malleolus across the front of the ankle, sloping at 45° towards the dorsum of the foot, to a point 1 cm below and 1 cm in front of the medial malleolus. Then bring the incision back to the starting point with a perpendicular incision around the plantar surface (Fig. 9.109).

Operative technique

1. With the foot plantar-flexed, deepen the incision to expose the extensor tendons which are pulled distally, divided with a knife and allowed to retract back. Ligate and divide the dorsalis pedis artery.

2. Further plantar flexion exposes the capsule of the ankle joint which is opened with a knife. Divide the calcaneofibular and deltoid (medial) ligaments carefully from the inside, taking care not to damage the posterior tibial artery which lies on the medial side at this level.

3. Further downward traction on the foot exposes the posterior capsule of the ankle joint (Fig. 9.110) which is incised with a knife to expose the achilles tendon and the upper surface of the posterior process of the calcaneum.

Division of structures in toe and metatarsal ray amputations

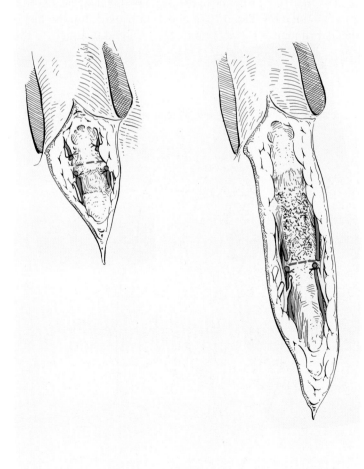

Fig. 9.108

Position of incision for Syme's amputation

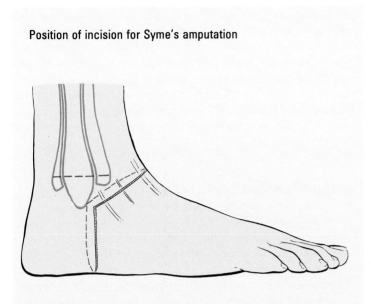

Fig. 9.109

Dissection in subperiosteal plane

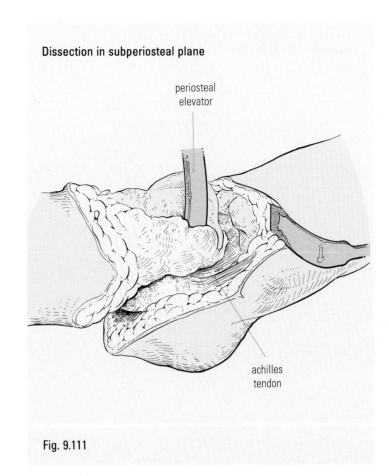

periosteal
elevator

achilles
tendon

Fig. 9.111

Exposure of posterior capsule

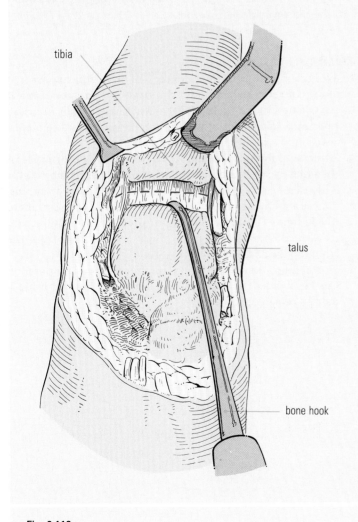

tibia

talus

bone hook

Fig. 9.110

4. Continue the dissection using a periosteal elevator in the subperiosteal plane of the calcaneum, with a bone hook in the talus to apply firm retraction and an extreme degree of equinus.

5. Separate the insertion of the achilles tendon from the calcaneum either by blunt dissection or using a knife, taking extreme care not to buttonhole the thin overlying skin.

6. Free the sides and inferior surface of the calcaneum with the periosteal elevator (Fig. 9.111) until the lower skin incision is reached, and then remove the foot by dividing the plantar fascia at the level of the skin incision with a clean sweep of a Syme's knife. Ligate and divide the posterior tibial artery at this level, and divide the medial and lateral plantar nerves under tension and allow them to retract.

7. Clear the medial and lateral malleoli of tissue with the periosteal elevator and transect the fibula and tibia horizontally with an oscillating saw at a level just above the deepest point of the ankle mortise (Fig. 9.112). Smooth the bone edges with a file.

Transected fibula and tibia

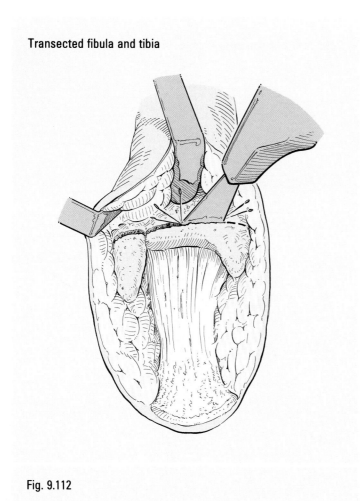

Fig. 9.112

Wound closure and dressing

Close the wound over a suction drain using an absorbable material (e.g. Vicryl) to oppose the deep fascia of the anterior flap to the divided plantar fascia. Use interrupted nylon mattress sutures for the skin. Dress the wound with gauze and orthopaedic wool and encase it in a below-knee plaster cast to keep the heel flap compressed against the divided tibia.

POSTOPERATIVE CARE

Following all these operations the limb is elevated, the drain is removed after 48 hours, and antibiotics should continue for 5–7 days. After the amputation of a toe or metatarsal ray heel walking is allowed as soon as the patient is comfortable and weight bearing gradually resumed as healing proceeds. The sutures are removed after 14 days. If a Syme's amputation has been performed the plaster is changed after 14 days when the sutures are removed. The patient is strictly non-weight bearing and mobilized on crutches; weight bearing is gradually reintroduced. The second plaster is removed and a prosthesis is fitted after 4–6 weeks.

SPECIAL OPERATIVE HAZARDS

1. Gross sepsis, in which case consider placing gentamicin impregnated ceramic beads into the wound, or performing a two-stage procedure with delayed primary closure.
2. Damage to the sensory nerve supply of the adjacent toes in a ray amputation.
3. Prominent metatarsal head when performing a disarticulation of the big toe. This can lead to ulceration of the overlying skin, so obliquely divide the shaft of the first metatarsal if the bone is prominent.
4. Damage to the posterior tibial neurovascular bundle in a Syme's amputation.
5. Buttonholing the skin over the achilles tendon insertion when performing a Syme's amputation.
6. Trimming of 'dog ears' can lead to necrosis of part of the heel flap in a Syme's amputation. Prominent 'dog ears' tend to remodel spontaneously with compression from the plaster and the prosthesis.

COMPLICATIONS

1. Wound infection. Minor degrees of infection are treated along conventional lines with drainage and antibiotics, but if persistent or if the wound fails to heal this generally indicates poor case selection and too timid a clearance and demands revision to a higher level amputation.
2. After amputation of a single toe secondary deformities of the adjacent toes and particularly hallux valgus may occur. The use of a spacer postoperatively will help to prevent this.
3. Amputation neuromas can be very painful. It is important to divide nerves under tension as far proximal as possible, and to allow the cut end to retract so it is kept away from the wound edge and areas of pressure.
4. Dorsal migration of the heel flap after a Syme's amputation can be avoided by not leaving excess skin and by using a patella-bearing prosthesis.

10

Peripheral Surgery

Excision of a Ganglion

A ganglion is a mucoid cyst related to the synovial membrane of a joint or tendon sheath, and is attached by a deep connection to the joint capsule or tendon sheath. The diagnosis of a ganglion is made on clinical grounds; the most common sites are the wrist joint and the flexor tendon sheath in the finger. A small ganglion feels solid on palpation while a large ganglion on the dorsum of the wrist may display fluctuance. Occult dorsal ganglia of the wrist are only palpable with the wrist in full volar flexion. These are best treated by splintage and hydrocortisone injection in the first instance.

PREOPERATIVE ASSESSMENT
1. Distinguish a ganglion from the lumps around the wrist produced by chronic tenosynovitis by the presence of a positive 'tuck' sign. This represents the tethering of skin to the underlying tendon sheath which becomes apparent on trying to move the skin over the tendon.
2. Perform an Allen's test where dissection around the radial artery is anticipated to check the patency of the ipselateral ulnar artery and the palmar arch anastomosis.

RELEVANT ANATOMY
Ganglia on the dorsum of the wrist commonly overlie the scapholunate ligament. The body of the ganglion may appear at various points between the extensor tendons, usually between extensor pollicis longus, extensor carpi radialis longus and extensor carpi radialis brevis on the radial side and extensor digitorum communis and extensor indicis towards the ulnar side. Even where the ganglion emerges towards the ulnar side of the wrist, a careful search should be made for a pedicle connecting the ganglion to the scapholunate ligament.

On the volar aspect of the wrist ganglia generally emerge between the tendons of abductor pollicis longus and flexor carpi radialis. Extension of a ganglion into the carpal tunnel or thenar muscles is possible and the skin incision must allow for this.

Ganglia may also arise in association with the flexor tendon sheath of the fingers, and do so at the level of the A1 pulley volar to the metacarpophalangeal joint; the flexor sheath comprises a series of annular and cruciate pulleys denoted A1, C1 etc.

In addition ganglia occur on the dorsum of the terminal phalanx arising from the distal interphalangeal joint.

OPERATION
Preparation
This procedure may be performed under general anaesthetic or a regional block. Local anaesthetic infiltration should not be used. The limb is exsanguinated by elevating the arm, applying an Esmarch bandage from the distal to the proximal part of the limb, and applying a pneumatic tourniquet. The tourniquet is then inflated and the bandage removed.

Dissection of communication with synovium

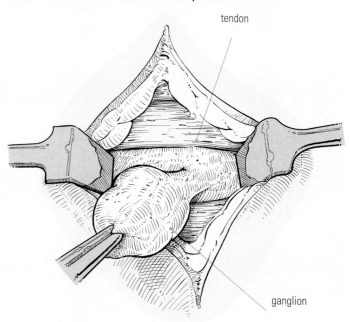

tendon

ganglion

Exposure of ganglion

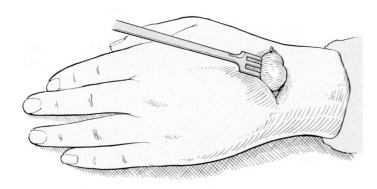

Fig. 10.1

Fig. 10.2

The limb is prepared and draped to expose the hand. A 'lead hand' may be of use keeping the fingers and thumb extended.

Incision
Make a skin crease incision overlying a dorsal wrist ganglion. A volar wrist ganglion should be approached through a longitudinal incision which may be extended along the thenar skin crease as required. Deepen the incision with care through the subcutaneous layer to expose the ganglion, which has a shiny surface (Fig. 10.1).

Operative technique
1. Retract the tendons on either side and expose the ganglion by sharp dissection.

2. It is important to see the attachment of the ganglion to the joint capsule and the dissection on the wall of the ganglion continues until it is fully displayed (Fig. 10.2). The ganglion may be multilocular.

3. Excise the ganglion in its entirety to include the body, pedicle, and base of the ganglion. The base is excised along with a cuff of joint capsule to ensure effective clearance and minimize the chance of recurrence (Fig. 10.3). Do not attempt to close the defect (Fig. 10.4).

4. Secure haemostasis by coagulating visible vessels using bipolar diathermy before and after release of the tourniquet.

Wound closure and dressing
Close the subcutaneous layer with an absorbable suture (e.g. 3/0 Vicryl) and the skin using simple interrupted, 4/0 or 5/0 nylon sutures. Apply an adhesive dressing directly over the wound and then wrap the hand with gentle compression using a wool and crepe bandage.

POSTOPERATIVE CARE
Elevate the hand in a roller towel for 24 hours. Early mobilization of the hand is encouraged, with emphasis on volar flexion of the wrist. The bulky dressing is reduced on the second day and the adhesive dressing and sutures removed after 7–10 days.

SPECIAL OPERATIVE HAZARDS
1. Damage to the radial artery or its branches is a hazard when removing ganglia from the volar aspect of the wrist.
2. Damage to cutaneous nerves and tendons which should be repaired if divided.
3. Puncturing the ganglia at an early stage of dissection makes it more difficult to define and hence remove.

COMPLICATIONS
1. Incomplete excision leading to recurrence.
2. Keloid scarring and scar contracture which may impede joint movement can occur on the dorsum of the wrist if a longitudinal incision is used.

Division of communication, excising a cuff of joint capsule

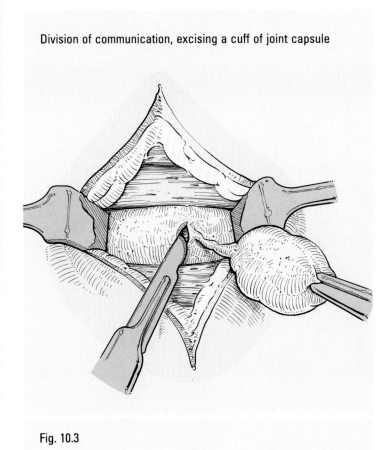

Fig. 10.3

Defect in joint capsule

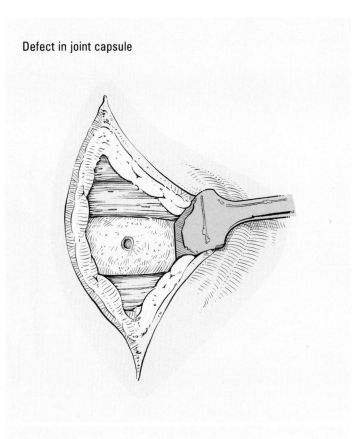

Fig. 10.4

Carpal Tunnel Decompression

Median nerve entrapment in the carpal tunnel is usually idiopathic, but may occur in association with chronic renal failure and dialysis, myxoedema, rheumatoid arthritis and pregnancy; the latter tends to be self-limiting and reversible. The condition is often bilateral.

PREOPERATIVE ASSESSMENT

1. Ensure that the clinical diagnosis is correct by differentiating it from other causes of sensory and motor dysfunction in the hand, especially cervical spondylosis. This may require electromyography.
2. Choose the appropriate type of anaesthesia (i.e. general, regional or local).
3. Forewarn patients that neurological recovery may be slow and it is often incomplete.

RELEVANT ANATOMY

The carpal tunnel is enclosed on three sides by the concavity of the carpal bones. The 'roof' is made of unyielding fibrous tissue, the flexor retinaculum, which stretches between the scaphoid tubercle and trapezoid ridge laterally to the pisiform and hook of the hamate medially. The flexor retinaculum is a well-defined tough layer that begins quite abruptly at the level of the distal wrist skin crease, and merges distally with the palmar fascia with no definite 'end'. The palmaris longus tendon merges with it anteriorly.

Through the carpal tunnel run the eight flexor tendons within a synovial sheath, the flexor pollicis longus tendon in a separate synovial sheath, and the median nerve which lies superficial to the tendons. Lateral to the carpal tunnel lies the flexor carpi radialis tendon in a separate tunnel (Fig. 10.5).

In the distal forearm the median nerve gives rise to its sensory

Relevant anatomy

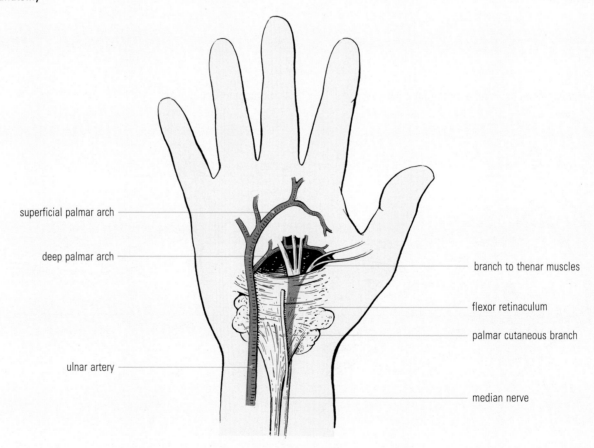

superficial palmar arch

deep palmar arch

ulnar artery

branch to thenar muscles

flexor retinaculum

palmar cutaneous branch

median nerve

Fig. 10.5

palmar branch which enters the palm superficial to the flexor retinaculum in the midline of the wrist. Distally in the carpal tunnel, the important motor branch to the muscles of the thenar eminence arises laterally. At the level of the web space between the thumb and index finger the superficial palmar arch artery crosses the palm.

OPERATION
Preparation
Once the chosen anaesthetic has been administered, a pneumatic tourniquet is placed around the upper arm, and the limb elevated and exsanguinated with an Esmarch bandage before inflating the tourniquet to 200mmHg. The time of inflation is noted and an assistant is instructed to monitor the tourniquet pressure continuously to prevent gradual deflation.

Place the patient supine with the arm abducted to 90° on an arm board. The forearm and hand are then cleansed and draped. Ensure that the palm is uppermost, and it is useful to immobilize the fingers and thumb in the extended position with a 'lead hand' (Fig. 10.6).

Incision
Locate the midpoint between the scaphoid tubercle and pisiform bone and make an incision through this point from the distal transverse crease of the wrist to the level of the carpometacarpal joint of the thumb. Note that since the scaphoid tubercle is medial to the lateral border of the scaphoid, this is medial to the midpoint of the wrist and is actually in line with the inner border of the ring finger. In some cases such as renal dialysis patients where a wide neurolysis is necessary due to the thickened perineural tissues, the incision may have to be extended proximally into the forearm. If the transverse wrist creases are crossed it is important to avoid a straight incision as this produces a thickened, uncomfortable scar; an 'S' or 'Z' shaped incision is used (Fig. 10.6).

Operative technique
1. Deepen the incision through the subcutaneous fat to expose the flexor retinaculum and insert a small self-retaining retractor (e.g. Arms) (Fig. 10.7).

2. Make a small incision in the middle of the flexor retinaculum which will characteristically spring open revealing the underlying tendons and median nerve (Fig. 10.8).

Exposure of flexor retinaculum

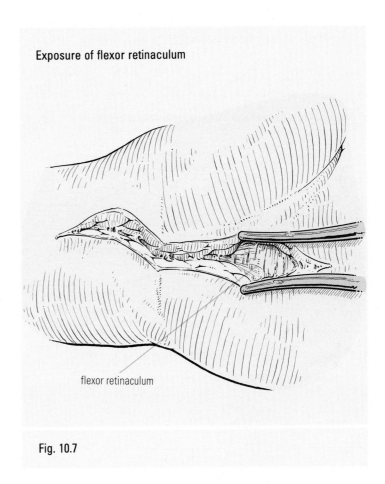

flexor retinaculum

Fig. 10.7

Incision for median nerve decompression with fingers immobilized in 'lead hand'

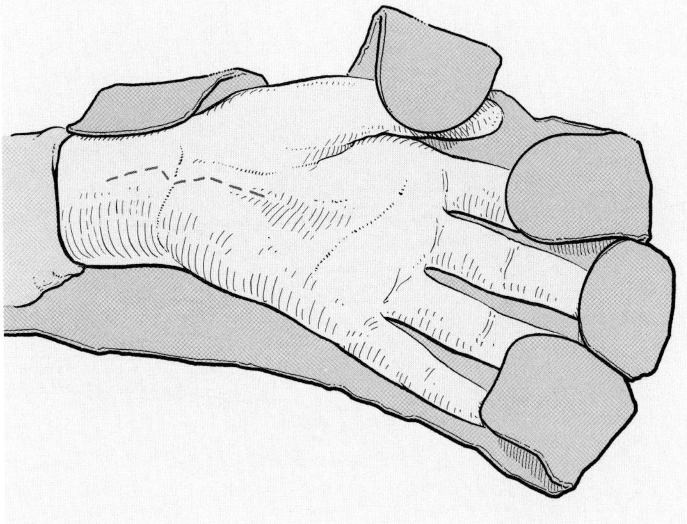

Small incision made in flexor retinaculum

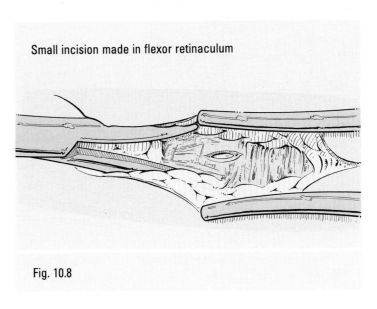

Fig. 10.6

Fig. 10.8

10.5

3. Pass a Macdonald dissector along the tunnel distally (Fig. 10.9), and run a knife with the blade upwards along the surface of the Macdonald to divide the flexor retinaculum (Fig. 10.10). The Macdonald protects the underlying nerve and tendons. Repeat proximally.

4. Incise the retinaculum to the proximal limit of the skin incision dividing all the tight bands. It should be possible to insert a little finger into the forearm along the nerve and tendons. The distal limit of the carpal tunnel can be recognized where the underlying bones become concave and slope away into the palm, and the nerve and tendons are no longer in a tight compartment. Look for and preserve the thenar branch of the median nerve which arises laterally in this part of the tunnel (Fig. 10.11). Decompression too far distally must be avoided as this endangers the palmar arch vessels.

5. Inspect the contents of the tunnel to ensure that they are fully decompressed and that the nerve is free from surrounding structures; avoid retracting the nerve medially as this may damage the thenar branch. In dialysis patients the nerve may have to be freed from the thickened perineural tissues (neurolysis). In rheumatoid arthritis perform a synovectomy if there is a florid overgrowth of the synovium.

6. Release the tourniquet and secure haemostasis.

Wound closure and dressing

The skin alone is closed using 4/0 nylon sutures. Cover the wound with a waterproof plaster and wrap the hand and forearm in a bulky wool and crepe dressing.

POSTOPERATIVE CARE

The arm is initially elevated in a roller towel at the bedside, and then in a high arm sling when the patient is ambulant. The bulky outer dressing is removed after 48 hours, and the stitches after 7 days.

SPECIAL OPERATIVE HAZARDS

1. Damage to the superficial branch of the medial nerve may lead to the loss of feeling in the skin over the thenar eminence.
2. Damage to the motor branch to the thenar muscles.
3. Bleeding due to damage to the superficial palmar arch.

COMPLICATION

Failure to recover function may reflect irreversible damage to the median nerve from entrapment, but it is important to exclude nerve entrapment elsewhere (e.g. at the elbow).

Macdonald's dissector introduced into carpal tunnel

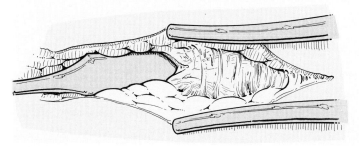

Fig. 10.9

Division of carpal ligament with median nerve protected

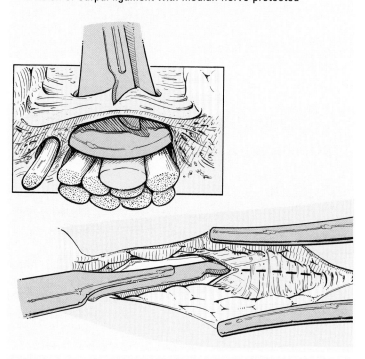

Fig. 10.10

Check thenar branch

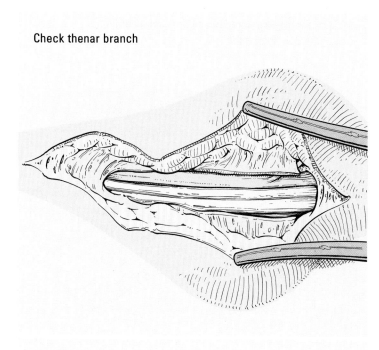

Fig. 10.11

Skin Grafting

PREOPERATIVE ASSESSMENT

1. A suitable donor area is chosen (e.g. front of the upper thigh or arm).
2. Do not attempt to place a split-skin graft onto exposed tendon, ligament or bone; a vascularized graft must be used under these circumstances.
3. If the defect to be grafted is already present, ensure that the recipient area is suitable for grafting (i.e. covered with healthy granulation tissue and free from gross infection). If infected or oozing, dress the recipient site with paraffin gauze and delay grafting until the surface is clean.
4. If the defect is to be created at the same operation, warn the patient that it may be necessary to take skin from a donor area for grafting.

RELEVANT ANATOMY

The skin is composed of two distinct structural layers; the epidermis which is superficial, and the dermis which is deep and lies on the loose connective tissue of the superficial fascia (Fig. 10.12).

The epidermis consists of keratinizing stratified squamous epithelium which is produced by the germinal layer. Its thickness varies in different regions of the body, and it gives rise to and lines the adnexa of the skin (i.e. the hair follicles with their associated sebaceous glands and the sweat glands). These structures protrude into the dermis which consists of tough connective tissue and contains cutaneous nerve endings and blood vessels.

The junction between the epidermis and dermis is undulating, and composed of rete pegs from the germinal layer of the epidermis which interdigitate with papillae from the dermis containing vascular loops. It is crossed by the ducts of sebaceous and sweat glands, and by hair follicles. Regeneration of the skin occurs from the germinal layer of the epidermis. If a split-skin graft is taken, the rete pegs remain in the dermis, as do the secretory glands and hair follicles, and the donor area will regenerate from these persisting islands of germinal epithelium.

OPERATION

Preparation

Cleanse the shaved donor site with aqueous chlorhexidine solution. Aim to take too much rather than too little skin; excess can be stored refrigerated for up to 3 weeks and used later. Drape the donor area and lubricate the skin surface with paraffin oil.

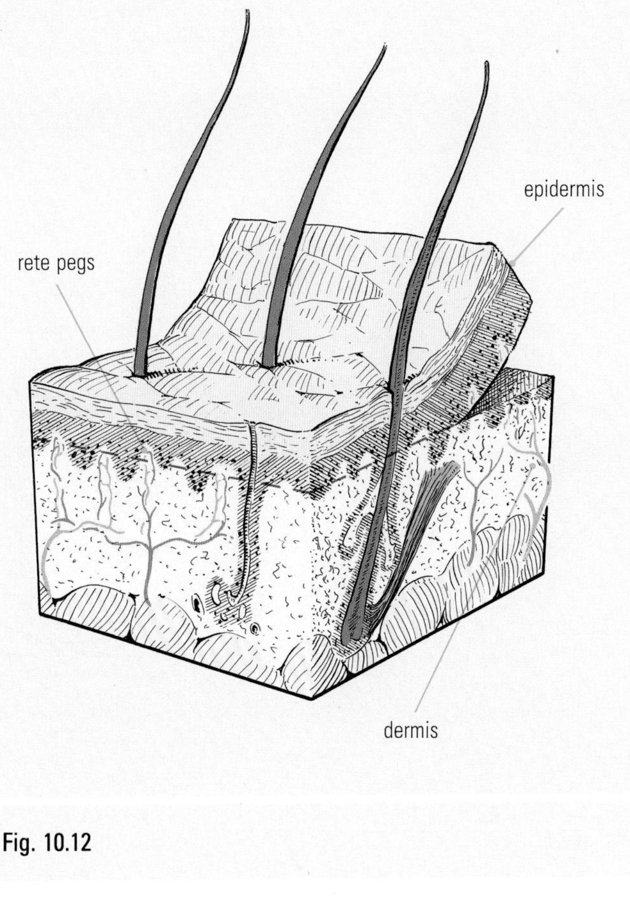

The most popular donor site is the front of the thigh (Fig.

Relevant anatomy

rete pegs

epidermis

dermis

Fig. 10.12

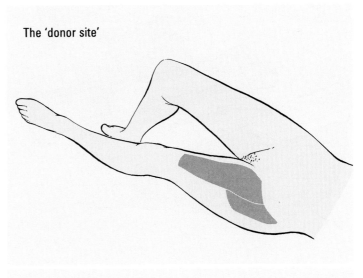

The 'donor site'

Fig. 10.13

10.7

10.13), where an assistant can keep the skin taut by exerting traction with sterile blocks. However, occasionally the skin cannot be taken from the thigh, and an adhesive dermatome (such as a Padgett dermatome) must be used. The following description applies to the use of a non-adhesive dermatome (a Humbly knife) for taking a split-skin graft.

Operative technique

1. Set the blade of the Humbly knife; in an adult a setting of 1.5 spaces will give a graft of the desired thickness (0.3 mm). By holding the instrument up to the light any distortion of the blade, causing an uneven gap between the blade and the body of the instrument, can be seen.

2. With the skin held taut, take the skin graft using a rapid back-and-forth sawing action, proceeding down the long axis of the limb, working towards yourself (Fig. 10.14). Punctate haemorrhage will occur from the donor site, from the divided vascular loops in the dermal papillae (Fig. 10.15).

3. Carefully remove the skin graft from the knife and unfold it onto a piece of paraffin gauze, with the raw side exposed (Fig. 10.16). It should be transparent.

Wound closure and dressing

1. Dress the donor site with a calcium alginate dressing which is soaked with 0.5% marcaine, a long acting local anaesthetic (Fig. 10.17). This can rapidly enter the circulation but is not dangerous if the maximum safe dosage is not exceeded.

2. If the graft is to be used straight away, and the defect is

Punctate bleeding from donor site

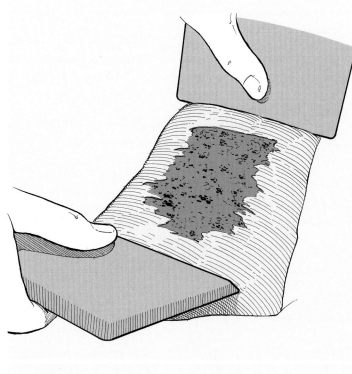

Fig. 10.15

Skin graft taken using a dermatome

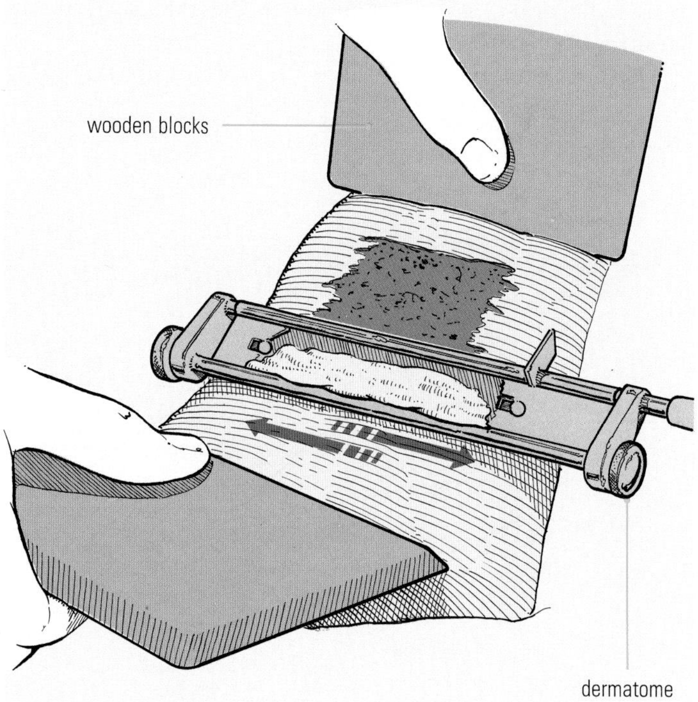

wooden blocks

dermatome

Fig. 10.14

Skin graft spread out, face down, on paraffin gauze

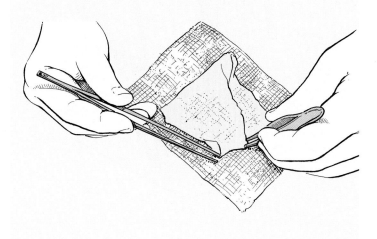

Fig. 10.16

moist but not bleeding, simply lay it on still adherent to the paraffin gauze, either intact or in postage stamp size pieces. Otherwise suture it with interrupted nylon stitches to the edges of the defect. If these sutures are left long they can be tied over the top of a foam pad, cut to the shape of the defect, which will apply gentle pressure to the graft. If the graft is to be stored, or if there is surplus to the immediate needs, it is folded (raw side to raw side), rolled up in a swab soaked with sterile physiological saline and placed in a labelled airtight container in a refrigerator.

3. Dress the recipient site with paraffin gauze, wool and crepe bandage.

POSTOPERATIVE CARE

If the defect was created and grafted at the same operation, the recipient site is checked after 24 hours to ensure that a haematoma has not lifted the graft from the defect. If a haematoma is present it should be aspirated and a dressing which results in slight pressure reapplied. It is redressed after 10–14 days, and the paraffin gauze peeled off. The shed epidermis is adherent to the gauze and often gives the impression that the graft has lifted off, but this is rarely the case. The excess stored skin can be applied to other raw areas.

Where practical, a wire cage is used to protect the donor site which is left undisturbed for 14 days. Great care is then taken when the dressing on the donor site is soaked off in warm water, to avoid damage to the delicate new epidermis; it can be left exposed thereafter.

Massaging the grafted area with lanolin will help to keep it supple and mobilization is encouraged.

SPECIAL OPERATIVE HAZARDS

1. Full thickness excision of skin from the donor area reflects incorrect setting of the dermatome or inadequate tension on the skin by the assistant.
2. Bleeding from the donor site.

COMPLICATIONS

1. Failure of the graft to take is generally due to an unsatisfactory recipient site rather than a poor skin graft, and is usually due to infection, ischaemia, or an unrecognized haematoma or seroma lifting the graft away from the defect. In an ischaemic area a vascularized flap, either on a pedicle or as a free flap with microvascular reconstruction, is an alternative. This should be performed by a specialized plastic surgeon.
2. Contractures; split-skin grafts tend to shrink and this can lead to both cosmetic deformity and loss of function (e.g. restriction of movement).

OTHER TYPES OF SKIN GRAFT
Pinch grafts

To repair a defect on the end of a digit, a donor site on the ventral surface (non-hairy) of the forearm is selected, picked up with a needle, and cleanly cut free with a scalpel. The donor site is closed by primary suture with fine interrupted nylon stitches, and the graft is tacked onto the defect and dressed. It should remain undisturbed for 14 days.

Wolfe grafts

These non-vascularized full thickness grafts are used on the face and hands. Non-hairy areas such as postauricular skin can be used for repairing the eyelid; abdominal skin is suitable for the hand or cheek. The defect is traced onto the donor site and the graft taken. It consists of the full thickness of skin, cleaned of all adherent fat, and it is sutured to the margins of the defect with fine sutures (e.g. 5/0 nylon). If the site allows it, a dressing is applied which exerts gentle uniform pressure. After 10 days the dressings are removed and the stitches taken out. The donor site is closed by direct suture or, if it is too large to allow this, it can be grafted with a split-skin graft.

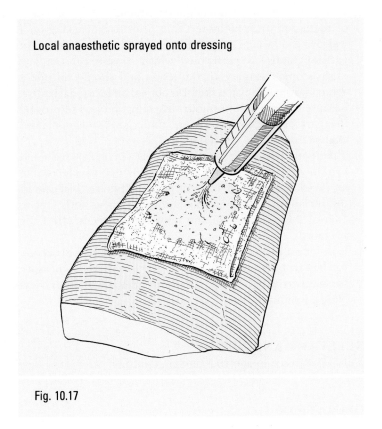

Local anaesthetic sprayed onto dressing

Fig. 10.17

Treatment of Skin Melanoma

The aim of surgery for skin melanoma is to completely clear the local disease which is accomplished by wide excision of the lesion. In specific instances block dissection of the regional lymph nodes is indicated. The patient's progress is related to the sex of the patient, the site of the lesion, the histological type (superficial spreading, nodular, lentigo maligna or acral lentiginous), the level of invasion into the dermis (Clarke's level), the thickness of the tumour (Breslow thickness), and to the presence or absence of metastases to the regional lymph nodes or distant organs.

PREOPERATIVE ASSESSMENT

1. Make a clinical assessment to establish the extent of the disease and carefully examine the regional lymph nodes, supplemented with investigations including chest X-ray, liver ultrasound and CT.
2. If doubt exists as to the diagnosis, histological examination of the lesion must be undertaken prior to embarking on a wide excision which is inevitably a mutilating procedure. An excision biopsy is performed which consists of complete macroscopic clearance of the lesion and should include a 2 mm margin of normal skin. Do not use an incisional biopsy, because of the risk of tumour dissemination and of missing the part of a lesion which has undergone melanomatous change.
3. Traditionally it was recommended that a 5 cm margin should be removed with the lesion. There is now good evidence that an excision margin of 1 cm for each millimetre thickness of the melanoma, up to a maximum of 3 cm, is sufficient to control the local disease and does not adversely affect the prognosis.
4. Consider subsequent lymph node excision by block dissection for lymph node involvement or as a prophylactic measure for patients with a lesion 1.5–3 mm thick, or a lesion overlying a lymphatic bed.

RELEVANT ANATOMY

This is covered on page 10.8 on Skin Grafting.

OPERATION
Preparation

The procedure may be performed under general anaesthesia or regional block. The area bearing the melanoma and the area from which the split-skin graft (the method usually used to cover the defect) is to be taken are prepared and draped in the usual way, the donor site having been shaved. A sterile ruler and mapping pen with Bonney's blue are used to measure and accurately mark the margin of excision. It may be necessary to compromise the excision margins in order to preserve the integrity of vital structures particularly on the face.

Incision

Incise the skin along the marked line, keeping the knife blade at 90° to the skin in order to avoid shelving the incision and thus reducing the effective margin of clearance (Fig. 10.18).

Operative technique

1. Continue the excision down to and through the deep fascia, where this exists in the limbs and neck, and down to muscle where it does not.

2. Working from one edge and maintaining the previously defined plane remove the disc of tissue (Fig. 10.19). Skin hooks are used to lift the edge of the specimen as work proceeds. A 'no-touch' technique should be used to avoid handling the tumour.

Skin incision

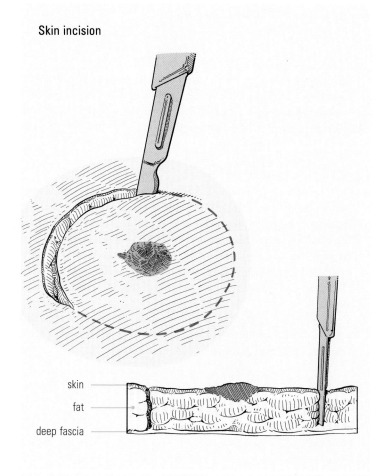

skin

fat

deep fascia

Fig. 10.18

Excision of disc of skin

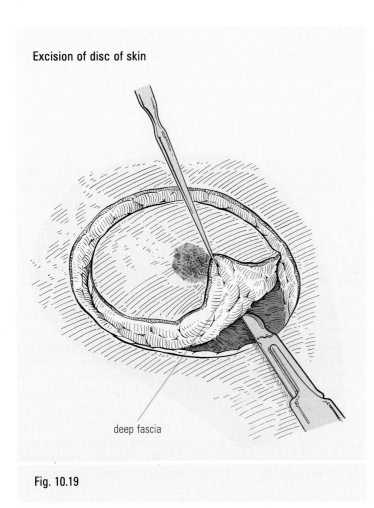

deep fascia

Fig. 10.19

Secure haemostasis

skin   fat

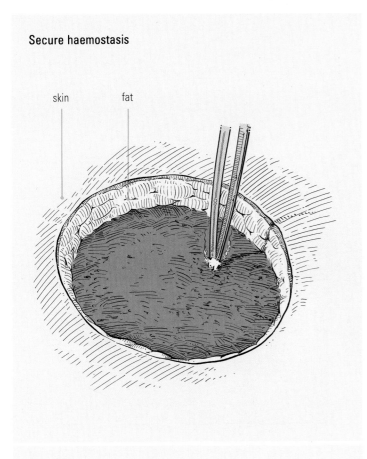

Fig. 10.20

3. Mark one point of the excised specimen (conveniently the superior pole) with a marker stitch and identify this orientation marker on the histology request form. This information is important when studying the clearance margins.

4. Secure haemostasis. This must be meticulous if a skin graft is going to be placed onto the area (Fig. 10.20).

Wound closure or covering and dressing
1. Where a deep defect has been created the ultimate contour may be improved by approximating the deep fascia and subcutaneous fat with several absorbable sutures if this can be done without tension.
2. Using the method described on page 10.8 on Skin Grafting take a split-skin graft from the anteromedial aspect of the thigh or upper arm. The surgeon should regown and use fresh instruments for this part of the operation to avoid possible tumour dissemination. Remember that the area to be covered will be larger than the area of skin excised due to the normal tension in the skin causing the wound to gape.
3. Dress the donor site with paraffin gauze and dressing gauze.
4. Apply a split-skin graft to the wound (see page 10.8) immediately, or after 24–48 hours on the ward if inspection of the wound shows it to be clean and dry. Secure the graft with a few peripheral sutures which are left long and tied over a foam pad, cut to the shape of the graft, or wrap the area with a firm crepe bandage. Store any excess skin in saline-soaked gauze in a refrigerator.

POSTOPERATIVE CARE
See page 10.8.

SPECIAL OPERATIVE HAZARDS
1. Local implantation of tumour cells. Direct handling of the tumour should not occur, and the same gloves and instruments should not be used on the excision site and the skin graft donor site.
2. Avoid shelving the excision margins.
See also the hazards on page 10.9.

COMPLICATIONS
1. Inadequate margin of clearance of the melanoma. Where the histological report shows the margin of excision to have been inadequate for the thickness of the lesion a further margin of skin should be excised. This may be done within 2 weeks of the original procedure without compromising the patient's prognosis.
2. Wound contracture.
See also the complications on page 10.9.

Block Dissection of the Groin

Block dissection of the groin is usually performed for clinically diagnosed inguinal lymph node recurrence after the previous removal of a malignant melanoma from a distal site in that limb. Occasionally the primary melanoma may have been in the lower back, buttock or perineum. Other indications are rare, but include squamous malignancy of the anal margin.

Prophylactic block dissection is only indicated if the primary tumour is situated immediately over the lymph node bed, when subsequent postoperative changes prejudice the reliability of clinical assessment of the nodes, or if other circumstances will preclude adequate follow-up.

The objective is to remove the contents of the femoral triangle preserving only the major vessels and nerves. No advantage has been demonstrated, and considerable morbidity is incurred, if the dissection is extended to include the iliac nodes.

PREOPERATIVE ASSESSMENT
1. Exclude proximal disease through clinical examination and chest X-ray as it is a contra-indication to this operation.

2. Consider performing a CT scan of the abdomen and chest. Using lymphangiography does not usually provide additional information.

RELEVANT ANATOMY
The femoral triangle is contained by the inguinal ligament, the sartorius muscle and the medial border of the adductor longus muscle (Fig. 10.21). The floor is formed by the iliacus, psoas and pectineus muscles. It contains, from lateral to medial, the femoral nerve, artery and vein and their various branches including the long saphenous vein. The nodes in the triangle are divided into those that are superficial and those that are deep to the fascia lata. They are separated by the cribiform fascia. The former are described as lying in three groups: the vertical group lies beside the long saphenous vein and drains almost all of the skin and superficial tissues of the lower limb, while the groups that are medial and lateral to the saphenous opening drain the anterior abdominal wall and perineum, and the lower back and buttock respectively. Efferent vessels pass through

Relevant anatomy

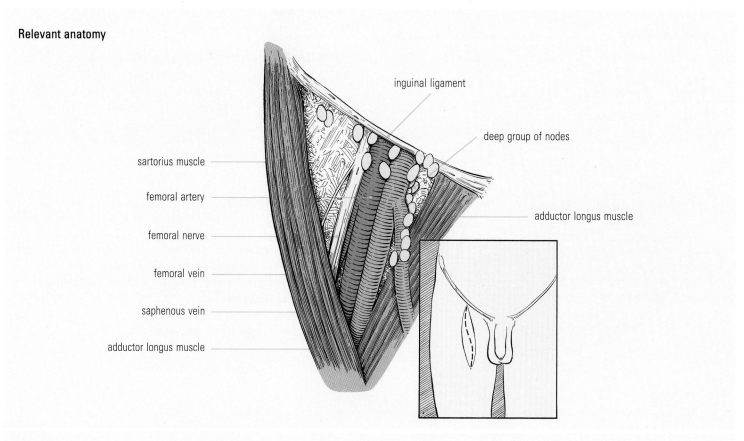

inguinal ligament

deep group of nodes

sartorius muscle

femoral artery

femoral nerve

adductor longus muscle

femoral vein

saphenous vein

adductor longus muscle

Fig. 10.21

the cribiform fascia on the medial side of the femoral vein to the deep group, and thence through the femoral canal to the external iliac nodes.

Preparation

The patient is shaved on the day of surgery, and under general anaesthesia with full muscle relaxation positioned supine with the leg in external rotation. Bipolar diathermy is recommended because of the proximity to vessels of the vulnerable skin flaps. The skin is cleansed and draped to expose the pubic tubercle, anterior superior iliac spine, and almost all of the anterior aspect of the thigh.

Mark a 'lazy S' incision which passes from 2 cm below the midpoint of the inguinal ligament to the apex of the femoral triangle and a long ellipse just enclosing the incision (see inset to Fig. 10.21). This incision will allow good exposure of the femoral triangle, has the theoretical advantage of avoiding a linear incision across the groin crease, and permits adjustment of the skin edges if vascularity is in doubt.

Incision

Incise the skin with a knife, lift the edges of the incision using skin hooks or 'catspaw' retractors, and raise medial and lateral skin flaps to reach the boundaries of the femoral triangle with a knife. It is essential to leave a thin layer of fat beneath the flaps, thus preserving the subdural plexus of vessels.

Operative technique

1. Beginning at the inferior apical end, clear the contents of the femoral triangle and identify the long saphenous vein which is tied in continuity and divided. Divide the deep fascia at the margins of the triangle, and elevate it from the muscles of the base by sharp dissection with a knife (Fig. 10.22).

2. Working cranially, lift the specimen and clear the underlying femoral artery, vein and nerve of all surrounding tissue. Branches of vessels are ligated and divided. The lateral cutaneous nerve of the thigh usually pierces sartorius and is therefore preserved, but other cutaneous nerves are removed. Carefully ensure haemostasis throughout this procedure to maintain a clean and unbloodied field.

3. Continue the dissection proximally to the saphenofemoral junction where the proximal saphenous vein is ligated and divided.

4. Free the upper limit of the specimen as far as the inguinal ligament, until it is attached by only a lymphatic 'pedicle' passing into the femoral canal. Draw the pedicle down to deliver the lymph nodes in this region and attach a haemostat to the specimen at this point before it is divided. This haemostat is later replaced with a marking suture to aid the pathologist in the orientation of the specimen. Check haemostasis.

5. Simple closure at this stage would leave the major vessels immediately below the wound, the skin flaps of which are vulnerable following the removal of their usual feeding vessels from the femoral triangle. It is therefore prudent

Elevation of deep fascia from muscles of base

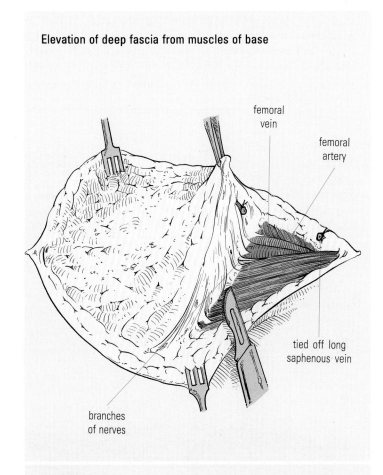

Fig. 10.22

Transposition of sartorius muscle

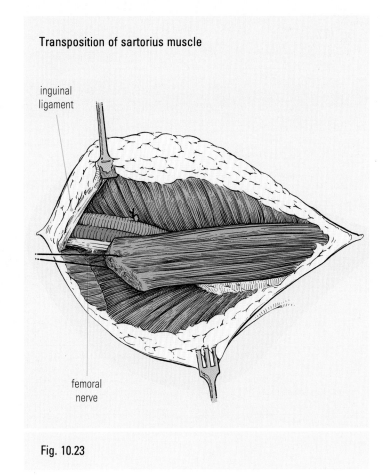

Fig. 10.23

to protect the vessels by transposing the sartorius muscle medially; this requires the division of the upper end of the muscle and then re-attaching it to the inguinal ligament with absorbable sutures (e.g. 3/0 Vicryl). In order to preserve the muscle's own blood supply do not dissect it laterally or inferiorly (Fig. 10.23).

Wound closure and dressing
1. Insert a closed suction drain so that it lies subcutaneously and emerges below the inferior end of the wound.
2. Examine the edges and flaps for vascularity and, if there is any doubt, the flaps are trimmed back to the elliptical lines marked around the incision (Fig. 10.24). Bleeding from the

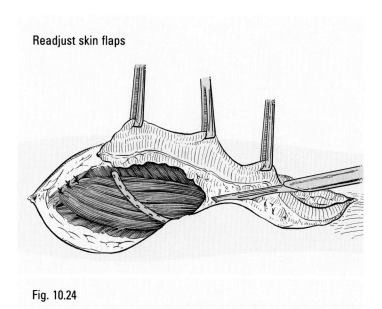

Readjust skin flaps

Fig. 10.24

skin edges confirms viability. There is generally sufficient skin laxity to permit closure without tension, which would compromise wound healing.
3. Closure is in two layers with subcutaneous interrupted catgut, and continuous nylon is used for the skin. Apply a self-adhesive padded dressing.

POSTOPERATIVE CARE
The foot of the bed is elevated to avoid venous congestion. The daily drainage is noted, and the drain is removed when this is less than 15 ml on 2 successive days, which seldom occurs before 5 days. The skin edges are watched to confirm viability. Sutures are removed after 7–10 days.

SPECIAL OPERATIVE HAZARDS
1. Skin flaps which are too thin and ischaemic or buttonholed. This can occur easily, particularly on the medial side where the skin rolls around the thigh.
2. Damage to the femoral vessels and motor branches of the femoral nerve.

COMPLICATIONS
1. Sloughing of the skin flaps and breakdown of the wound.
2. Prolonged drainage of lymph, and the development of a seroma after removal of drain is a relatively common problem. Eventually the drain is removed, as there is always a fear that the drain itself will generate discharge. Intermittent aspirations may be necessary. Pressure dressings are difficult to maintain.
3. Some swelling of the ankle occurs in 30% of patients, and is helped by an elasticated stocking and elevation of the limb whenever practical.
4. Numbness of the upper anterior thigh is inevitable.

This condition is predisposed to by incorrectly fitting footwear, and it is important to advise the patient on this as well as providing instruction on the correct technique for cutting nails (i.e. horizontally).

PREOPERATIVE ASSESSMENT

1. Determine if there is peripheral vascular disease, because in such cases sepsis is very serious and wound healing is impaired.
2. Warn patients undergoing Zadik's operation (radical excision of the nail root) that the nail will never regrow.
3. Plan to simply avulse the nail in the presence of gross sepsis and as a first line of treatment for ingrowth, but proceed to wedge excision or Zadik's operation if it recurs.
4. Onychogryphosis, where the nail grows with a thickened ram's horn deformity, is best treated by Zadik's operation.

RELEVANT ANATOMY

The nail consists of a dense, thick layer of cornified cells (Fig. 10.25) which only grow from the germinal matrix or nail root (a transverse strip of epidermis which has infolded into the dermis) without a contribution from the nail bed.

The tendon of extensor hallucis longus is inserted into the dorsal surface of the distal phalanx, and the digital nerves and arteries run along the medial and lateral sides of the phalanx just under the thick plantar skin.

With an ingrowing toenail, incurving of the distal end of the nail's lateral margin traumatizes the underlying skin and leads to recurrent infection. Toes other than the hallux are rarely affected.

OPERATIONS

Preparation

Operations for an ingrowing toenail can be carried out under local anaesthetic, using a ring block. This is performed by injecting a local anaesthetic (e.g. 1% lignocaine) into the region of the digital nerves by introducing the needle through the softer dorsal skin at the base of the digit, and advancing it to one side of the proximal phalanx until the tip is just palpable through the thick plantar skin (Fig. 10.26). After injecting 2–3 ml of local anaesthetic, the process is repeated for the other

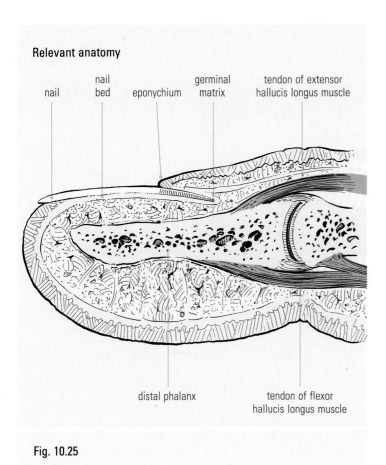

Relevant anatomy

nail | nail bed | eponychium | germinal matrix | tendon of extensor hallucis longus muscle

distal phalanx | tendon of flexor hallucis longus muscle

Fig. 10.25

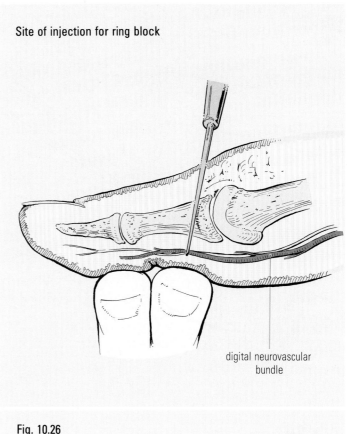

Site of injection for ring block

digital neurovascular bundle

Fig. 10.26

neurovascular bundle. The use of adrenaline in the local anaesthetic is avoided because of the risk of digital ischaemia. Apply a tourniquet of rubber tubing to the base of the hallux.

REMOVAL OF NAIL
Operative technique

1. Lift the nail by gently pushing a pair of small, blunt-ended scissors (e.g. Kilner's) between the nail and the nail bed and opening the blades. Then push the scissors between the nail and eponychium and open the blades again.

2. Grasp the nail with Kocher's tissue-holding forceps and avulse it by traction and rotation (Fig. 10.27).

3. Pare down 'proud' granulation tissue with a scalpel. If only one side of the nail is ingrowing, the nail can be divided longitudinally with a scalpel which is held with the cutting edge facing upward to protect the nail bed (Fig. 10.28). Remove the affected part of the nail.

Wound dressing

The bare nail bed is dressed with paraffin gauze and a crepe bandage.

Simple avulsion of nail

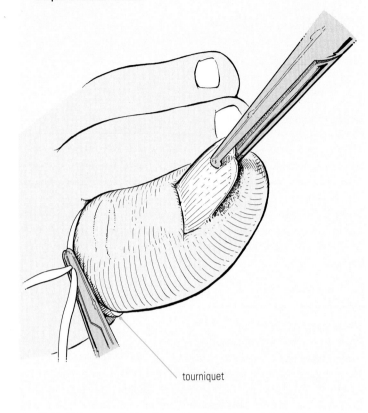

tourniquet

Fig. 10.27

Division of the nail

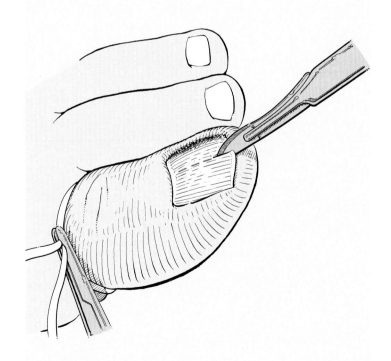

Fig. 10.28

Line of incision for wedge excision

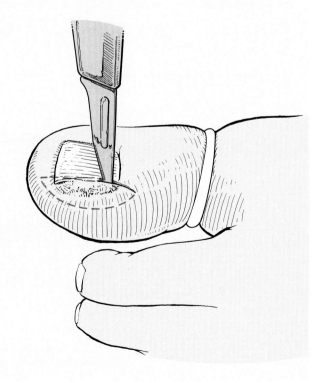

Fig. 10.29

Excision of wedge from germinal matrix

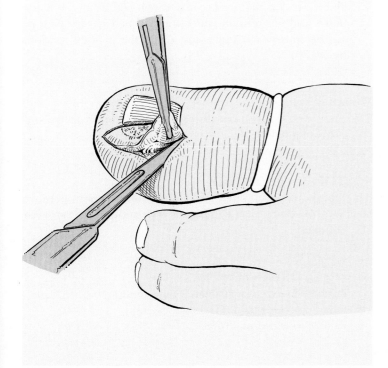

Fig. 10.30

Currettage of cavity after wedge resection

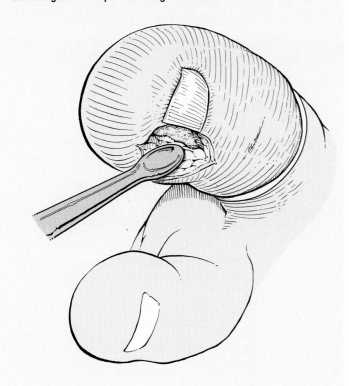

Fig. 10.31

WEDGE RESECTION (WINOGRAD 1929)
Operative technique

1. Make an incision down the nail at a position one-third of the width of the nail across from the affected margin, and then a curved, laterally placed incision as shown in Fig. 10.29.

2. Remove the ingrowing margin of the nail and accompanying granulation tissue in a wedge extending proximally to the base of the distal phalanx (Fig. 10.30). The wedge must be deep enough to ensure complete removal of the lateral portion of the germinal matrix, since inadequate excision will be followed by regrowth of a troublesome nail spike.

3. Use a Volkmann's spoon to curette out any remaining granulation tissue or germinal matrix (Fig. 10.31).

Wound closure

Close the wedge by suturing the skin margin to the cut edge of the nail with 2/0 nylon on a cutting needle (Fig. 10.32).

RADICAL EXCISION OF THE NAIL ROOT (ZADIK 1950)
Operative technique

1. Avulse the nail as described earlier in this chapter.

2. Make two oblique incisions from the corner of the nail to the crease of the distal interphalangeal joint (see Fig. 10.33).

3. Dissect the skin flap from the underlying germinal matrix (Fig. 10.33); a lacrimal duct probe in the nail fold will show the extent of the matrix.

Completed wedge resection

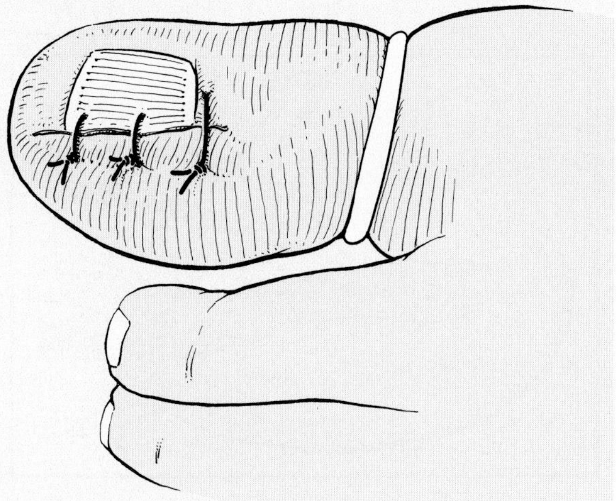

Fig. 10.32

10.17

Defining the germinal matrix

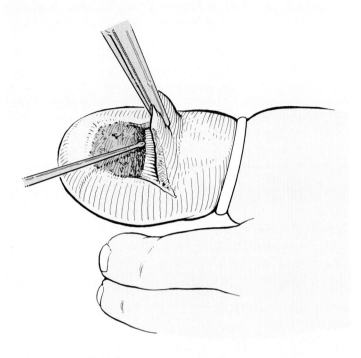

Fig. 10.33

Reflection of the skin to expose the germinal matrix

Extent of excision
of germinal matrix

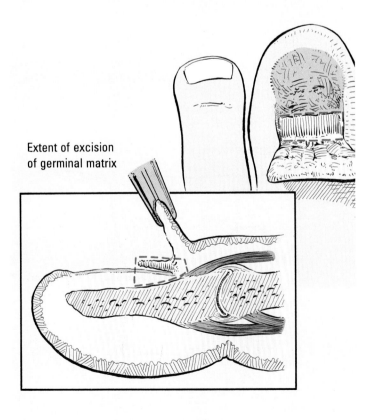

Fig. 10.34

4. Incise the nail bed down to the distal phalanx at the level of the lunula and mobilize it proximally off the periosteum so that the entire germinal matrix can be removed as an 'envelope' of tissue (Fig. 10.34).

5. Suture the skin flap to the incised nail bed using 3/0 nylon stitches without tension, since the nail bed is very delicate and the sutures cut out easily. Close the oblique incisions (Fig. 10.35).

Wound dressing

The toe is dressed with paraffin gauze and a bulky gauze and crepe dressing before the tourniquet is removed.

POSTOPERATIVE CARE

The foot should be elevated for 24 hours and any postoperative bleeding treated by firm bandaging. The sutures are removed after 14 days.

SPECIAL OPERATIVE HAZARDS
1. Damage to extensor hallucis longus tendon.
2. Opening the distal interphalangeal joint.
3. Failure to excise nail root.

COMPLICATIONS
1. Infection of the soft tissues, and on rare occasions osteomyelitis.
2. Haemorrhage resulting from damage to digital vessels.
3. Recurrence of nail growth with spikes; this invariably occurs from the corners of the germinal matrix following failure to appreciate its full extent.

Closure following Zadek's operation

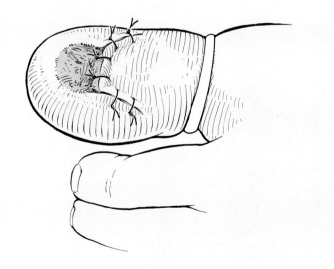

Fig. 10.35

11

Urological Surgery

Circumcision

The indications for circumcision are phimosis, recurrent balanoposthitis, balanitis xerotica obliterans, religious reasons and prior to radiotherapy for carcinoma of the penis.

PREOPERATIVE ASSESSMENT
1. Treat active balanoposthitis prior to surgery.
2. Do not undertake a circumcision in a child with hypospadias, since the skin may be required for urethral reconstruction.

Stretching the prepuce

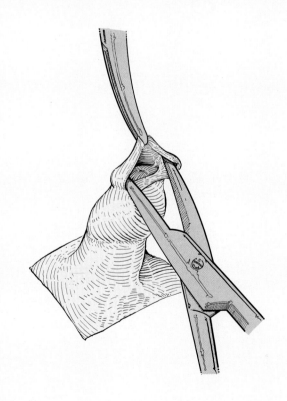

Fig. 11.1

11.2

3. Avoid circumcising children who are not toilet-trained since the foreskin protects the glans from ammoniacal dermatitis (nappy rash).
4. Whilst a relatively minor operation in the child, it is more distressing for an adult.
5. If a retracted tight foreskin causes a paraphimosis which cannot be reduced, perform a dorsal slit of the prepuce, followed by an elective circumcision at a later date.

RELEVANT ANATOMY
The glans of the penis is covered by the prepuce (foreskin) which has an inner and outer epithelial lining. The base of the glans has a circumferential groove called the corona, which is continuous with the inner layer of the prepuce. The outer layer of the prepuce is continuous with the skin of the body of the penis.

The frenulum is a ventral midline fold of skin connecting the inner layer of the prepuce to the external urethral meatus. It contains the frenular artery. The prepuce is adherent to the glans at birth but is usually free by the age of 2 years. In some children the prepuce remains adherent and the opening very narrow (phimosis), which may impede the urinary flow and cause recurrent infection of the space between the glans and prepuce (balanoposthitis).

OPERATION
Preparation
Although local anaesthesia may be used for this operation, general anaesthesia is preferred. A caudal block or a dorsal penile nerve block is also given to reduce postoperative pain.

Operative technique
1. Pick up the foreskin on its dorsal edge in the midline with an artery forceps and carefully stretch it open with the blades of a second artery forceps to allow it to be retracted (Fig. 11.1). Separate any adhesions between the foreskin and glans gently using a blunt probe to expose the corona (Fig. 11.2) and clean it of inspissated secretion (smegma).

2. With one finger, firmly press on the skin over the symphysis pubis, and mark the level of the corona on the penile skin by grasping it with toothed dissecting forceps (Fig. 11.3). This prevents excising too much skin.

3. Stretch the prepuce over the middle finger of the left hand and cut through the skin only with a scalpel, curving the incision slightly distally towards the frenulum (Fig. 11.4). Grasp the end of the prepuce with two pairs of artery forceps and open it dorsally with scissors to within 5 mm of the corona (Fig. 11.5).

Separation of prepuce and glans

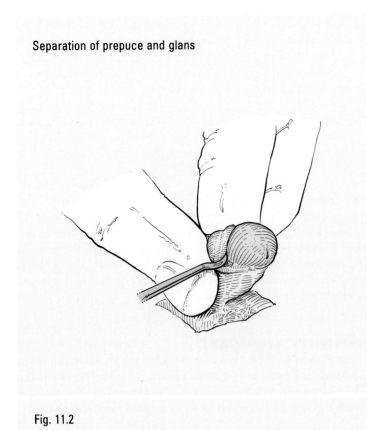

Fig. 11.2

Skin incision

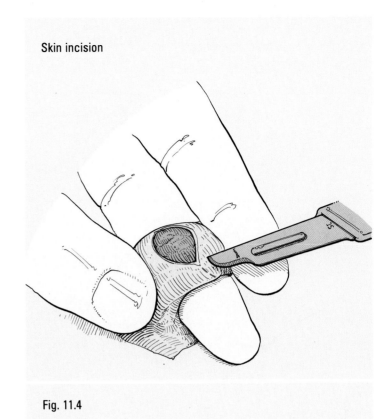

Fig. 11.4

Mark level of corona on penile skin

pressure from finger

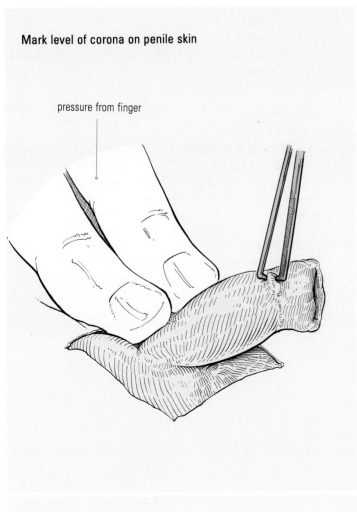

Fig. 11.3

Dorsal slit

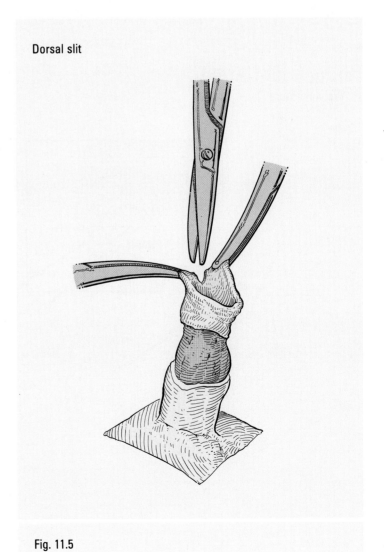

Fig. 11.5

Division of inner layer of prepuce

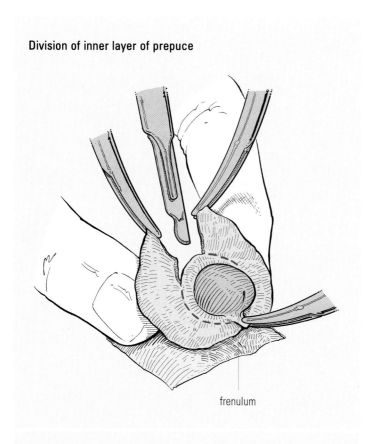

frenulum

Fig. 11.6

Wound closure

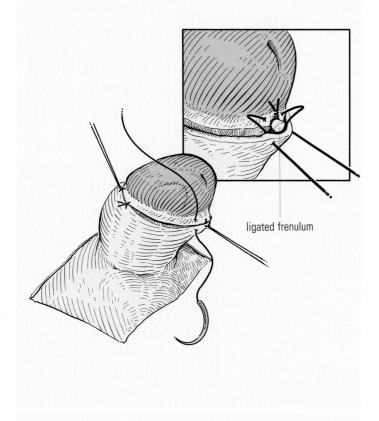

ligated frenulum

Fig. 11.7

4. With traction on the artery forceps, expose the inner layer of the prepuce and grasp the frenulum with artery forceps. Divide the inner layer of the prepuce circumferentially on either side, from the dorsal slit to the frenulum and remove the redundant prepuce (Fig. 11.6).

5. Apply fine artery forceps to bleeding points and ligate them with fine catgut ligatures. Ligate the frenulum and its contained frenular artery. Diathermy must not be used.

Wound closure and dressing

Suture the cut edges together with interrupted catgut sutures; this is facilitated by inserting anterior and posterior sutures first and leaving the ends long as stay sutures (Fig. 11.7). The bulky ligated frenulum is buried as shown (see inset to Fig. 11.7). Apply vaseline around the corona and cover the wound loosely with gauze.

POSTOPERATIVE CARE

The patient is usually kept in hospital for 24 hours although children can be discharged home on the same day provided they have been able to micturate. The parents are instructed to keep the wound clean and to return if there is bleeding.

SPECIAL OPERATIVE HAZARDS

1. Inserting artery forceps or scissors into the urethra when stretching the phimosis.
2. Adhesions must be separated gently to avoid trauma to the glans with the danger of ulceration, scarring and meatal stenosis.
3. Removing too much skin.

COMPLICATIONS

1. Urinary retention in children if the pain is not controlled.
2. Penile haematoma.
3. Secondary haemorrhage. This is usually controlled by pressure with a dental roll soaked in 1:1000 adrenaline solution, but if not it is necessary to re-explore the wound, ligate the bleeding point and evacuate haematoma.
4. Wound infection.
5. Meatal stenosis (see Special Operative Hazards).
6. Painful erections can be prevented with regular diazepam.

Management of Hydrocele

Surgery is advised in adults with large hydroceles. Two techniques are described, the Jaboulay and the Lord's procedures. The latter is more appropriate for a large hydrocele, as the risk of scrotal haematoma is less.

PREOPERATIVE ASSESSMENT

1. In the elderly or unfit consider aspiration with or without sclerotherapy, although this carries a significant risk of infection. The recurrence rate after aspiration is high.
2. In children the underlying defect is a patent processus vaginalis which should be ligated in the inguinal canal.

RELEVANT ANATOMY

The testis and epididymis are enclosed within the tunica vaginalis which extends proximally along the spermatic cord for a short distance; it then reflects to form a parietal layer lining the scrotal cavity.

A hydrocele is a collection of serous fluid within the tunica vaginalis. This may be primary (due to a defect in the reabsorption of fluid) or secondary (due to increase in the production of fluid). The latter is associated with epididymo-orchitis and less commonly malignant disease of the testis.

OPERATIONS

Preparation

Anaesthetize the patient with either a general or spinal anaesthetic. Cleanse the lower abdomen, upper thighs and genitalia, and place drapes to expose the scrotum.

Incision

Make a transverse incision in the scrotum over the hydrocele between the easily visible skin vessels. The length of the incision is tailored according to the size of the hydrocele. Deepen the incision through the dartos muscle (Fig. 11.8).

1. Dissect free the surface of the tunica vaginalis and deliver the hydrocele and the contained testicle into the wound (see Fig. 11.9).

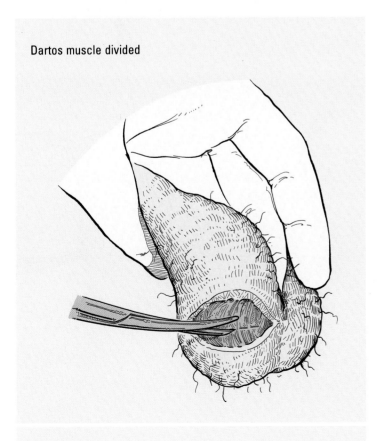

Dartos muscle divided

Fig. 11.8

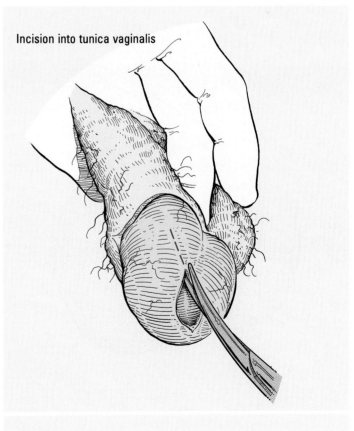

Incision into tunica vaginalis

Fig. 11.9

Eversion of the incised tunica vaginalis

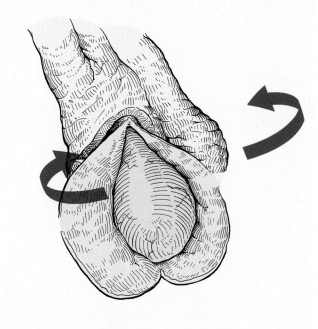

Fig. 11.10

Completion of Jaboulay repair

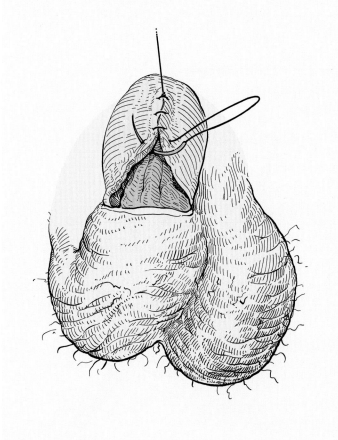

2. Divide the tunica vaginalis longitudinally toward the spermatic cord (Fig. 11.9) and fold it around behind the testis. The hydrocele sac will now be lying inside-out (Fig. 11.10).

3. Trim away excess tunica and suture its cut edges together behind the testis and spermatic cord with a running chromic catgut suture. Avoid strangulating the cord (Fig. 11.11).

4. Check carefully for haemostasis.

Operative technique – Lord's procedure

1. Incise through the dartos and tunica vaginalis in the line of the skin incision and empty the hydrocele. Do not separate the dartos from the tunica.

2. Hold the tunica widely open with an artery forceps and insert a series of sutures from the cut edge of the tunica vaginalis to the tunica albuginea, taking a succession of small bites from the intervening tunica vaginalis (Fig. 11.12).

3. With all the sutures in place, tie each in turn so as to plicate tunica vaginalis and obliterate the hydrocele space (Fig.11.13).

4. Check for haemostasis.

Plicating sutures in tunica vaginalis

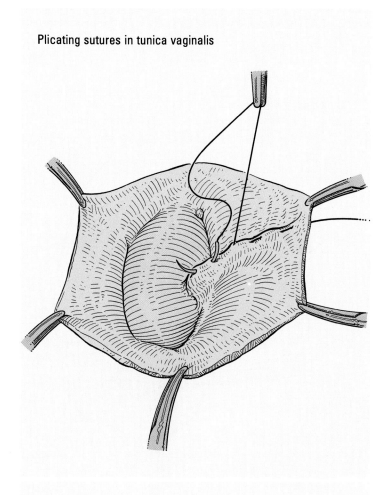

Fig. 11.11

Fig. 11.12

Sutures ready for tying for Lord's plication

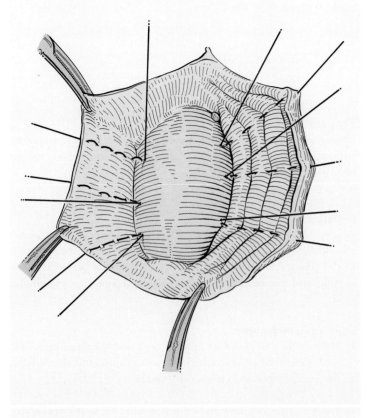

Fig. 11.13

Wound closure and dressing

Close the dartos with a running catgut suture and the scrotal skin with subcuticular absorbable sutures (e.g. Vicryl). Apply a gauze dressing and a scrotal support or a scrotal turban-type bandage.

SPECIAL OPERATIVE HAZARDS

1. Strangulation of the cord in a Jaboulay procedure if the tunica is sutured too tightly.
2. Underlying testicular neoplasm. If the testis is bivalved, there is a risk of tumour implantation into the scrotum when inspecting its contents (see page 11.23).
3. Incorrect diagnosis.

COMPLICATIONS

1. Scrotal haematoma.
2. Wound infection.
3. Recurrent hydrocele.
4. Testicular atrophy if the cord is strangulated.

Excision of Epididymal Cyst

Epididymal cysts are often multiple and multiloculated and frequently bilateral. Conservative treatment by aspiration is usually followed by recurrence.

PREOPERATIVE ASSESSMENT
1. Epididymal cysts are usually bilateral and multiple. Differentiate from other scrotal swellings. Both an epididymal cyst and a hydrocele transilluminate, but cysts are felt as distinct from the testis, unlike a typical hydrocele. The two conditions often coexist.
2. Surgery on an epididymal cyst may result in interruption of the passage of spermatozoa into the vas. In view of this risk of infertility surgery should be avoided in young patients.

RELEVANT ANATOMY
Epididymal cysts contain serous fluid and are believed to be due to cystic degeneration of the paradidymis, appendix epididymis or appendix testis, and arise from the head of the epididymus. The anatomy of these structures is described in the chapter on testicular torsion (see page 11.20). Spermatoceles, on the other hand, are more likely to be retention cysts arising from blocked tubules.

OPERATION
Preparation
Under a general or spinal anaesthetic the patient is placed supine, and the skin cleansed and draped so as to leave just the scrotum exposed.

Incision
A scrotal approach is used, although an inguinal approach should be considered if an inguinal hernia repair is also to be undertaken. The scrotum is incised transversely between visible vessels, and the incision deepened through the tunica vaginalis.

Operative technique
1. Deliver the testis and its appendages into the operative field and identify the cysts, which are usually around the head of the epididymis and covered by fascia.

2. Dissect the cysts free by a combination of blunt and sharp dissection with round-ended scissors (Fig. 11.14), starting away from the epididymis (Fig. 11.15). Keep close to the cyst wall. Ensure that all the cyst is removed to minimize the chance of recurrence.

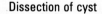

Dissection of cyst

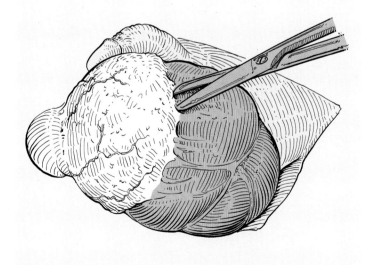

Fig. 11.14

Cyst excised intact

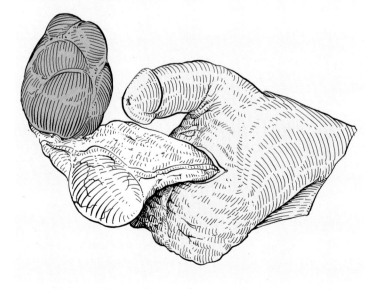

Fig. 11.15

3. Once excised meticulous haemostasis is essential. Sew the cut edge of the tunica vaginalis behind the cord, as in a Jaboulay hydrocele procedure (see page 11.5).

Wound closure and dressing
Close the scrotum with two layers of chromic catgut, closing the dartos layer and skin separately. Apply a gauze dressing and scrotal support.

POSTOPERATIVE CARE
The patient can usually go home the following day but should continue to wear either an athletic support or tight Y-front-type underpants.

SPECIAL OPERATIVE HAZARDS
1. Damage to the vas or the testicular vessels.
2. Rupture of the cyst, which makes complete removal more difficult. This is particularly likely where the cyst is adherent to the epididymus.

COMPLICATIONS
1. Scrotal haematoma.
2. Recurrence of cyst.

Vasectomy

Preoperative counselling should be given to both partners and patients with infants should be advised to defer the procedure until their children are at least 1 year old, when the risk of infant mortality is reduced. The risk of either immediate or late failure of the operation (1:3–4000) must be explained, as should the fact that the operation should be considered irreversible. That this is clearly understood must form part of the patient's and the wife's informed consent and both should sign the consent form. Vasectomy is the commonest urological procedure subject to litigation.

PREOPERATIVE ASSESSMENT
1. The scrotum should be examined for any coexisting pathology, such as a varicocele.
2. Identify both vasa deferentia by palpation.
3. Ensure that there is no history of reaction to local anaesthetic agents.

RELEVANT ANATOMY
The vas deferens (or ductus deferens) is the continuation of the duct of the epididymis which passes from the testis, through the neck of the scrotum, along the inguinal canal, and through the internal ring to join the seminal vesicle duct and form the ejaculatory duct (Fig. 11.16). Aberrant ductules also occur which are remnants of mesonephric tissue; they are blind ending and open into the epididymis.

Within the scrotum the vas lies in the posterior part of the spermatic cord, covered by the internal, cremasteric and external spermatic fascia. It has a thick muscular wall and is easily palpated between finger and thumb as a firm cord distinct from other structures within the spermatic cord. It is usually closely associated with the artery to the vas, a branch of the superior vesical artery, and its accompanying small veins. These vessels must be carefully teased from the vas when a segment is excised as they are responsible for large scrotal haematomas if damaged and not coagulated.

OPERATION
Preparation
The operation is usually performed under local anaesthesia, but if difficulty is anticipated it is best performed using a general anaesthetic. The patient is positioned lying with his legs apart and with the scrotum fully prepared. He is draped to exclude the penis from the operative field.

Incision
The operation is usually performed via incisions at the neck of the scrotum, but both vasa can be approached through one transverse incision made across the median raphe, high on the scrotum, about 2 cm long. The incision is extended through the dartos.

Operative technique
1. Identify the vas on the first side, along with its coverings, and deliver it into the wound where it is held with a tissue forceps.

2. Make a longitudinal incision through the fascial coverings with a scalpel until the thick, white vas, which feels like a piece of string, is reached (Fig. 11.17). Grasp only the vas and deliver it through the overlying incised fascia.

3. When delivered, the vas is seen to be surrounded by vascular connective tissue, which is dissected off to free a segment 2–3 cm in length (Fig. 11.18). Coagulate any bleeding vessels at this stage, because once a segment of vas is excised the ends retract into the scrotum rendering any bleeding vessels very difficult to find.

4. Place a clip at both ends of the isolated vas. The intervening

Relevant anatomy

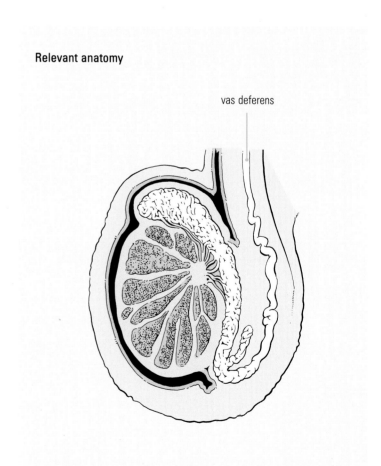

vas deferens

Fig. 11.16

segment is then excised and sent for histological verification. Ligate the free ends or transfix them with non-absorbable ligatures (Fig. 11.19).

5. Various techniques are available to try to prevent recanalization: the ends may be either looped back on themselves and secured, or replaced in different fascial layers. The latter is done by closing the original fascial incision (step 2, above) over one end with 3/0 chromic catgut (Fig. 11.20), leaving the other end outside the fascia (Fig. 11.21).

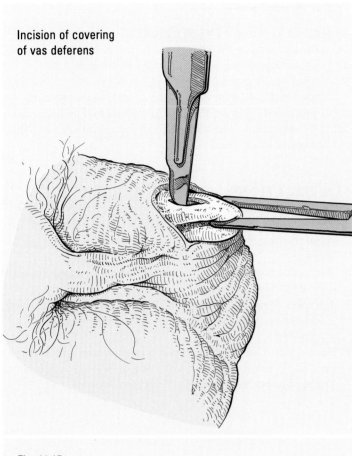

Incision of covering of vas deferens

Fig. 11.17

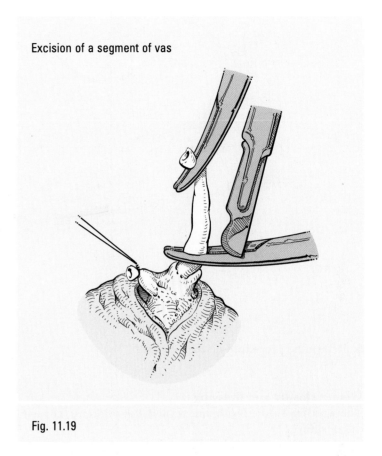

Excision of a segment of vas

Fig. 11.19

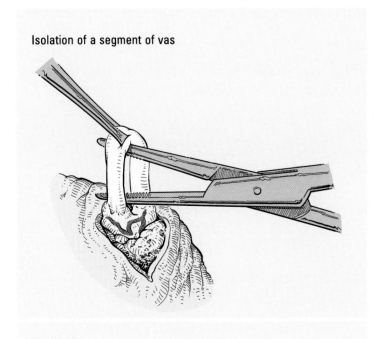

Isolation of a segment of vas

Fig. 11.18

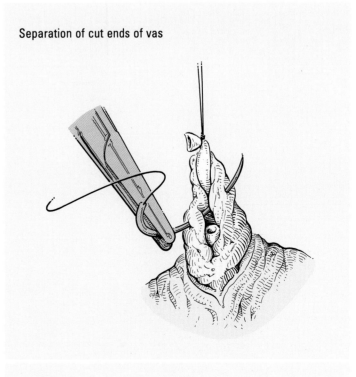

Separation of cut ends of vas

Fig. 11.20

11.11

Separation of cut ends of vas

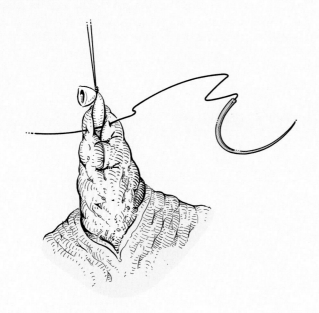

Fig. 11.21

6. Repeat the procedure on the other vas.

Wound closure and dressing
The scrotum is closed with interrupted, full-thickness, chromic catgut sutures.

POSTOPERATIVE CARE
Postoperative discomfort is lessened by supporting the scrotum with either close-fitting underpants or a scrotal support. Semenal analysis should be performed 10–12 weeks after the operation, and repeated until no motile sperm are seen in consecutive samples. The patient should be advised to abstain from unprotected intercourse until this point has been reached.

SPECIAL OPERATIVE HAZARDS
1. When a midline incision is used, care is needed to avoid removing both segments of vas from the same side.
2. Although congenital absence of the vas can occur, the inability to identify the vas preoperatively is an indication for a more extensive exploration under general anaesthesia.
3. The testicular artery should not be confused with the firmer, thicker, white vas.

COMPLICATIONS
1. Wound infection.
2. Haematomas can be severe, resulting in gross scrotal enlargement. If this occurs the testis is best re-explored through the groin.
3. Recanalization and re-anastomosis occur in approximately 1:3–4000 cases.
4. Excision of a 2cm segment of vas should be adequate. Excessive excision renders subsequent reversal technically impossible.
5. Sperm granuloma formation is a later sequel which results in a painful nodule in the distal vas or epididymis. It is the result of a local foreign body reaction to sperm.

Ligation of Varicocele

Varicoceles occur in 5–10% of the normal adult male population and are usually on the left. Surgical intervention is indicated for the scrotal discomfort of a large varicocele and for subfertility, where a raised scrotal temperature impairs spermatogenesis, as demonstrated by scrotal thermography.

PREOPERATIVE ASSESSMENT
1. Examine the patient while he is standing. A varicocele feels like a bag of worms and usually has a cough impulse. The ipselateral testis is usually smaller than the contralateral one.
2. Explain to the subfertile patient that 30% of patients have no improvement in their sperm count after the operation.
3. A varicocele appearing in later life is sometimes associated with a left-sided renal carcinoma spreading along the renal vein and occluding the gonadal vein.

RELEVANT ANATOMY
A varicocele is a varicosity of the testicular veins. These veins drain the testes and receive tributaries from the epididymis to

Relevant anatomy

Fig. 11.22

form the pampiniform plexus in the spermatic cord (Fig. 11.22). This plexus forms a counter-current heat-exchange mechanism which lowers the temperature of the testicular arterial blood by about 3°C in normal subjects.

Just below the external inguinal ring the plexus coalesces to become three or four veins which traverse the inguinal canal before uniting as paired testicular veins running on either side of the testicular artery on the posterior abdominal wall. These veins contain valves. The right testicular vein enters the inferior vena cava at an acute angle which will tend to act as a valve if the caval pressure increases, whereas the left testicular vein enters the left renal vein at a right angle and any increase in pressure in the inferior vena cava will be transmitted directly into the left testicular vein. In addition, the left testicular vein may become compressed by a loaded left colon. These two facts may partially explain the condition's predilection for the left side.

An underlying abnormality of the valves in the venous system is suggested by the association of the condition with varicose veins in the lower limb.

Following ligation of a varicocele the testis drains via the cremasteric veins.

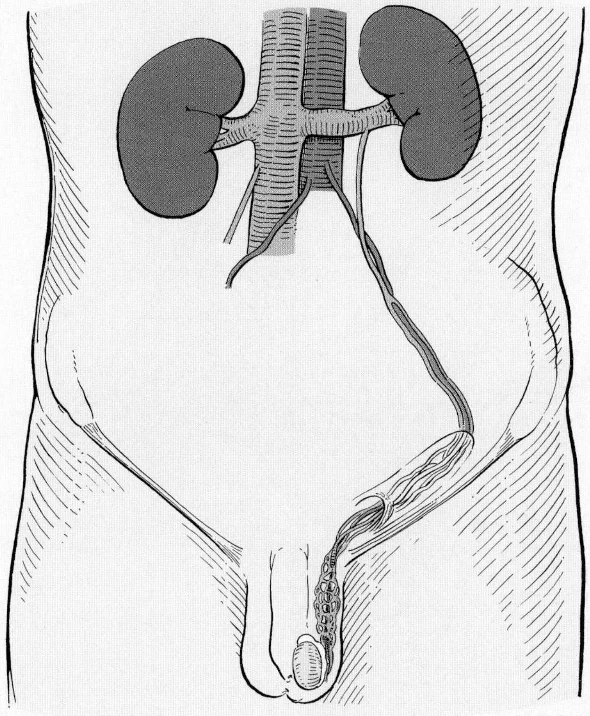

OPERATION
A scrotal, inguinal or supra-inguinal approach can be used to ligate the testicular veins. The scrotal approach, in which the tributaries of the pampiniform plexus are directly ligated, risks damage to the intimately related adjacent arteries, leading to testicular atrophy. The inguinal approach is simplest, and aims to ligate the veins as they traverse the inguinal canal; this approach is described. The supra-inguinal (Palomo) approach is more difficult than the inguinal approach, although it does give good results.

Preparation
Under a general anaesthetic place the patient supine with 10% head-up tilt to distend the veins of the pampiniform plexus. Cleanse and drape the groin of the affected side.

Incision
Make a 5–10 cm incision in the skin crease overlying the inguinal canal on the affected side and deepen the incision through the fascia to expose the external oblique aponeurosis.

Operative technique
1. Using scissors incise the external oblique aponeurosis from the superficial ring in the line of its fibres to open the inguinal canal.

2. Identify and preserve the ilio-inguinal nerve and then

11.13

Cord mobilized from cremasteric vessels

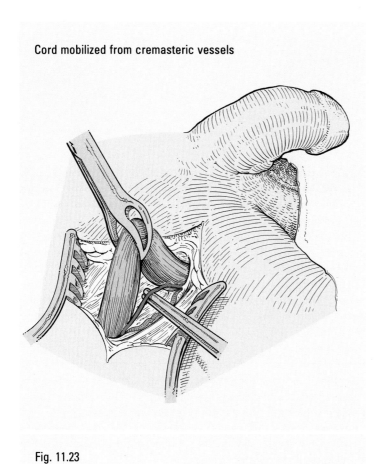

Fig. 11.23

mobilize the spermatic cord (Fig. 11.23). The cremasteric veins lie posteriorly on the floor of the inguinal canal and the testicular veins lie within the coverings of the cord. Only ligate and divide the cremasteric veins if they are varicose.

3. Open the cremaster and internal spermatic fascia with scissors in the line of the cord and identify the cord structures (i.e. vas deferens, testicular artery and pampiniform plexus) (Fig. 11.24).

4. Taking care to avoid damage to the testicular artery or vas deferens, pick up each venous tributary in turn and individually ligate and divide them with fine ligatures such as 4/0 catgut (Fig. 11.25).

5. Check for haemostasis.

Wound closure and dressing
Close the external oblique aponeurosis with continuous 2/0 chromic catgut, the fascia with interrupted 2/0 chromic catgut, and the skin with interrupted or subcuticular nylon. Apply a waterproof dressing.

Opening the coverings of the cord

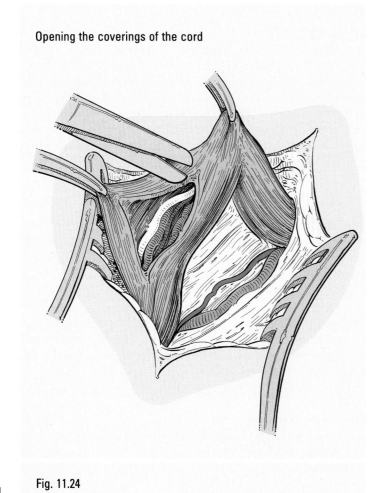

Fig. 11.24

Venous tributaries ligated and divided

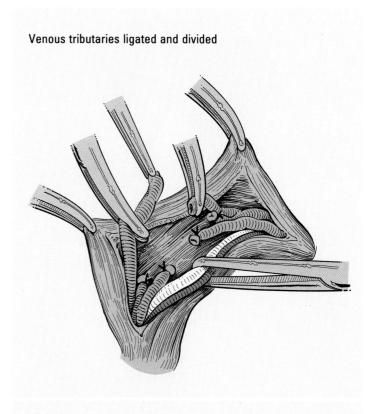

Fig. 11.25

11.14

POSTOPERATIVE CARE

Postoperative discomfort is minimized with a firm scrotal support. The patient is encouraged to mobilize the following day and allowed home. The sutures are removed after 7 days. For cases of subfertility arrange for follow-up analysis of the semen.

SPECIAL OPERATIVE HAZARDS

1. Damage to the testicular artery.
2. Damage to the vas deferens. Having the patient head-up facilitates identification of the veins.

COMPLICATIONS

1. Testicular atrophy resulting from damage to the testicular artery.
2. Painful thrombosed varicosities resulting from inadequate postoperative scrotal support.
3. Recurrence which may follow failure to ligate all the pampiniform plexus, or a varicose cremasteric vein.
4. Failure to improve the sperm count.

Orchidopexy

Orchidopexy should be performed before the age of five but is generally not undertaken during the first year of life. The incidence of malignancy is increased in maldescended testicles and this persists to some extent despite orchidopexy.

The parents should be warned that the testis may not be located and if found it may be too atrophic to have any function and may need to be excised. Consent for this action must be obtained.

PREOPERATIVE ASSESSMENT

1. Differentiate an incomplete descent and ectopic testis from a retractile testis (a testis which can be brought down into the scrotum but due to cremaster muscle contraction, normally lies above the scrotum). An orchidopexy is unnecessary in the latter condition as the testis will come to lie in a normal position with growth of the child. The scrotum is always well-developed in the child with a retractile testis, but under-developed in cases of undescent.
2. A pelvic CT or ultrasound scan may demonstrate the position of the testis if it is not palpable.
3. Fully assess a child with bilateral cryptorchidism to exclude an underlying endocrine or chromosomal abnormality.
4. Obtain consent for orchiectomy, which is appropriate if a unilateral maldescended testis is too atrophic to be able to function usefully.

RELEVANT ANATOMY

The testis develops from the germinal ridge in the germinal epithelium adjacent to the mesonephros on the posterior abdominal wall. It descends during the seventh and eighth months of gestation, partly by contraction of the gubernaculum, and brings with it a tube of peritoneum (the processus vaginalis) which becomes the tunica vaginalis clothing the anterior surface and sides of the testis.

The process of testicular descent is not fully understood, but the testis may be arrested during the course of its descent and lie in the abdomen, in the inguinal canal, at the superficial ring or high in the scrotum, or it may stray outside the normal line of descent (ectopic testis). The usual site for an ectopic testis is the superficial inguinal pouch, which lies lateral to the superficial inguinal ring and deep to Scarpa's fascia; less commonly an ectopic testis is situated in the femoral or perineal region or by the base of the penis. (Fig. 11.26). Ninety percent of maldescended testes will have an associated indirect inguinal hernial sac.

OPERATION
Preparation

Under a general anaesthetic take this opportunity to carefully examine the child to locate the testis. Cleanse and drape the lower abdomen including the groin and scrotum.

Incision

Make a skin crease incision 1 cm above the inguinal ligament, over the inguinal canal.

Operative technique

1. Lift the subcutaneous tissues with two pairs of toothed forceps (one held by an assistant) and divide between them with diathermy (Fig. 11.27). An ectopic testis may lie immediately deep to Scarpa's fascia and should therefore be located at this stage.

2. Define the superficial ring and open the inguinal canal by dividing the external oblique aponeurosis with scissors. An undescended testis in the canal will become apparent at this stage.

3. Divide the gubernaculum.

4. Hold the testis gently between thumb and forefinger and ascertain the length of the vessels and the presence or

Relevant anatomy

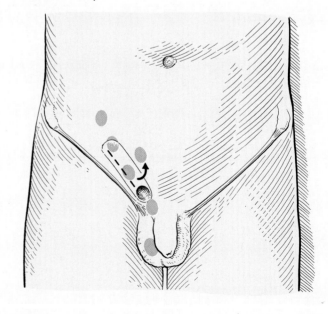

Fig. 11.26

Mobilization of ectopic testis

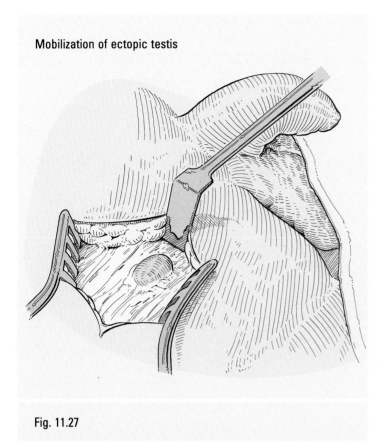

Fig. 11.27

Dissection of vessels and vas deferens

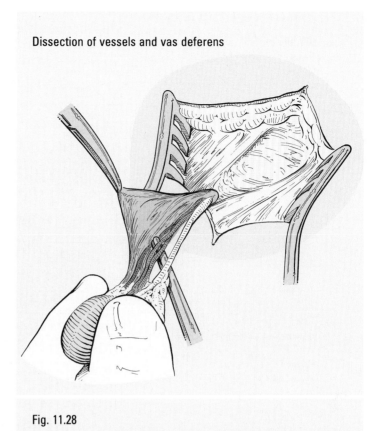

Fig. 11.28

absence of a hernial sac. Incise the tunica vaginalis to reveal the shiny surface of the tunica albuginea. Excise a hydatid if present.

5. Separate the vas and testicular vessels from the coverings and hernial sac as far as the deep ring (Fig. 11.28). Ligate the coverings and sac with an absorbable suture such as catgut. Sufficient length should now be available to allow the testis to lie in the scrotum without tension. If additional length is required, insert a retractor into the deep ring and dissect the vessels further cranially, and the vas inferomedially, dividing the inferior epigastric vessels between ties to facilitate this.

6. Insert the left index finger into the inguinal wound and pass it down into the scrotum, breaking through any fascial barriers which are encountered. Stretch the scrotal wall over the finger tip.

7. Make a 1 cm incision in the skin over this point (Fig. 11.29) and, by opening the blades of a pair of scissors immediately deep to the skin, create a subcutaneous pouch between the skin and the dartos for the testis to lie in (see inset to Fig. 11.29).

8. Press the tip of an artery forceps against the tip of the left

index finger via the scrotal incision and withdraw the finger keeping the forceps firmly applied so as to follow along the same track. Push the tip of the artery forceps through the dartos and grasp the testis by the incised tunica or the gubernaculum.

9. Draw the testis through the scrotum by withdrawing the artery forceps, ensuring the cord is not twisted (Fig. 11.30), and ease the testis through the hole in the dartos muscle and out through the skin incision.

10. Holding the testis with a non-toothed forceps, slip it into the pouch by easing the skin flaps over it.

11. Close the scrotal skin with two or three interrupted 4/0 chromic catgut sutures, taking a small bite of the tunica albuginea with each stitch to secure the testis in position.

Wound closure and dressing
Close the wound with interrupted absorbable sutures (e.g. Vicryl) to the external oblique aponeurosis and fascia and a subcuticular stitch for the skin. Apply a waterproof dressing to the groin and a plastic spray to the scrotal wound.

11.17

Incise skin of scrotum over fingertip

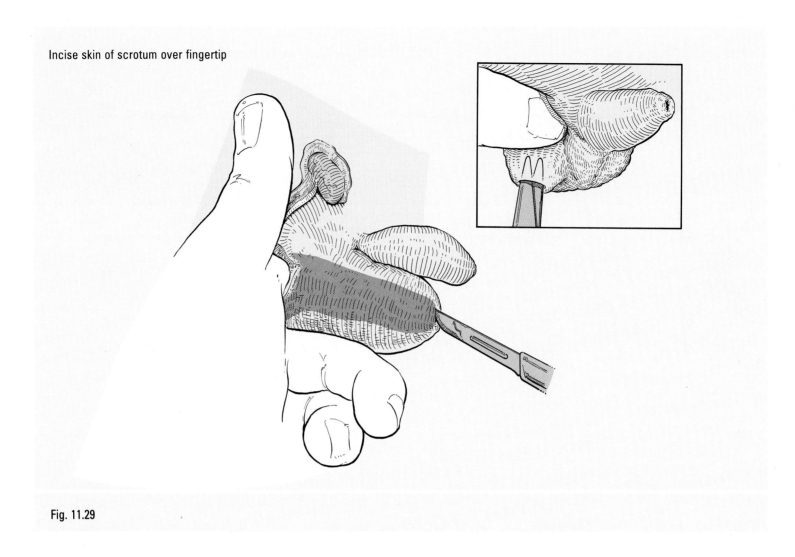

Fig. 11.29

Deliver testis into scrotum

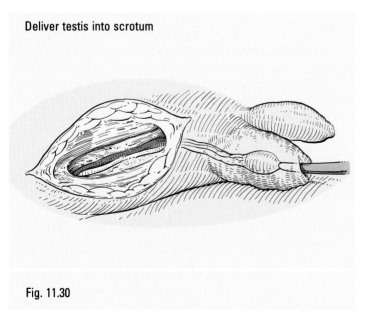

Fig. 11.30

POSTOPERATIVE CARE

The child can usually be discharged home the same day. The skin sutures will dissolve. The child should not be allowed to ride a bicycle or to do sports for four weeks.

SPECIAL OPERATIVE HAZARDS

1. Damage to the vas deferens or testicular vessels.
2. Twisting the cord when delivering the testis into the scrotum.
3. If the testis is grossly atrophic and the other side normal, ligate the cord and excise it.
4. If the testis will not reach the scrotum despite dissection into the retroperitoneum, this is usually due to inadequate length on the vessels rather than the vas. Fix the testis at the neck of the scrotum and elect to re-explore it at a later date.

COMPLICATIONS

1. Wound infection.
2. Scrotal haematoma.
3. Testicular atrophy due to damage to its blood supply.
4. Malignant change in the testis. The increased risk is not abolished by orchidopexy. The risk of malignancy in the contralateral testis is also increased.

Torsion of the Testis

The surgical intervention for testicular torsion is a true emergency. Tubule damage from ischaemia occurs within an hour of a complete torsion, and infarction of the testis will follow within 6–12 hours. The differential diagnosis of the sudden onset of pain or swelling in the scrotum of a young male is between torsion of the testis (or its appendages), epididymo-orchitis and idiopathic scrotal oedema. The diagnosis in a male under 18 years of age must be made by exploration. Torsion may follow either exposure to cold (cremaster reflex) or intercourse. There is often an existing abnormality, such as maldescent or horizontal lie, and therefore the contralateral testis should be examined for a similar abnormality.

PREOPERATIVE ASSESSMENT

1. A torted testis lies high in the scrotum.
2. Epididymo-orchitis is common in the sexually active male and is associated with microscopic pyuria. If in doubt it is wiser to explore.

3. Idiopathic scrotal oedema occurs in young children and is characterized by a painless, red swollen scrotum, with the swelling extending across the midline, to the penis and across the perineum. It may be recurrent.
4. Torsion of a testicular appendage is not uncommon. A torted hydatid of Morgagni (appendix testis) may be diagnosed by the presence of a pea-sized blue swelling adjacent to the epididymal head lying within the scrotum; it may be obvious when transilluminated. If present, it may be left to infarct and drop off; if painful then exploration and excision is indicated. They are usually bilateral, but twist on the contralateral side in only 2% of cases.
5. Consent must be obtained to explore both testes and for an orchidectomy if the delay in presentation is long; consider a prosthetic testis in such cases. An attempt to untwist a torsion preoperatively is worthwhile.
6. Radionucleotide tests to confirm torsion are available. However, they must not delay exploration.

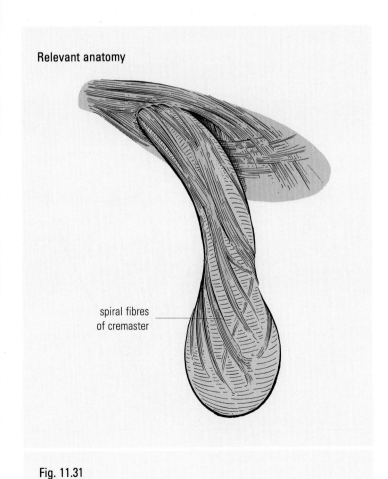

Relevant anatomy

spiral fibres of cremaster

Fig. 11.31

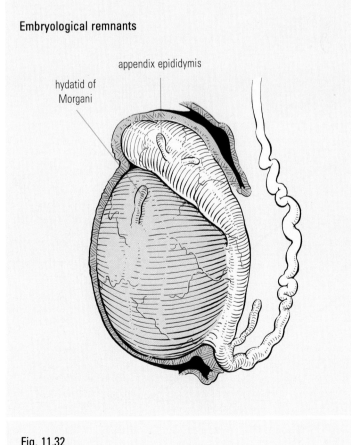

Embryological remnants

appendix epididymis

hydatid of Morgani

Fig. 11.32

RELEVANT ANATOMY

The testis lie obliquely within the scrotum, the upper border tilted anterolaterally and the lower border posteriomedially. Cremasteric muscle fibres spiral around the spermatic cord and upper tunica vaginalis anteromedially (Fig. 11.31). When contracting, these muscles tend to rotate the testis.

The testis itself is covered by a tough, blue-white fibrous membrane called the tunica albuginea, except posteriorly where it forms the mediastinum testis from which the vessels and nerves arise. The head and tail of the epididymis are also applied to this posterior surface and are covered by the visceral layer of tunica vaginalis (Fig. 11.32). If the investment of the tunica vaginalis is higher, the testis tends to lie horizontally (the 'bell-clapper' testis) and is more prone to undergo torsion (Fig. 11.33). Similarly, a long mesentery between testis and epididymis predisposes to torsion around this axis.

In embryological development, the paramesonephric and mesonephric ducts regress. Occasional vestiges remain, namely the appendix testis, a remnant of the upper end of the paramesonephric duct (the Hydatid of Morgagni), and the appendix epididymis, a remnant of the mesonephric duct (Fig. 11.32).

OPERATION

Preparation

Under a general anaesthetic place the patient supine, cleanse the skin and place the drapes so as to cover the penis but expose the scrotum.

Incision

Make a transverse incision over the affected side of the scrotum, with the skin stretched over the testis. Incise the skin and dartos muscle to expose the tunica vaginalis (Fig. 11.34).

Operative technique

1. Deliver the testis out of the scrotum. A reactive hydrocele will usually be present within the tunica vaginalis.

'Bell-Clapper' testis

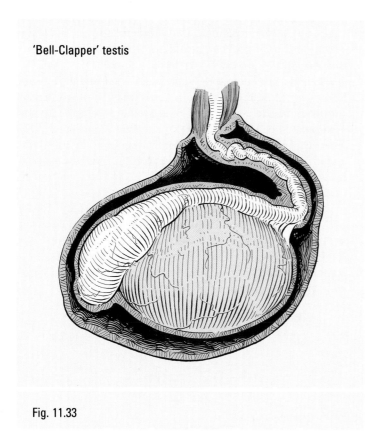

Fig. 11.33

Scrotal incision

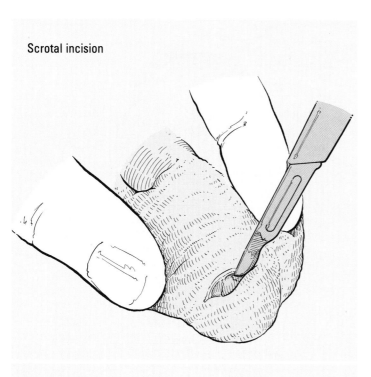

Fig. 11.34

Torted testis delivered

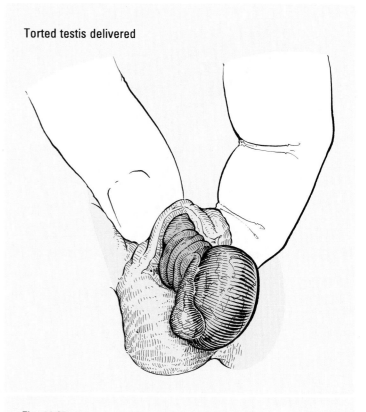

Fig. 11.35

11.20

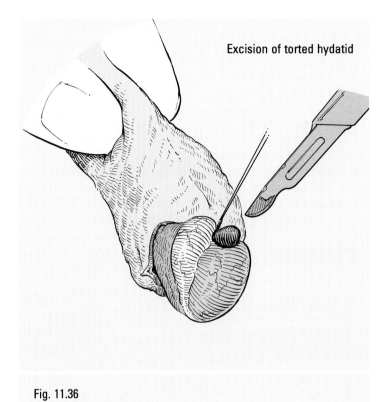

Excision of torted hydatid

Fig. 11.36

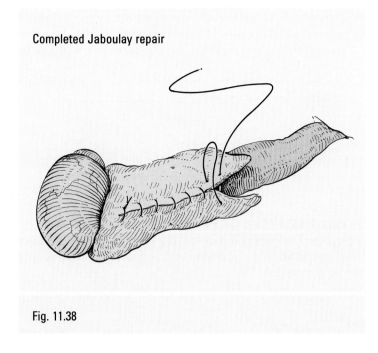

Completed Jaboulay repair

Fig. 11.38

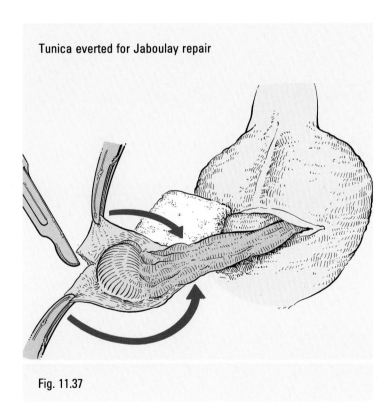

Tunica everted for Jaboulay repair

Fig. 11.37

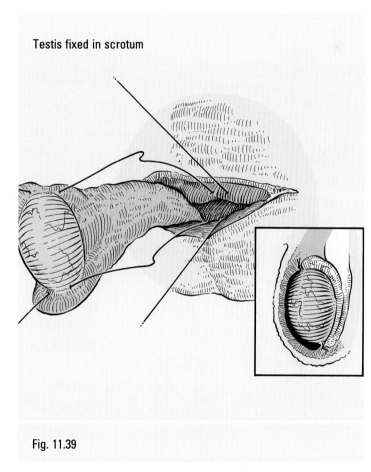

Testis fixed in scrotum

Fig. 11.39

2. Carefully incise the tunica vaginalis. Once opened, a glistening bead of hydrocele fluid appears which may be blood-stained. The incision should be completed with scissors to avoid damage to the underlying tunica albuginea (Fig. 11.35).

3. Reduce a torsion, if present, and wrap the testis in a warm, damp swab. If there is a torted appendix (Fig. 11.36), it should be ligated and excised.

4. If a torsion is confirmed, expose the contralateral testis by extending the transverse scrotal incision.

5. Incise the tunica vaginalis of the second testis and either suture it loosely back over the cord, inside out as in a Jaboulay procedure (Figs 11.37 and 11.38), or fix the testis to prevent further torsion with non-absorbable sutures at two points on the antimesenteric border, securing it to the septal wall (Fig. 11.39).

6. Now return to the torted testis. If its colour has improved and it is pink, it may be returned to the scrotum and fixed as above, but if it remains blue/black or is necrotic it should be removed (see page 11.23) and a prosthesis inserted if this has been considered and discussed. A dubious testis should be left rather than excised.

Wound closure and dressing
Close the scrotum in two layers with chromic catgut, taking care to secure haemostasis from the wound edge.

POSTOPERATIVE CARE
The patient will be up and mobile the next day. He should use a firm scrotal support to minimize haematoma formation and discomfort.

SPECIAL OPERATIVE HAZARDS
1. When fixing the testis, care must be taken to minimize damage caused by the needle.
2. Incorrect diagnosis.

COMPLICATIONS
1. Haematoma formation.
2. Atrophy of the previously torted testis.
3. Impaired fertility is usually due to a pre-existing abnormality, which may predispose the testis to torsion. It is no longer thought to be due to an auto-immune reaction initiated by the presence of an ischaemic or infarcted testis.

Orchidectomy

An inguinal orchidectomy is performed for testicular tumour. If the indication is for benign disease or hormonal control of a prostatic carcinoma, then a scrotal approach is less traumatic. If a tumour is explored through the scrotum, this may result in malignant cells being introduced into the skin and dermal lymphatics which drains to the inguinal nodes, and necessitates subsequent irradiation of the scrotum including, inevitably, the contralateral testis.

PREOPERATIVE ASSESSMENT

1. An ultrasound scan of the testes will identify a testicular tumour and distinguish it from an epididymal mass.
2. Blood should be taken preoperatively to screen for tumour markers, in particular α-fetoprotein (AFP) and human chorionic gonadotrophin (ß-HCG).

3. If a solitary testis is to be removed in a young patient, he should be offered sperm bank storage preoperatively and counselled regarding postoperative testosterone replacement.
4. A testicular prosthetic replacement should be considered in young adults.
5. The side of operation must be checked and marked pre-operatively.

RELEVANT ANATOMY

The testis lies within the scrotum suspended by the spermatic cord, which transmits its blood supply and lymphatic drainage. The lymphatics pass with the testicular vessels on the psoas major muscle to drain into the para-aortic nodes of the same side. Hence testicular tumours metastasize to the ipsilateral nodes, which is a helpful indicator if the primary tumour is impalpable.

The scrotum, by contrast, drains along the external pudendal vessels into the superficial inguinal nodes and will be involved with tumour only if there has been either previous trans-scrotal testicular surgery, such as an orchidopexy, or an injudicious scrotal orchidectomy.

The spermatic cord comprises the testicular and cremasteric arteries, the artery to the vas, the accompanying veins and lymphatics and the vas deferens. Therefore particular care is required when transfixing the cord to ensure full haemostasis.

OPERATION
INGUINAL ORCHIDECTOMY
Preparation
Confirm the side upon which the operation is to be performed. The patient is placed supine, the skin is cleaned, and drapes are applied, to expose the inguinal region.

Incision
An inguinal approach similar to that used for inguinal hernia repair (see page 7.10) should be used.

Operative technique
1. Open the external oblique aponeurosis from the external (superficial) ring to the internal (deep) ring.

2. Mobilize the proximal part of the spermatic cord and lifting it with Lane's tissue forceps, place a non-crushing bowel clamp across it at the internal ring (Fig. 11.40).

3. Only now should the testis be mobilized, delivering it through the neck of the scrotum by a combination of cord traction and pressure on the scrotum below. Dissect the intact tunica free of the inverted scrotum (Fig. 11.41).

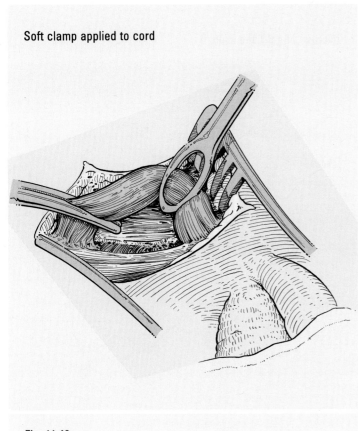

Soft clamp applied to cord

Fig. 11.40

11.23

Testis mobilized from scrotum

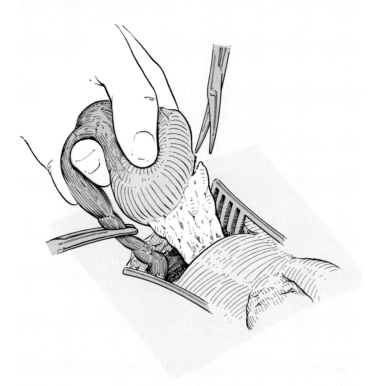

Fig. 11.41

Transfixion of the cord

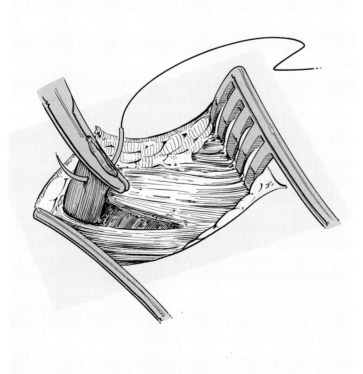

Fig. 11.42

Insertion of gel-filled implant

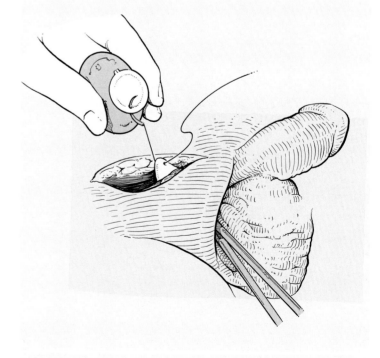

Fig. 11.43

4. At this point some authorities advocate aspirating cord venous blood for tumour marker assay. If the systemic concentration of the marker proves to be higher than that in the cord, extragonadal disease is indicated.

5. The testis may now be bivalved as follows: the wound is covered with swabs, and then a longitudinal incision is made along the antimesenteric border of the testis. This allows the testis to be opened like a book and frozen section histology to be performed on any lesion. It is not uncommon for small primary tumours to be missed by this technique and pre-operative ultrasound localization is preferable.

6. Once the decision to remove the testis has been made, place crushing clamps across proximal and distal cord and divide it between them.

7. Transfix the cord with heavy 00 catgut ensuring an indirect hernial sac containing viscera is not present (Fig. 11.42). Haemostasis must be checked before allowing the cord to retract into the internal ring, which is subsequently closed with catgut.

8. If a prosthesis is to be inserted, hold the base of the scrotum in forceps and invaginate it into the inguinal canal. Suture the sewing collar of the prosthesis to the dartos muscle with non-absorbable sutures (Fig. 11.43), taking care not to breach the scrotal skin or to puncture the gel-filled implant. It can then be reduced into the scrotum, and the neck of the scrotum sutured with chromic catgut.

Scrotal orchidectomy

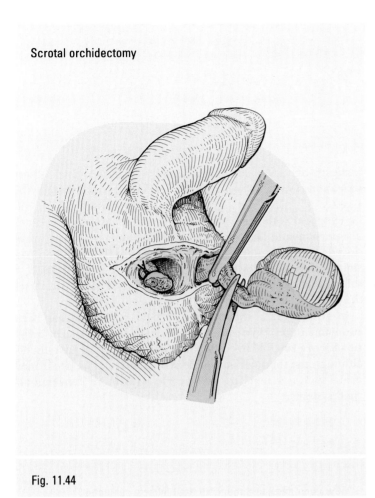

Fig. 11.44

Wound closure and dressing
A drain is not necessary. Close the external oblique muscle with chromic catgut and the skin with interrupted nylon. A dressing is then applied.

POSTOPERATIVE CARE
The patient will be up and mobile the next day. Full staging investigations are best performed in conjunction with the oncology department.

SPECIAL OPERATIVE HAZARDS
1. Damage to the contents of an unrecognized hernial sac.
2. Puncture of a prosthetic testis.

COMPLICATIONS
1. Bleeding from the transected cord can be severe but can be prevented if the cord is checked for haemostasis before it is allowed to retract through the internal ring.
2. Scrotal haematoma.
3. Tumour seeding resulting from bivalving must be avoided if possible. If the testis is bivalved, the wound must be protected with swabs, and gloves and instruments changed before continuing.
4. Division of the ilio-inguinal nerve resulting in anaesthesia over the pubis and the neck of the scrotum.

SCROTAL ORCHIDECTOMY
A scrotal orchidectomy is most often used for hormonal manipulation of prostatic cancer. A 'subcapsular' orchidectomy leaves a significant amount of hormone secreting tissue and a total orchidectomy is to be preferred.

Preparation
Similar to that described for inguinal orchidectomy, except the drapes are applied to expose the scrotum.

Incision
Make a transverse incision in the scrotum.

Operative technique
1. Deliver the testes as for a torsion repair (see page 11.20).

2. Clamp each cord in turn and excise the testes by dividing the cord distal to the clamp (Fig. 11.44).

3. Transfix the cord with heavy chromic catgut.

Wound closure and dressing
A drain is not necessary. Close the external oblique aponeurosis with chromic catgut and the skin with interrupted nylon. A dressing is then applied.

COMPLICATIONS
1. Infertility is inevitable but rarely a problem as this operation is usually performed in elderly men. However, sperm bank storage can be offered in suitable cases.
2. Scrotal haematoma.

Cystoscopy

Cystoscopy is the single most commonly performed urological procedure, which is testament to its value as a diagnostic tool. It can provide information regarding the urethra, the prostate and the bladder, and by means of retrograde ureterography can also provide X-ray visualization of the ureter and pelvic-alyceal collecting system.

Rigid cystoscopy was revolutionized by the introduction of rigid rod-lens optics which provides a clear image from the end of the telescope. The distal lens (objective) may be set at a variety of angles to the axis of the cystoscope, though the 30° telescope is the most commonly used and is also the most useful. 0° telescopes are useful for urethroscopy and ureteric intubation, while 70° telescopes are of value in the assessment of the bladder neck region. A fibreoptic cable attached to a socket on the cystoscope provides the light source. Around the telescope there is

a sheath of varying diameter (usually 17–27 Fr) which allows irrigation through a separate channel. With wider sheaths the passage of guidewires and catheters is also possible. As would be expected with the wider sheaths, faster irrigant flow rates are possible and larger catheters or instruments may be introduced. In a diagnostic procedure normal saline solution is a suitable irrigant; however, when diathermy is to be used, a solution of glycine (1.5%) is necessary, since saline disperses the electrical current.

In recent years, the traditional rigid cystoscope has been supplemented by narrower flexible endoscopes, which, being smaller are suitable for outpatient use under local anaesthetic, although the therapeutic manoeuvres which can be performed using such a system are fewer than with more conventional rigid systems.

Insertion of cystoscope

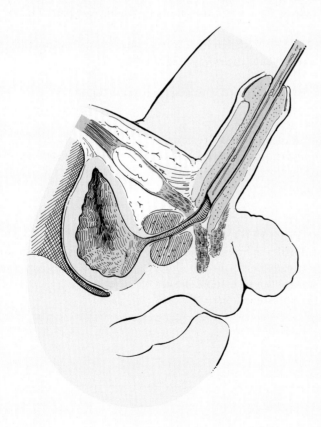

Fig. 11.45

View upon passing through striated muscle sphincter

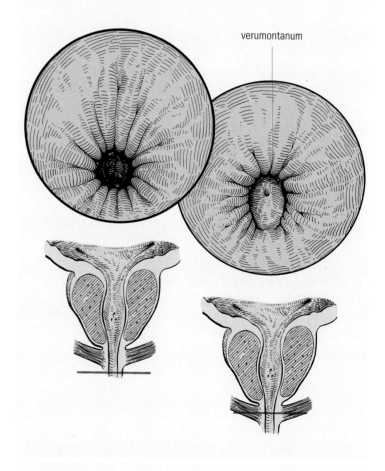

verumontanum

Fig. 11.46

PREOPERATIVE ASSESSMENT

1. Consider antibiotic prophylaxis when there is documented evidence or a strong suspicion of urinary tract infection.
2. If hip movement is limited (e.g. due to osteoarthritis) then full examination of the bladder with a rigid cystoscope may be impossible. Under these circumstances, flexible cystoscopy is of great value.
3. Use cystoscopy as an adjunct to other investigative techniques such as intravenous pyelography when pursuing symptoms such as haematuria.
4. Urinary cytology can be usefully combined with cystoscopy in the follow-up of transitional cell carcinoma.

RELEVANT ANATOMY

The male urethra is at its narrowest just proximal to the urethral meatus, so that in some patients, a urethrotomy is necessary to allow introduction of the cystoscope. Further along the urethra, in its bulbar region, the urethra bends through almost 90°. Unless the surgeon is aware of this, he may push the cystoscope too posteriorly, thereby producing a false passage.

PROCEDURE

Preparation

Under general or spinal anaesthesia, the patient is placed in the lithotomy position. In men, 20ml of lignocaine gel is inserted into the urethra to provide lubrication, local anaesthesia and some antiseptic protection. The genitalia are cleansed and draped, keeping the penis or vagina exposed.

Operative technique

1. While standing, hold the penis with thumb and index finger in the groove between the corpora cavernosa and the corpus spongiosum, pull the penis out straight in order to straighten the penile urethra, and introduce the cystoscope into the urethral meatus (Fig. 11.45). The penile urethra may thus by traversed, until the bulbar urethra is entered and the external striated sphincter is seen (Fig. 11.46). In women there is usually little difficulty in setting the cystoscope directly into the bladder.

2. The urethra then bends ventrally, so while gently advancing the cystoscope, gradually sit down, thereby rotating the tip of the cystoscope ventrally. In this way the sphincter is traversed, although there is often some resistance at this point. Upon entry into the prostatic urethra, the verumontanum may be seen and then the bladder neck is encountered (Fig. 11.47). At this point it is usual to move the cystoscope tip even further ventrally to get over the circular smooth muscle fibres of the bladder neck.

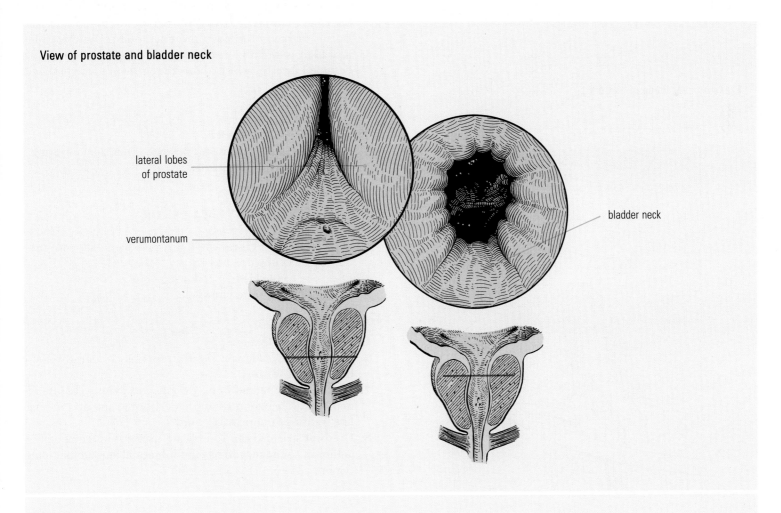

View of prostate and bladder neck

lateral lobes of prostate

verumontanum

bladder neck

Fig. 11.47

View of the trigone

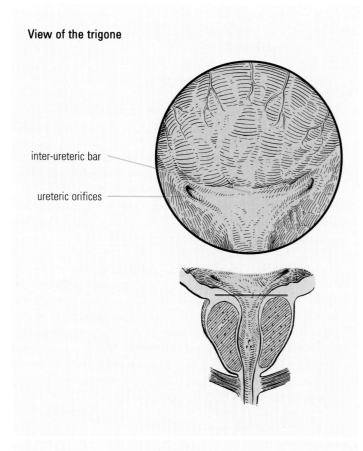

inter-ureteric bar

ureteric orifices

Fig. 11.48

Pressure over dome of bladder

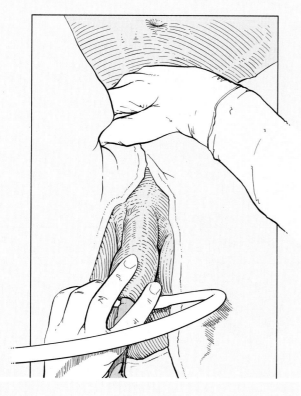

Fig. 11.49

3. Upon entry into the bladder, remove the telescope to allow the residual urine to drain from the bladder. A thorough examination of the bladder then follows.

4. Using the 30° telescope examine the base of the bladder. By regular sweeping of the cystoscope backwards and forwards, it should be possible to identify the trigone, the ureteric orifices and the interureteric bar (Fig. 11.48).

5. In a similar fashion, systematically examine the side walls and dome of the bladder. The dome of the bladder usually contains a small air bubble (introduced with the irrigation fluid). The visualization of this area is often made easier by pressure on the lower abdomen (Fig. 11.49) or by using a 70° scope (Fig. 11.50) instead of a 30° scope (Fig. 11.51).

6. Bladder biopsy is the commonest procedure necessary during cystoscopy. Specially-designed biopsy forceps may be introduced down the cystoscope sheath, allowing cup biopsies of any suspicious area to be taken. It is generally wise to diathermy these points following biopsy and a coagulating diathermy cable can also be passed down the instrument channel to achieve this.

7. When the examination is complete, drain the bladder through the cystoscope sheath and remove the cystoscope.

8. Other procedures may be performed if indicated (e.g. optical urethrotomy, diathermy of small bladder tumours, insertion of ureteric stents, retrograde ureterography and Dormia basketry for lower ureteric stones). Ureteric catheterization is aided by use of a 0° telescope and a specially designed director which allows the surgeon to angle the tip of a guidewire.

POSTOPERATIVE CARE

There are no specific measures needed, other than ensuring a high fluid intake by the patient.

SPECIAL OPERATIVE HAZARDS
1. Creation of a false passage. This most commonly occurs in the bulbar urethra where it is possible to advance the tip of the cystoscope posteriorly.
2. Rupture of the bladder following biopsy/cautery.
3. Haemorrhage from biopsy site.

COMPLICATIONS
1. Septicaemia occasionally occurs, especially if a urethrotomy has been performed.
2. Acute urinary retention may occur postoperatively (usually in men with benign prostatic hypertrophy) and may necessitate transurethral prostatectomy.
3. Urethral stricture can complicate urethral instrumentation and most commonly affects the submeatal and membranous regions.

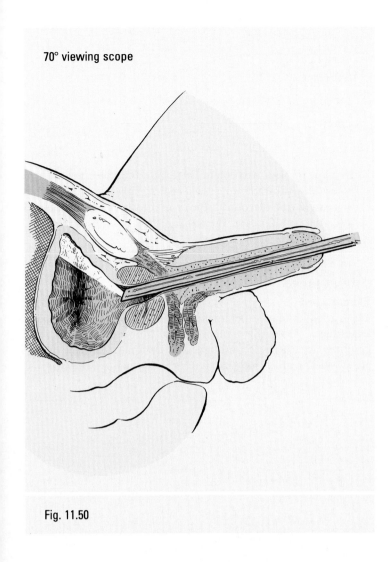

70° viewing scope

Fig. 11.50

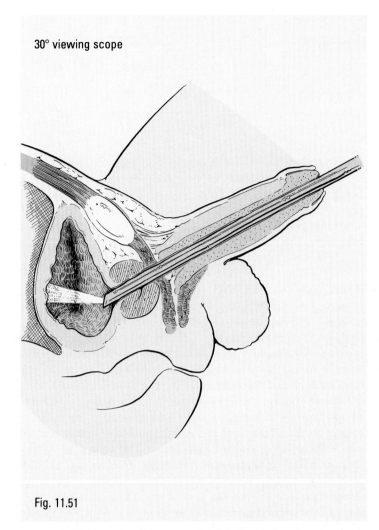

30° viewing scope

Fig. 11.51

Transurethral Prostatectomy

Over the past thirty years, transurethral prostatectomy (TURP) has become the mainstay of treatment for most patients with benign prostatic hypertrophy, superceding open methods of prostatectomy, because of its reduced mortality and morbidity. Technological advances in the fields of optics and diathermy have aided the effectiveness of this operation.

RELEVANT ANATOMY

Benign prostatic hypertrophy arises in the central zone of the prostate, and may lead to a gradual obstruction of the urinary flow. Rectally, the benign prostate feels to have two lateral lobes separated by a midline groove, but when viewed endoscopically there is commonly seen a third (median) lobe lying under the bladder neck and often approaching the ureteric orifices.

Urinary continence depends upon both the proximal sphincter mechanism, where the bladder neck musculature is the most important structure, and the distal sphincter mechanism, of which the striated urethral sphincter is the main component. Transurethral prostatectomy inevitably destroys the bladder neck mechanism, so it is vital that the striated urethral sphincter is not damaged during the procedure. The endoscopic landmark of the striated sphincter is the verumontanum (Fig. 11.52), and accordingly it is essential that resection is not carried distal to this point.

Surrounding the prostatic adenoma is a capsule composed of compressed prostatic tissue, which has a different consistency to the adenoma itself. Beyond this lies a venous plexus, which if damaged by over aggressive resection may result in profuse haemorrhage.

PREOPERATIVE ASSESSMENT

1. Confirm the clinical diagnosis of benign prostatic hypertrophy with urinary flow measurements, and ultrasound to assess the post-voiding residual volume and the prostate itself.
2. Measure serum acid phosphatase in cases suspicious of malignancy. TURP will still relieve the obstructive symptoms due to prostatic malignancy.
3. Correction of electrolyte abnormalities. In long-standing bladder outflow obstruction associated with chronic urinary retention, there may be impaired renal function. This is best dealt with by catheterization and fluid replacement until the renal function has stabilized.
4. Warn patients of the risks of the operation and in particular, the likelihood of retrograde ejaculation.
5. Prophylactic antibiotics are necessary if there is proven urinary infection and where infection is likely (e.g. those patients with an indwelling urinary catheter).
6. If the patient is unable to achieve the lithotomy position, usually due to arthritis of the hips, an open prostatectomy is necessary.

7. In patients with extremely large glands, where the time to resect the prostate would exceed 90 minutes, there is an increased risk of complications related to extravasation of irrigating solution and fluid absorption; open prostatectomy is usually safer.

OPERATION
Preparation

The operation may be performed under either general or spinal anaesthesia. With the patient in the lithotomy position, the genitalia are cleansed and specially designed surgical drapes are applied with a finger stall attached which can be inserted

View through cystoscope

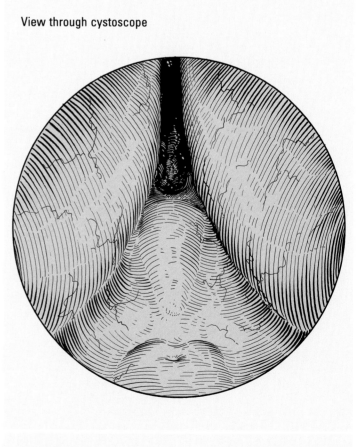

Fig. 11.52

11.30

into the rectum, thus allowing the surgeon to examine the prostate during the operation, in order to assess the amount of residual tissue and also to ease the resection of the apex of the prostate. Preliminary cystoscopy is performed to exclude other causes of bladder outflow obstruction (such as urethral stricture) and to identify coexistent bladder pathology.

Squirt 20 ml 2% lignocaine gel into the urethra. This provides lubrication, some degree of local anaesthesia and also some local antisepsis, since the gel also contains cetrimide.

Operative technique
Many different techniques of transurethral resection of the prostate exist, but the method described here is similar to that popularized by Blandy.

1. The resectoscope is enclosed within an external sheath with an external diameter of either 24 or 27 Fr (the smaller is more commonly used). Irrigation is with a 1.5% solution of glycine or mannitol in water by intermittent filling and emptying of the bladder or continuous irrigation into the bladder with continuous suction to remove the intravesical fluid via two separate channels in the resectoscope sheath. Both cutting and coagulating current should be available. A 30° telescope is used which is connected to a fibreoptic light source.

2. With a succession of sweeping movements of the resectoscope loop resect the bladder neck and the median lobe (if prominent). Carry the resection distally to the verumontanum in the midline. Avoid undermining the bladder neck. The multiple small arteries seen in this region should be coagulated. When resecting the median lobe it is important not to encroach upon the ureteric orifices.

3. Starting at the 10 o'clock position, cut a groove from the bladder neck back to the level of the verumontanum and deepen this groove until the capsular fibres are seen. Because the prostate is round it is important to make curved runs with the resectoscope loop. Resection then proceeds downwards (in an anticlockwise direction) until the floor of the prostatic cavity is reached (Fig. 11.53). Take care not to resect distal to the verumontanum and it is vital to check repeatedly the position of the resectoscope loop relative to this landmark.

4. Resect the other side of the prostate in a similar fashion, although this is often found to be more difficult because contraction of the capsule rotates the verumontanum towards the unresected side. Accordingly it is important to dig deeper into the substance of the prostate with each run of the resectoscope loop. This leaves prostatic tissue remaining only in the roof of the cavity and at the apex of the prostate.

5. Inevitably, blood vessels will be encountered during resection, but most are small and easily diathermied. However, there are usually several larger arteries which pierce the capsule at 10 and 2 o'clock; take care to ensure adequate haemostasis at these points. If accumulating resected chips of prostate interfere with both vision and with the irrigation, remove them with an Ellik evacuator (Fig. 11.54) attached to the end of the resectoscope sheath and perform a bladder washout.

6. Resect prostatic tissue in the roof of the cavity. Here the prostatic tissue is usually thin, and again, care is needed to avoid resecting either distal to the verumontanum or through the capsule.

7. Finally, resect the apical prostatic tissue. It is the tissue closest to the striated urethral sphincter, so the utmost care is needed when resecting in this region. It is often helpful at this stage to insert a finger into the rectum and push up the apical prostatic tissue.

8. Check haemostasis, remove residual prostatic fragments, and insert a catheter (usually an irrigating three-way 22 or 24 Fr). Immediately commence irrigation with normal saline.

POSTOPERATIVE CARE
Continue irrigation for 24–48 hours. It is usually possible to remove the catheter 24 hours later. Patients can eat and drink on the first postoperative day, when it is usual to check the postoperative haemoglobin.

Resection of lateral lobe

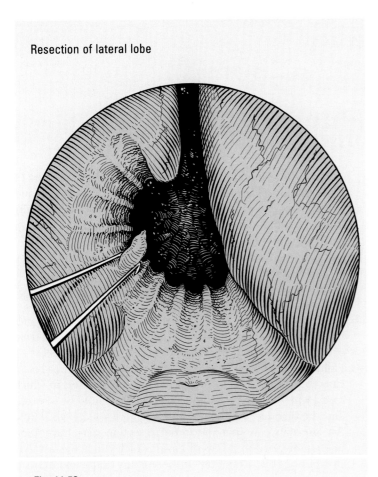

Fig. 11.53

Use of Ellik evacuator

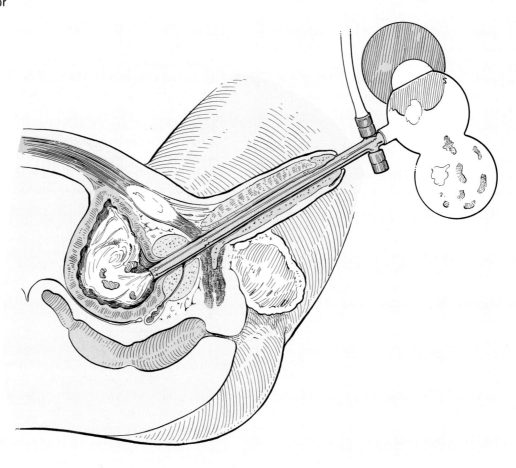

Fig. 11.54

SPECIAL OPERATIVE HAZARDS
1. Damage to the ureteric orifice which may lead to stenosis or reflux.
2. Damage to the urethral sphincter from resecting distal to the verumontanum.
3. Perforation of capsule.
4. Bleeding.

COMPLICATIONS
1. Bleeding is common following TURP but is not usually severe. If significant, it should be treated in the first instance by transfusion and applying traction to the catheter by pulling the catheter balloon down onto the bladder neck and then tying a swab around the catheter at the level of the glans penis to prevent the catheter slipping back. This traction should not be continued for more than 6 hours. If profuse bleeding continues despite this, check and correct clotting. Further cystoscopy may be necessary, with coagulation of any visible bleeding points. Occasionally open exploration with packing of the prostatic fossa may be necessary.

Secondary haemorrhage typically occurs after 10–14 days, usually as a result of infection; it is usually minor and may be treated with oral antibiotics. However, occasionally it may require catheterization with irrigation; and, rarely, cystoscopy and bladder washout is necessary.
2. Confusion and hypotension associated with hyponatraemia, and occasionally with pulmonary oedema due to excessive absorption of hypotonic irrigant fluid. It is usually managed by fluid restriction and diuretics.
3. Septicaemia is rare providing that prophylactic antibiotics have been used appropriately. Take blood cultures and treat with fluid resuscitation and antibiotics.
4. Failure to pass urine may result from retention due to blood clots or prostatic chips retained within the bladder, in which case a wide-bore rigid catheter (22–24 Fr) should be inserted and the bladder washed out and irrigated for 24–48 hours. An alternative is that the initial resection may have been inadequate, or left a flap of tissue which can act as a valve, preventing free urine flow. If there is any doubt about this, a second cystoscopy is necessary, perhaps with a further resection. Finally the bladder may be relatively atonic as a

result of longstanding bladder outflow obstruction. Administration of a cholinergic agent may be of value, but it is often necessary to recatheterize the patient for 4–6 weeks which gives the bladder time to recover some motor function prior to catheter removal. If the patient is unable to pass urine at this stage, then intermittent self-catheterization or an indwelling catheter is necessary.

5. Urinary incontinence, can be treated conservatively in the first instance. If, however, there is persistent incontinence at six months, further investigation is necessary. The two main causes are stress incontinence due to sphincter damage, and detrusor instability. Urodynamic studies are necessary to differentiate these two conditions, so that appropriate treatment can be instituted. For sphincteric incontinence, an artificial sphincter may be needed, while for detrusor instability, anticholinergic drugs are the mainstay of treatment.

6. Retrograde ejaculation is extremely common following a TURP (present in over 80% of cases). Patients must be warned of this danger preoperatively.

7. Urethral stricture will occur in a small proportion of patients (approximately 2–5%) following a TURP. The commonest sites are the submeatal region and the membranous urethra, since these are the sites of maximum leverage and compression by the resectoscope sheath during TURP.

With the advent of transurethral surgery the indications for open prostatectomy in the treatment of benign prostatic hypertrophy are few, but include very large glands in excess of 60–100g, where transurethral surgery would be prolonged with all the attendant risks of extravasation, fluid absorption and haemorrhage. The exact prostatic size which will require open surgery will depend upon the skill and experience of the individual surgeon. In addition, patients unable to be positioned in the lithotomy position (e.g. due to severely stiff hips) and those where benign prostatic hypertrophy is to be treated in association with a large bladder calculus or a large bladder diverticulum may require open prostatectomy.

PREOPERATIVE ASSESSMENT

1. Counsel the patient about the risks of surgery and in particular the likelihood of postoperative retrograde ejaculation.

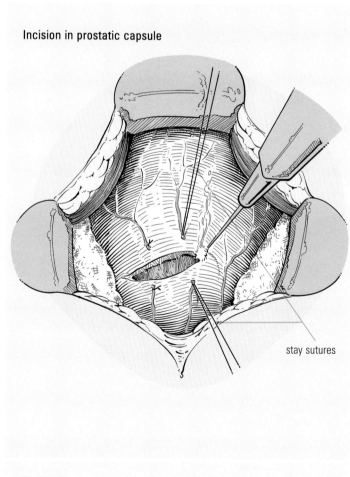

Incision in prostatic capsule

stay sutures

Fig. 11.55

2. Preoperative catheter drainage is necessary in patients with acute or chronic urinary retention. In cases of chronic urinary retention with impaired renal function, surgery should not be undertaken until the serum urea and creatinine are stable.
3. Cross-match two units of blood.
4. Commence prophylactic antibiotics with the premedication. The choice of antibiotic is based on the results of preoperative urine culture and sensitivity, but in the absence of this information gentamicin is usually effective.

RELEVANT ANATOMY

Benign prostatic hypertrophy arises in the central portion of the prostate gland and typically grows to compress the peripheral prostate, which forms the pseudocapsule of the prostate. Open prostatectomy involves the removal of only the central 'adenoma', and there is usually a clear plane of cleavage between it and the false capsule.

OPERATION

The most commonly used technique is that of retropubic prostatectomy which is safer than the older technique of transvesical prostatectomy.

Preparation

Use cystoscopy to exclude the presence of a urethral stricture which may interfere with peroperative catheterization, and to identify any other intravesical pathology (e.g. calculus or a bladder tumour). The patient is then placed supine on the operating table, with a slight head-down tilt, and the skin is prepared from the xiphisternum to the upper thigh, including the external genitalia.

Incision

Make a Pfannenstiel incision (see page 6.53); separate the recti in the midline from the pubis to just below the umbilicus but do not enter the peritoneum.

Operative technique

1. Insert a self-retaining retractor (e.g. Millins) and expose the prostate by careful blunt dissection in the retropubic space. It is helpful to push a small swab down into the space on either side of the prostate gland. Care must be taken to avoid damage to the large veins which lie on the dorsal surface of the gland.

2. Place and tie two stay sutures in the capsule in the midline so that some of the veins which lie over the surface of the prostate are picked up; the proximal suture should be 1–2 cm

Enter the plane between adenoma and false capsule

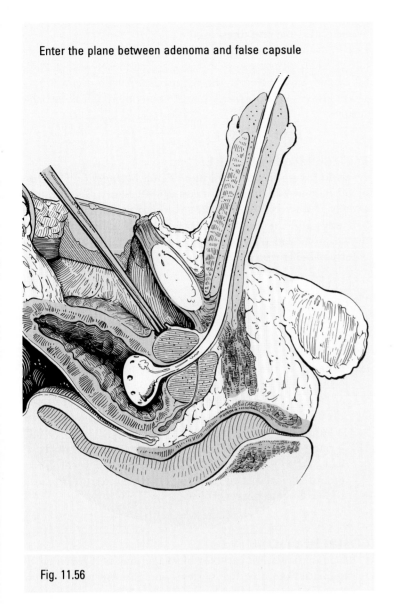

Fig. 11.56

Enucleation of adenoma

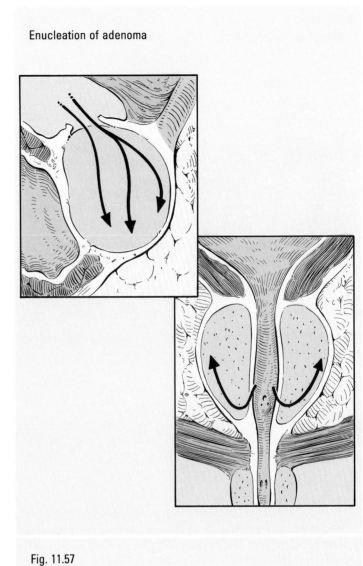

Fig. 11.57

distal to the bladder neck, with the distal suture just below this. Using cutting diathermy, make a transverse incision in the capsule across the full dorsal surface of the gland between the stay sutures (Fig. 11.55). This typically encounters small capsular arteries which should be diathermied, before deepening the incision until the glistening surface of the adenoma is seen. Then use scissors to gently open the plane between the adenoma and the capsule (Fig. 11.56).

3. Insert an index finger through the prostate in the midline until the urethra has been entered. Then after identifying the verumontanum, develop the plane between the capsule and the adenoma. Starting distally, at the apex of the prostate, this plane is then developed laterally down the sides of the gland and then finally posteriorly until the urethra is re-entered (Fig. 11.57). Mobilize each lobe of the prostate in this way, so that only a small connection is left proximally around the bladder neck and the median lobe.

4. Insert a bladder neck spreader into the bladder to expose the trigone and the median lobe and make a wedge-shaped

incision in the bladder mucosa, taking care not to damage the nearby ureteric orifices (Fig. 11.58). Through this incision dissect the median lobe free. By now it should be possible to remove the prostatic adenoma. Although it is occasionally possible to remove the whole adenoma in one piece, it is more usual to remove the two lateral lobes separately.

5. At this stage of the operation there is often profuse haemorrhage and it may be useful to insert a pack into the prostatic fossa to control the bleeding. The main source of this bleeding is arterial and can be secured by placing an absorbable suture (e.g. 2/0 Vicryl) at each extremity of the capsular incision where the main arterial supply to the prostate enters. The needles are left on the sutures.

6. Remove the pack in the prostatic cavity and use diathermy or underrun other large arterial bleeding points with an absorbable suture. If there are ragged edges of bladder mucosa, these may be sutured to the floor of the prostatic cavity with interrupted absorbable sutures (e.g. 2/0 Vicryl).

11.35

Resection of median lobe

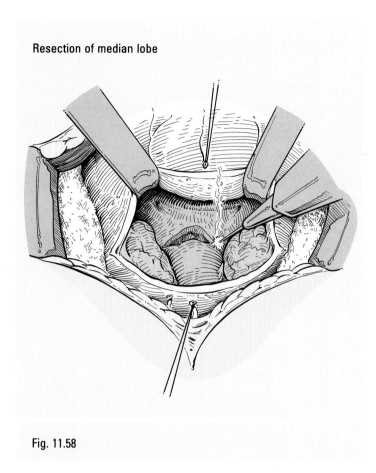

Fig. 11.58

7. Insert a 22 Fr Foley catheter transurethrally into the bladder, and then pass a nylon stitch through one of the eyes of the catheter, through the bladder and the abdominal wall to the outside. This stitch is left long and at the end of the operation is secured to the abdominal wall using a button. Occasionally it is necessary to change the urethral catheter postoperatively and the nylon stitch allows a new catheter to be railroaded into the bladder. Also insert a 22 Fr suprapubic catheter through the abdominal wall into the bladder.

8. Use the stitches at the lateral corners of the capsular incision to reconstitute the prostatic capsule with two continuous running sutures which meet each other in the midline. Ensure that this closure is watertight to prevent extravasation of urine and irrigating fluid.

9. At this point it is useful to inflate the urethral catheter balloon and gently pull it down into the prostatic cavity, before commencing irrigation with saline. This is most easily achieved by infusing through the suprapubic catheter and collecting the irrigation fluid through the urethral catheter. Should there be any difficulty in drainage a bladder wash-out may be performed.

Wound closure and dressing

Leave a tube drain in the retropubic space, remove the swabs lateral to the prostate and oppose the recti loosely with a single 00 catgut suture. Repair the rectus sheath with a continuous nylon suture and close the skin with interrupted non-absorbable sutures.

POSTOPERATIVE CARE

Irrigation is continued until the irrigant becomes only slightly bloodstained. This typically takes 36–48 hours. The drain is usually removed after 48 hours, the suprapubic catheter after 3–4 days and the urethral catheter 24–48 hours later. Early mobilization and physiotherapy is especially important in the elderly patients who typically undergo this operation.

SPECIAL OPERATIVE HAZARDS

1. Haemorrhage is the major operative hazard which can be profuse. However the access given by this approach usually permits adequate control of any bleeding.

2. Damage to the external striated urethral sphincter may occur while mobilizing the distal part of the prostatic adenoma. It is minimized by commencing with an intra-urethral dissection after first identifying the verumontanum.

3. Ureteric damage may occur while removing the median lobe. To avoid this the ureteric orifices should be carefully identified and if at risk, the insertion of ureteric catheters should help to prevent injury.

COMPLICATIONS

1. Haemorrhage and catheter blockage may be prevented by adequate operative haemostasis and the use of irrigation. However, on occasions bladder wash-outs are necessary, and rarely it may be necessary to re-explore the patient to control the bleeding. Adequate replacement of blood volume is of course necessary. Some degree of secondary haemorrhage is common, usually 10–14 days postoperatively. Only occasionally does severe bleeding with clot retention occur and this should be treated by catheterization, transfusion if necessary, and antibiotics.

2. Urinary fistula can occur but should be avoided by removing the suprapubic catheter before the urethral catheter.

3. Urinary incontinence may develop due to detrusor instability or to sphincter damage. Initial management is conservative since most cases resolve spontaneously.

4. Retrograde ejaculation resulting from damage of the normal bladder neck sphincter is to be expected.

5. Bladder neck stenosis occurs in about 5% of cases.

6. Regrowth of the prostate following inadequate prostatectomy.

Open Cystostomy

In recent years the development of commercially available types of percutaneous suprapubic catheter has made the need for open cystostomy for urinary drainage less common. However, there are situations where percutaneous insertion of a suprapubic catheter is contra-indicated, and in these situations open cystostomy is necessary. It is sometimes necessary to perform an open cystostomy in order to perform some other urological procedure such as the removal of a large bladder stone.

PREOPERATIVE ASSESSMENT

1. Are there contra-indications to percutaneous suprapubic catheterization in cases requiring suprapubic urinary drainage, such as a previous midline incision to which bowel loops may be adherent, or a non-palpable bladder (e.g. following pelvic fractures and urethral injury)?
2. In cases with pelvic trauma, ensure adequate resuscitation and exclude other injuries.
3. Prescribe prophylactic antibiotics.

RELEVANT ANATOMY

The distended bladder rises out of the pelvis to become palpable suprapubically. As it does so, a fold of peritoneum is carried with it so that no part of the peritoneal cavity interposes between the most anterior part of the dome of the bladder and the abdominal wall. The reflection of peritoneum is highest in the midline at the attachment of the median umbilical ligament. It is important to site the cystostomy in this part of the bladder, rather than have the catheter traverse the peritoneal cavity; this ensures that on catheter removal leakage of urine into the peritoneal cavity is avoided (Fig. 11.59).

OPERATION
Preparation

The anaesthetized patient is placed supine with slight head-down tilt. The skin is prepared from the xiphisternum to the upper thighs and towels are placed to square off the lower abdomen and to cover the external genitalia.

Relevant anatomy

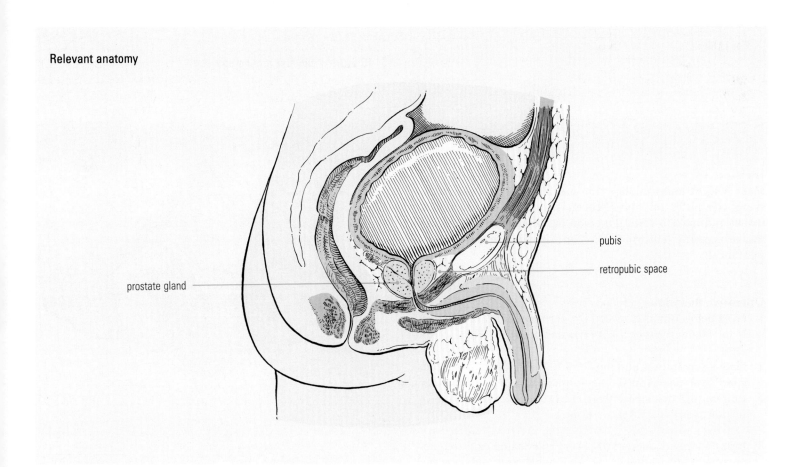

prostate gland

pubis

retropubic space

Fig. 11.59

Exposure of the bladder

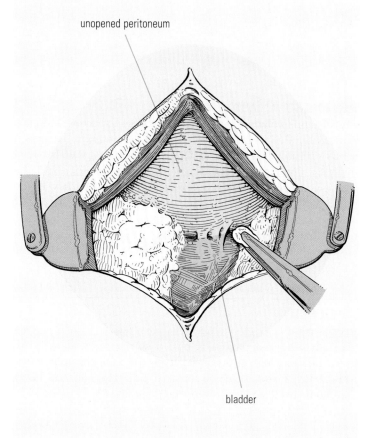

unopened peritoneum

bladder

Fig. 11.60

Opening the bladder

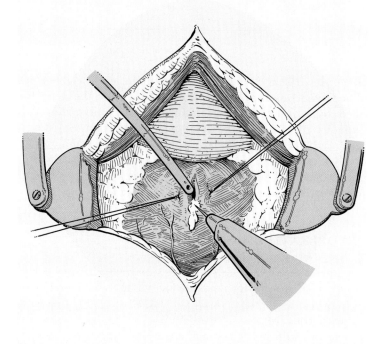

Fig. 11.61

Closure of bladder around catheter

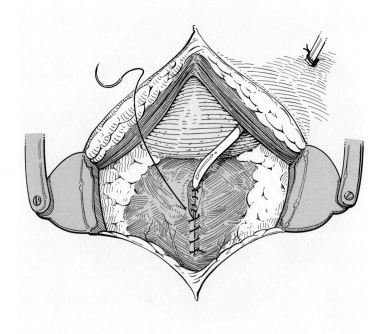

Fig. 11.62

Incision

Make a short lower midline skin incision from just above the symphysis pubis for about 10cm. Divide the subcutaneous tissues and make a vertical incision in the linea alba. Separate the recti gently, ensuring that the dissection remains extra-peritoneal.

Operative technique

1. From below upwards, sweep the peritoneum off the surface of the bladder. Insert a self-retaining retractor (Fig. 11.60).

2. Place 2 stay sutures into the dome of the bladder, about 2cm apart, and make a small longitudinal incision in the bladder with cutting diathermy (Fig. 11.61). It is advisable to have suction available to aspirate urine.

3. Insert a large diameter (20–24Fr) Foley catheter through a separate stab wound in the abdominal wall and into the bladder, and inflate the balloon. Close the vesical incision in two layers with a continuous absorbable suture (e.g. 2/0 Vicryl) to leave the catheter sitting snugly at the upper end

of the wound (Fig. 11.62); the first layer consists of full thickness stitches, and the second layer catches only the outer layers of the bladder, so as to invert the deeper layer.

Wound closure and dressing
Leave a tube drain in the retropubic space and then close the linea alba with a continuous 00 nylon mass closure and the skin with interrupted nylon. Cover the wound with a dry dressing. Secure the suprapubic catheter and the drain to the skin with single silk stitches.

POSTOPERATIVE CARE
The post-operative management depends upon the indications for the cystostomy. In general the drain can be removed after 24–48 hours and the sutures after 8–10 days.

SPECIAL OPERATIVE HAZARDS
1. Entry into the peritoneal cavity. It is important to ensure that the catheter remains extraperitoneal.
2. Bleeding is occasionally troublesome and usually arises from the venous plexus on the surface of the prostate and the bladder. In cases associated with pelvic trauma, there may be severe distortion of the normal anatomy and care is needed to minimize the dissection and thus avoid excessive bleeding.

COMPLICATIONS
Although some urinary leakage is common following catheter removal, the formation of a persistent suprapubic urinary fistula is uncommon. It is best treated by transurethral bladder drainage but if this is impossible re-exploration is necessary to close the defect in the bladder.

Cystectomy and Urinary Diversion

Invasive carcinoma of the bladder is treated initially with radiotherapy. Cystectomy is performed as a salvage procedure for recurrent tumour or for severe symptoms due to a fibrotic shrunken bladder following radiotherapy or intractable haemorrhage. Urinary diversion alone is indicated for a neurogenic bladder or bladder incompetence (with loss of continence or failure of the bladder neck mechanism to relax during voiding).

PREOPERATIVE ASSESSMENT

1. Use an intravenous urogram, cystoscopy with bladder biopsy and bimanual examination, chest X-ray, bone scan and CT scan to assess patients with malignant disease.
2. A stoma nurse should explain the nature of a urinary stoma to the patient.
3. Sympathetically discuss the loss of male potency which will occur after the operation.

Division of ureters

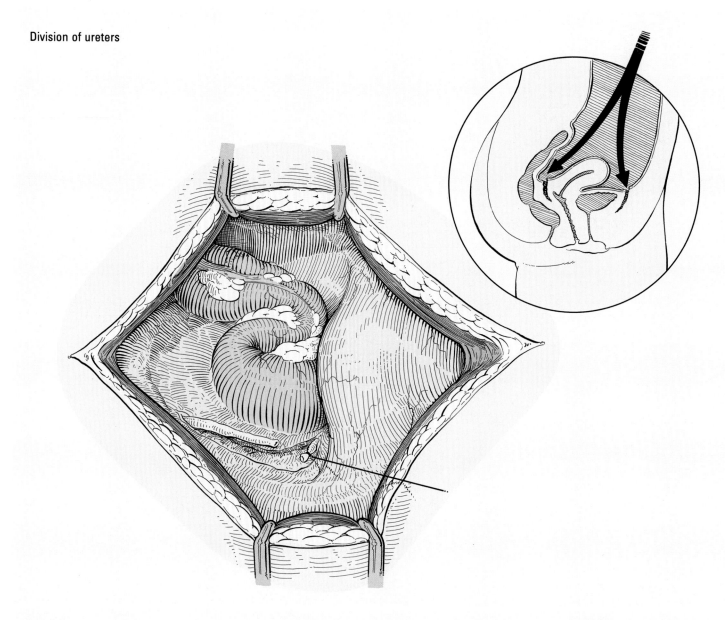

Fig. 11.63

11.40

4. Prepare the bowel and mark a suitable site for the stoma in the right iliac fossa.

RELEVANT ANATOMY

The fundus of the bladder is covered by peritoneum and lies behind the body of the pubic bones. The bladder is separated from the pubic bones by the retropubic space (or cave of Retzius), containing loose areolar tissue. The base of the bladder is separated from the rectum in the male by the vas, seminal vesicles and the fascia of Denonvilliers, and by the uterus in the female.

The blood supply of the bladder is from the superior and inferior vesical arteries, the obturator and pubic branches of the inferior epigastric artery. The lymphatic drainage follows the arteries and is mostly alongside the internal iliac artery and to nodes alongside the obturator vessels. The vesical veins drain into the vesical plexus which lies at the base of the bladder. This plexus communicates with the prostatic plexus and middle rectal veins in the male and drains into the internal iliac veins. The plexus drains across the floor of the broad ligament to the internal iliac veins in the female.

OPERATION
Preparation

The patient is placed supine with a Trendelenberg tilt and is catheterized. A nasogastric tube is passed and, in women, the vagina is swabbed with a sponge soaked in iodine (e.g. Betadine). The abdomen is cleansed and draped, leaving the stoma site exposed.

Incision

Make a lower midline incision (see the Introduction).

Operative technique

1. Perform a full laparotomy (see page 5.2) in cases of bladder tumours to exclude intra-abdominal metastases, particularly to the iliac and obturator lymph nodes. If there is gross local invasion or distant spread, the cystectomy is not generally appropriate.

2. Insert a self-retaining retractor and pack the small bowel into the upper part of the abdomen.

3. Mobilize the sigmoid colon. Identify the distal end of each ureter and divide the overlying peritoneum. Mobilize the ureters upward from this level taking care not to damage the blood supply by stripping their adventitia.

4. Divide the ureters close to the bladder (Fig. 11.63) and check the proximal ends to ensure that they are healthy, bleeding and free of tumour. Ligate the distal ends of the ureter and tuck the proximal ends safely away; these are returned to later.

5. The cystectomy is performed next; this involves both opening the retropubic and retrovesical (male) or retro-uterine (female) spaces (see inset to Fig. 11.63) by incising the overlying peritoneum, as the first step.

Division of vesical pedicles

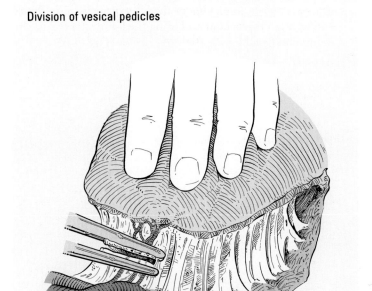

Fig. 11.64

6. In males, ligate and divide the vas deferens on each side and dissect the bladder from the rectum posteriorly. In females, ligate and divide the ovarian and uterine vessels and the round ligaments (see page 6.59). Transect the vagina, below the fornix, and close the distal end with a continuous, haemostatic, absorbable suture.

7. The bladder is now attached by the urethra inferiorly and vesical vessels laterally. Starting at the bifurcation of the common iliac artery and vein, dissect the fatty tissue including the iliac and obturator lymph nodes free from the pelvic side wall and ligate and divide the vesical vessels encountered close to their origins from the internal iliac vessels until the lateral sides of the bladder are completely free (Fig. 11.64).

8. Clamp a Roberts' forceps across the urethra distal to the prostate in males and the bladder neck in females, and divide the urethra (including the Foley catheter). Remove the specimen and remaining catheter. The surgical specimen should consist of the bladder, ureteral stumps and the iliac and obturator lymph nodes in both sexes. In males it also includes the prostate and seminal vesicles, while in females the uterus, ovaries, fallopian tubes and a cuff of vagina are also attached.

9. Insert a 24 Fr Foley catheter into the urethra, inflate the balloon with 30 ml water, and place on traction. Insert a warm pack into the pelvis to control bleeding whilst the ileal conduit is constructed.

10. The ileal conduit is performed as follows: using a Roberts' forceps, create a tunnel under the inferior mesenteric vessels and sigmoid mesocolon and bring the left ureter across the midline to lie alongside the right ureter (Fig. 11.65).

11. Isolate and mobilize a loop of ileum 20cm in length and approximately 50cm from the ileocaecal valve on its vascular pedicle (the vessels can be seen clearly in the mesentery by having a lamp shining from behind) (Fig. 11.66). Divide

Ureter tunnelled under peritoneum

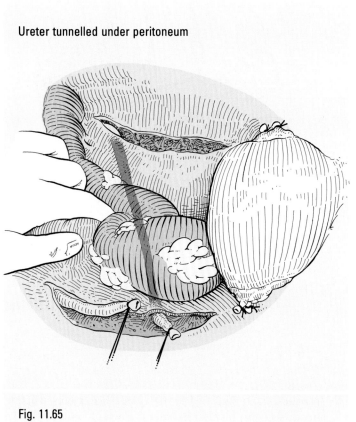

Fig. 11.65

Creation of a single orifice

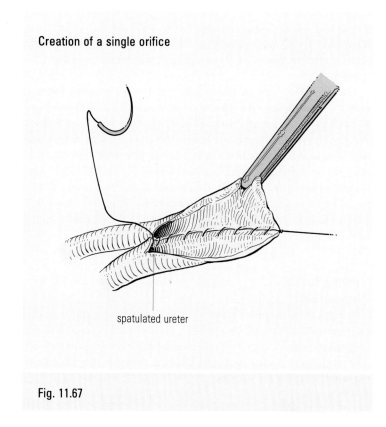

spatulated ureter

Fig. 11.67

Mobilized loop of ileum

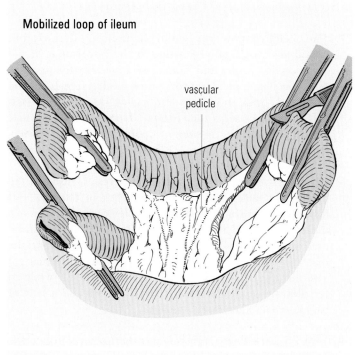

vascular pedicle

Uretero-ileal anastomosis

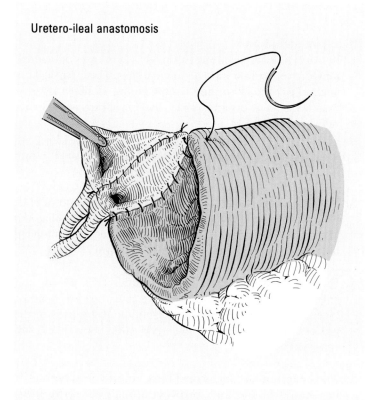

Fig. 11.66

Fig. 11.68

Completed conduit

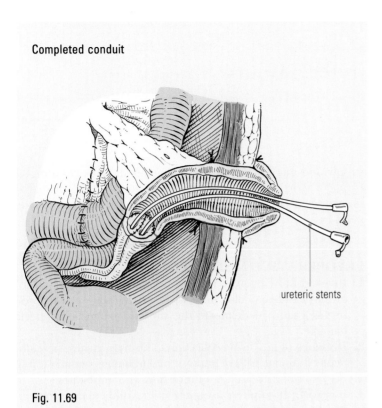

ureteric stents

Fig. 11.69

the bowel between clamps. Restore the continuity of the bowel with an end-to-end anastomosis (see the Introduction).

12. Spatulate the ends of the ureters, suture them together along one edge to create a common orifice (Fig. 11.67) which is then anastomosed to the proximal end of the ileal loop with a single layer of continuous Vicryl or catgut (Fig. 11.68). Ureteric catheters are inserted into each ureter before the anastomosis is completed and the other ends passed out through the ileal conduit (Fig. 11.69). Secure the catheters to the inside of the loop with a 4/0 catgut suture.

13. Secure the ileal loop by passing several interrupted sutures through the serosa of the bowel and the peritoneum of the posterior abdominal wall.

14. Bring the distal end of the ileal loop through the abdominal wall at the preselected site and fashion a spout as for an ileostomy (see page 5.69).

15. If a urethrectomy is to be performed, in males this involves mobilization of the bulbar urethra via a perineal incision. Dissect the rest of the urethra and excise it as the penis invaginates with traction. In females, excise the urethra with a strip of vagina via two vertical parallel incisions in the anterior vaginal wall.

16. Remove the pack from the pelvis and ensure haemostasis is complete. Leave the Foley catheter in place to control venous oozing and insert a silicone drain.

Wound closure and dressing
Close the wound with loop nylon and interrupted skin sutures. Apply a dry dressing to the wound, and a urostomy bag to the conduit.

POSTOPERATIVE CARE
Remove the silicone drains when there is minimal drainage, the Foley catheter after 48 hours, and the nasogastric tube when bowel function returns and oral fluids are tolerated. Antibiotics are continued for 48 hours. The ureteric catheters should be gently pulled each day from the 10th day until they come out.

SPECIAL OPERATIVE HAZARDS
1. Rectal damage whilst dissecting the bladder off the anterior wall of the rectum especially after irradiation to the pelvis.
2. Bleeding. Usually this is a venous ooze and responds to packing.
3. Ureteric ischaemia due to tension or adventitial stripping.

COMPLICATIONS
1. Prolonged ileus is common after this operation.
2. Urinary leak from, or stenosis of, the uretero-ileal anastomosis.
3. Pelvic abscess formation. This usually follows pelvic haematoma.
4. Retraction, stenosis, or infarction of the ileal conduit. These are usually due to tension.
5. Problems relating to the bowel anastomosis, such as stricture or leakage with fistula or abscess formation. These are not uncommon since the bowel has frequently been irradiated.
6. Transitional carcinoma occurring in the renal pelvis or ureter.
7. Urinary sepsis and calculi.
8. Psychological stigmata of a urinary stoma and impotence.

Management of Ureteric Injury

Ureteric damage is uncommon, but when it occurs, it may lead to obstruction and progressive renal damage, urinary fistula and urinoma formation.

The commonest cause of ureteric injury is peroperative damage during endoscopic manipulation of the ureter (e.g. ureteroscopy) but damage may also result from open pelvic surgery, such as radical hysterectomy, aorto-iliac surgery or resection of the rectum. The injury may be noticed at the time of operation, in which case immediate repair is usually possible, or it may become apparent in the postoperative period.

Injudicious placement of an artery clip or a ligature may stenose the ureter, and result in hydronephrosis, which may be silent or may be accompanied by loin pain or a swinging fever. Ischaemic damage due to excessive stripping of the ureteric blood supply may result in similar problems or may result in urinary leakage and fistula formation. Ureteric damage most typically presents 5–10 days postoperatively.

If the ureteric damage is localized and there is little or no devascularization, then it is usually feasible to anastomose the ends of the ureter directly. However, should the damage be more extensive and accompanied by significant devascularization then alternative manoeuvres may be necessary.

Injuries to the lower third of the ureter are probably best treated by ureteric reimplantation (see below) with a psoas hitch and/or a Boari flap. Occasionally the ureter is damaged by external trauma (usually a penetrating injury), when the principles of management are similar.

If the ureter is damaged during ureteroscopy, the operation should be terminated, a urethral catheter inserted and antibiotics commenced. If the patient develops loin pain or a fever, perform an ultrasound to look for hydronephrosis or a urinoma. If present, insert a percutaneous nephrostomy which can be removed after 7–10 days if a nephrostogram shows that the ureter has healed.

RELEVANT ANATOMY

The ureter descends from the kidney on the psoas muscle (where it may be at risk during aortic aneurysm surgery) to pass over the sacro-iliac joint and enter the pelvis. It passes over the bifurcation of the common iliac artery and round the side wall of the pelvis to enter the bladder posteriorly. At this point it lies anterior to the rectum, and may be damaged during rectal surgery. In women its course is posterior to the uterine arteries, where it may be damaged at hysterectomy.

The ureter is normally narrowed at the pelvi-ureteric junction, at the point where it passes over the pelvic brim and at the vesico-ureteric junction. These points are where ureteric calculi most commonly lodge and are also the commonest sites of endoscopic ureteric damage.

The ureter receives a rich blood supply from many sources (including the renal, gonadal, iliac and vesical arteries). However, excessive mobilization of the ureter may compromise this supply and increase the risk of ischaemic damage resulting in fistula or stricture. In general the blood supply arises medial to the ureter above the pelvic brim and lateral to it within the pelvis.

PREOPERATIVE ASSESSMENT

1. Investigation involves ultrasound and intravenous pyelography, and may also necessitate retrograde or antegrade ureterograms to delineate the site and extent of ureteric damage.
2. Drainage of any urine collection. This may involve percutaneous drainage with or without percutaneous nephrostomy.
3. Prevention or treatment of infection with antibiotics.
4. It is worth attempting an endoscopic solution to the problem, which may involve either retrograde or antegrade insertion of a double-J stent. Under antibiotic cover and with X-ray support a joint approach from above and below is often helpful. If this approach fails (as occasionally happens), then under the same anaesthetic it is possible to proceed to an open operation.

OPERATIONS

If the ureter is divided and the injury recognized at the time of surgery, it can be dealt with by primary repair.

DIRECT ANASTOMOSIS OF URETER

1. A double-J stent is inserted into the divided ureter so that one end of the stent lies within the bladder and the other end lies within the renal pelvis. If there is any doubt as to the position of the stent, then an on-table X-ray may be used to confirm this.

2. The ends of the ureter are spatulated and anastomosed with 4–6 interrupted 4/0 Vicryl sutures. The anastomosis should be drained externally with a tube drain and a bladder catheter is also necessary.

URETERIC REIMPLANTATION

1. The ureter is mobilized above the site of the injury, taking care not to further compromise the blood supply. A fine stay suture (4/0 chromic catgut) may be used to mark the end of the ureter. The patency of the upper ureter should be checked by passing up a 6Fr ureteric catheter. The lower portion of the damaged ureter is then dissected down to the bladder wall, where it is transfixed with a heavy suture.

2. The bladder is opened between stay sutures. It is often helpful to open the bladder obliquely, so that if it is closed in a 'pyloroplasty' fashion, the bladder is 'funnelled' up towards

the damaged ureter (Fig. 11.70). At this point a decision must be made as to where the ureter is to be reimplanted. Ideally a submucosal tunnel should be formed across the trigone of the bladder, but in cases of ureteric damage, loss of ureteric length may make this impossible, and it is usually necessary to bring the ureter through somewhere above the original ureteric orifice.

Occasionally there is insufficient ureteric length even for this, and in these cases the bladder may be 'hitched' up extraperitoneally on to the psoas muscle using one or two 00 Vicryl sutures (Fig. 11.71).

3. An artery forceps is pushed through the bladder from within at a point 4–5 cm above the original ureteric orifice. Grasping the tie on the end of the ureter, the ureter is pulled through into the bladder. It is important that this hole is large enough to take the ureter without constricting it.

4. A site 2–3 cm above the undamaged ureteric orifice is chosen as the site for the new orifice, and a small disk of mucosa is excised at this point.

5. Perform a careful submucosal dissection with sharp pointed scissors which are opened progressively along the line of the proposed tunnel until the neocystostomy is reached. Care is taken to ensure that the tunnel only has a mucosal covering and that it is of adequate width to allow the ureter to slide freely within it.

6. An artery forceps is pushed through the tunnel from the site of the new ureteric orifice and by grasping the marking suture the ureter is pulled through the tunnel (Fig. 11.72). The end of the ureter is then sutured to the margins of the new orifice with 4–8 interrupted 4/0 Vicryl sutures. The same material is used to close the mucosa over the neocysto-

'Psoas hitch'

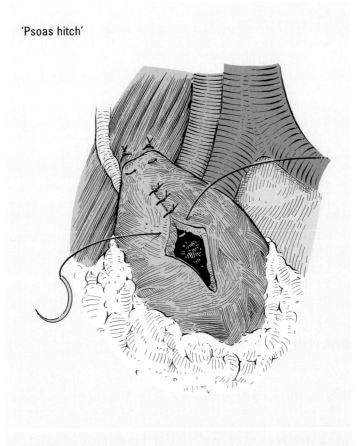

Fig. 11.71

Leadbetter-Politano type reimplantation

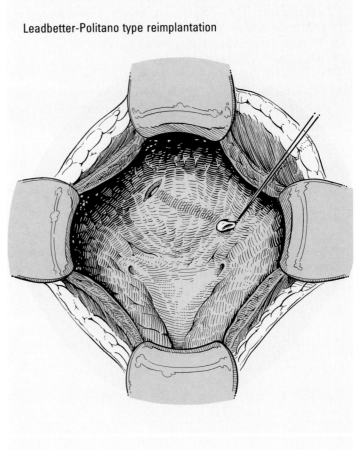

Oblique vesicostomy

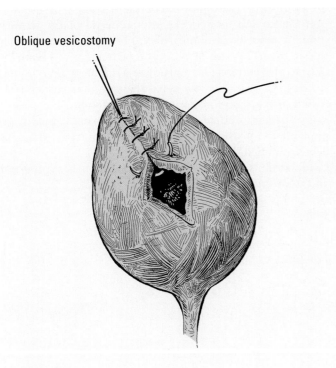

Fig. 11.70

Fig. 11.72

11.45

stomy in the bladder wall. If the end of the ureter is markedly oedematous then a 6 Fr ureteric catheter should be inserted into the ureter and brought out to the skin through the bladder and abdominal wall.

7. The bladder is closed in two layers around a suprapubic catheter (see page 11.38) and a drain is left to the retropubic space.

OTHER PROCEDURES

Injuries to the middle third of the ureter may be amenable to reimplantation with a psoas hitch and/or a Boari flap, but in some cases a transuretero-ureterostomy is necessary.

Injuries to the upper third of the ureter may need autotransplantation of the kidney onto the iliac vessels, or interposition of a section of small intestine between the damaged ends of the ureter. In some cases, however, nephrectomy is a more appropriate solution.

POSTOPERATIVE CARE

The drain can be removed after 48 hours if the drainage has ceased. The urethral catheter should remain for at least 5 days. If used for a reimplantation, a ureteric catheter is removed after 5 days following a ureterogram. If a double-J stent has been used to splint a ureteric repair this can be removed cystoscopically after 6 weeks following an intravenous urogram.

SPECIAL OPERATIVE HAZARDS
1. In some cases of attempted reimplantation a psoas hitch will not suffice to bring the bladder to the ureter and in such cases a Boari flap is necessary (Fig. 11.73).
2. Twisting of ureter in reimplantation tunnel.
3. Repairing ureter under tension.
4. Devascularization of the ureter during mobilization.
5. Long segment damaged. If following mobilization the ureter cannot be repaired without tension consider an alternative treatment.

COMPLICATIONS
1. Persistent urinary leakage is common with direct repairs to the ureter, but providing a stent is *in situ*, and there is an external drain down to the anastomosis, then an expectant policy may be followed and the patient comes to little harm.
2. Ureteric stricture may be a late complication, with ischaemic damage to the ureter, or due to undue narrowing of the

Boari flap

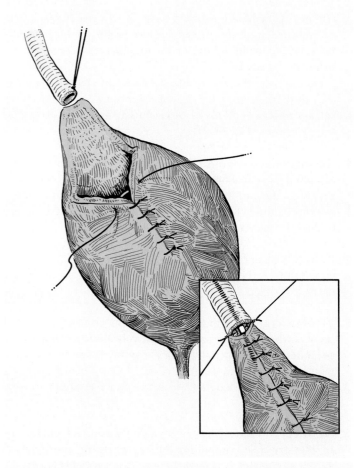

Fig. 11.73

ureter during anastomosis. For this reason it is usual to perform an IVP 6–8 weeks after removal of the ureteric stent. If there is an abnormality, obstruction may be confirmed by a DTPA (or MAG 3) isotope renogram. Treatment may involve endoscopic insertion of a double-J stent or open surgery. Occasionally the renal damage that ensues from such a stricture may necessitate nephrectomy.
3. Vesico-ureteric reflux is a rare complication of ureteric reimplantation provided that an adequate mucosal tunnel has been fashioned.
4. Complications from an indwelling stent such as infection and stone encrustation.

Percutaneous Surgery for Renal Calculi

Even with the advent of extracorporal shock wave lithotripsy (ESWL), percutaneous nephrolithotomy (PCNL) is still useful for the treatment of larger calculi and especially for the removal of staghorn calculi as a preliminary debulking procedure prior to ESWL. This technique allows stone removal through a small incision, with few complications and with a shorter hospital stay than is necessary following conventional open surgery.

RELEVANT ANATOMY
The anatomy of the kidney is discussed on page 11.49.

PREOPERATIVE ASSESSMENT
1. Check the clotting status of the patient since a bleeding diathesis is one of the few contraindications to PCNL.
2. Group and save serum.
3. Administer prophylactic antibiotics.
4. Determine which is the most appropriate calcyx to be punctured in order to gain direct access to the calculus. An intravenous pyelogram (IVP) is essential.
5. A preoperative X-ray is necessary to check the position of the stone.

OPERATION
Preparation
Anaesthetize and examine the patient with a cystoscope.

Operative technique
1. Cystoscopically insert a 6 Fr catheter into the ipselateral ureteric orifice. Catheterize the patient with a 14 Fr Foley catheter and tape the two catheters together, and secure to the patient. Turn the patient over into the prone position, with a foam wedge under the affected loin: this will improve access to the kidney.

2. Inject via the ureteric catheter a solution of urografin and methylene blue in saline (usually 500 ml normal saline with 10 ml methylene blue and 50 ml 30% urografin) so that the pelvicalyceal system may be visualized under image intensification. Initially 30–50 ml is sufficient but regularly top up throughout the procedure.

3. Choose the most appropriate route to the kidney. Under image intensifier control, choose a point in the area bounded by the erector spinae, the twelfth rib and the iliac crest, which gives the best access to the target calcyx (Fig. 11.74). Enter laterally so that the track passes through renal substance (which will tamponade any bleeding), rather than medially where the renal pelvis might well be punctured. It is usual to gain access below the twelfth rib, but occasionally

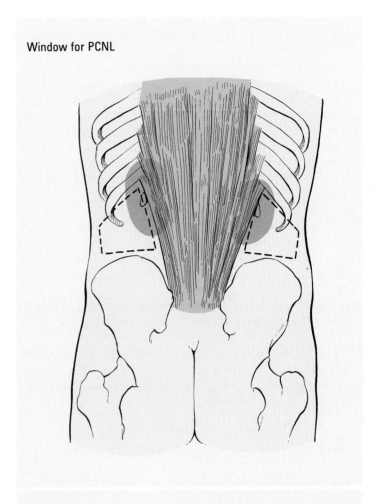

Window for PCNL

Fig. 11.74

puncture above the twelfth rib is necessary to gain appropriate access. Inevitably, the risk of pneumothorax is greater in these cases.

4. Make a 1–2 cm skin incision and introduce a narrow gauge skinny needle under X-ray control into the tip of the target calcyx. If this is difficult, slight rolling of the patient will demonstrate whether the needle is either too superficial or too deep. Moreover, if the collecting system has been punctured, blue stained contrast solution may be gently aspirated confirming a direct hit.

5. Use the skinny needle to assess the direction and the depth of the kidney prior to insertion of the more substantial needle which has an outer plastic sheath, through which a guidewire may be introduced.

11.47

6. Insert the larger needle alongside the skinny needle until the collecting system is punctured, and then withdraw the metal inner portion and advance the outer plastic cannula slightly into the collecting system. Blue contrast solution should flow freely from the kidney.

7. After removal of the skinny needle introduce a guidewire down the plastic cannula into the kidney. While rigid for most of its length, the terminal 5–10 cm should be floppy, allowing the guidewire to curl inside the collecting system.

8. Remove the plastic cannula and introduce a series of graduated dilators over the guidewire to dilate the track into the kidney. To overcome any resistance while dilating through the lumbar fascia, gently twist the dilator. Do not let the guidewire come out of the collecting system and ensure the dilators are not advanced too far, as puncturing the opposite side of the collecting system may occur. Increase the size of the dilator in 4 Fr intervals until a track diameter of 26–30 Fr is produced.

9. Over the largest dilator, advance a plastic tube (Amplatz sheath) and remove the dilator. With the guidewire still *in situ*, this produces a 28 or 30 Fr conduit into the collecting system of the kidney.

10. Insert a nephroscope while continuously irrigating with normal saline. Remove any blood clots with forceps.

11. Negotiate the collecting system until the stone is visualized. Intermittent squirting of blue contrast up the ureteric catheter and/or X-ray screening will help to identify the pelvic–ureteric junction.

12. Upon visualization of the stone, if it is small enough to fit through the Amplatz sheath remove it intact with stone grabbing forceps (Fig. 11.75) which are introduced through the instrument channel.

13. If the stone is large it must be disintegrated *in situ* by either ultrasonic or electrohydraulic lithotripsy. Ultrasonic lithotripsy produces a fine dust which is collected by suction while large fragments are removed piecemeal with stone grabbing forceps; it is more commonly used as there is less risk to the pelvis and calcyx unless the stone is extremely hard. This portion of the operation should not normally exceed 2 hours duration so as to avoid excessive extravasation of irrigant solution.

14. When all fragments have been removed check the pelvicalyceal system for any residual stone, and then remove the nephroscope.

15. Through the Amplatz sheath insert a wide bore (24 Fr) nephrostomy tube, remove the sheath and the guidewire and secure the nephrostomy tube to the skin. Finally, remove the ureteric catheter.

POSTOPERATIVE CARE

A postoperative X-ray will confirm complete stone removal and the nephrostomy tube may be clamped after 48 hours or when significant bleeding has ceased. If there is no pain or fever the tube may be removed 24 hours later.

The urethral catheter can usually be removed after 24 hours.

SPECIAL OPERATIVE HAZARDS
1. Failure to enter correct calyx.
2. Inability to remove or fragment a calculus.
3. Bleeding from the track. If significant haemorrhage occurs terminate the procedure and insert a nephrostomy tube.
4. Perforation of collecting system.

COMPLICATIONS
1. Reactionary haemorrhage. Postoperative bleeding through the nephrostomy tube is rarely profuse. Clamp the tube and commence blood transfusion. For severe continued bleeding, consider embolization or open exploration.
2. Paralytic ileus. Some degree of ileus is common though short-lived following PCNL. If there is marked extravasation of irrigant during the operation, the ileus may persist for 48–72 hours. Intravenous fluids are necessary, occasionally with a nasogastric tube.
3. Sepsis.
4. Retained stones. It is not usually possible to remove the whole of a staghorn calculus at the first operation. Insert a nephrostomy tube and deal with any residual fragments at a second operation, one week later. Alternatively, if the fragments are small, ESWL may be of value.

Removal of stone

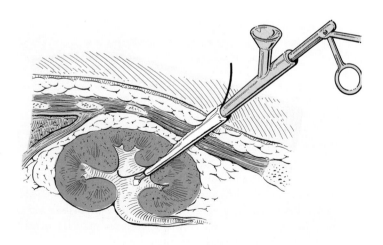

Fig. 11.75

Open Surgery for Urinary Calculi

Percutaneous stone surgery, upper tract endoscopy and extra-corporeal lithotripsy, have markedly reduced the indications for open stone removal, which can be summarized as the failure of the above mentioned techniques and the need for surgical correction of an underlying abnormality of the urinary tract (e.g. pelvi-ureteric junction obstruction, ureteric stenosis).

PREOPERATIVE ASSESSMENT
1. The function of each kidney must be assessed. An IVU is sufficient in most circumstances; a renogram will quantify differential function and confirm obstruction.
2. The position of the stone must be documented with a recent IVU (or ureterogram) and is confirmed with a plain film in the operating theatre.
3. Antibiotic prophylaxis should be used, and treatment continued postoperatively in cases of infective stones.
4. The patient must be positioned on a radiolucent operating table, and X-ray facilities must be available.
5. Perform metabolic studies in an attempt to define the cause of stone formation in recurrent stone formers.
6. Consider nephrostomy drainage and antibiotics as the initial treatment in cases of pyonephrosis with obstruction.

RELEVANT ANATOMY
The renal pelvis lies posterior to the vascular pedicle. A posterior branch of the renal artery runs from the upper pelvis down in close relation to the renal sinus. Lower polar vessels may run on either side of the PUJ. A relatively avascular plane (of Gil Vernet) can be found between the adventitial and muscular layers of the pelvis, in the renal sinus and up to the necks of the calices.

The upper ureter courses in the retroperitoneum on a fat plane on the psoas muscle. It is crossed anteriorly by the gonadal vessels which run almost parallel to it. The ureter has the specific property of showing peristalsis when gently touched with a pair of forceps (vermiculation) and this assists with its identification. Upon entering the pelvis the ureter passes over the bifurcation of the common iliac artery. It continues on the lateral wall of the pelvis, on the inside of the superior vesical pedicle. As it approaches the trigone of the bladder it crosses below the vas deferens in the male and uterine vessels in the female.

The segmental vessels in the kidney run in a radial pattern, and a nephrotomy along this line is the least damaging. A watershed plane exists between the posterior two-thirds and the anterior one-third of the kidney, which are perfused by the respective branches of the renal artery. An incision along this line (anatrophic nephrotomy) is the best means of bivalving the kidney.

The renal artery can be clamped for up to 15 minutes with impunity. For longer periods a cooling system is needed.

OPERATIONS
STONES IN THE KIDNEY AND RENAL PELVIS
Preparation
The patient is placed in the lateral position as for a simple nephrectomy.

Incision
An approach is used through the bed of the twelfth rib as described for a simple nephrectomy (see page 11.57).

SIMPLE PYELOLITHOTOMY
1. Retract the peritoneum anteriorly and enter the retro-peritoneal space.

2. Palpate the kidney through the perirenal fat and identify the upper ureter and pass a silastic sling around it. Extensive mobilization of the ureter is not necessary and can be harmful by interfering with the blood supply.

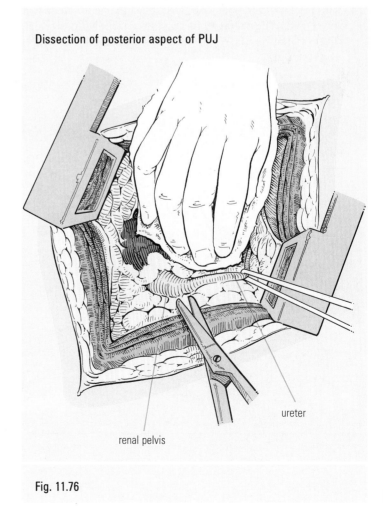

Dissection of posterior aspect of PUJ

ureter

renal pelvis

Fig. 11.76

3. Sharply dissect along the ureter to reach the PUJ (Fig. 11.76).

4. Lift the kidney forwards and dissect the overlying fat and fascia from the posterior aspect of the renal pelvis and lower pole of the kidney.

5. Palpate the stone and place catgut stay sutures either side of the proposed pyelotomy, which is made longitudinally in the posterior pelvis onto the stone, or just proximal to it if it is impacted at the PUJ (Fig. 11.77). Be ready with the sucker to collect spillage of stagnant urine, a specimen of which should be sent for culture.

6. Tease the stone out with a MacDonald dissector and stone forceps. Carefully remove all fragments and flush the pelvis with normal saline through a fine catheter. Stone fragments must be sent for biochemical and microbiological analysis.

7. Sound and probe the calices with curved stone forceps (Fig. 11.78) but only if calculi are suspected within them. A nephroscope will allow direct inspection.

8. Pass a ureteric catheter into the bladder to make sure that no stone fragments have passed into the ureter.

9. Approximate the edges of the pyelotomy with interrupted 4/0 catgut sutures (Fig. 11.79).

PYELONEPHROLITHOTOMY

1. Enter Gerota's fascia with scissors, and clean the whole kidney of perirenal fat, exposing the renal pelvis posteriorly and vascular pedicle anteriorly as described for simple nephrectomy.

Removal of stone from calyx

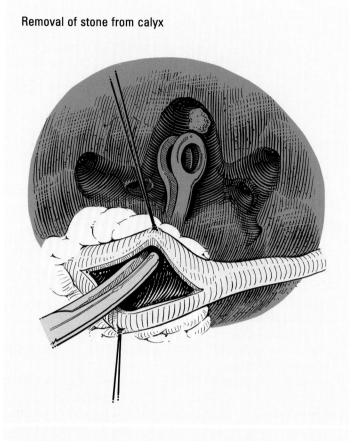

Fig. 11.78

Pyelotomy

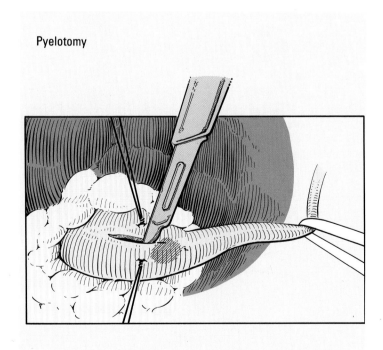

2. Identify the renal artery and pass a tape around it.

3. Lift the kidney anteriorly and ask the assistant to hold it between slings or with a purpose-designed Tubegauze mesh.

4. Develop a plane under the adventitial layer of the posterior renal pelvis, deep into the renal sinus, which is retracted with Blandy retractors (Fig. 11.80).

5. Insert stay sutures into the renal pelvis and fashion a pyelotomy parallel to the convex margin of the kidney, exposing the pelvic component of the stone.

6. Gently tease the stone free with a Watson–Cheyne or MacDonald dissector. If it is large it is better to fragment it with sturdy forceps or scissors and to remove it piecemeal.

7. If the intrarenal component of the calculus is extensive, with multiple branches, remove as much of the stone as possible through the pelvis. This will leave several discrete fragments in the calices, the presence and position of which can be confirmed by probing the kidney with a needle.

8. Clamp the renal artery with a bulldog clip, and if a prolonged procedure is anticipated, the kidney is cooled with special plastic cooling coils through which nitrous oxide is

Fig. 11.77

Closure of pyelotomy

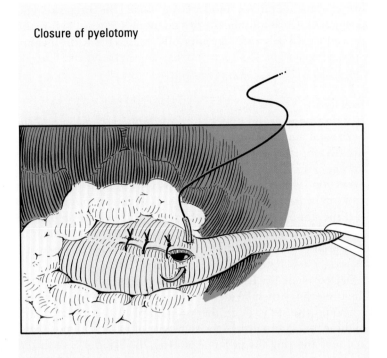

Fig. 11.79

Dissection into renal sinus

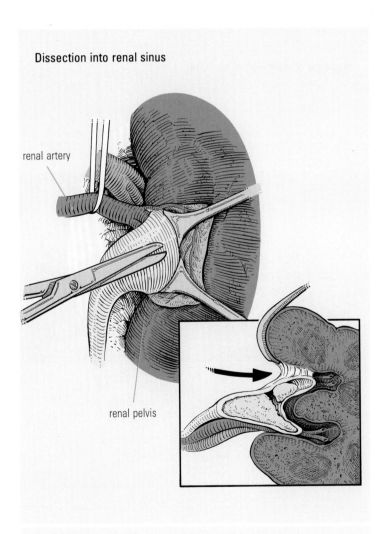

renal artery

renal pelvis

Fig. 11.80

run. A temperature probe in the renal substance confirms that the appropriate temperature (10–20°C) is reached.

9. Perform radial nephrotomies directly over the stones (previously identified by needle probing) by incising the capsule and the cortex, and deepening the incision with sinus forceps until the caliceal fat and the stone are recognized. Hold the margins apart with catgut stay sutures and then remove fragments (Fig. 11.81). The calyx is then irrigated with a catheter.

10. After ensuring that no residual calculi are left behind with an intra-operative contact X-ray, the arterial clamp is removed. Major intrarenal branches which may have been incised are transfixed and ligated with catgut sutures.

11. Close the nephrotomies with catgut, and insert a 16 Fr Malecot or Cumming's catheter as a nephrostomy and suture it to the capsule with catgut.

12. Close the pyelotomy with 4/0 catgut sutures and close the renal sinus fat over it.

Wound closure and dressing
Place a medium silicone tube drain in the renal bed near the pyelotomy and close the wound as for a simple nephrectomy (see page 11.58).

POSTOPERATIVE CARE
Obtain a plain abdominal film or a nephrostogram to confirm the complete removal of all fragments. The drain is removed when drainage has ceased. The nephrostomy tube is left for 10 days, then clamped for 24 hours and removed if no temperature or pain develop. An IVU is performed after 3 months.

SPECIAL OPERATIVE HAZARDS
1. Blood loss can be significant with accidental injury to major vessels. Arterial clamping with cooling is used to prevent haemorrhage when operating on the renal parenchyma.
2. Injured lower polar vessels when dissecting the PUJ.
3. Accessory arteries, if not identified and controlled, can prevent effective cooling of the kidney when performing a pyelonephrolithotomy.
4. Situating a pyelotomy too close to the PUJ can lead to scarring and a degree of stenosis.
5. Damage to the necks of the calices and the delicate plexus of veins surrounding them by forcible extraction of too large an intrarenal component of a stone through the renal pelvis. Under these circumstances it is better to proceed to a radial nephrotomy.
6. Deposition of mineral and the formation of calculi when suturing in the urinary tract with slowly absorbable or non-absorbable materials.
7. Residual fragments of calculi.

COMPLICATIONS

1. Leakage of urine from the drain is common but usually self-limiting. If drainage does not decrease after 10 days a nephrostogram or an IVU must be obtained to exclude distal obstruction.
2. Stenosis at the PUJ. This can be prevented by attention to the details already mentioned.
3. Retained stones are best referred for lithotripsy, or percutaneous extraction under X-ray control down the nephrostomy tract.
4. Sepsis is always a threat when handling potentially infected urine and particularly in operations on struvite staghorn calculi. It can be prevented by appropriate antibiotic prophylaxis, and treatment should be guided by pre- and peroperative cultures.
5. Postoperative ileus from the retroperitoneal dissection.

URETEROLITHOTOMY FOR URETERIC CALCULI
Preparation

The patient is anaesthetized and placed supine with a sandbag under the ipselateral loin. The incision and approach to the ureter depend on the level of the stone, the presence and position of which must be confirmed by an X-ray just before the procedure. Ideally an image intensifier is used to site the incision appropriately. The abdomen and loin are prepared and draped.

Incision

If the stone is in the upper third of the ureter, make a 10cm horizontal muscle-cutting incision anterior to the tip of the twelfth rib. It is important to stay in the extraperitoneal plane by stripping the peritoneum forwards with finger and blunt dissection. The ureter normally strips away with the peritoneum and can be found adherent to the back of the membrane.

If the stone is in the middle third of the ureter use an oblique muscle-splitting incision in the appropriate iliac fossa similar to that used for an appendicectomy (see page 5.56). Deepen the incision to reach the peritoneum which is kept intact and bluntly reflected medially. By dissecting in the extra-peritoneal plane the ureter may then be identified.

Should the stone lie in the lower third of the ureter, a low midline or Pfannenstiel incision will offer adequate access. Without entering the peritoneal cavity, the bladder is retracted

Nephrotomy incision

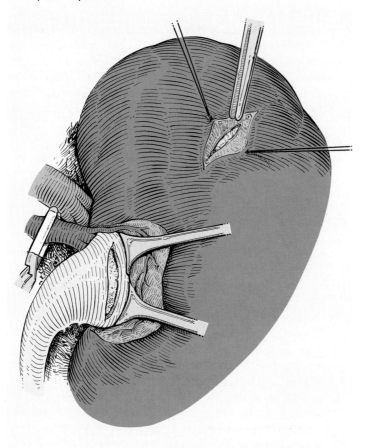

Exposure of middle third of ureter

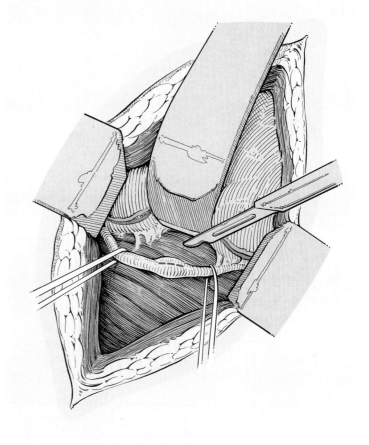

Fig. 11.81

Fig. 11.82

to the opposite side. The superior vesical pedicle is identified by following the obliterated umbilical artery down to the lateral wall of the bladder and is divided between ligatures. The ureter is then exposed just before it enters the bladder. If it is difficult to identify the ureter, it can be located at the pelvic brim, overlying the bifurcation of the common iliac artery, and a sling passed around it. Gentle traction will display its course.

Operative technique

1. Locate the stone taking care not to dislodge it up or down, and pass right angle forceps under the ureter and thread two silastic slings above and below the stone to prevent migration of the calculus. It is not usually necessary to mobilize the ureter extensively.

2. Incise the ureter with a scalpel longitudinally directly on to the stone (Fig. 11.82).

3. Express the stone from the ureter with a gentle squeezing action of the index finger and the thumb, or with the help of a Watson–Cheyne dissector if necessary (Fig. 11.83).

4. Once the stone is removed, pass a ureteric catheter proximally and distally and flush with saline to make sure that no fragments are left behind.

5. If there is a lot of ureteric oedema or the procedure has been traumatic, it is best to introduce a double-J ureteric stent.

6. Approximate the lips of the incision with fine interrupted catgut stitches, which should bite no deeper than the adventitial layer (Fig. 11.83). Some surgeons prefer to leave the ureterotomy open.

Wound closure and dressing

Place a drain near the ureterotomy and close the muscle layers with a continuous 00 nylon mass closure and the skin with interrupted nylon. Cover the wound with a dry dressing. Secure the drain to the skin with a silk stitch.

POSTOPERATIVE CARE

Following a ureterolithotomy if a stent has been inserted, a plain abdominal X-ray is obtained the following day to document its position. The drain is removed when drainage has ceased and the stent is removed cystoscopically after 6 weeks. An IVU and a DTPA renogram are performed 1 month after the removal of the stent to exclude obstruction at the site of the ureterotomy.

SPECIAL OPERATIVE HAZARDS
1. The stone can easily slip into the renal pelvis if the surgeon is not careful to stabilize its position between slings.
2. Excessive mobilization of the ureter may impair its blood supply.
3. Opening the peritoneum. If this occurs, close the defect with catgut before the peritoneal cavity fills with air and obstructs the view of the operative field.

COMPLICATIONS
1. Persistent leakage of urine is unusual and is dealt with by performing a retrograde ureterogram and passing a ureteric stent.
2. Stenosis of the ureter. This is often due to rough handling and/or ischaemia. It can be treated endoscopically in specialized centres (either by balloon dilatation or ureterotomy and intubation).
3. Sepsis.

Ureterotomy

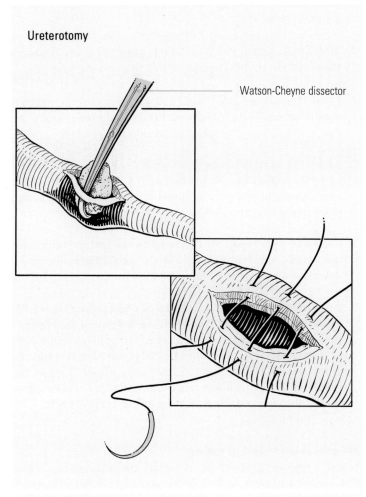

Watson-Cheyne dissector

Fig. 11.83

Pyeloplasty

This operation is indicated for pelvi-ureteric junction obstruction. The majority of cases are idiopathic; an aberrant lower pole artery is not infrequently found in this condition, but only in a small number of cases is it the cause of the obstruction (Fig. 11.84).

The principle of the operation is to fashion a new pelvi-ureteric junction (PUJ) which is wide, dependent and funnel shaped so that urine can pass easily into the ureter. The operation described is the Anderson–Hynes pyeloplasty in which the abnormal PUJ is excised and any aberrant lower pole vessels, if present, are displaced behind the reconstructed PUJ.

PREOPERATIVE ASSESSMENT
1. Perform an intravenous urogram to confirm and to visualize the dilated renal pelvis and calyces to see whether bilateral obstructions are present and to exclude hydroureters.
2. Use a DTPA renogram to assess parenchymal function and the degree of obstruction present.
3. Use a micturating cystogram if vesico-ureteric reflux cannot be excluded.

RELEVANT ANATOMY
This is covered on page 11.61 in Renal Transplantation.

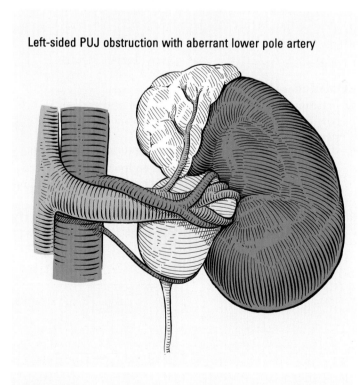

Left-sided PUJ obstruction with aberrant lower pole artery

Fig. 11.84

OPERATION
Preparation and incision
For a child

Place the patient in a supine position with a sandbag under the loin. A transverse abdominal incision is made and the muscles are divided in line with the skin incision taking care not to enter the peritoneum (Fig. 11.85). The peritoneum is displaced medially and Gerota's fascia is incised to expose the kidney and renal hilum.

For an adult

A 'supra-12' exposure above the twelfth rib is generally employed, as for a simple nephrectomy (see page 11.57), with the patient on their side and the table angulated to open up the space.

Operative technique
1. Identify the ureter and gently mobilize it, taking care not to damage its blood supply (Fig. 11.86). A nylon tape is placed around the ureter.

2. Mobilize the renal pelvis and PUJ, preserving any accessory renal vessels, by clearing the adherent connective tissue.

3. Place a stay suture into the medial wall of the ureter, which is divided between the narrowed PUJ and the stay suture. Its end is spatulated along the lateral side (Fig. 11.88).

4. Excise the renal pelvis as shown in Fig. 11.87. It is important to retain a flap of the lower part of the renal pelvis for anastomosis to the ureter. Insert a stay stitch into this flap prior to excising the pelvis.

5. Close the upper part of the renal pelvis with a continuous absorbable suture, such as 3/0 chromic catgut, leaving a defect of similar size to the spatulated ureter.

6. Anastomose the ureter to the flap of renal pelvis (Fig. 11.88) using a continuous absorbable suture, in front of an accessory polar vessel if present. Having completed the posterior layer of the anastomosis, a double-J stent is inserted to splint the anastomosis, and positioned such that upper 'J' is in the renal pelvis and the lower one is in the bladder. The anterior wall of the anastomosis is then completed (Fig. 11.89).

Wound closure and dressing
Insert a silicone drain to lie alongside the anastomosis. Close the wound in layers with a continuous monofilament nylon, subcutaneous catgut, and interrupted or subcuticular sutures for the skin. A dry dressing is applied.

Incision in a child

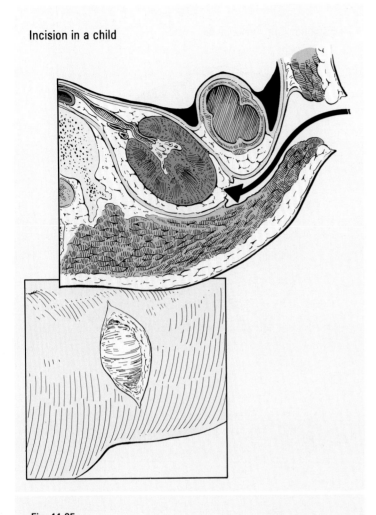

Fig. 11.85

Resection of PUJ

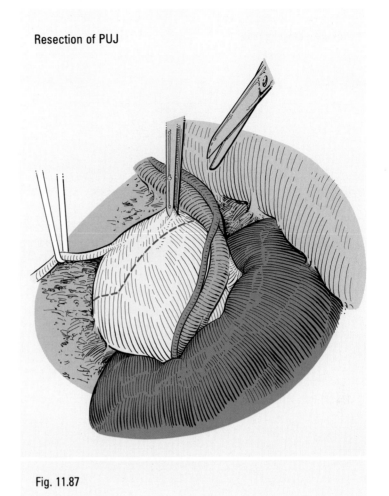

Fig. 11.87

Mobilization of upper ureter

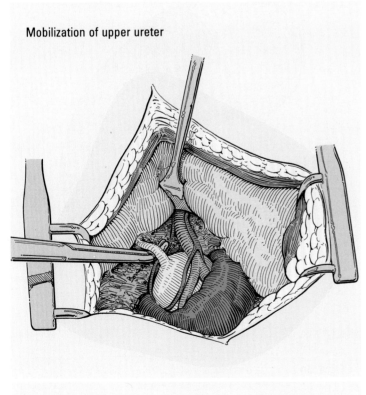

Fig. 11.86

Spatulation and anastomosis of ureter

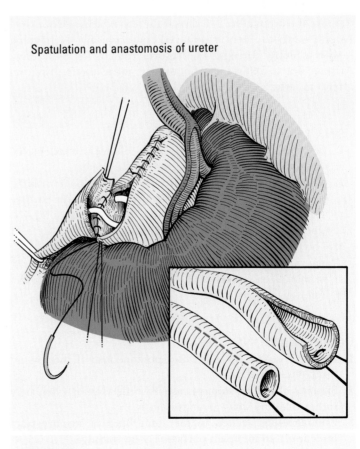

Fig. 11.88

Completed pyeloplasty

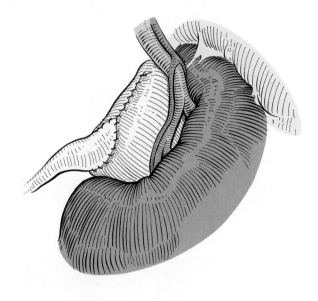

Fig. 11.89

Incision for Culp pyeloplasty

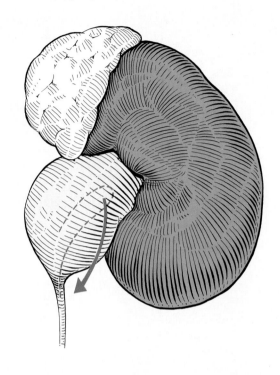

Fig. 11.90

POSTOPERATIVE CARE
Remove the drain after 2–3 days if there is no leakage of urine. After 2 weeks the stent is removed cystoscopically by grasping it with a biopsy forceps. The sutures remain for 8–10 days. Arrange for a follow-up renogram or intravenous pylogram after 3 months.

SPECIAL OPERATIVE HAZARDS
1. Devitalization of the ureter; this follows overextensive mobilization too close to the wall of the ureter.
2. Damage to a polar artery which can lead to a polar infarct of the kidney and compromise the blood supply to the ureter.
3. Opening the pleura or peritoneum.
4. The renal pelvis is unsuitable for Anderson–Hynes pyeloplasty, for example the obstruction is largely intrarenal. In such cases, consider a Culp (Figs 11.90 and 11.91) or a Foley (V–Y) pyeloplasty.

COMPLICATIONS
1. Urinary fistula; this will close spontaneously if there is no distal obstruction.
2. Stenosis of the anastomosis usually reflects poor vascularity rather than too small an anastomosis.
3. Complications related to the stent, such as urinary tract infection, and loin pain particularly on voiding.

Completed Culp pyeloplasty

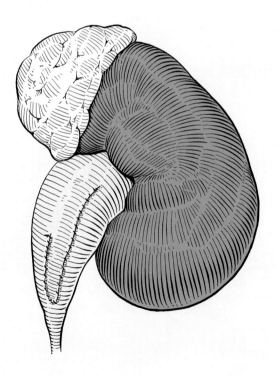

Fig. 11.91

Nephrectomy

A nephrectomy can be performed through a lateral or an anterior approach; some surgeons prefer the latter for renal carcinoma since it allows early control of the vessels and access to the inferior vena cava. For papillary carcinoma of the renal pelvis the kidney is mobilized through the loin, and the patient then turned supine and the ureter excised in continuity through a lower abdominal muscle-cutting incision.

PREOPERATIVE ASSESSMENT
1. Intravenous urography and ultrasound will demonstrate renal pathology on the diseased side and visualize the other kidney. A renogram is used to give a quantitative estimate of the differential function.
2. Measure serum urea, electrolytes and creatinine to assess overall renal function and the need for dialysis in patients with renal failure.

3. Treat urinary tract infection with antibiotics and correct hypertension which may be due to renal disease. Renal adenocarcinoma can cause polycythaemia which must be corrected.
4. In cases of renal carcinoma use radiology including CT scanning, MRI and a cavogram to look for metastases and for growth of the tumour into the renal vein and inferior vena cava.
5. In patients with transitional cell carcinoma of the renal pelvis or ureter perform a cystoscopy to check the bladder since the epithelial instability affects the entire urothelium.

RELEVANT ANATOMY
This is covered on page 11.61 in Renal Transplantation.

OPERATIONS
LOIN APPROACH
The twelfth rib loin approach is described.

Preparation
The catheterized patient is placed in the full lateral position with the side to be operated uppermost (Fig. 11.92). The back is brought to the edge of the table which has a 'break' under the lower ribs. The lower leg is flexed at the hip and knee and separated from the extended upper leg with a pillow. The position can be held with table-mounted padded supports and adhesive strapping. The trunk is now flexed laterally by 'breaking' the operating table. The lower arm is flexed so as not to be compressed and the upper one is supported on a rest in front of the face. The skin is cleansed from the axilla to the trochanter and drapes applied to expose the loin from the midline anteriorly to the midline posteriorly.

Position for nephrectomy

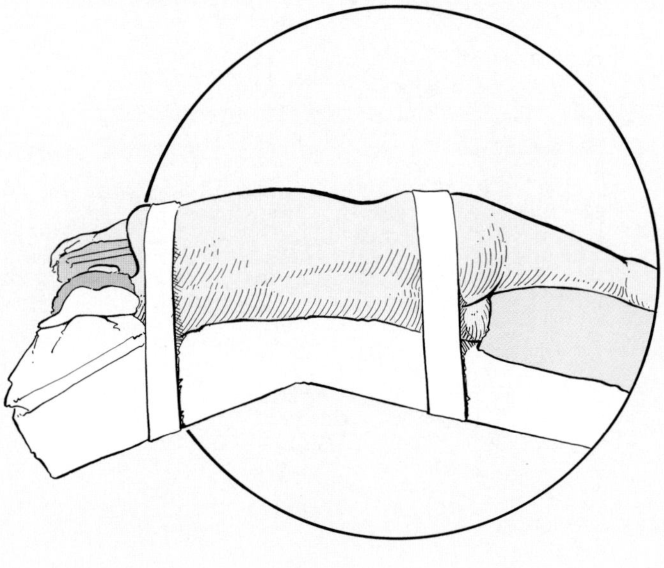

Incision
Make an incision over the twelfth rib and continue it anteriorly toward the umbilicus. Divide latissimus dorsi and serratus posterior with cutting diathermy and incise the periosteum of the twelfth rib with a diathermy point (Fig. 11.93). Strip the periosteum from the upper border of the rib with a periosteal elevator, taking care not to damage the underlying pleura. The anterior two-thirds of the twelfth rib can be resected, or the costotransverse ligament divided to allow the eleventh and twelfth ribs to be widely separated. Incise the bed of the twelfth rib to reveal retroperitoneal fat. The peritoneum is bluntly swept forward off the inner surface of the abdominal wall musculature and the incision extended anteriorly by dividing the abdominal wall musculature with a diathermy point. Take care at the edge of the rectus sheath to avoid opening the peritoneum.

Fig. 11.92

11.57

Operative technique

1. Insert a self-retaining retractor and have an assistant retract the peritoneum medially. For cases of malignancy, dissection proceeds around the intact renal fascia which encases the kidney and adrenal gland until the hilum is reached (radical nephrectomy), whereas for benign disease the renal fascia is incised (Fig. 11.94) and the surface of the kidney identified within the peri-nephric fat and the capsule of the kidney cleared using a mixture of blunt and sharp dissection (Fig. 11.95).

2. Proceed with the dissection in the chosen plane over the anterior and posterior surfaces and around the poles of the kidney towards the renal hilum.

3. Draw the kidney forward and medially to allow identification of the renal artery which is divided between strong ties, doubly ligating the vessel on the aortic side (Fig. 11.96). Some authorities recommend ligation of the renal vein first in cases of malignancy to prevent embolization of the tumour, although this causes the kidney to become congested.

4. Doubly tie the renal vein in a similar way from the front and ligate and divide any accessory vessels on the medial aspect of the kidney if they are present. In a radical nephrectomy the adrenal gland is removed with the kidney; on the right side the adrenal vein is ligated and divided where it joins the vena cava; on the left the renal vein is divided proximal to the adrenal and gonadal veins, and the latter ligated and divided.

5. Divide the ureter at a convenient point and ligate the distal end with an absorbable tie and remove the kidney and secure haemostasis.

Wound closure and dressing

Insert a silicone drain into the renal bed and have the 'break' taken off the operating table to close the loin. In a simple nephrectomy the renal fascia is closed with chromic catgut. Close the muscle layers with monofilament nylon and the skin with interrupted nylon sutures and apply a dry dressing.

ABDOMINAL APPROACH
Preparation

Place the patient supine with a sandbag under the affected side. Cleanse and drape the abdomen.

Division of latissimus dorsi and serratus posterior

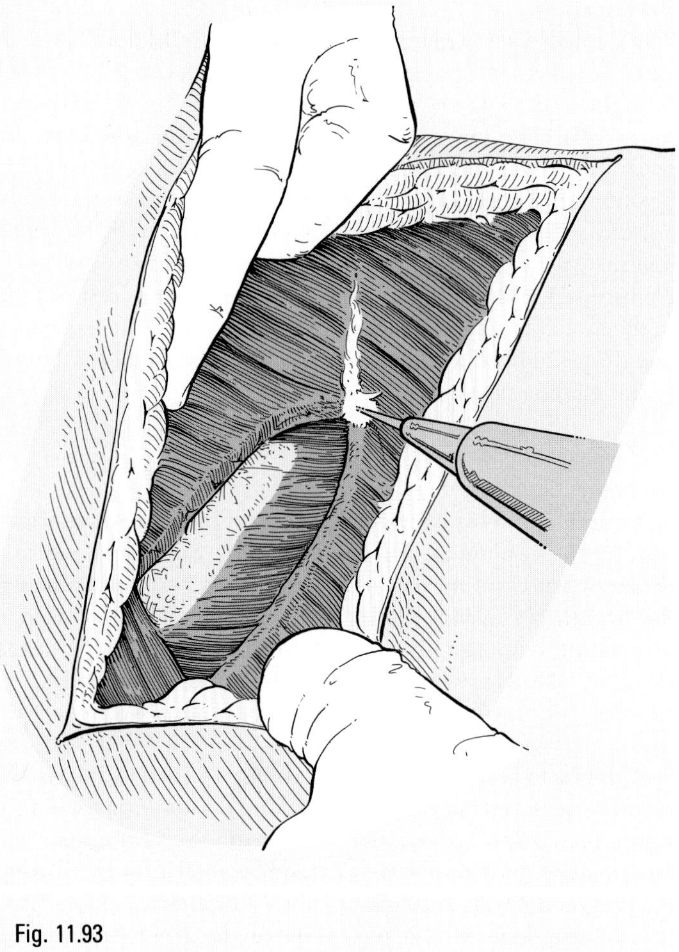

Incision of renal fascia

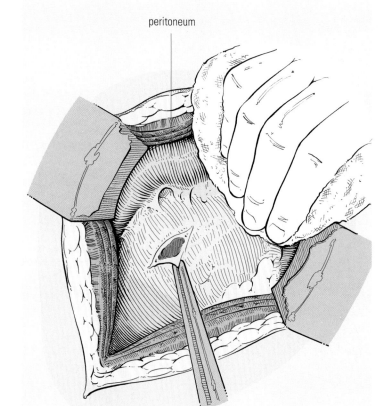

peritoneum

Fig. 11.93

Fig. 11.94

Dissection of peri-nephric fat

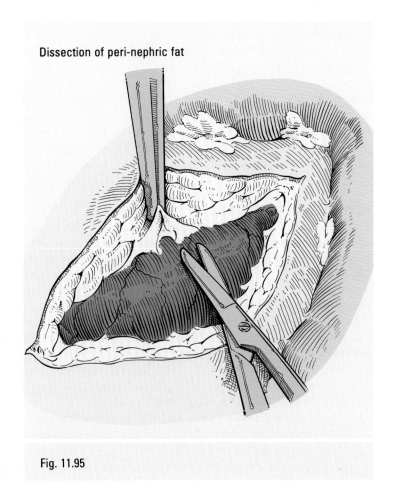

Fig. 11.95

Retraction of colon to expose right kidney

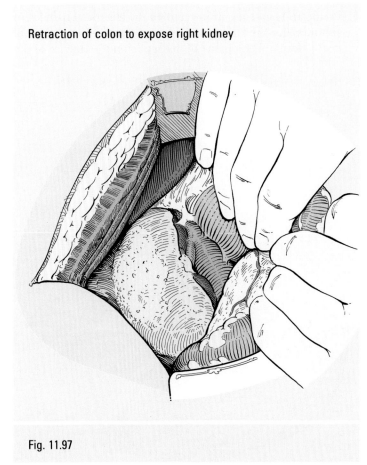

Fig. 11.97

Ligation of renal artery

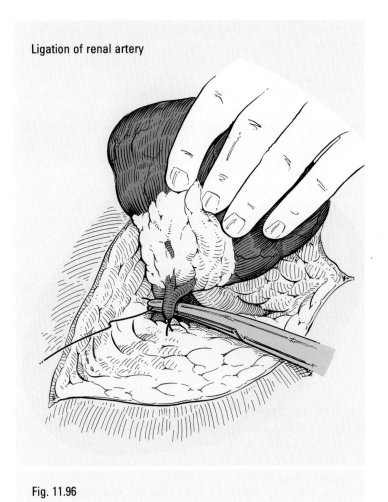

Fig. 11.96

Incision

Enter the abdomen with a paramedian, midline, or an upper transverse incision (see the Introduction).

Operative technique

1. Insert a self-retaining retractor and perform a full laparotomy noting any metastases. Pack the bowel away to the opposite side of the abdomen from the kidney to be removed.

2. Expose the kidney to be removed within its fascia by mobilisation of the overlying bowel (i.e. caecum, ascending colon and hepatic flexure on the right, and splenic flexure and descending colon on the left) (Fig. 11.97).

3. Gerota's fascia should not be disturbed. Identify the renal vein and place an untied ligature around it proximal to any tumour involvement. Any accessory veins are ligated and divided at this stage.

4. Identify the renal artery behind the vein and doubly ligate and divide it (Fig. 11.98) as far proximal as possible. Accessible enlarged para-aortic nodes are removed.

5. Doubly ligate and divide the renal vein proximal to any tumour growth along the vein, if need be establishing control of the inferior vena cava to allow excision of the entire vein (Fig. 11.99).

11.59

6. Divide and ligate the ureter and on the left the gonadal vein and mobilize the kidney and adrenal gland within the renal fascia, developing a plane of dissection on the surface of the muscles of the posterior abdominal wall. As the kidney is freed it is drawn further medially until the divided vessels are encountered from behind.

Control of renal vessels

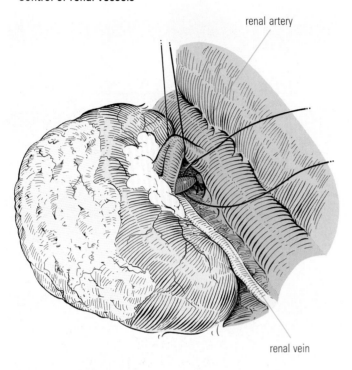

renal artery

renal vein

Fig. 11.98

Control of inferior vena cava

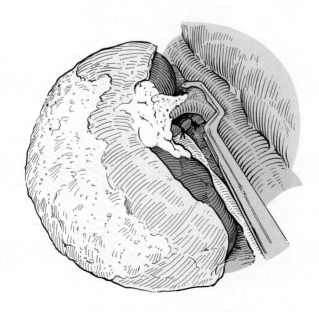

Fig. 11.99

Wound closure and dressing

Insert a silicone drain. Close the muscles in one layer with monofilament nylon and the skin with interrupted nylon sutures and apply a dry dressing.

POSTOPERATIVE CARE

The patient is given intravenous fluids and nursed with a naso-gastric tube until bowel function returns and wind is passed, even if the peritoneum has not been entered since the retroperitoneal dissection can lead to an ileus. Pain relief can be supplemented by intercostal blocks. The catheter is removed as soon as the patient is mobile and sutures after 8–10 days.

In cases of transitional cell carcinoma it must be remembered that the entire urinary epithelium is potentially unstable and the remaining urinary tract must be kept under surveillance.

SPECIAL OPERATIVE HAZARDS

1. Opening the pleura. This is not uncommon when performing a nephrectomy through the loin. Ask the anaesthetist to forcibly expand the lung holding open the hole to act as a vent. When the lung is fully re-expanded close the hole with a running catgut stitch. If the hole is large it is wise to insert a chest drain which can be removed after 24 hours if the lung is fully expanded.
2. Opening the peritoneum in the lateral approach. The hole should be closed at once or air will be drawn into the peritoneal cavity and the peritoneum will billow into the operative field.
3. Dense adhesions around the kidney. Consider placing a single clamp across the pedicle and either transfixing it or dissecting the vessels after removing the kidney. Alternatively an intracapsular removal can be performed, stripping the capsule off the kidney until the hilum is reached. This can lead to considerable bleeding.
4. Locally invasive tumour. Radical *en bloc* excision of abdominal muscles and adjacent bowel may be worthwhile.
5. A large hydronephrotic kidney is easier to remove if it is aspirated with a syringe and needle first.
6. Damage to the inferior vena cava or avulsion of an unrecognized polar artery.
7. Bleeding. Apply pressure with packs for 5–10 minutes before attempting to locate the bleeding point if it is not immediately obvious. Never blindly apply haemostats.
8. Embolization of tumour from the renal vein. Always establish proximal control before approaching tumour growth within the renal vein.

COMPLICATIONS

1. Pneumothorax.
2. Paralytic ileus.
3. Haemorrhage from the renal bed, which may require re-exploration.
4. Arteriovenous fistula from mass ligation of the renal pedicle.

Renal Transplantation and Allograft Nephrectomy

Renal transplantation is the treatment of choice for suitable patients with end-stage renal disease.

PREOPERATIVE ASSESSMENT

1. Check the haemoglobin level as anaemia is a feature of chronic renal failure, but is generally well-tolerated. Blood transfusions can lead to antibody production.
2. Aim to place the graft ipselaterally, although either kidney can be placed on either side. Note any previous surgery, including failed transplants and arterial reconstruction, when planning the operation.
3. Determine if removal of the patient's own kidney is indicated at the same operation (e.g. polycystic disease with chronic infection). In general, removal of the patient's own kidney(s) is best performed as a separate operation.
4. Check serum electrolytes to ascertain if preoperative dialysis is indicated (e.g. for hyperkalaemia or overhydration).
5. Take care of any arteriovenous fistula (e.g. Cimino fistula) to avoid thrombosis. Fully drain out dialysate from patients on peritoneal dialysis.
6. If the donor kidney has been removed by another surgeon, carefully check all available information supplied with the kidney (especially concerning vascular anatomy of the graft). Note the ischaemia time and ensure that any delays are kept to a minimum.
7. Some centres commence preoperative immunosuppression (e.g. with azathioprine).
8. Confirm that the white cell cross-match is negative.

RELEVANT ANATOMY

The kidneys measure 10 by 5 by 2 cm and are situated high up on the posterior abdominal wall, are retroperitoneal and are largely protected by the costal margin (Fig. 11.100). The hilum faces forward and medial. It is the point of entry and exit of the renal vessels and the renal pelvis, which receives the urine and is continuous with the ureter. The left kidney lies higher than the right. The hilum of the right kidney is overlain by the second part of the duodenum, the left by the tail of the pancreas.

The renal arteries arise from the aorta, oppose the second lumbar vertebra, lie behind the corresponding renal veins and may be multiple. The right renal artery crosses behind the inferior vena cava. Each renal artery gives off branches to the ureter and adrenal gland, and at the renal hilum divides into three branches, two passing in front of the renal pelvis and one behind. Each branch divides into several smaller branches, each one of which supplies a 'renule' as an endartery (i.e. without anastomosis with other branches). Accessory arteries, which are not uncommon, do not usually enter at the hilum but pierce the renal capsule. The accessory arteries usually arise directly from the aorta, sometimes at some distance from the main artery, although a lower pole artery may come off the common iliac

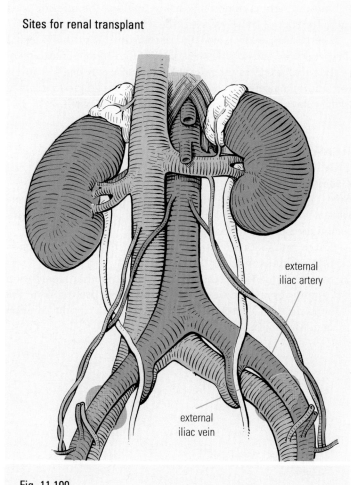

Sites for renal transplant

external iliac artery

external iliac vein

Fig. 11.100

artery. Failure to recognize and vascularize an aberrant artery can lead to a polar infarct, and in the case of the lower pole vessel can also render the donor ureter ischaemic.

The renal veins arise from the confluence of about half a dozen tributaries at the hilum. The main renal vein is usually single, but may be multiple. Unlike the arteries, there is free venous anastomosis within the kidney. Both the left and right renal veins drain into the inferior vena cava at the level of second lumbar vertebra with the left side receiving adrenal, gonadal and usually lumbar veins.

The ureter arises from the renal pelvis and crosses the sacro-iliac joint and the bifurcation of the iliac vessels to reach the bladder. The ureter usually derives its blood supply from branches of the renal, gonadal, common iliac and vesical arteries, but in a transplanted kidney it relies on the branch from the renal artery alone for its blood supply.

The aorta divides at the level of the fourth lumbar vertebra, to the left of the midline, into the common iliac arteries. These cross the sacro-iliac joints and divide into the internal and external iliac arteries; the bifurcation is crossed by the ureter.

The external iliac artery runs along the pelvic brim on the surface of psoas before entering the femoral sheath by passing under the inguinal ligament. It gives off two branches, the inferior epigastric artery and the deep circumflex iliac artery. The iliac arteries carry lymphatic channels around their adventitia. The external iliac vein runs medial to the external iliac artery and is joined by the internal iliac vein over the sacro-iliac joint to form the common iliac vein on each side. These join behind the right common iliac artery to form the inferior vena cava. In front of these vessels is the parietal peritoneum.

A renal transplant is usually vascularized from the external iliac vessels by end-to-side anastomosis. End-to-end anastomosis of the renal artery to the internal iliac artery may be used and is the author's preferred technique for transplantation from a living related donor, where there is no arterial patch.

RENAL TRANSPLANTATION
PRINCIPLES OF DONOR NEPHRECTOMY
Cardiac arrest donor
Speed is of the essence since the kidneys rapidly suffer irreversible ischaemic damage following cardiac arrest. The operative technique can be summarized as follows:

1. Enter the abdomen of a non-beating heart donor rapidly using midline incision.
2. Swift cannulation of the lower aorta with either a perfusion cannula or a Foley catheter is essential. Perfusion of the aorta is then commenced with cold preservation solution (e.g. Marshall's solution).

3. Insert a large bore tube into the inferior vena cava to drain the blood and perfusate that has passed through the kidneys.
4. Cross clamp the aorta at the diaphragmatic hiatus.
5. Once perfused, remove the kidneys (see below).

Beating heart donor
With a brain-dead, beating heart donor, kidney retrieval may be combined with removal of other organs such as heart and liver. Perfusion is effected in the same way as above, although this must be co-ordinated with the perfusion of the other organs (see Liver Transplantation on page 4.21). Some surgeons favour dissection of the kidneys prior to perfusion but it is safer to perfuse them first. The technique of dissection is summarized below.

1. Following heparinization and having checked that no accessory renal arteries arise from the iliac vessels, dissect the lower abdominal aorta and encircle it with two strong ligatures.

2. Tie off the aorta just above the bifurcation using the lower of the two ligatures, and control higher up with a Burkett clamp (Fig.11.101).

3. Incise the aorta horizontally, insert the perfusion cannula and slide the cannula up the aorta following release of the clamp. Secure it with the second tie (Fig.11.102).

Aortotomy for cannulation

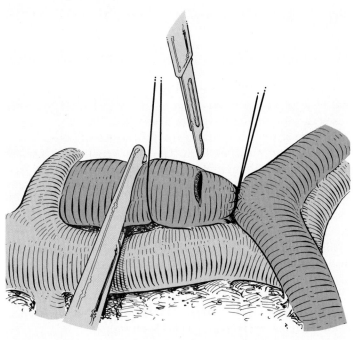

Fig. 11.101

Insertion of perfusion and drainage cannulae

vent in vena cava

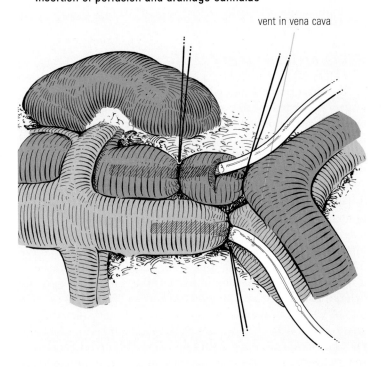

Fig. 11.102

4. Cross-clamp the upper abdominal or thoracic aorta with a Roberts' forceps and commence perfusion via the lower aorta.

5. Vent the vena cava in a similar manner to the aorta (Fig. 11.102) with a wide-bore tube, connected to a suitable collection apparatus.

6. Incise the inferior vena cava vertically and then reflect the renal veins to each side with a patch of vena cava. Care should be taken to avoid damage to the right renal artery which lies behind the vena cava. The branches entering the renal veins (e.g. adrenal and gonadal veins) are ligated with silk.

7. Once the kidneys are fully perfused and cooled, divide the aorta vertically; this reveals the renal artery orifices on each side.

8. Divide the ureters as close to the bladder as possible, and mobilize them with a generous covering of connective tissue to prevent devascularization.

9. Remove the kidneys by incising Gerota's fascia, drawing the kidneys medially, and dividing their attachment to the posterior abdominal wall. The kidneys are dissected with the full length of renal artery and vein, including patches of aorta and vena cava on each side (Fig. 11.103). On the left side this requires careful dissection of the vessels from under the root of the left mesocolon.

10. Once removed, check the kidneys for damage and pack each one separately in a bag of cold preservation solution (e.g. Marshall's solution) within another bag. They are then packed in ice, and the containers carefully labelled left and right.

11. Samples of spleen/lymph nodes are removed for tissue typing.

Living donor

A living donor nephrectomy can be performed through the loin or transperitoneally as for a normal nephrectomy (see page 11.57). As much of the vessels as possible is taken, but without any patches. Similarly, as much ureter as possible is removed with the kidney. Following removal, the kidney is perfused 'on the bench'. Ideally the recipient operation should already be in progress in an adjoining operating theatre to keep ischaemia times to a minimum.

RECIPIENT SURGERY
Preparation

The patient is placed supine and a urinary catheter inserted. The bladder is drained, if necessary, and the catheter connected to a 1 litre bag of sterile normal saline via an intravenous giving set. This will be used to inflate the bladder. This account describes an extravesical technique of ureteric reimplantation, similar to the methods described by Lich and Gregoir. An alternative, the Leadbetter–Politano technique, is described on page 11.44.

Dissected donor kidneys

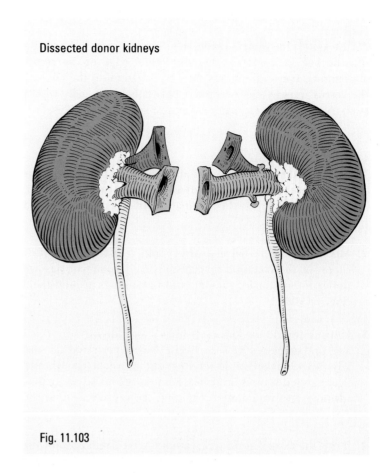

Fig. 11.103

Exposure of vessels for renal transplant

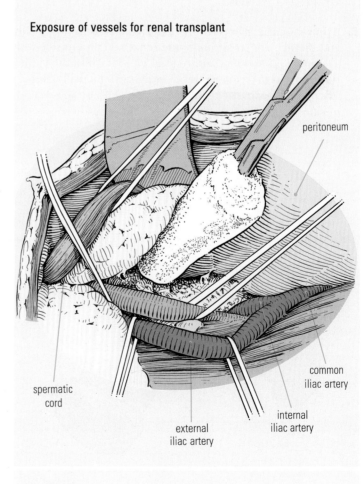

peritoneum

spermatic cord

external iliac artery

internal iliac artery

common iliac artery

Fig. 11.104

Incision

An Alexandre incision is made. This skin incision is the shape of a hockey stick and overlies the lateral edge of the rectus abdominus. Incise the rectus sheath just lateral to the edge of the rectus muscle and sweep the peritoneum medially with a swab to allow an extraperitoneal exposure of the iliac vessels.

Operative technique

1. Carefully dissect the external iliac artery and vein. Access is improved in the female by division of the round ligament. In the male, identify the spermatic cord and control it with a tape.

2. Mobilize the external iliac artery and vein from the bifurcation of the common iliac vessels to the point of passage under the inguinal ligament, and place slings around them (Fig. 11.104).

3. Unpack the donor kidney from ice and identify the renal and any accessory vessels. Excise excess perirenal fat and any other unwanted adherent tissue (adrenal gland), and ligate untied venous branches. Some surgeons advocate performing a capsulotomy by incising the capsule around the convex outer border of the kidney.

4. Trim the donor aorta to create a Carrel patch around the vessel origin (i.e. a cuff of arterial wall to produce a sewing ring, see Fig.11.105). For multiple arteries, keep them all on one patch if possible.

5. Apply vascular clamps to the external iliac vein proximally and distally, and anastomose the renal vein end-to-side with a running 5/0 vascular suture (Fig. 11.106) whilst the kidney is supported in a cold wet swab and drawn medially. Repeat this procedure for the renal artery which is anastomosed end-to-side to the external iliac artery (Fig. 11.107). Accessory

Anastomosis of donor renal vein to external iliac vein

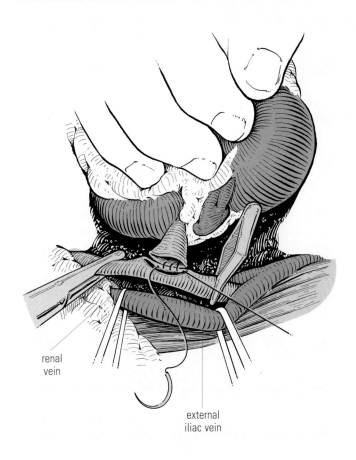

renal
vein

external
iliac vein

Fig. 11.106

Anastomosis of donor renal artery to external iliac artery

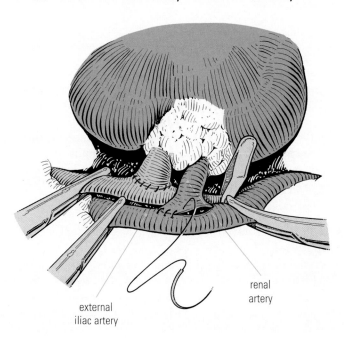

external
iliac artery

renal
artery

Fig. 11.107

Carrel patch on artery

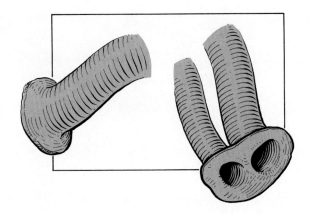

Fig. 11.105

Preparation of bladder

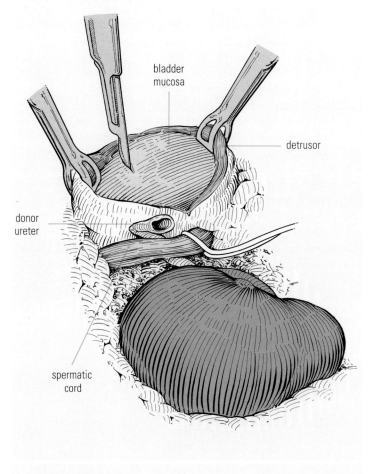

Fig. 11.108

Anastomosis of ureter to bladder

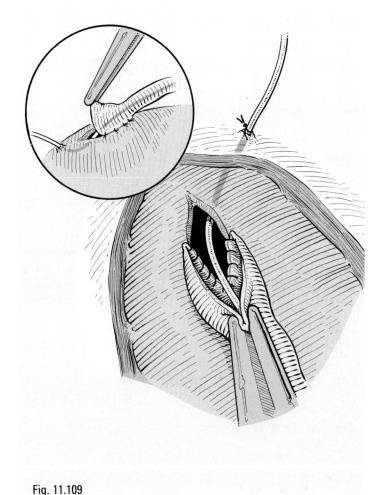

Fig. 11.109

vessels are commonly on the same patch of aorta, but if not they must be implanted separately into the external iliac artery using a 6/0 vascular suture (e.g. Prolene). An accessory lower pole artery can be anastomosed end-to-end to the inferior epigastric artery. The times of application and removal of all clamps are carefully recorded. Just prior to completion of the arterial anastomosis it is the policy of the author's unit to administer intravenous bolus doses of methyl prednisolone, mannitol and frusemide.

6. Remove the proximal venous clamp, followed immediately by the proximal arterial clamp, the distal venous clamp, and finally the distal arterial clamp. Check the anastomoses for bleeding; this requires inspection of their medial aspect by gently drawing the graft laterally. Place swabs around the vascular anastomoses and observe graft perfusion which should be rapid and uniform; compression of the renal vein should produce swelling and pulsation of the graft (Hume's test).

7. Inflate the bladder with saline via the catheter and expose the upper lateral wall of the bladder by blunt dissection through the perivesical fat. Create a submucous tunnel valve by dividing the detrusor muscle for 2.5 cm until the mucosa bulges and make a small incision at the distal extremity of mucosa (Fig. 11.108). Empty the bladder by placing the catheter bag on the floor.

8. Trim the donor ureter to the length required, spatulate it and then implant it into the bladder (Fig. 11.109) by anastomosis with interrupted absorbable 5/0 P.D.S. sutures. It is the author's policy to splint this anastomosis over a Tizzard catheter which is brought out through a separate small stab incision in the bladder and secured with a catgut purse-string suture. Mucosa-to-mucosa opposition between the ureter and bladder is important. Following completion of the anastomosis, reinflate the bladder with saline to test for leaks and insert additional sutures if necessary.

9. Loosely suture the bladder muscle over the distal ureter with interrupted catgut sutures. Interpose a Moynihan forceps between the ureter and detrusor muscle whilst these sutures are being placed to keep it loose (Figs 11.110 and 11.111). Carefully inspect the vascular anastomoses, and if there are bleeding points, insert additional 5/0 sutures with care. Take a minute open biopsy from the upper pole of the graft.

Wound closure and dressing

Insert a large silicone drain and close the wound with loop nylon, and interrupted nylon or staples for the skin. A dry dressing is applied.

POSTOPERATIVE CARE

Commence immunosuppressive therapy; the author's policy is to use triple therapy of azathioprine, cyclosporin and prednisolone. Perform a renogram on the first postoperative day to assess graft perfusion, and a 'Tizzardogram' on day 5, removing the Tizzard catheter if there is no leak at the ureteric anastomosis. Just prior to discharge, perform an intravenous urogram.

SPECIAL OPERATIVE HAZARDS

1. Poor perfusion of the graft which may be due to:
   i. vascular spasm which may respond to papaverine placed topically onto and also injected into the artery;
   ii. twisting or intimal damage and intimal dissection in the donor vessels;
   iii. arterial disease in the donor;
   iv. acute tubular necrosis due to long preservation times or prolonged warm ischaemia.
   v. overlooked polar vessels.
2. Bleeding from anastomoses. Avoid reapplying clamps to the vessels; use packs and carefully inserted additional sutures to control.
3. No arterial patch. Consider mobilizing and dividing the internal iliac artery with end-to-end anastomosis to the renal artery.
4. Opening the peritoneum. Any defect should be closed with catgut.
5. Retrieval damage to the kidney such as divided polar vessels and devascularized ureter.

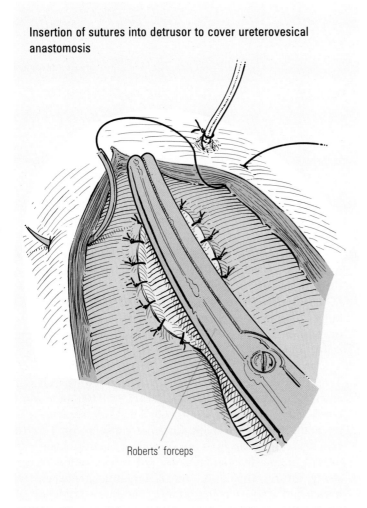

Insertion of sutures into detrusor to cover ureterovesical anastomosis

Roberts' forceps

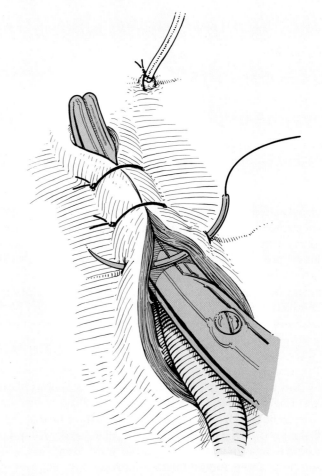

Creation of submucosal tunnel

Fig. 11.110

Fig. 11.111

COMPLICATIONS

1. Ureteric stricture/leak/necrosis which may be due, in some cases, to an overlooked lower pole artery. It may be possible to salvage this situation by reimplantation, or anastomosis of the recipient's own ureter to the renal pelvis of the graft.
2. Lymphocoele formation. This can be percutaneously aspirated under ultrasound guidance, but if persistent is best treated by laparotomy through a midline incision and 'fenestration' into the peritoneal cavity.
3. Haematoma/urinoma due to anastomotic leakage.
4. Hyperacute, acute and chronic graft rejection.
5. Recurrence of original disease (e.g. IgA nephropathy and oxalosis).
6. Testicular damage in the male due to damage to the cord.
7. Complications of immunosuppression such as opportunistic infection.
8. Renal artery stenosis, suggested by deteriorating renal function, hypertension and sodium retention.

ALLOGRAFT NEPHRECTOMY

PREOPERATIVE ASSESSMENT

1. Identify the indication for operation (e.g. hypertension).
2. Correct acid base, electrolyte and fluid balance disorders with preoperative dialysis.
3. Withdraw immunosuppression but ensure steroid cover with intravenous hydrocortisone.

Preparation
This is similar to that described for the transplant.

Incision
Reopen the old incision.

Operative technique

1. If early graft failure necessitates graft nephrectomy, it is usually possible to reconstruct the external iliac vessels with 5/0 vascular sutures after having established proximal and distal control of the iliac vessels and removing the graft. Stenosis is avoided by leaving a cuff of graft vessel.

2. In a longer established graft, fibrosis exacerbated by cyclosporin therapy means it is not usually possible to define the anastomoses, and the graft will be densely adherent to the surrounding tissue. In such cases use an intracapsular approach and secure the renal pedicle close to the kidney. Ligate the artery and vein individually whenever possible, as mass ligature can lead to arteriovenous fistula formation.

3. It is best to remove the ureter at the bladder. Close the defect with interrupted absorbable sutures and test for leaks by introducing sterile saline into the bladder via the urinary catheter.

Wound closure
Insert a drain and close the wound in a similar manner to renal transplantation.

POSTOPERATIVE CARE
The patient is likely to require dialysis in the postoperative period and will need fluid, salt and protein restriction. The drain is removed after 24–48 hours and sutures taken out at 14–21 days as wound healing is impaired in the presence of renal failure.

SPECIAL OPERATIVE HAZARDS
1. Blood loss, which may be considerable during this operation.
2. Damage to the iliac vessels.
3. Entering the peritoneum which means that a patient cannot to straight back onto peritoneal dialysis after the operation.

COMPLICATIONS
1. Fistula from the bladder.
2. Arterovenous fistula.
3. Secondary haemorrhage and aneurysm/pseudo-aneurysm formation from the anastomotic sites.

Adrenalectomy

The most common indication for adrenal surgery is a primary adrenal tumour now that bilateral adrenalectomy is no longer performed for advanced breast carcinoma. The three approaches to the adrenals are the anterior, posterior and lateral. The anterior transperitoneal approach is described since this is applicable to almost all indications for adrenalectomy.

PREOPERATIVE ASSESSMENT

1. Use imaging techniques such as ultrasound, CT scanning, I^{131} MIBG and iodocholesterol scanning to identify the involved side. Bilateral examination is seldom required except when Cushing's syndrome or Conn's syndrome is due to bilateral hyperplasia.
2. In Cushing's syndrome: image using iodocholesterol scintigram. Control hypertension, cardiac failure, hypokalaemia and diabetes prior to operation.
3. In Conn's syndrome: control hypokalaemia and hypertension with spironolactone and potassium supplements.
4. Phaeochromocytoma. Detect with I^{131} MIBG scan or selective venous sampling for catecholamines. Control hypertension with alpha blockers and arrhythmias with beta blockers.

RELEVANT ANATOMY (Fig.11.112)

The adrenals are situated over the upper poles of the kidneys deep to fascia and, although surrounded by perirenal fat, are readily recognizable by their chrome yellow colour and firm granulated appearance. On the right the pyramidal shaped adrenal lies partly on the diaphragm, alongside the inferior vena cava (IVC) and under the liver. On the left the adrenal is crescentic in shape and extends more around the medial side of the kidney and lies beneath the tail of the pancreas on the left crus of the diaphragm. The arterial supply is by a variable number of small vessels. Venous drainage is more consistent, but sometimes duplicated. On the left there is a single vein running from the inferior medial surface of the gland downwards to the left renal vein, and on the right a very short vein drains from the anteromedial surface of the gland to the adjacent IVC.

OPERATION

Preparation

The anaesthetized patient is placed supine with the table tilted 15° to the right and tilted 15° feet down. The surgeon stands on the right of the patient. The abdomen is prepared and draped.

Incision

For unilateral adrenalectomy, use a subcostal incision (see the Introduction) which is extended across the midline if the right adrenal is to be approached. For bilateral adrenalectomy a

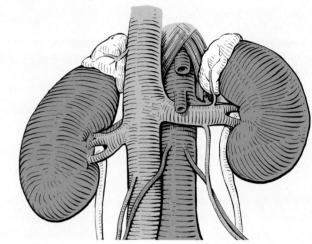

Relevant anatomy

Fig. 11.112

transverse subcostal incision is employed. The rectus muscle is divided with cutting diathermy and the transverse and oblique muscles split along their fibres.

Operative technique

LEFT SIDE

1. Retract the left costal margin upwards, place the left hand over the spleen and pull it downwards and medially to expose the lienorenal ligament. Divide the peritoneum of the posterior part of the ligament with scissors laterally and continue the incision superiorly around the spleen so that the spleen and tail of pancreas can be drawn downwards and medially. This exposes the perinephric fat over the upper pole of the kidney (Fig. 11.113).

2. In thin patients the adrenal and upper pole of the kidney may be seen; in obese patients the upper pole of the kidney should be palpated and the overlying fat dissected by an assistant on the patient's left until the adrenal is identified by its chrome yellow colour and firm consistency. The assistant holds up the fat with dissecting forceps and diathermizes any small vessels.

3. Even small tumours within the adrenal can usually be palpated as hard round lesions. Commencing along the lateral border, with dissection close to the surface of the gland, gradually

mobilize it on all aspects except medially. To facilitate dissection grasp the gland and lift with Duvall's forceps (Fig. 11.114). Use diathermy to divide the small arteries.

4. When the gland is mobilized, the main vein is seen on the medial aspect and can be divided between clips or ties. The gland is then removed.

5. Confirm haemostasis and then allow the spleen to fall back over the area.

RIGHT SIDE

1. Retract the right costal margin upwards and, by dividing the peritoneum above the hepatic flexure, partially mobilize the colon downwards.

2. The assistant on the left of the patient retracts the kidney inferiorly with a gauze pack to bring the adrenal inferiorly. A second assistant gently retracts upwards the undersurface of the right lobe of the liver.

3. At this stage the IVC should be identified running up to and under the liver edge. The adrenal gland is sometimes visible closely applied to the IVC after incising the overlying peritoneum, but in obese patients can be found by careful dissection into the perinephric fat alongside the IVC.

4. If exposure of the adrenal gland, especially its upper pole, is inadequate due to overlying of the right lobe of the liver resist attempts to remove the gland using this approach because of haemorrhage control and potential damage to the IVC. In such cases mobilize the right lobe of the liver and retract anteromedially (Fig. 11.115). To facilitate this enlarge the incision. Adequate costal retraction is important and a fixed retractor (e.g. Thompson or Omnitract) is preferred. The assistant places a gauze pack over the right lobe of the liver and retracts it medially and anteriorly, so that the right triangular and coronary can be divided lateral to the IVC.

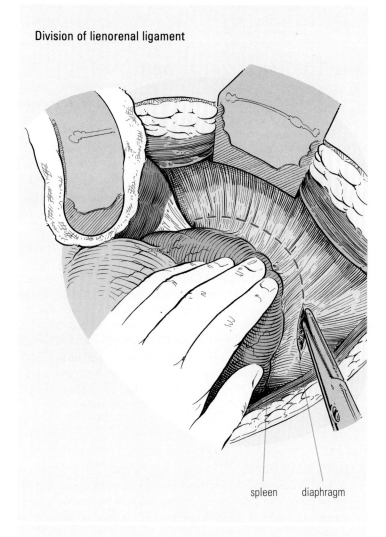

Division of lienorenal ligament

spleen   diaphragm

Fig. 11.113

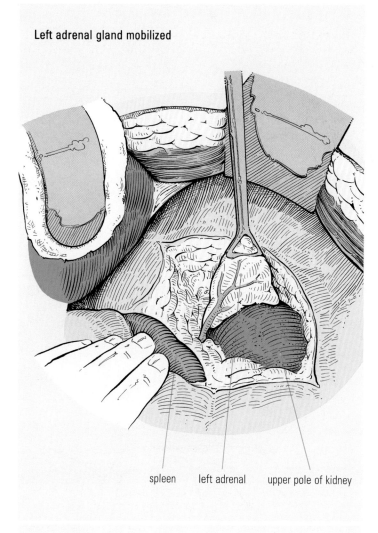

Left adrenal gland mobilized

spleen   left adrenal   upper pole of kidney

Fig. 11.114

Mobilization of right lobe of liver

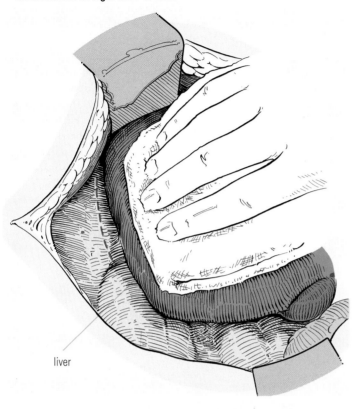

liver

Fig. 11.115

Mobilization of right adrenal gland, grasping the gland with Duvall's forceps

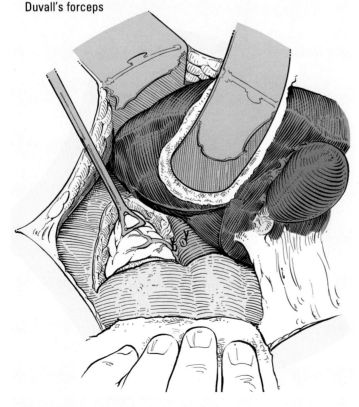

Fig. 11.116

5. Identify the adrenal and divide its vein between ties or ligaclips prior to mobilization of the gland, as this avoids the risk of tearing the vein or avulsing it from the IVC. As with the left side the gland can be mobilized by grasping it with Duvall's forceps, dissecting close to the gland and diathermizing the small arteries, but clip and divide any vessel in close relation to the IVC (Fig. 11.116). Divide the fascial attachments to the kidney last as they prevent upward displacement of the adrenal. After removal of the adrenal the liver can be allowed to lie over the area once haemostasis has been secured.

Wound closure and dressing
Drainage is not necessary. Close the abdomen with looped monofilament nylon and the skin with sutures or staples. Cover the wound with a light non-occlusive dressing.

POSTOPERATIVE CARE
Ensure there are daily electrolyte estimations, and regular (every 30 minutes) monitoring of postoperative blood pressure until it has been stable for 24 hours.

Following bilateral adrenalectomy or operations for Cushing's syndrome patients should receive perioperative hydrocortisone and long-term cortisone and fluorocortisone.

Remove skin sutures or clips 7 days after surgery for most patients, but after 10 days for those with Cushing's syndrome.

SPECIAL OPERATIVE HAZARDS
1. Carcinomas of adrenals are often large, vascular and invade local structures including the IVC. At least 3 units of blood should be cross-matched.
2. Haemorrhage from the adrenal vein can usually be controlled by oversewing the vein end. On the right side avulsion of the vein or laceration of the IVC is more serious. Small holes may be oversewn whilst the blood is removed by suction. For larger holes initially control the haemorrhage by packing for 5 minutes whilst the anaesthetist prepares a blood transfusion. Optimize retraction and ensure suction is available. Remove the pack and as the edge of the laceration appears grasp the IVC with forceps, lift and apply a Cooley or Satinsky clamp along the IVC. Perform repair with continuous 5/0 Prolene.
3. Phaeochromocytoma. During surgery continuously monitor the blood pressure. Care must be taken to handle the gland gently. During the mobilization divide the vessels as early as possible. Treat hypertensive crises with intravenous phentolamine and arrhythmias with propranolol and lignocaine. On removal of the gland administer intravenous colloids to maintain the blood pressure.
4. Damage to the spleen or liver.

COMPLICATIONS
1. Acute circulatory failure may be due to adrenocortical insufficiency and should be treated with intravenous hydrocortisone, colloid fluid load and if necessary inotrophic support.
2. Delayed wound healing in Cushing's syndrome.

Index